LESLEY PAINE
GIRAFFE WARD.

LESLEY PAINE
GIRAFFE WARD.

NURSING CARE OF THE CHILD WITH CANCER

NURSING CARE OF THE CHILD WITH CANCER

Second Edition

ASSOCIATION OF PEDIATRIC ONCOLOGY NURSES
Richmond, Virginia

Editors

Genevieve V. Foley, RN, MSN, OCN, CNAA
Director of Nursing Practice
Memorial Sloan-Kettering Cancer Center
New York, New York

Dianne Fochtman, RN, MN, OCN, CPNP
Pediatric Nurse Practitioner, Pediatric Oncology
Kapiolani Medical Center for Women and Children
Honolulu, Hawaii
FORMERLY:
Clinical Specialist, Pediatric Oncology
The Children's Memorial Hospital
Chicago, Illinois

Kathleen Hardin Mooney, RN, PhD, FAAN
Professor
University of Utah College of Nursing
Salt Lake City, Utah

W.B. SAUNDERS
A Division of Harcourt Brace & Company

PHILADELPHIA LONDON TORONTO MONTREAL SYDNEY TOKYO

W.B. Saunders Company
A Division of
Harcourt Brace & Company

The Curtis Center
Independence Square West
Philadelphia, PA 19106-3399

Library of Congress Cataloging in Publication Data
Nursing care of the child with cancer / Association of Pediatric Oncology Nurses : edited by Genevieve V. Foley, Dianne Fochtman. Kathleen Hardin Mooney.—2nd ed.
p.   cm.
Includes bibliographical references and index.
ISBN 0-7216-4006-0
1. Tumors in children—Nursing.   I. Foley, Genevieve V. II. Fochtman, Dianne.   III. Mooney, Kathleen Hardin. IV. Association of Pediatric Oncology Nurses (U.S.)   [DNLM: 1. Neoplasms—in infancy & childhood. 2. Neoplasms—
nursing.   WY 156 N9733 1993]
RC281.C4N87 1993
610.73'62—dc20
DNLM/DLC   93–5015

NURSING CARE OF THE CHILD WITH CANCER   ISBN 0-7216-4006-0

Printed in the United States of America

Last digit is the print number: 9   8   7   6   5   4   3   2   1

To the children and their families
and
To past, present, and future pediatric oncology nurses

CONTRIBUTORS

ARLENE L. ANDROKITES, BSN, CPNP
Pediatric Oncology Nurse Practitioner, Dana Farber Cancer Institute, Children's Hospital, Boston, Massachusetts
Malignant Tumors of Childhood and Adolescence: Wilms' Tumor

ELIZABETH A. BERRO, RN, MA
Pediatric Nursing Instructor, New York Hospital, Cornell Medical Center, New York, New York
Malignant Tumors of Childhood and Adolescence: Retinoblastoma

PATRICIA BENSON, RN, MN
Director of Pediatric Oncology/Bone Marrow Transplant Nursing, Egleston Children's Hospital, Atlanta, Georgia
Home and Hospice Care for the Child or Adolescent With Cancer

DONNA BETCHER, RN, MSN
Pediatric Nurse Practitioner, Mayo Clinic, Rochester, Minnesota
Malignant Tumors of Childhood and Adolescence: Bone Tumors

EDITH D. BURKEY, PA, BA
Assistant Director of Home Care, The Children's Hospital of Philadelphia, Philadelphia, Pennsylvania
Home and Hospice Care for the Child or Adolescent With Cancer

JANE C. CLARK, RN, MN, OCN
Clinical Nurse Specialist, Oncology, Emory University Hospital, Atlanta, Georgia
Home and Hospice Care for the Child or Adolescent With Cancer

DEBRA GADDY COHEN, RN, MSN, PNP
Clinical Nurse Specialist, Pediatric Oncology, North Carolina Baptist Hospital, Winston-Salem, North Carolina
Leukemia in Children and Adolescents: Acute Lymphocytic Leukemia

CONSTANCE COLTER, RN, MS, PNP
Pediatric Nurse Practitioner, Division of Immunology, Schneider Children's Hospital at Long Island Jewish Medical Center, New Hyde Park, New York
FORMERLY: Pediatric Clinical Nurse Specialist, Memorial Sloan-Kettering Cancer Center, New York, New York
Biologic Response Modifiers

ROSEMARY DRIGAN, RN, MEd, CRNP
Pediatric Oncology Nurse Practitioner, Dana Farber Cancer Institute, Children's Hospital, Boston, Massachusetts
Malignant Tumors of Childhood and Adolescence: Wilms' Tumor

JANET DUNCAN, RN, BSN
Staff Nurse III, Children's Hospital, Boston, Massachusetts
Nursing Management of Physical Care Needs

JEAN H. FERGUSSON, RN, EdD, CRNP
Adjunct Assistant Professor, School of Nursing, University of Pennsylvania, Philadelphia, Pennsylvania; Nurse Practitioner and Coordinator of Patient Education, Divisions of Pediatric Hemotology and Oncology, Children's Hospital of Philadelphia, Philadelphia, Pennsylvania
History, Issues, and Trends

DIANNE FOCHTMAN, RN, MN, OCN, CPNP
Associate Clinical Professor of Nursing, University of Hawaii, Honolulu, Hawaii; Pediatric Nurse Practitioner, Pediatric Oncology, Kapiolani Medical Center for Women & Children, Honolulu, Hawaii
FORMERLY: Clinical Specialist, Pediatric Oncology, The Children's Memorial Hospital, Chicago, Illinois
The Terminally Ill Child or Adolescent

GENEVIEVE V. FOLEY, RN, MSN, OCN, CNAA
Director of Nursing Practice, Memorial Sloan-Kettering Cancer Center, New York, New York
History, Issues, and Trends

MARY KAY FOLEY, RN, MS

Clinical Nurse Specialist, Pediatric Hematology/Oncology, Wyler Children's Hospital, The University of Chicago Medical Center, Chicago, Illinois

Nursing Management of the Child or Adolescent With Blood Component Deficiencies

BETH FREDERICK, RN, MS

Clinical Nurse Specialist, Autologous Bone Marrow Transplant-Solid Tumors, Childrens Hospital Los Angeles, Los Angeles, California

Bone Marrow Transplantation

MARY JO HANIGAN, RN, MN, OCN

Clinical Nurse Specialist, formerly of Pediatric Hematology/Oncology and Bone Marrow Transplant, University of Nebraska Medical Center, Omaha, Nebraska

Bone Marrow Transplantation

SUE P. HEINEY, RN, MN, CS

Adjunct Faculty, College of Nursing, University of South Carolina; Manager, Psychosocial Oncology, Center for Cancer Treatment and Research, Richland Memorial Hospital

Nursing Management of Psychosocial Care Needs

WENDY HOBBIE, RN, MSN, PNP

Project Director, TEEN Survivorship Study, University of Rochester School of Nursing, Rochester, New York

Late Effects in Long-Term Survivors

DEBRA P. HYMOVICH, RN, PhD, FAAN

Professor, University of South Florida College of Nursing, Tampa, Florida

Nursing Management of Psychosocial Care Needs

MARCIA LEONARD, RN, BSN, PNP

Clinical Nurse IV, University of Michigan, Ann Arbor, Michigan

Nursing Implications of Diagnostic and Staging Procedures

PATRICIA LIEBHAUSER, RN, MSN

Staff Nurse, Egleston Children's Hospital at Emory University, Atlanta, Georgia

Malignant Tumors of Childhood and Adolescence: Hodgkin's Disease

PATSY McGUIRE, RN, MS, CPNP

Pediatric Nurse Practitioner, Childhood Hematology-Oncology Associates & the Rocky Mountain Children's Cancer Center, Presbyterian-St. Luke's Medical Center, Denver, Colorado

Radiation Therapy

LESLIE WAGNER McMAHON, RN, MSN

Nursing Director of the Center for Cancer and Blood Disorders, Children's Medical Center of Dallas, Dallas, Texas

FORMERLY: Nursing Director, Pediatrics/Bone Marrow Transplant Services, H. Lee Moffitt Cancer Center and Research Institute, Tampa, Florida

Interdisciplinary Management of the Child or Adolescent With Cancer

BELINDA MARTIN MITCHELL, RN, MS, FAAN

President and Chief Executive Officer, Childrens Home Health Care, Los Angeles, California

FORMERLY: Coordinator for Home Care Program for Children with Catastrophic Diseases, Childrens Hospital, Los Angeles, California

Home and Hospice Care for the Child or Adolescent With Cancer

KATHLEEN HARDIN MOONEY, RN, PhD, FAAN

Professor, University of Utah College of Nursing, Salt Lake City, Utah

Biologic Basis of Childhood Cancer

IDA (KI) MOORE, RN, DNS

Associate Professor, Family and Community Nursing, College of Nursing, University of Arizona, Tucson, Arizona

Late Effects in Long-Term Survivors

CHERYL PANZARELLA, RN, MS

Oncology Clinical Nurse Specialist, Children's Hospital, Boston, Massachusetts

Nursing Management of Physical Care Needs

MARY McELWAIN PETRICCIONE, RN, MS, CPNP

Pediatric Nurse Practitioner, Neuro-Oncology Service, Memorial Sloan-Kettering Cancer Center, New York, New York

Malignant Tumors of Childhood and Adolescence: Central Nervous System Tumors

NOREEN McGOWAN QUINLAN, RN, MA, CPNP

Clinical Nurse Specialist, Children's Mercy Hospital, Kansas City, Missouri

FORMERLY OF Memorial Sloan-Kettering Cancer Center, New York, New York

Malignant Tumors of Childhood and Adolescence: Non-Hodgkin's Lymphoma

ALICE RENICK-ETTINGER, RN, MSN, CPNP

Adjunct Clinical Instructor of Pediatrics, Program Coordinator, Division of Pediatric Hematology-Oncology, University of Medicine & Dentistry of New Jersey, Robert Wood Johnson Medical School, New Brunswick, New Jersey; Robert Wood Johnson University Hospital, New Brunswick, New Jersey

Chemotherapy

KATHLEEN RUCCIONE, RN, MPH

Assistant Clinical Professor, University of California-Los Angeles School of Nursing, Los Angeles, California

Late Effects in Long-Term Survivors

MARY C. SULLIVAN, RN, MSN, CRNP

Adjunct Faculty Member, University of Alabama in Birmingham, Birmingham, Alabama

Malignant Tumors of Childhood and Adolescence: Neuroblastoma

JACQUIE TOIA-MARINO, RN, MS

Clinical Nurse Specialist, Oncology Long Term Follow-up Program, Children's Memorial Hospital, Chicago, Illinois

Malignant Tumors of Childhood and Adolescence: Histiocytosis

SUSIE TRUESDELL, PA

Physician Assistant, Division of Cardiology, University of Rochester Medical Center, Rochester, New York

Late Effects in Long-Term Survivors

GERI VanWEZEL-BOLEN, RN, MSN

Clinical Nurse Specialist, Pediatric Hematology/Oncology, Children's Hospital of Illinois, St. Francis Medical Center, Peoria, Illinois

Malignant Tumors of Childhood and Adolescence: Rhabdomyosarcoma

CAROLYN L. WALKER, RN, PhD

Associate Professor and Graduate Advisor, School of Nursing, San Diego State University, San Diego, California

Nursing Management of Psychosocial Care Needs

MARY J. WASKERWITZ, BSN, CPNP

Pediatric Nurse Practitioner, DeVos Children's Hospital at Butterworth, Division of Pediatric Hematology/Oncology, Grand Rapids, Michigan

Malignant Tumors of Childhood and Adolescence: Unusual Tumors

DeLOIS P. WEEKES, RN, DNSc

Assistant Professor, University of California, San Francisco, School of Nursing, Department of Family Health Care Nursing, San Francisco, California

Nursing Management of Psychosocial Care Needs

MEREDITH HAPP WEINTRAUB, RN, MSN, PNP

Nurse Practitioner, Hematology/Oncology Division, The Children's Hospital of Alabama, Birmingham, Alabama

Nursing Management of the Child or Adolescent With Infection

LINDA WELLS, RN, MA, CNA

Administrative Manager, Children's Center for Cancer and Blood Disorders of Richland Memorial Hospital, Columbia, South Carolina

Nursing Management of Psychosocial Care Needs

ELIZABETH HANNIGAN WHITTAM, RN, C, MSN, FNP

Family Nurse Practitioner, Department of Pediatrics, Memorial Sloan-Kettering Cancer Center, New York, New York

Nursing Management of the Child or Adolescent in Pain

FRANCES McKINNEY WILEY, RN, MN

Professor of Pediatrics, School of Medicine, University of California-Los Angeles, Los Angeles, California; Clinical Nurse Specialist, University of California-Los Angeles, Los Angeles, California

Leukemia in Children and Adolescents: Acute Myelogenous Leukemia

LINDA WOFFORD, RN, MSN, PNP

Houston, Texas

Malignant Tumors of Childhood and Adolescence: Introduction

MYRA WOOLERY-ANTILL, RN, MN

Pediatric Clinical Nurse Specialist, Cancer Nursing Service, Nursing Department, Warren Grant Magnuson Clinical Center, National Institutes of Health, Bethesda, Maryland

Biologic Response Modifiers

PREFACE

The first edition of *Nursing Care of the Child With Cancer* was published 10 years ago. The changes occurring over the ensuing decade have resulted in the need for a second edition that is substantially different from the first. This book is, in essence, a new book.

The most exciting and gratifying changes are those related to improved outcomes for the children and their families. Pediatric cancer, once considered a death sentence, is now thought of as a potentially curable chronic disease. Advances in the biologic sciences have resulted in new treatment modalities, refinements and improvements in established strategies, and greater understanding of side effects and long-term sequelae. Advances in the social sciences have resulted in more accurate assessments of the psychosocial needs of children, adolescents, and families. Research findings now guide practice much more frequently than in the past. More effective interventions to assist children, adolescents, and families living with cancer have emerged. The outcome of survivorship has mandated greater emphasis on psychosocial adaptation, and research findings regarding bereavement have prompted changes in understanding this complex psychologic challenge.

The role of nursing has also changed dramatically in the past 10 years. Pediatric oncology's pioneering use of pediatric nurse practitioners to care for chronically ill children has become a firmly established model for other areas of nursing specialization. New practice roles such as the combined clinical nurse specialist–nurse practitioner role are being explored. The multidisciplinary team has expanded to include health care providers in schools, occupational health settings, and adult medicine, to cite but a few. This change has been necessitated by the reality of children living into adulthood with all the resultant needs for physical and psychosocial monitoring and follow-up. Nursing research has responded to the challenges of more complex care requirements in both the physical and psychosocial domains. Advances in research-based practice have fostered more effective clinical nursing practice in all care settings.

The second edition of *Nursing Care of the Child With Cancer* has been developed to address the changes of the past decade. New chapters cover important material essential to those practicing in the field today, including the pathophysiology/epidemiology of pediatric cancers, bone marrow transplantation, and biologic response modifiers. These reflect the advances of the biologic sciences that have led to new treatment approaches. Outcome changes are explored in new chapters dealing with the dying child and late effects, and the addition of a chapter on home and hospice care acknowledges the key roles now being played by nonhospital care settings. All remaining chapters have been extensively revised and most have been expanded. Chapters on the malignant diseases of children and adolescents, diagnostic interventions, chemotherapy, and radiation have all been updated. The psychosocial chapter has been expanded through the use of a stress-coping framework and by emphasis on the needs of the entire family. Chapters on the multidisciplinary team and on history, issues, and trends focus on the contributions of pediatric oncology nurses to the care of children with cancer.

This book will be useful to a wide variety

of nurses. It is an indispensable reference for new practitioners in the field, students, school nurses, community-based nurses, and nurses caring for adolescents in adult units. Experienced practitioners will find advanced content related to pathophysiology and genetics.

The development of a book of this scope and size is an arduous labor of love. Neither the authors nor the editors received monetary compensation for their efforts. This generosity of resources was matched by generosity of time. Our thanks to the chapter authors who worked diligently to provide the most accurate, up-to-date, relevant information. Their intelligence, dedication, and good humor made a difficult job easier. Several individuals graciously provided consultation services. Particular thanks to Ralph Vogel, RN, MSN, of the University of Tennessee School of Nursing; Jo Ann Belle Isle, RN, MSN, University of Rochester School of Nursing; and Margaret Fracaro, RN, MA, Columbia University Hospitals.

The staff of W.B. Saunders Company provided us with support, encouragement, and gentle guidance. Our thanks to Michael Brown, our original editor and former editor-in-chief, and to Thomas Eoyang, current editor-in-chief who helped guide the book through the final stages of preparation. Tom masterfully dealt with our anxiety about changing editors so late in the process. Much appreciation to Cass Stamato and to Marilyn Marcella and to the W.B. Saunders production staff. Joy Moore of Cracom Corporation and Kitty McCullough, our free-lance editor, were patient, knowledgeable, goal-directed, and fun to work with.

In each of our offices, certain heroic staff members assisted us. In New York City, Isabelle Margle coordinated, cajoled, and patiently listened while typing, mailing, and faxing. Pat Piano in Chicago and Susan Chamberlain assisted by Deb Bacham in Salt Lake City provided expert support services, graciousness, and diligence.

We are indebted to the nursing leadership of our institutions: Patricia Mazzola Lewis, Chairman, Division of Nursing at Memorial Sloan-Kettering Cancer Center; Jamie O'Malley, former Vice President of Nursing at Children's Memorial Hospital in Chicago; Cora Freitas, former Vice President of Nursing at Kapiolani Medical Center for Women and Children; and Dean Linda Amos of the University of Utah College of Nursing. The staff and students, patients and families with whom we work provided inspiration and kept us goal oriented. To our families, friends, and coworkers, our fondest and most grateful thanks; they were patient with the limited time we had available for them, forgiving our preoccupation with writing and editing, and resourceful as they struggled to clarify whether the dining room table was for eating or for manuscript development. Without their love and steadfast support, this second edition would not have been possible.

CONTENTS

History, Issues, and Trends

Genevieve V. Foley
Jean H. Fergusson

"... I believe there is merit in looking at the past in order to have a perspective of accomplishments, challenges, trends and future needs. Moreover, I think it can give us courage and determination to pursue our ideas and ideals."

—Renilda Hilkemeyer[50]

The emergence of oncology as a distinct discipline began during the Renaissance but was not completed for centuries.[90] This languid maturation pace resulted from complex historical causes, many of which influenced the general development of medicine and others of which directly affected oncology. Not surprisingly, the subspeciality of pediatric oncology took even longer to appear since it also was affected by factors relating to the care of children. Indeed it was not until the early nineteenth century that the first cases of childhood malignancies were reported in scientific literature.[24]

The history of pediatric oncology nursing as a distinct subspeciality begins soon after the end of World War II. The complex factors prompting the emergence of pediatric oncology nursing are rooted in the histories of pediatrics, oncology, and nursing. This chapter examines the resulting mosaic of traditions, beliefs, values, and practices that influenced the past, shaped the present, and suggest the future of pediatric oncology nursing.

LEGACY OF HIPPOCRATES AND GALEN

Determining the existence and prevalence of malignancies before the time of Hippocrates (460–370 BC) has proved challenging and controversial.[12,65,83] The technical problems of studying fossil and skeletal remains thousands of years old and the complex issues involved with accurate translation of ancient manuscripts combined to cast doubt on whether cancer has been known since the earth's earliest days. Further study is needed to answer this question.

The influence of Hippocrates on oncology is significant. Hippocrates was the first to use the term *karkinos* to describe a cancer. The Hippocratic writers of the fifth and fourth century BC used *karkinos* and *karkinoma* interchangeably. Both meant *crab*; neither was precisely defined; and both were used to describe a variety of conditions, some of which correspond to the present definition of *malignant neoplasm*.[53] Hippocrates mentions neck growths in children, but it is not known whether these growths were cancers.[23] Often a swelling was considered a cancer if the patient died.[65] Thus, although true malignancies did exist during this time, the occurrence and prevalence remain unknown.[81]

Hippocrates suggested that cancer was caused by an excess of black bile, or melanchole,[90] a humoral theory reaffirmed and elaborated by Galen (130–200 AD), who described an unhealthy swelling arising from a single or multiple humor as *oncos*.[53] Galen, the medical authority of the Western world for the next 13 centuries, listed cancer among the "Tumors Contrary to Nature." Ulcers, fistulas, and carbuncles also were so classified.[90] Both these men believed that advanced cancer was best left alone. Superficial tumors located on visible parts of the body were treated with caustic pastes and various herbal preparations, excision, or cautery.[83]

The opinions of Hippocrates and Galen were unchallenged for nearly 2000 years, and little progress was made in medicine until the Renaissance when the process now known as the *scientific method* was introduced. This new approach, characterized by reliance on observation and induction and by refusal to accept unquestionably the views of the past, slowly led to new discoveries, theories, and inventions.

PEDIATRICS

As in other fields of medicine, pediatrics relied on the views of the ancients, and few advances were made for many centuries.[39] From the 1470s a small but steady number of publications dealt with the diseases of children. These writings, published in several European countries, usually included information on pregnancy, newborns, and infants, a pattern that persisted for several hundred years and hampered the development of separate disciplines.

For centuries ill children received care in their homes. Children began to be admitted to hospitals during the sixteenth century in France.[39] Specialized facilities for children came into existence when the Hôpital des Enfants Malades opened in Paris in 1802. The first pediatric hospital in an English-speaking country was The Hospital for Sick Children in Great Ormond Street, London, founded in 1852. The Children's Hospital of Philadelphia, America's first hospital devoted exclusively to children, was established in 1855.[47]

In 1880 pediatrics became a speciality when the American Medical Association (AMA) established a separate section on diseases of children. Abraham Jacobi (1830–

1919) became the section's president.[20] Eight years later the first medical speciality society in the United States, the American Pediatric Society, was founded.[76]

L. Emmett Holt (1855–1924) succeeded Jacobi as Professor of Pediatrics at the College of Physicians and Surgeons. Holt's milestone textbook, *The Diseases of Infancy and Childhood*, contributed to pediatrics what Osler's *Principles and Practice of Medicine* gave to internal medicine.[77] With funds from the Rockefeller Foundation, Holt developed a laboratory at Babies Hospital in New York, which used the biochemical methods then known to study diseases of children. John Howland (1873–1926) shared Holt's funding to implement physical and chemical measurements of children treated at the Harriett Lane Home of the Johns Hopkins University Hospital, Baltimore. These activities were pioneering efforts in the use of quantitative research in pediatrics.[71]

Jacobi, Holt, and Howland were influenced by German and Viennese medical schools that used autopsy to confirm clinical evaluations and diagnosis. This acceptance of pediatric autopsy was an important element in the advancement of American pediatrics.[71]

Controversy surrounding proposals to reduce the infant mortality rate by improving infant nutrition eventually led to the establishment of the American Academy of Pediatrics. In 1921 the Sheppard-Towner Act established the nation's first federal formula grant program. The AMA vigorously opposed the original act and its extension. The defeat of the act prompted many members of the pediatric section to break away from the AMA. Thus in 1930 the American Academy of Pediatrics cast its fate with the child welfare movement, a course it has maintained to the present.[20]

The introduction of sulfonamides and penicillin and key discoveries pertaining to the fluid and electrolyte disorders of children combined to change childhood morbidity and mortality rates in the 1940s and 1950s.[47] New and perhaps more difficult challenges emerged, engendered by chronic illnesses such as cancer, social diseases, and psychologic problems resulting from changes in the child's and adolescent's environments.

Across cultures and throughout the centuries, the fate of children has been linked with the major societal values and problems of the time.[59] In virtually all cases, whatever the societal malady, the impact on children is more adverse than on other groups.[39,58] In response to the realities of children's needs, it has been customary for many of those caring for children to assume a broad mandate.[17] Pediatrics has been concerned not only with the ill child but also with health education, preventive health guidance, and child-rearing practices. To better the lives of children, advocacy and social activism have been accepted elements of pediatric practice through the centuries.[58]

PEDIATRIC ONCOLOGY

The first documented account of cancer in children appeared in 1809 when James Wardrop described 24 cases of malignant eye tumors, 20 of which occurred in children less than 12 years of age. This report represents the first collection of childhood cancer cases.[24] In 1876 C.J. Duzan published a tabulation of 182 pediatric malignancies reported in the literature between 1832 and 1875. Duzan's work represents the first publication devoted exclusively to cancer in children.[23]

Procedures for collecting and reporting statistics in the United States made it difficult to assess the incidence and mortality of pediatric cancers primarily because data for persons less than 30 years of age were presented in a single-age category. James Ewing, the pathologist for whom Ewing's sarcoma is named, objected strongly to that reporting system. He believed that juvenile cancers ". . . are so peculiar that properly they may not be compared with any adult tumors, and that this entire subject deserves to be treated as a special department in the descriptive history of neoplastic disease."[31]

The leading causes of death in children 1 to 14 years of age in 1936, 1966, and 1988 are compared in Table 1–1. Leukemia and Hodgkin's disease were included with other cancers in the 1936 statistics after being classified separately for many years. Their inclusion provided a more accurate picture of cancer deaths in children. Differences in the causes of death between 1936 and 1966 were also due to advances in general pediatric care, particularly the control of infectious disease. Sidney Farber (1903–1973) believed that these advances "unmasked" the problem of pediatric cancer. Indeed, by the end of World War II, cancer was identified as the leading cause of death from disease in the 1- to 15-year-old age group.[32] Although indicating the persistence of cancer as a major childhood health prob-

TABLE 1–1. *Leading Causes of Death in the United States in 1936, 1966, and 1988 for Children 1 to 14 yr: Rate per 100,000 Children, Age Adjusted*

RANK	CAUSE	1936	CAUSE	1966	CAUSE	1988
1	Accidents	40.1	Accidents	23.7	Accidents	14.0
2	Pneumonia	38.6	Cancer	7.0	Cancer	3.3
3	Diarrhea and enteritis	16.1	Congenital malformations	4.9	Congenital anomalies	2.6
4	Influenza	11.0	Influenza and pneumonia	4.5	Homicide	1.7
5	Appendicitis	10.6	Meningitis	0.8	Heart diseases	1.3
6	Tuberculosis	9.7	Heart diseases	0.8	Influenza and pneumonia	0.6
7	Heart Diseases	8.8	Homicide	0.8	Cerebral palsy	0.5
8	Diphtheria	7.6	Gastritis	0.7	Suicide	0.6
9	Cancer	5.3	Cerebral hemorrhage (stroke)	0.7	Meningitis	0.3
10	Scarlet fever	5.1	Meningococcal infections	0.7	Benign neoplasms	0.3
11	Diseases of the ear and mastoid	4.7	Cystic fibrosis	0.7	Human immunodeficiency (HIV) infection	0.3
12	Diseases of buccal cavity and pharynx	4.5	Cerebral spastic infantile paralysis	0.6	Diseases of infancy	0.3

From Vital Statisics of the United States, Washington, D.C.: U.S. Government Printing Office.

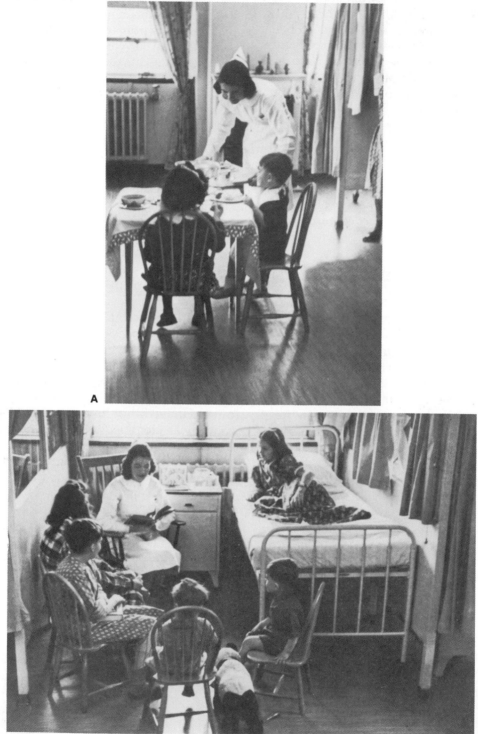

FIGURE 1–1.   **A,** Luncheon and, **B,** story hour in children's ward, Memorial Hospital, New York City, 1939. For many years only surgery and radiation were available to treat childhood cancers. Nurses monitored the effects of these treatments while focusing on providing care and comfort. *(Courtesy Memorial Sloan-Kettering Cancer Center, New York.)*

lem, data from 1988 also depict the results of improved cancer treatments.

Advances in pediatric hematology were necessary prerequisites for the development of pediatric oncology. An early need, to establish normal blood values according to age groups, proved a formidable task. For example, attempts began in 1919 to determine the life span of fetal and mature red blood cells; the question was not settled until the 1950s.[106]

The importance of bone marrow as a diagnostic tool was neglected in the United States.[106] Thomas Cooley (1871–1945) and colleagues published a series of papers on thalassemia yet never examined the bone marrow of those patients with the disease. Kenneth Blackfan and Louis Diamond's *Atlas of the Blood in Children* (1944) did not contain a single illustration of bone marrow. The difficulty of obtaining bone marrow led to much reliance on surgical biopsy. Katsuji Kato published a definitive study of the results of bone marrow aspirations from the sternums of 51 healthy infants and children in 1937. Possibly because Kato used the sternum as the aspiration site, few followed his lead. European hematologists were more inspired by Kato's work, and a series of European papers helped to define marrow characteristics in a variety of diseases. By the late 1940s the techniques of marrow aspiration including sternal aspirations were established and in wide use.[27]

Before 1950 pediatric hematology was concerned with diseases such as iron deficiency anemia, thalassemia, erythroblastosis fetalis, and aplastic anemia. Correcting these and other blood diseases was a frustrating experience because of the technical limitations involved. Small-caliber butterfly needles were not available in the 1940s.[78] Blood transfusions were uncommon,[106] partially because blood group subtypes were unknown, resulting in transfusion reactions with some frequency and intensity. Transfusions often were administered in the operating room, both for safety and for ensuring freshness of the blood. Administration routes included intravenous infusion, intramuscular injection, or subcutaneous clysis. Diamond, in the late 1940s, developed the technique of umbilical artery catheterization. Modern blood administration techniques were commonplace only after World War II.

The contributions of Sidney Farber and his colleagues at Boston Children's Hospital pioneered the era of chemotherapy as an effective primary and adjuvant therapy. Their work with folic acid antagonists was a milestone in the history of pediatric cancer. As other advances were made, the need to establish specialized clinical facilities was identified.[96] The first children's cancer unit, a four-bed ward, was established in 1934 at Memorial Hospital in New York City. It was enlarged to 26 beds in the early 1950s. St. Jude Children's Research Hospital, founded in the early 1960s in Memphis, was the first hospital devoted exclusively to pediatric malignancies.

The organization of pediatric oncology has been essential to its success.[32] Sidney Farber is credited with formulating the concept of the multidisciplinary team. The idea of making treatment decisions after receiving the input of all relevant specialists has greatly aided the quest for optimal treatment and end results. The National Wilms Tumor Study (NWTS), the first nationwide cooperative oncology group, was an outgrowth of Farber's multidisciplinary model.[16]

Board certification developed relatively soon after the emergence of the speciality.[103] The first certification examination was given in 1974, a milestone for American oncology in that no other country offered such an examination. In recognition of the historical links between pediatric hematology and pediatric oncology, expertise in both areas was required for board certification. A section on oncology-hematology was established within the American Academy of Pediatrics in 1975.[79] Accreditation for training programs in hematology-oncology was first required in 1987.[103]

The impact of pediatric cancer is far greater than might be expected from a relatively uncommon disease. The use of the multidisciplinary team and the pervasiveness of national cooperative trials are two examples of how pediatric oncology has led the way and influenced adult oncology.[16,103] As early as 1955 the Children's Leukemia Study Group A, later the Children's Cancer Study Group,

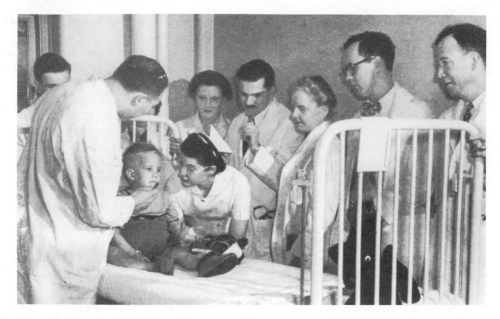

Figure 1–2. At Boston Children's Hospital the small patient's soft toys are laid aside as he is visited by nurse Lisa Blumenthal and Dr. Sydney Farber and his staff. *(Reprinted from the Saturday Evening Post © 1951.)*

formed. The Pediatric Oncology Group (POG) was established in 1979, the result of a merger between the Pediatric Division of the Southwest Oncology Group (SWOG) and the pediatric section of the Cooperative Acute Leukemia Group B (CALGB), both of which had formed in the late 1950s.[96]

Pediatric oncology has also influenced adult oncology as the result of clinical and laboratory investigations of rare pediatric tumors that have led to important discoveries about the role of genetics in adult and pediatric malignancies. The identification of long-term sequelae of treatment and the development of the concept of survivorship were pioneered in pediatric oncology.

FORMATIVE YEARS: ONCOLOGY

Advances in oncology were made slowly and unevenly and were dependent on the development of the sciences of anatomy, physiology, and histology.

A central problem throughout the first 18 centuries was the generally held belief that cancer was a local disease.[19] Thus discoveries made in one era often were not understood

for hundreds of years. For example, Gaspare Aselli (1581–1625) accidentally discovered lymphatic vessels and lymph fluid during an experimental study of visceral dog nerves.[95] The thoracic duct was pointed out by Jean Pecquet (1622–1674). Neither man understood the relationship of these findings to the spread of cancer.[83] Henri Francais Le Dran (1685–1770) postulated that cancer began as a local disease that spread through the lymphatic system to the lymph nodes and then to the general circulation. Le Dran's work was a key factor in putting aside the concept of cancer as a local problem.[9] Finally in 1829 Joseph Claude Anselme Récamier (1774–1852) used the term *metastasis* to describe what he believed were secondary tumors in the brain of a woman with breast cancer.[90]

Awareness of occupational and environmental carcinogens developed relatively early.[90] In 1700 Bernardini Ramazzini published *Diseases of Tradesmen* (English translation), the first systematic compilation of occupational diseases. He noted that nuns had a high incidence of breast cancer and postulated that this was due to their celibate lifestyle. This association between an occupation and a specific cancer is considered the first of its kind. Other important contributions were John Hill's association in 1761 between the use of snuff and nasal cancer and Samuel von Soemmering's identification in 1795 of the correlation between pipe smoking and lip cancer. Percivall Pott in 1775 documented the first occupational exposure to carcinogenic materials' resulting in clinical disease when he linked cancer of the scrotum with the occupation of chimney sweep.

Throughout much of oncology's history, surgery stood virtually alone as a treatment for cancer. Surgeons were limited by the difficulties of operating on a conscious patient struggling in pain as the surgeon worked.[95] The introduction of anesthesia in 1846,[30] coupled with the slowly advancing doctrines of Lister,[7] enabled surgeons to excise internal cancers. Since surgery was the only effective treatment available for cancer at the time, the expanded possibilities for surgery were critical to improved patient outcomes.[11]

SPECIALITY YEARS: AMERICAN ONCOLOGY

Oncology as a distinct discipline emerged slowly during the years leading up to World War II, then rapidly in the years following (Table 1–2). Although oncology continued to benefit from advances in other disciplines, it began to make original contributions, often linked with the work of laboratory and basic sciences.

Specific accomplishments of the twentieth century in treatment modalities are detailed in the appropriate chapters. However, surgery remained the cornerstone of therapy for many patients—the best hope for those whose ultimate outcome depended on adequate surgical removal of disease.

Lack of adequate radium sources slowed the early development of radiation therapy. The first division of radium therapy was not established until 1916.[21] The radium source

TABLE 1–2. *Selected Milestones—Maturation of Oncology as a Speciality*

MILESTONE	DATE
The New York Cancer Hospital is established (later called Memorial Hospital). First private facility in the United States treating cancer patients.[21]	1884
Wilhelm Conrad von Röntgen discovers x-rays.[19]	1895
Pierre and Marie Sklodowska Curie identify and isolate radium.[95]	1898
Bertillon classification of the causes of death is issued for international use. United States Death Registration System is set up, with 10 states participating.[90]	1900
Rockefeller Institute for Medical Research is established in New York City (first of its kind).[33] Karl Landsteiner discovers blood types.[19]	1901
American Association for Cancer Research (AACR) is established. Compiling cancer statistics is major priority.[11]	1907
F. Peyton Rous describes a filterable substance that causes chicken sarcoma (now called Rous sarcoma virus).[19]	1911
American Society for the Control of Cancer and the American College of Surgeons are founded.[15]	1913
Journal of Cancer Research begins publication as official journal of AACR.[90]	1916
U.S. Public Health Service sets up Office of Cancer Investigations, which issued Public Health Bulletin 155. Appreciable 20-year increase in cancer deaths is documented.[11]	1922 1925
Connecticut sets up first population-based tumor registry in United States.[71] International Union Against Cancer is established.[90]	1935
National Cancer Institute Act of 1937 is passed.[15]	1937
Journal of the National Cancer Institute begins publication.[90]	1940
American Society for the Control of Cancer is reorganized and renamed the American Cancer Society.[15]	1944
Cancer begins publication.[90]	1948
Austin Hill and Richard Doll report cancer-cigarette connection.[86]	1956
The surgeon general issues landmark report, "Smoking and Health."[86]	1964

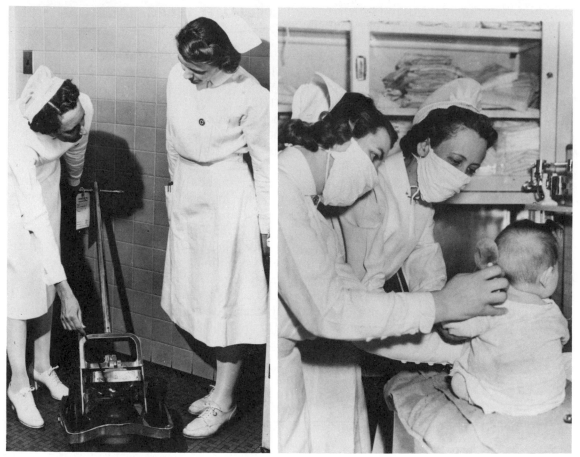

A

B

FIGURE 1–3. Katherine Nelson of Columbia University, New York City, received an American Cancer Society grant in the late 1940s for continuing education of nurses caring for cancer patients. Here she instructs a nurse about transporting radium, **A,** and caring for a pediatric patient, **B.** *(Courtesy Memorial Sloan-Kettering Cancer Center, New York.)*

for the facility at Memorial Hospital in New York City was donated by a bereaved parent. James Douglas, a physician and philanthropist, tried unsuccessfully to have his daughter treated in the United States with radium. In her memory Douglas established a mining operation in Colorado that yielded a significant supply of uranium. Clinical uses for radium expanded quickly, leading the way for recognition of radiation therapy as an important treatment option. Over the years improvement in the techniques, technologies, and delivery systems of radiation therapy have ensured advancement of the speciality.

The introduction of hormonal therapy influenced therapy strategies and care delivery systems.[11] For much of the time before World War II decisions about treatment for a partic-

ular patient were made by the patient's doctor in consultation with other physicians, usually a pathologist, then a surgeon and/or a radiation therapist. The need for a tumor expert, or oncologist, gained impetus in 1939 when Dr. Charles A. Huggins at the University of Chicago successfully demonstrated that orchiectomy, followed by administration of female sex hormones, was a way to treat advanced cancer of the prostate.

The emergence of chemotherapy was an event closely linked to the war effort.[11] Nitrogen mustard gas had been used with lethal effect during World War I. In 1919 E.B. Khrumbaar noted bone marrow aplasia and lymph tissue destruction among the deleterious attributes of the gas. Interest in the potential of nitrogen mustard gas reemerged during World War II. As part of a classified, chemical-warfare–type project, a group of investigators at Yale University in New Haven, Connecticut, Louis Goodman, Alfred Gilman, T.F. Dougherty, and Fredrick S. Philips, demonstrated that the nitrogen analogue of the gas was capable of shrinking lymphoma in laboratory animals.[90] Clinical trials were authorized at Yale, the University of Chicago, and Memorial Sloan-Kettering Hospital in New York. In 1946 when the war ended, the results of these studies were declassified and published. The subsequent introduction of other antineoplastic medications reinforced the usefulness of chemotherapy to improve outcomes.[11]

Another treatment modality, use of the biologic response modifiers, can trace its roots to the beginnings of immunology in the 1890s. For immunology to develop, many technical and conceptual discoveries were required. Most of the needed advances took place after World War II and were heralded by James Watson and Francis Crick's elaboration of double-helix DNA in 1953. This development accelerated the impetus to explore cell physiology, an event critical to the emergence of biologic response modifiers.[19]

The capabilities of all treatment modalities have been enhanced by the maturation of pathology and histology. Early attempts to assess the efficacy of treatment were impaired by uncertainty about whether like conditions were being compared. The establishment and refinement of a classification system was, and is, a cornerstone of modern, effective treatment.

Unlike today, cancer research at the turn of the century did not have public support, an understandable situation given that controlling infectious diseases and improving the public's health preoccupied the nation. The notion of cancer control as a public health responsibility likewise received little support. In 1926 the Massachusetts legislature took the unusual step of authorizing the state health department to devise care and treatment plans for persons with cancer "with or without the cooperation (of) . . . local physicians."[14]

Support for research came initially from the private sector and voluntary organizations. Their efforts encouraged government participation in cancer research. An early leader in philanthropic giving was John D. Rockefeller, who established the Rockefeller Institute. The American Cancer Society (ACS), known as the American Society for the Control of Cancer from 1913 to 1944, was founded to educate the public.[75] Support for research was accomplished through influencing public policy and legislation. The society played a key role in securing passage of the National Cancer Institute Act of 1937 authorizing establishment of the National Cancer Institute (NCI) and a National Advisory Cancer Council. Physician reaction to these initiatives was mixed, with concern expressed about governmental intrusion into research.[15]

In 1944, under the leadership of Mary Lasker, the society was reorganized and was named the American Cancer Society. Although a strong emphasis on education and patient services was maintained, a financial commitment to research was made.[86]

Undoubtedly the most important piece of legislation affecting cancer in the latter decades of the twentieth century was the National Cancer Act of 1971,[15] which upgraded the National Advisory Cancer Council to the National Cancer Board and which guaranteed by-pass budget approval, a special privilege enjoyed by no other component of the National Institutes of Health. The National Cancer Act also provided for the development of regional cancer centers, a critical element in enhancing availability of optimal treatment to all citizens, and reaffirmed cancer control activities as part of the national agenda.

Although many advances in cancer research, care, and treatment have been made in the United States, it would be an error to assume total American leadership.[83] Significant contributions have been made by scientists worldwide. Through the efforts of the International Union for Cancer Control (UICC) and other international agencies, global achievements and advances are shared on a regular basis.

FORMATIVE YEARS: NURSING

Little documentation exists about the beginnings of nursing.[4,26,52] Evidence from diverse sources such as Greek mythology, religious manuscripts, and medical texts indicates that the roles of caretaker of the sick, reliever of suffering, and conservator of health existed from mankind's earliest days. These roles were implemented through activities carried out in homes, usually by women as part of everyday life. Another common role of nursing was that of wet nurse or caretaker of children. Early Greek literature, for example, contains numerous references to nurses who were primarily children's nurses and not attendants of the sick.[4]

The advent of Christianity was a critical event in the history of nursing,[28,29] for it provided the altruistic basis needed to extend caring and service beyond the home, the neighborhood, and the tribe. Christianity elevated care of the sick, homeless, and imprisoned to acts of nobility. Men and women, some wealthy and well educated for the time, joined religious organizations or communities dedicated to the care of the sick and suffering. No longer were such activities commonplace and unworthy of notice.

Ensuing centuries witnessed the rise of military nursing orders and the formation of several Catholic and Protestant religious communities that provided the finest nursing care for centuries.[28] The Reformation, and later the Industrial Revolution, fostered societal changes that altered the role of religion, the status of women,[26] and attitudes toward children. The care of the sick, the young, and the poor was most adversely affected by these changes.[29]

MATURATION OF NURSING

Modern nursing begins in the mid-nineteenth century. Nursing at that time was in urgent need of reform. Most hospitals were dirty, overcrowded, and poorly ventilated. Nursing was an undesirable occupation, a view reinforced by the women employed as attendants to the sick. These women were poorly paid, lacked education, and often were of disreputable character.[52]

Florence Nightingale (1829–1910) responded to the pressing need to reform nursing. Nightingale was born into an upper-class English family. Her parents believed in edu-

cation for women, and her father personally taught her several classical subjects. Always devoutly religious, Nightingale felt called to care for the sick from her teen years. Because nursing was not suitable for a woman of her social class and moral character, her father refused her permission to become a nurse.[89] Finally she prevailed by going to Kaisersworth Institute for the Training of Deaconesses in Germany. The institute was a model center for learning for the time and taught what was then known about care of the sick.[88]

Almost single-handedly Florence Nightingale addressed key barriers to establishing nursing as a profession. She established a system of education for nurses, used specific measures of patient outcome to demonstrate the correctness of her interventions, and implemented systems of record keeping. A gifted writer, she used prose and statistics to document her many accomplishments.[73,88] Through Nightingale's efforts the value of education to prepare a trained nurse was recognized by the beginning of the twentieth century. Although many specifics of her program were not implemented in the United States, her philosophy of caring and excellence endures.

The care of children was not Nightingale's main concern, although she wrote regularly about their welfare. She understood the special problems of children and commented that ". . . (they) are much more susceptible than grown people to all noxious influences. They are affected by the same things, but much more quickly and seriously. . . ."[73]

With the establishment of children's hospitals, speciality nursing started to develop. One of the earliest nursing textbooks, *How to Nurse Sick Children*, was published in London in 1855. It reflected the nurse's predominant role of child caretaker, concerned with maintaining physical care and comfort.[68] Toward the end of the nineteenth century, Harvard University in Cambridge, Massachusetts, established the nation's first Department of Pediatrics. Academic pediatrics entered a new era, a development that supported the need for special preparation for nurses to care for children.[101]

The roles assumed by nurses caring for children reflected the needs of the times. As the twentieth century began, most pediatric nurses were experts in infectious diseases. These nurses cared for children in many settings, including the floating hospitals, ships anchored at some distance from the shore that often served as isolation centers.[28]

Care of well children was the prime responsibility of the public health nurse. Many Nightingale schools were located in the large cities of the East, which often had active public health departments. Lillian Wald, founder of the Henry Street Settlement House, and other socially conscious nurses were active participants in the struggle to improve sanitation, decrease morbidity and mortality, and improve the infant mortality rate.[13,29]

The segregation of patients by disease entities began in the 1920s and encouraged the emergence of staff dedicated to a specific clinical problem.[28] The explosion of knowledge and technology that occurred after World War II further hastened the trend toward specialization. Although the roles of nurse midwife and nurse anesthetist had existed since the early part of the century, other expanded and extended roles gradually developed as specialization increased.

Resistance to undergraduate and graduate education for nurses prevented these early efforts from gaining momentum. A parallel issue was the struggle to develop a knowledge base for nursing through nursing research.[72] Without nurses educationally prepared in institutions of higher learning, nursing research could not flourish. Although Florence Nightingale used clinical research to improve patient outcomes, it has taken more than 100 years for nursing research to establish itself firmly.[42]

Collegiate education for nurses, specialization of nursing practice, and nursing research have provided the impetus for sustained progress of the profession of nursing. Table 1–3 highlights selected milestones in the maturation of American nursing.

PEDIATRIC ONCOLOGY NURSING

The emergence of pediatric oncology nursing as a distinct subspeciality occurred in the late

TABLE 1–3. *Selected Milestones—Maturation of American Nursing*

MILESTONE	DATE
American Society of Superintendents of Training Schools for Nurses forms (eventually known as National League for Nursing).[26]	1893
American Journal of Nursing begins publication.[54]	1900
North Carolina, New Jersey, New York, and Virginia adopt licensing requirements for nursing.[54]	1903
M. Adelaide Nutting is appointed America's first Professor of Nursing, Teacher's College, New York.[30]	1907
National Association for Colored Graduate Nurses is established.[28]	1908
University of Minnesota offers first university-based nursing program.[72]	1909
American Nurses Association (ANA) founded.[26]	1911
National Organization for Public Health Nursing is established.[30]	1912
Sigma Theta Tau, national honor society of nursing, is founded at Indiana University.[28]	1922
The Goldmark Report is released (called for upgrading of nursing education).[54]	1923
Teacher's College, Columbia University, offers Doctor of Education for nurses preparing to teach at the college level.[72]	1924
Sigma Theta Tau begins funding nursing research.[72]	1936
Esther Lucille Brown publishes *Nursing for the Future*, and recommends collegiate education for nursing.[54]	1948
Nursing Research begins publication.[80]	1952
American Nurses Foundation established.[72]	1955
Lysaught Report is issued (urges funding for nursing research).[54]	1970
Department of Nursing Research is established within ANA.[80]	1972
Center for Nursing Research is established.[80]	1983
National Center for Nursing Research is set up within the National Institutes of Health.[72]	1985

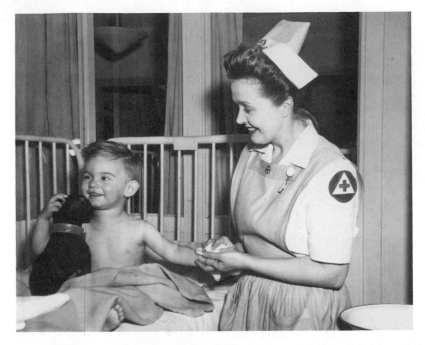

FIGURE 1–4. Child being bathed, Children's Ward, Memorial Hospital, New York City, 1943. Parents were excluded from participating in the everyday care of their children in most hospitals during the 1940s and 1950s. *(Courtesy Memorial Sloan-Kettering Cancer Center, New York.)*

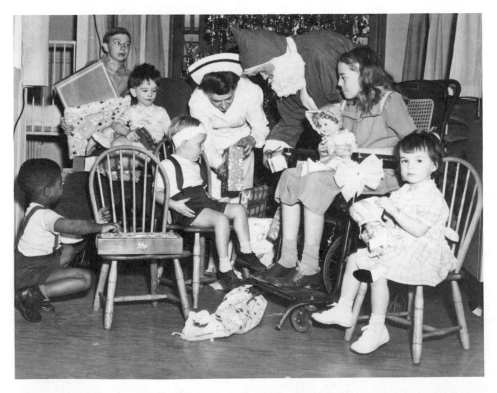

FIGURE 1–5. Christmas party, Children's Ward, Memorial Hospital, New York City, 1945. Even during holiday times, parental visitation was limited. *(Courtesy Memorial Sloan-Kettering Cancer Center, New York.)*

1940s. At that time the diagnosis of cancer in childhood was a metaphor for death. Nursing care consisted of providing comfort measures and skillfully using analgesics. Keeping a child clean, comfortable, and out of pain was the primary nursing goal. In contrast to the present, complete disclosure was not the norm. Protecting the child from the knowledge of his or her diagnosis was mandatory, as was supporting the family's denial. It was a time of strained silences and incomplete communication that was difficult for staff and families.[33]

In the 1940s care for children with cancer was provided by private duty nurses as "specials." Most often nurses gained skill and expertise through self-instruction and on-the-job training. Educational opportunities were limited.[22,61] There was little in the literature to inform the specialist nurse. Continuing education as it is known today did not exist.

In the late 1940s children began receiving chemotherapy. At that time the treatment was directed by a tumor therapist, now called a *pediatric oncologist*, who worked in association with a tumor therapy nurse. Many of the clinical functions of the tumor therapy nurse—administration of chemotherapy, teaching about the disease and treatment, coordinating hospital services for families, home visiting, school visiting, and involvement in research—are similar to ones performed today. All of these functions were learned by discussing and working with a tumor therapist. For example, triage skills were taught and monitored by the tumor therapist. Patient management decisions were based on joint decisions about treatment. In sum, most of the earlier nurse's "advanced clinical practice skills" were developed through clinical practice and close association with the tumor therapist who treated children with cancer. Jean Fergusson, an early pioneer in oncology nursing, worked with Dr. Sidney Farber and his associates at Children's Hospital in Boston and helped develop one of the first tumor

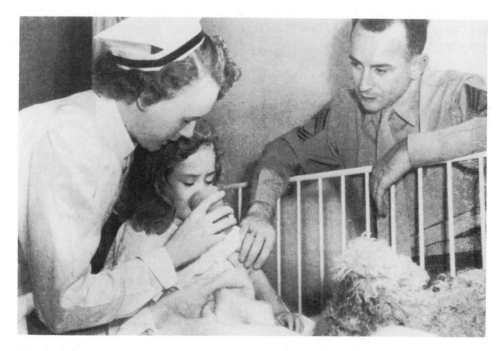

FIGURE 1–6. Great care was taken in the 1950s to keep the children unaware of what was wrong with them. This father must avoid betraying his feelings to his daughter, who is being given a drink by nurse Lois Jenkins, Head Nurse, Inpatient Tumor Therapy Service, Children's Hospital, Boston. *(Reprinted from the Saturday Evening Post © 1951. Thanks to Thomas Coates, M.D., an oncologist from the Division of Oncology at Children's Hospital of Los Angeles (CHLA), who found this issue of the Saturday Evening Post in a thrift-shop in Big Bear California. He brought it back to Kathy Ruccione at CHLA who sent it east to Jean Fergusson, who will treasure it forever.)*

therapy clinics in this country for children with cancer. From 1948 to 1953, working both full- and part-time, she enjoyed a clinical practice that included all of the aforementioned responsibilities.

Much of the history of pediatric oncology nursing during the 1950s is lost. A generation of nurses provided undocumented, unheralded care during what was one of the most difficult eras of pediatric oncology. In those days administering chemotherapy to children was considered cruel by some because the remissions were brief, the side effects devastating, and the supportive interventions limited. Family-centered care was almost unknown. Stringent hospital policies prevented parents from visiting their children more than a few hours per week unless the child was critically ill, and siblings were forgotten.

By the 1960s physical outcomes for the child began to improve substantially. More effective treatment strategies were developed, and advances in blood banking, infection control, and pediatric intensive care provided essential supportive care. Psychosocial care became more family centered,[57] partially in response to research findings and partially because of consumer pressure for change. Pediatric oncology nurses established new relationships with parents, which included more emphasis on parent and family participation and education.

In the 1960s pediatric oncology nurses began to assume new roles. Physician mentorship was a key factor in educating nurses for these roles. Once a cadre of nurses was established, continuing education programs often led by these nurses provided the necessary instruction and support. As the roles matured, preparation for them moved into academic institutions.

Research and practice roles followed this general pattern. In the 1960s nurses were recruited to assist with clinical research in pediatric oncology. They received on-the-job training that included physical assessment skills and basic knowledge about medical research methodology. This training was conducted by a pediatric oncologist who was primarily interested in cancer research and who needed a nurse to assist with data collection and patient evaluation. Initially many of these nurses were employed by the Clinical Cancer Research Branch of the National Institutes of Health. Today almost all pediatric oncology nurses play a vital role with pediatric oncologists in the management of medical protocols. In addition, some nurses design and implement nursing research studies.

The 1960s also were an important period for the development of advanced practice roles. The role of pediatric nurse practitioner developed early and exerted a significant influence on pediatric oncology nursing.

To prepare nurses to function in this new role, a Pediatric Nurse Practitioner Program was established at the University of Colorado in Denver by Dr. Henry Silver, a pediatrician, and Dr. Loretta Ford, a nurse educator.[36,92] This continuing education program prepared candidates to provide comprehensive well-child care and identify, assess, and manage both common disorders of childhood and developmental issues associated with each age group. The program modeled the realignment of the functions performed by pediatric nurses and pediatricians.

The nurse practitioner program at the University of Colorado came to the attention of Dr. Donald Pinkel, the first medical director of St. Jude Children's Research Hospital in Memphis. Dr. Pinkel and other physician leaders at St. Jude's adapted the Colorado model and developed a program that provided selected nurses with training in physical assessment skills and advanced technical skills such as bone marrow aspirations and spinal taps.[93] First Andi Wood, then Ellen Shanks, Clara Mason, and Shirley Stagner achieved nurse practitioner status through this program. These women were pioneers in oncology nursing.[43]

The nurse practitioner program at St. Jude's Hospital was in place when Robbie Simpson, a much-respected staff nurse, died of hepatitis.[44] In her honor the Robbie Simpson Fellowship was created in 1972 to commemorate exceptional nursing practice. The program focused on learning assessment and advanced technical skills, which were taught through direct participation in care and through educational conferences, seminars, and/or symposia offered by the institution. Those completing the fellowship were awarded a certificate from St. Jude's and were called *nurse practitioners in pediatric oncology.* Patricia E. Greene was the first graduate of the program.[43]

The nurse practitioner program at St. Jude's Hospital and the Robbie Simpson Fellowship influenced the development of pediatric oncology nursing throughout the country. The early leaders of the program emphasized nursing as the central component of the role. These nurses, beginning with Andi Wood, stressed a tradition of nurse mentorship that has characterized the speciality.[93]

Jean Fergusson took the next step in the maturation process. In 1976 Jean, who was prepared as a nurse practitioner by Northeastern University in Boston, designed a two-semester educational program in pediatric oncology at Children's Hospital of Philadelphia (CHOP). The program offered continuing education for pediatric oncology nurses seeking advanced clinical practice skills, particularly in the ambulatory care setting. Curriculum for the program followed the guidelines developed by the American Nurses Association (ANA) and the American Academy of Pediatrics (AAP), with didactic and clinical focus in pediatric oncology. The first two students in the program were Mary Waskerwitz from Mott Children's Hospital in Ann Arbor, Michigan, and Betsy Becker from CHOP. Within a year this pioneering program was approved by the National Association of Pediatric Nurse Associates and Practitioners (NAPNAP) and the Pennsylvania State Board of Nursing.

The CHOP program provided a select group of pediatric oncology nurses with practitioner skills and knowledge about the most recent advances in pediatric oncology. Eventually the program became associated with Widener University Graduate School of Nursing in Chester, Pennsylvania, and was changed from continuing education to graduate education, with ongoing sponsorship by the cancer center at CHOP. The influence of the CHOP program was enormous. Ninety-four nurses completed the program, and most are practicing in cancer centers throughout this nation and Canada, with many becoming leaders in pediatric oncology nursing.

By the mid-1980s continuing education programs to prepare nurses as practitioners were phased out. Education for the role became part of graduate nursing programs that award a master's degree and enable graduates to obtain specific practitioner licensure in those states requiring it.

Pediatric oncology nursing was a pioneer in the development and use of expanded nursing roles.[43] The idea that nurse practitioners could provide ambulatory care for chronically ill children was tested and validated in pediatric oncology. That contribution is part of the speciality's lasting legacy.

Other advanced roles such as that of the nurse clinician[35] and clinical nurse specialist[49] have contributed to the development of pediatric oncology nursing. These roles have been based primarily in the inpatient setting. Each role has been characterized by the ability to use advances in medical and nursing research and in clinical practice, to exhibit a high level of professional accountability, and to function both independently and interdependently with other providers.[46] Individuals in these advanced roles understand that accountability flows from an adequate knowledge base and a lifelong commitment to learning.[74]

The emergence of speciality nursing organizations also influenced the development of pediatric oncology nursing. The ACS's National Nursing Advisory Committee, established in 1951, provided the sole national forum for cancer nurses for decades.[50] As oncology nursing developed and specialized, more specific opportunities for networking and education were needed.[6]

The Association of Pediatric Oncology Nurses (APON) was instrumental in meeting the communication and support needs of pediatric oncology nurses. Once organized, APON established formal relationships with other nursing organizations, particularly the Oncology Nursing Society, the ANA, and the Federation of Nursing Speciality Organizations. Pediatric oncology nurses have made significant and varied contributions to the ACS throughout its organizational structure. Strong ties with the national parent group, The Candlelighters, and other parent groups have matured throughout the years and constitute a significant source of support for both groups. Improvements in physical and psy-

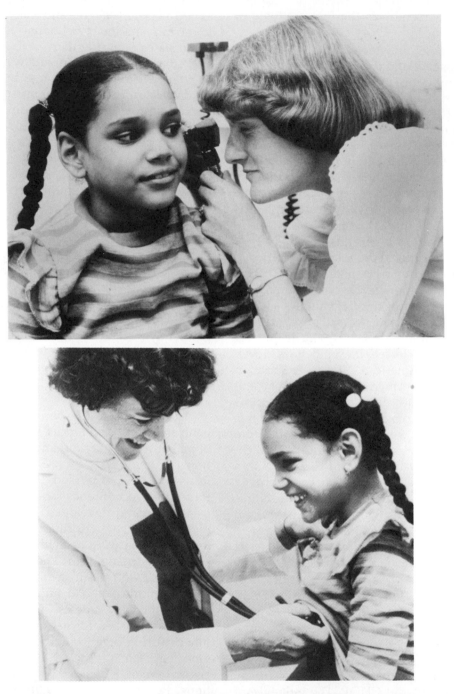

Figure 1–7.   The Pediatric Nurse Practitioner program developed by Jean Fergusson at Children's Hospital of Philadelphia educated a cadre of advanced practitioners who provided pediatric oncology nursing throughout the country. *(Photographs of Judy Lea* (top) *and Barbara Carroll* (bottom) *courtesy Jean Fergusson, R.N., and Children's Hospital of Philadelphia.)*

chosocial aspects of care have been facilitated by these relationships.

Table 1–4 depicts selected milestones in the history of pediatric oncology nursing.

ISSUES AND TRENDS

Pediatric oncology nurses are proud of their historical contributions to the care of children and families, the multidisciplinary team, the profession of nursing in general, and cancer nursing in particular. They have facilitated advances in the biologic and social sciences by their own scholarship and research and by participation in the scholarly and research activities of other professionals. These accomplishments provide a strong foundation from which to face future challenges.

What are the actual and potential concerns that will test pediatric oncology nursing in the years ahead, influence practice, education, and research, compel the establishment or renewal of alliances, and require the assessment and development of more effective strategies for action? Although prediction is always a risky business, it is likely that the following will be of importance.

Maintaining and Improving Outcomes of Care

The therapies of the last 40 years have resulted in significant advances in lives saved. Since 1973 overall survival has improved yearly. For some diseases, an upward survival curve has existed even longer.[18,66] So dramatic are these improvements that by the year 2000 it is estimated that one in 900 persons 15 to 45 years of age will be a survivor of childhood cancer.[10] Despite this substantial progress,

TABLE 1–4. *Selected Milestones in Pediatric Oncology Nursing*

MILESTONE	DATE
Pediatric Oncology Nurse Practitioner role created at St. Jude Children's Research Hospital. Andi Wood, Ellen Shanks, Clara Mason, and Shirley Stagner are first to implement role.[43]	1969
Candlelighters forms under leadership of Grace Powers Monaco.	1970
Eugenia Waechter publishes landmark study on children's awareness of fatal illness.[100]	1971
St. Jude Hospital institutes Robbie Simpson Memorial traineeship. Patricia E. Greene is first graduate.	1972
American Cancer Society's First National Cancer Nursing Conference is held. Session on childhood cancer nursing included.[43] Association of Pediatric Oncology Nurses (APON) is founded.	1973
Patricia E. Greene elected first APON president.	1974
Oncology Nursing Society (ONS) is incorporated in the state of Illinois.[105]	July 1, 1975
APON is incorporated in the state of Tennessee.	April 15, 1976
Jean Fergusson develops pediatric nurse practitioner (PNP) in oncology program at Children's Hospital of Philadelphia.	1976
Liaison is established with ONS.	1978
Ida Martinson publishes pioneer research on home care for children dying of cancer.[64]	1978
Standards of Care is published in cooperation with ANA. Provides first subspecialty standards in oncology nursing.[50]	1979
First textbook of pediatric oncology nursing is published, with Dianne Fochtman and Genevieve Foley as editors.[34]	1982
Journal of the Association of Pediatric Oncology Nursing (JAPON) is established, with Dianne Fochtman as editor.	1984
Marilyn Hockenberry and Deborah Coody publish *Pediatric Oncology and Hematology: Perspectives on Care.*[51]	1986
First issue of the *Journal of Pediatric Oncology Nursing* (JOPON) is published by W. B. Saunders with Dianne Fochtman continuing as editor.	1989

more must be done for the average years of life lost to pediatric cancer remains unacceptably high.[85]

Although the distribution of pediatric cancers has been relatively constant within age groups, overall incidence has increased slightly. Projections of data from the Surveillance Epidemiology and End Results (SEER) program of the National Cancer Institute estimate an annual U.S. incidence of 14 cases per 100,000 children younger than 15.[85] This increase appears related to higher incidence of acute lymphoblastic leukemia (ALL) and brain and central nervous system tumors.

Throughout the history of pediatric oncology, compilation of accurate statistics has been problematic. Current concerns center on adolescent data. Most pediatric statistics end at age 14 years, some extend to age 19, and others group 15 to 24 year olds together. Obtaining accurate data describing cancer in the teen years is important for several reasons, the most important of which is survival. Evidence suggests that some adolescents are not receiving state-of-the-art physical and psychosocial care.[18] Adolescents apparently are not entered in either pediatric or adult cooperative group trials; therefore they less frequently receive the benefits of multidisciplinary involvement in planning and carrying out treatment strategies. Adolescents may receive care on adult units from staff members who are not aware of the appropriate spectrum of psychosocial supports and interventions required. The ACS maintains that adolescent care outcomes require further study and action if outcomes of care are suboptimal. Pediatric oncology nurses need to assist in the fact-finding effort, to offer consultation services to adult units caring for adolescents, and to advocate adolescent registration in clinical trials.

Two other significant areas involved in maintaining and improving outcomes of care are psychosocial wellness and late effects. The concept of the truly cured child[99] is a goal for all children. As physical cure is attained for more children, challenges and opportunities to enhance psychosocial outcomes become more numerous and complex. Likewise the needs of the dying child and bereaved family

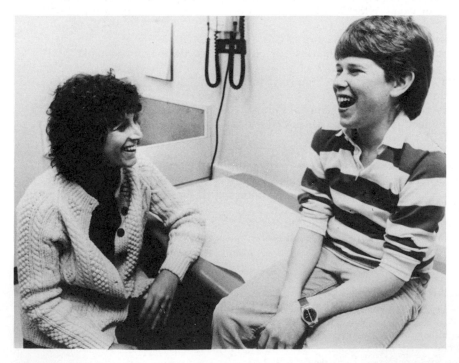

FIGURE 1–8. Physical and psychosocial evaluation of childhood cancer survivors is an important new role for the pediatric oncology nurse. *(Photograph of Wendy Hobbie courtesy Jean Fergusson, R.N., and Children's Hospital of Philadelphia.)*

must occupy a more prominent place in providing expert psychosocial care.

The emergence of long-term or late effects of pediatric cancer and its treatment has redefined and refocused care outcomes. The pediatric oncology nurse must be ready to respond to refinements in treatment that facilitate improved quality of life while maintaining curative potential. In addition, the concept of rehabilitation must guide care from the earliest days of treatment. The recognition and prevention of late effects have become the responsibility of all pediatric oncology nurses.

Ensuring Access to Appropriate Care

The high success rate of pediatric cancer therapy has been enhanced by the treatment of children by a multidisciplinary team in specialized facilities in which the children are enrolled in clinical trials.[18,45] However, there are several worrisome signs that these critical care patterns are in danger.

The most important issue relating to ensuring access to appropriate care is that children are America's poorest age group.[55] In 1990 12.7 million children lived below the poverty level, an increase of 2.7 million children from 1979. Approximately one in seven white children is poor; thus most poor children are white. The percentage of poor children is greater in other races, however. More than one third of Hispanic children and almost one half of African-American children live in poverty.

Overall, children in poverty reside in two-parent households in which one or both parents work. Minority children are more likely than white children to live in one-parent households, a condition associated with intensifying the effects of poverty. Nevertheless virtually all families except the most wealthy have less income, for between 1979 and 1990, the real median income of families with children fell by 5%.

The issue of children and poverty is affecting all of pediatrics. In the general pediatric community access to care among children and adolescents is uneven and in some cases inadequate.[67,69,70,104] Absent or suboptimal health insurance is one of the most important factors contributing to this problem. Between 1987 and 1991 approximately one fifth of the nation's children had no health insurance.[48,55,62]

There is evidence that cancer care for adults is being adversely affected by impaired access and underfunding.[38,59] The ACS launched a major program initiative in 1988 to identify issues and develop solutions to the problem of cancer in the socioeconomically disadvantaged. The society's Children and Cancer Committee is studying whether economic and access factors are affecting care received by childhood cancer patients.

Pediatric oncology has experienced the economic pressure of decreased funding for cooperative group trials. Philanthropic funds from parents, grandparents, families, and friends of the pediatric oncology patient have provided some research monies. It is likely, however, that new dollars will be required for clinical care to ensure open access to all children regardless of their socioeconomic status. These funds may be even more difficult to obtain than research dollars.

Awareness of economic factors is essential for the pediatric oncology nurse. Also vital is knowledge of the resources available and not available in the child's particular community. Close working relationships with social workers and the personnel of community agencies are critical. Finally, alliances must be formed with those concerned with improving access. Organizations such as the American Academy of Pediatrics,[2] Candlelighters, and the Children's Defense Fund have advocacy programs for children. The pediatric oncology nurse, individually and through APON and ANA,[3] must work to forge improvements in children's health. As the 1990 to 1991 measles epidemic demonstrated, unsolved general pediatric problems pose a risk to the child or adolescent with cancer. Likewise the reality of inadequate access to care poses an even greater risk.

Mitigating the Effects of Demographic Changes

The most important demographic reality for children and families is the aging of the population.[84] The evolution of the contemporary view of childhood as a period of special concern and investment is a result of the gradual decrease in child mortality rates and the rise in adult life expectancy. The increased likelihood that a child will live to adulthood makes it easier for parents to become emotionally invested in individual children and to plan for their future. Indeed, emotional and financial investment in children began in earnest only after childhood mortality rates fell. In addition, with a steady increase in the number of years Americans expect to live after reaching adulthood, it became more appropriate to view childhood as a preparation for adult life and to allot more of an individual's early years for that preparation.

It is ironic that the same demographic forces contributing to a special social status for children have created an aging society in which that status may be threatened.[37,91,102] Since 1960 when children under age 18 made up 35.7% of the total U.S. population, the percentage has fallen dramatically. By 1980 the percentage was 27.9, and by the first quarter of the twenty-first century it is projected to be 21.6%. In 1970 there were approximately 6 million more children in the population than in 1990. At the same time the population over 65 is growing much more rapidly than the population as a whole.[37,91,102] From a mere 8% in 1950, the percentage of elderly climbed to 12% in 1984 and is projected to reach 17% of the population in the first quarter of the new century. That proportion is the same as in today's most "elderly" state, Florida.

In the aging society America's children may be viewed as either a treasured resource or a needy minority.[84,87,97] The optimistic view holds that society will recognize the increasing need for healthy, well-motivated, and properly educated young people capable of becoming the workers, providers, innovators, and defenders of the aging society.[82] The pessimistic view argues that the trends of the last 20 years suggest that children will be perceived as a needy minority. Americans have not been particularly committed to supporting children as a group with growing needs. The absence of appropriate day care, despite an expanding number of women in the work force, attests to a national lack of will or lack of understanding or both.

Perhaps more important than the declining concern for the needs of *all* children is that the basic economic support for *needy* children, never generous in the first place, is declining even further. Unlike programs for the elderly, public assistance initiatives for children and families are not indexed to inflation, are not available to all children within a specific age group regardless of income level, and do impose criteria for living arrangements. Aid to Families With Dependent Children usually provides only for children of single parents. State-by-state variations in eligibility criteria and benefits are another difference. Programs for the elderly, social security retirement and medicare, are national in scope and generally more comprehensive.

Children and adolescents receiving treatment for cancer or experiencing survivorship may be needy in other ways.[87] At least some cancer survivors will be physically, intellectually, or emotionally challenged. These young people may be competing for scarce financial and health care resources with the aged. Individuals over 65 years old use approximately 30% of all health services despite their comprising approximately 12% of America's total population.

Given the pervasiveness of the aging society phenomenon and its potential detrimental effect on children and families, pediatric nursing must take an active role in advocating for children and in forming alliances with the elderly. The ingenuity of pediatric oncology nursing must be used to devise win-win strategies based on the concern about cancer that unites the aged and the young.

Managing the Impact of Changes in the Family Life of Pediatric Oncology Patients

By 1995 it is estimated that the total number of two-parent, never-divorced families in the United States will be less than the total of single-parent and remarried families. Single parenting may occur as the result of death, divorce, or separation and out-of-wedlock births. More than 25% of American children are now involved in a single-parent situation, and more than 60% may have the experience by the end of their high school years.[60]

In addition to divorce, remarriage is a

long-term American trend. Men commonly remarry 1 year after divorce and women closer to 1½ years after divorce. Approximately 80% of divorced persons remarry,[60] often giving rise to the creation of a blended family in which children from each marriage live with the remarried couple. Other family patterns that may affect the child, either positively or negatively, are the multiple generation family, the multiple wage earner family, and partners of the same or opposite sex sharing living quarters.[41]

In assessing the impact of these trends, the pediatric oncology nurse must understand that in periods of rapid social change, the problem of adjustment is especially great and leads to increasing signs of personal and family stress.[63] A significant stressor for children is that fewer children today than four decades ago know the benefits of lifelong dependable ties between themselves and their parents. In addition, nontraditional living patterns, although not necessarily detrimental to the child, do require extra effort by the adults in the child's world to mitigate negative consequences.

The diagnosis of cancer strains the most stable marriage and the strongest family. The pediatric oncology nurse likely will encounter more complex, less stable family situations, requiring greater theoretic knowledge and more sophisticated skills.

Retaining Nursing Focus on Humanizing the Cancer Experience

A key role of the pediatric oncology nurse is to humanize the cancer experience—to connect with the child and family in such a way that the dignity, uniqueness, and strengths of the child and family are enhanced. Technology is a potential force for dehumanization, and pediatric oncology is a technology-intense speciality. To focus beyond the disease, beyond the technology, is a constant challenge for the nurse.

Although there are many possible concerns, those relating to ethics are especially important.[8,25,98] Integrating ethical principles into nursing practice and research requires that the nurse be knowledgeable about specific issues relating to the care of minors. Consent for treatment, particularly if it is of limited or no benefit to the child, the need to obtain the child's assent for participation in research studies, and limits on parental decision making are all areas of special importance. Pediatric oncology first challenged existing ethical thought by using investigational agents on terminally ill children. Now broad ethical issues involve genetic engineering, whether it is ethical to conceive a child to be a transplant donor, and conflicts between parent and child about termination of treatment. It is clear that technology will continue to become available before society has reached consensus on the ethical issues involved. The long tradition of advocacy and social activism that has characterized pediatrics will demand that pediatric oncology nurses contribute to the societal dialogue and assist in achieving resolution.

Creating and Strengthening Alliances

The problems facing children with cancer and their families will be increasingly complex and will require new strategies. Alliances among the current pediatric team must be strengthened to provide the child and family with optimal care. Also important will be strengthening ties within pediatric nursing. As the pediatric community has become increasingly concerned about over-subspecialization,[1] there has been a call for renewed cooperation within pediatrics. Nurses caring for children with other chronic illnesses may be a valuable resource in areas such as adherence to treatment regimens, integration of growth and development concepts in psychosocial care and patient teaching, and bereavement interventions.

The creation of nurse-to-nurse networks with colleagues in adult nursing will be of greater importance. The emergence of a large group of pediatric cancer survivors will compel dialogue with nurses in college infirmaries, internal medicine practices, obstetric practices, and gynecology facilities. Such collaboration is essential to enhance understanding of late consequences of treatment and to ensure optimal care for the "pediatric graduate."[56,62]

Pediatric oncology nurses must also

broaden their role to encompass public and social advocacy. The time and energy required to provide nursing care to the children and families are extensive. Yet without a commitment to participate in legislative and public policy change, the work of the pediatric oncology nurse cannot achieve its full potential.

Developing New Practice Roles

In some settings the roles of pediatric nurse practitioner and clinical nurse specialist are coming together to provide care for hospitalized pediatric patients.[40] This trend may represent an opportunity to expand the definition of nursing practice. Nurse practitioner care of chronically ill children was a development of the role beyond well child care. Having nurse practitioners care for children sick enough to require hospitalization may be another plateau. The nurse practice act of each state may or may not accommodate such a change, but testing of that limit is likely.

As cancer prevention strategies mature, pediatric oncology nurses will assume more visible roles in educating young people about avoiding the cancers of adulthood. Prime opportunities involve informing young people about positive measures they can take to control their health. Areas of particular emphasis include use of sunscreens, prevention of obesity, selection of low-fat, high-roughage foods, and moderate use of alcohol. Of special importance are behaviors that support avoidance of tobacco in all its deleterious forms. In these and other areas of cancer prevention, the most basic role of the pediatric oncology nurse is that of exemplar.

REFERENCES

1. Alpert JJ. Primary care: The future for pediatric education. Pediatrics 1990; 7:653–659.
2. American Academy of Pediatrics. Children First. Washington, D.C.: Department of Government Liaison, 1990.
3. American Nurses Association. Nursing's Agenda for Health Care Reform. Washington, D.C.: The Association, 1991.
4. Austin AL. History of Nursing Source Book. New York: G.P. Putnam's Sons, 1957.
5. Ballabriga A. One century of pediatrics in Europe. In Nichols BL, Ballabriga A, Kretchmer N (eds). Nestle Nutrition Workshop Series, vol 22. New York: Raven Press, 1991, pp 1–21.
6. Barckley V. The best of times and the worst of times: Historical reflections from an American Cancer Society national nursing consultant. Oncol Nurs Forum 1982; 9:54–56.
7. Bender GA. Great Moments in Medicine. Detroit: Parke-Davis, 1961.
8. Benjamin M, Curtis J. Ethics in Nursing, 3rd ed. New York: Oxford Press, 1992.
9. Bett WR. Historical aspects of cancer. In Raven RW (ed): Cancer, vol 1. London: Butterworth & Co, 1957, pp 1–5.
10. Bleyer WA. The impact of childhood cancer on the United States and the world. CA 1990; 40:355–367.
11. Bordley J III, McGehee Harvey A. Two Centuries of American Medicine. Philadelphia: WB Saunders, 1976.
12. Brothwell D. The evidence for neoplasms. In Brothwell D, Sanderson AT (eds): Diseases in Antiquity. Springfield, Ill.: Charles C Thomas, Publisher, 1967, pp 320–345.
13. Buhler-Wilkerson K. Lillian Wald: Public health pioneer. Nurs Res 1991; 40:316–317.
14. California, University of at Los Angeles School of Public Health. A History of Cancer Control in the United States 1946–1971: Introductory Materials. Washington, D.C.: Department of Health, Education and Welfare, 1979.
15. California, University of at Los Angeles School of Public Health. A History of Cancer Control in the United States 1946–1971: Book Two, A History of Programmatic Developments in Cancer Control. Washington, D.C.: Department of Health, Education and Welfare, 1979.
16. Carter SK. Introduction. Front Radiat Ther Oncol 1982; 16:1–8.
17. Charney E. The field of pediatrics. In Oski FA, De Angelis CD, Feigin RD, et al. (eds): Principles and Practice of Pediatrics. Philadelphia: JB Lippincott, 1990, pp 4–10.
18. Children and Adolescents With Cancer: Report of an American Cancer Society Workshop. Atlanta: American Cancer Society, 1992.
19. Closing in on Cancer. Washington, D.C.: United States Department of Health and Human Services, 1987.
20. Cone TE Jr. History of American Pediatrics. Boston: Little, Brown & Co., 1979.
21. Considine B. That Many May Live. New York: Memorial Center for Cancer & Allied Diseases, 1959.
22. Craytor JK. Highlights in education for cancer nursing. Oncol Nurs Forum 1982; 9:51–59.
23. Dargeon HW. Malignant tumors in childhood. In Dargeon HW (ed): Cancer in Childhood. St. Louis: CV Mosby, 1940, pp 21–30.
24. Dargeon HW. Tumors of Childhood: A Clinical Treatise. New York: Paul B. Hoeber, 1960.
25. Davis AJ, Aroskar MA. Ethical Dilemmas and Nursing Practice, 3rd ed. Norwalk, Conn.: Appleton & Lange, 1991.
26. Deloughery GL. History and Trends of Professional Nursing, 8th ed. St. Louis: CV Mosby, 1977.
27. Diamond LK. Foreward. In Miller DR, Baehner R, Miller LP (eds): Blood Diseases of Infancy and Childhood. St. Louis: CV Mosby, 1989, pp ix–xiii.
28. Dolan JA. Nursing in Society: A Historical Perspective. Philadelphia: WB Saunders, 1978.
29. Donahue MP. Nursing. The Finest Art. St. Louis: CV Mosby, 1985.
30. Duffy J. The Healers: A History of American Medicine. Urbana, Ill.: University of Illinois Press, 1979.

31. Ewing J. A survey of cancer in children. In Dargeon HW (ed): Cancer in Childhood. St. Louis: CV Mosby, 1940, pp 13–20.

32. Farber S. The control of cancer in children. In Neoplasia in Childhood. Chicago: Year Book, 1969, pp 321–327.

33. Fergusson J. Pediatric oncology nursing: A historical perspective. Keynote address. Fifteenth Annual APON Conference. Boston, 1991.

34. Fochtman D, Foley GV. Nursing Care of the Child With Cancer. Boston: Little, Brown & Co, 1982.

35. Foley GV. The role of the pediatric nurse clinician in pediatric oncology. In Beal JA (ed): Issues and Advanced Practice in Pediatric Nursing. Reston, Va: Reston Publishing, 1983, pp 155–174.

36. Ford L. A nurse for all settings: The nurse practitioner. Nurs Outlook 1979; 27:516–521.

37. Frank-Stromborg ML. Population changes in the coming decade: Health care implications. In Issues in Cancer Care and Economics: Proceedings of the Sixth National Conference on Cancer Nursing. Atlanta: American Cancer Society, 1992, pp 1–20.

38. Freeman HP. Cancer in the socioeconomically disadvantaged. CA 1989; 39:266–288.

39. Garrison FH. History of pediatrics. In Abt-Garrison History of Pediatrics. Philadelphia: WB Saunders, 1965, pp 1–170.

40. Gleeson RM, McIlwain-Simpson G, Boos ML, et al. Advanced practice nursing: A model of collaborative care. MCN 1990; 15:9–12.

41. Glick PC. Fifty years of family demography: A record of social change. J Marriage Fam 1988; 50:861–873.

42. Grant MM, Padilla GV. Cancer Nursing Research, A Practical Approach. East Norwalk, Conn.: Appleton & Lange, 1990.

43. Greene P. The Association of Pediatric Oncology Nurses: The first ten years. Oncol Nurs Forum 1983; 10:59–63.

44. Greene P. Personal communication. Atlanta, 1992.

45. Hammond GD. The cure of childhood cancers. Cancer 1986; 58(suppl):407–413.

46. Hamric A, Spross J. The Clinical Nurse Specialist in Theory and Practice. New York: Grune & Stratton, 1983.

47. Harrison HE. The history of pediatrics in the United States. In Oski FA, De Angelis CD, Feigin RD, et al. (eds): Principles and Practice of Pediatrics. Philadelphia: JB Lippincott, 1990, pp 2–4.

48. Harvey B. Special report: A proposal to provide health insurance to all children and all pregnant women. N Engl J Med 1990; 323:1216–1220.

49. Henke C. Emerging roles of the nurse in oncology. Semin Oncol 1980; 7:4–8.

50. Hilkemeyer R. A historical perspective in cancer nursing. Oncol Nurs Forum 1982; 9:47.

51. Hockenberry MJ, Coody DK. Pediatric Oncology and Hematology: Perspectives on Care. St. Louis: CV Mosby, 1986.

52. Kalisch PA, Kalisch BJ. The Advance of American Nursing. Boston: Little, Brown & Co, 1978.

53. Keil H. The historical relationship between the concept of tumor and the ending—Oma. Bull Hist Med 1950; 24:352–375.

54. Kelly LY. Dimensions of Professional Nursing, 5th ed. New York: Macmillan, 1985.

55. Kids Count Data Book: State Profiles of Child Well-Being. Washington D.C.: Center for the Study of Social Policy and the Anne E. Casey Foundation, 1992.

56. Komp DM. The medical care of young adults: The practice of ephebiatrics. J Adolesc Health 1991; 12:291–293.

57. Koocher G, O'Malley E. The Damocles Syndrome. New York: McGraw-Hill, 1981.

58. Kretchmer N. Summary and conclusions. In Nichols BL, Ballabriga A, Kretchmer N (eds): Nestle Nutrition Workshop Series, vol 22. New York: Raven Press, 1991, pp 277–283.

59. Lerner M. Access to the American health care system: Consequences for cancer control. CA 1989; 39:289–295.

60. McGeady SMR. Disconnected kids: An American tragedy. America 1991; 164:639–645.

61. McGee RF. Oncology nursing: Five decades of growth. J Cancer Educ 1989; 4:167–173.

62. McManus MA, Newacheck JW, Greaney AM. Young adults with special health needs: Prevalence, severity and access to health services. Pediatrics 1990; 86:674–682.

63. Mancini JA, Orthner DK. The context and consequences of family change. Fam Relations 1988; 37:363–366.

64. Martinson J, Armstrong G, Geis D, et al. Facilitating home care for children dying of cancer. Cancer Nurs 1978; 1:41–45.

65. Micozzi MS. Disease in antiquity: The case of cancer. Arch Pathol Lab Med 1991; 115:838–844.

66. Miller RW, McKay FW. Decline in United States childhood cancer mortality 1950 through 1980. JAMA 1984; 251:1567–1570.

67. Moodie DS. Our children's health: Prospects for the 1990's. Clin Pediatr 1991; 30:357–362.

68. Mott SR, James SR, Sperhac AM. Nursing Care of Children and Families, 2nd ed. New York: Addison-Wesley Nursing, 1990.

69. Newacheck PW. Financing the health care of children with chronic illnesses. Pediatr Ann 1990; 19:60–63.

70. Newacheck PW. Improving access to health care for children, youth, and pregnant women. Pediatrics 1990; 86:626–634.

71. Nichols BL. The European roots of American pediatrics. In Nichols BL, Ballabriga A, Kretchmer N (eds): Nestle Nutrition Workshop Series, vol 22. New York: Raven Press, 1991, pp 49–53.

72. Nieswiadomy RM. Foundations of Nursing Research. Norwalk, Conn.: Appleton & Lange, 1987.

73. Nightingale F. Notes on Nursing, commemorative ed. Philadelphia: JB Lippincott, 1992.

74. Padilla GV, Padilla GJ. Nursing roles to improve patient care. In Padilla GV (ed): The Clinical Nurse Specialist and Improvement of Nursing Practice. Wakefield, Mass.: Nursing Resources, 1979.

75. Patterson JT. The Dread Disease. Cancer and Modern American Culture. Cambridge, Mass.: Harvard University Press, 1987.

76. Pearson HA. Centennial history of the APS. Pediatr Res 1990; 27(suppl):S4–S7.

77. Pearson HA. Pediatrics in the United States. In Nichols BL, Ballabriga A, Kretchmer N (eds): Nestle Nutrition Workshop Series, vol 22. New York: Raven Press, 1991, pp 55–63.

78. Pochedly CP. Biographical vignette: Dr. Lois Murphy. Am J Pediatr Hematol Oncol 1986; 8:58–62.

79. Pochedly CP. Emergence of pediatric hematology/oncology as an independent specialty. Am J Pediatr Hematol Oncol 1985; 7:183–190.

80. Polit DF, Hungler BP. Nursing Research: Principles and Methods, 4th ed. Philadelphia: JB Lippincott, 1991.

81. Rather LJ. The Genesis of Cancer: A Study in the History of Ideas. Baltimore: Johns Hopkins University Press, 1978.
82. Rauch J. Kids as capital. Atlantic Monthly August 1989; 265:56–61.
83. Raven RW. The Theory and Practice of Oncology: Historical Evolution and Present Principles. New Jersey: Parthenon Publishing Group, 1990.
84. Richman HA, Stagner MW. Children in an aging society: Treasured resource or forgotten minority. Daedalus 1986; 115:171–190.
85. Ries LAG, Hankey BF, Miller BA, et al. Cancer Statistics Review 1973–1988. NIH publication 91-2789. Bethesda, Md.: National Cancer Institute, 1991.
86. Ross W. Crusade: The Official History of the American Cancer Society. New York: Arbor House, 1987.
87. Ruccione K. Survivorship needs and issues after treatment for childhood cancer. In Surviving Cancer: Proceedings of the Sixth National Conference on Cancer Nursing. Atlanta: American Cancer Society, 1992, pp 9–31.
88. Sattin A (ed). Florence Nightingale: Letters from Egypt 1849–1850. New York: Weidenfeld & Nicolson, 1987.
89. Schuyler CB. Florence Nightingale. In Notes on Nursing, commemorative ed. Philadelphia: JB Lippincott, 1992, pp 3–17.
90. Shimkin MB. Contrary to Nature. Washington D.C.: U.S. Department of Health, Education and Welfare, 1977.
91. Siegel JS, Taeuber CM. Demographic perspectives on the long-lived society. Daedalus, 1986; 115:77–117.
92. Silver H, Ford L. The pediatric nurse practitioner program. JAMA 1968; 204:298–302.
93. Stagner S. Personal communication. Memphis, 1992.
94. Still GF. The History of Paediatrics: The Progress of the Study of Diseases of Children up to the End of the XVIII Century. London: Oxford University Press, 1931.
95. Talbott JH. A Biographical History of Medicine. New York: Grune & Stratton, 1970.
96. Taylor G (ed). Pioneers in Pediatric Oncology. Houston: The University of Texas MD Anderson Cancer Center, 1990.
97. Tice CH. Intergenerational initiatives past, present and future. Children Today 1985; 14:6–11.
98. Truman JT, van Eys J, Pochedly C. Human Values in Pediatric Hematology/Oncology. New York: Praeger, 1986.
99. van Eys J. The Truly Cured Child. Baltimore: University Park Press, 1976.
100. Waechter E. Children's awareness of fatal illness. Am J Nurs 1971; 71:1168–1172.
101. Waechter EH, Phillips J, Holaday B (eds). Nursing Care of Children, 10th ed. Philadelphia; JB Lippincott, 1985, pp 27–33.
102. Wetrogan SS. Projections of the population of states by ages. Stat Bull 1989; 70:3–10.
103. Wolff JA. History of pediatric oncology. Pediatr Hematol Oncol 1991; 8:89–91.
104. Wood DL, Hayward RA, Corey CR, et al. Access to medical care for children and adolescents in the United States. Pediatrics 1990; 86:666–672.
105. Yarbro CH. The early days: Four smiles and a post office box. Oncol Nurs Forum 1984; 11:79–85.
106. Zuelzer WW. Pediatric hematology in historical perspective. In Nathan DG, Oski FA (eds): Hematology of Infancy and Childhood, 3rd ed. Philadelphia: WB Saunders, 1987, pp 1–13.

BIOLOGIC BASIS OF CHILDHOOD CANCER

Kathleen Hardin Mooney

To nurses working in pediatric oncology, childhood cancer seems like a very common disease. In reality, cancer in childhood is quite rare. Nonetheless, what has been learned about the epidemiology, genetics, cellular biology, and responsiveness to treatment of these cancers has contributed significantly to understanding cancer in general and to the development of more effective treatment strategies for all cancers.

EPIDEMIOLOGY
Incidence

Although there is no national registry that accounts for every case of childhood cancer in the United States, estimates are projected based on data from population-based registries that record cancer incidence for a specific area. The most commonly cited registry for pediatric oncology statistics is the Surveillance Epidemiology and End Results (SEER) program of the National Cancer Institute. Since 1973 SEER has recorded approximately 12% of all cases of cancer in the United States. It is the largest source of data on children's cancer.

Based on SEER data, the 1992 incidence of childhood cancer in children 15 years of age and under is estimated as 7800 new cases,[20] reflecting a continued increase in incidence of approximately 0.7% per year.[30] The reason for this small but persistent increase is not known. There has been speculation that some environmental factors may play a role, but there is insufficient research to substantiate this possibility. The incidence of cancer in the adolescent years, 15 to 19 years of age, is increased over that of childhood. Fourteen childhood cancers per 100,000 children are diagnosed each year, compared to 20 adolescent cancers per 100,000.[15] This translates into approximately 3500 adolescent cancers diagnosed each year in the United States,[15] resulting in approximately 11,300 cancers diagnosed each year in children less than 20 years of age. Given these incidence figures, approximately 1 in 475 children will be diagnosed with cancer before the age of 15, and before the age of 20, approximately 1 in 333 children will be diagnosed.[15] These figures are in sharp contrast to the 1,100,000 total new cases of cancer reported on an annual basis in the United States and the cancer incidence of 1 in 3 for adults.[20] Thus childhood cancer represents less than 1% (0.6% to 0.7%) of cancers diagnosed in this country. Nevertheless, it is the second leading cause of death in childhood, second only to accidents and trauma among children less than 15 years of age.[89]

Mortality Rate

The mortality rates for childhood cancer have declined dramatically during the past three decades.[30] Initially in the 1960s improvements were seen for patients with the kidney tumor, Wilms' tumor, and Hodgkin's disease, a form of lymphoma. Over the past 20 years as multimodality therapy has been refined, survival rates have increased for children with acute lymphocytic leukemia (ALL), non-Hodgkin's lymphoma, bone tumors, and rhabdomyosarcoma (a soft tissue sarcoma). Survival rates for other tumor types have improved less dramatically. Although long-term survival rates vary among the different childhood cancers, overall more than 60% of children diagnosed with cancer will be cured.[30] Childhood cancer is more responsive to current treatment than cancer occurring during the adult years. The long-term survival rate for adult cancers is approximately 40%; when adjusted for normal life expectancy, the relative survival rate is closer to 50% for adults.[20]

TABLE 2–1. *Comparison of Usual Childhood and Adult Cancers*

FACTOR	CHILDHOOD CANCERS	ADULT CANCERS
Incidence	Rare; <1% of all cancers	Common; >99% of all cancers
Sites	Involves tissue (e.g., reticuloendothelial system, central nervous system, muscle, bone)	Involves organs (e.g., lung, breast, colon, prostate)
Histology	Most common type: nonepithelial—sarcomas, embryonal, leukemia, lymphoma	Most common type: epithelial—carcinomas
Latency (from initiation to diagnosis)	Relatively short period	Long period; can be well over 20 yr
Influence of environmental factors in causation	Some environmental factors; few life-style factors; overall, not strong influence shown; more likely interaction of genetic alterations and environmental factors (i.e., ecogenetics)	Strong relationship to environmental exposures and life-style factors
Prevention	Minimal strategies known to date	80% estimated as preventable
Early detection	Generally accidental; small percentage known as genetically at high risk can be followed more closely	Possible with adherence to early detection screening tests and examination recommendations
State at diagnosis	Metastatic disease present in 80%	Local or regional disease
Response to treatment	Very responsive to chemotherapy; tolerate higher doses	Less responsive to chemotherapy
Treatment side effects	Less difficulty with acute toxicity but more significant long-term consequences	More difficulty with acute toxicity but fewer long-term consequences
Prognosis	>60% cure	<60% cure

Modified from Fernbach DG, Vietti TJ. General aspects of childhood cancer. In Fernbach DJ, Vietti TJ (eds): Clinical Pediatric Oncology, 4th ed. St. Louis: Mosby—Year Book, 1991, p 2.

COMPARISON OF ADULT-ONSET CANCER WITH CHILDHOOD CANCER

Childhood cancers are quite different from the more common cancers of adults. Table 2–1 compares some of these differences. Approximately 92% of childhood cancers arise from the mesodermal germ layer, which in the embryo becomes connective tissue, bone, cartilage, muscle, blood, blood vessels, sex organs, kidney, lymphatic, and lymphoid organs. The resulting cancers are most commonly of primitive embryonal tissue, sarcomas, leukemias, or lymphomas. Some childhood cancers arise from neuroectodermal tissue, resulting in central nervous system (CNS) tumors.[23] The most frequent cancers in adults (approximately 87%) involve tissue of epithelial origin, called *carcinomas*, that are extremely rare in childhood. The disparity in adult and child tissue type continues until 15 years of age; the types then merge between 15 and 19 years of age to reflect equal frequency of epithelial and nonepithelial cancers. Thereafter epithelial cancers predominate.[63]

Arising from more deep-seated tissue than epithelial tumors, childhood cancers do not often present obvious visual, palpable, or functional abnormalities until they are very large, thus probably contributing to the observation that almost 80% of children with cancer have distant metastases at the time of diagnosis. However, some early stage childhood tumors such as rhabdomyosarcoma stage I may already have occult metastases at diagnosis. In such a case the biologic behavior of the cancer is more critical to metastasis. The biologic behavior of childhood tumors also favors rapid spread, even when tumors are small.

Childhood cancers demonstrate a pattern of occurrence that parallels peak times of physical growth and cellular maturation. As discussed later in this chapter, this key observation underlies the current understanding of the mechanisms of cancer in children and suggests that cellular development and growth are central to pediatric cancer formation, differing from common adult carcinomas in which environmental exposure is a primary component of carcinogenesis.

TYPES OF CHILDHOOD CANCER

Table 2–2 illustrates the estimated incidence and distribution of the most common child-

TABLE 2–2. *Estimated Annual Incidence of Childhood Cancer*

CANCER SITE OR TYPE	ESTIMATED TOTAL NUMBER/YEAR	PERCENT OF CHILDHOOD CANCER
Leukemia (Primary type: acute lymphocytic leukemia [ALL])	2257	33
Central nervous system (Primary type: gliomas)	1362	20
Lymphoma (Primary types: non-Hodgkin's and Hodgkin's diseases)	758	11
Sympathetic nervous system (Primary type: neuroblastoma)	526	8
Kidney tumors (Primary type: Wilms' tumor)	444	6.6
Bone tumors (Primary types: osteosarcoma and Ewing's sarcoma)	312	4.5
Soft tissue sarcoma (Primary type: rhabdomyosarcoma)	228	3
Other	994	14
All sites	6881	100

From Bleyer WA. The impact of childhood cancer on the United States and the world. CA 1990; 40:366.

hood cancers. (See Chapters 8 and 9 for detailed descriptions of these cancers.) The data indicate that the majority of childhood cancers involve the reticuloendothelial system (leukemias and lymphomas), representing nearly 43% of childhood cancers, followed by the CNS tumors that account for another 19%.

Age, Sex, Race, and Geographic Variations

There are considerable variations in age-at-onset among the childhood cancers. Some have unique gender, racial, and geographic patterns. Tables 2–3 and 2–4 illustrate these differences in age distribution, gender, and race. The data for these tables are taken from the 1973 to 1982 SEER program. Although more recent SEER data have been published (now through 1989), neuroblastoma has not been separated from CNS tumors. For this reason the earlier data were chosen to provide a perspective that includes neuroblastoma. However, there has been an overall increase in childhood cancer; therefore the actual rates may be slightly increased.

Awareness of the age variation in childhood cancer is important for understanding factors that may influence the cause of specific cancers and because some histologically identical cancers have different malignant potential and prognosis, depending on age. For example, neuroblastoma has a favorable prognosis in infants less than 1 year of age but a very unfavorable prognosis in older children. The tumors of embryonal origin such as neuroblastoma, Wilms' tumor, retinoblastoma, and the embryonal form of rhabdomyosarcoma have a peak age before 5 years, suggesting prenatal influences in their development or reflection of the rapid growth that occurs in the first 5 years of age. Other childhood cancers such as lymphomas and bone tumors have peak ages during middle childhood and adolescence, clearly reflecting possible postnatal influences.

There is a male predominance for childhood cancer, although the ratio is not large (male:female ratio of 1.2:1).[94] The increased risk for males is reflected in higher rates of ALL, lymphoma, and medulloblastoma (a CNS tumor). However, among African-American children between the ages of 5 and 14 years, females rather than males have a higher incidence rate. During these ages, African-American females have more leukemias, brain tumors, and bone tumors.[94] Overall, the cancer rate in the United States for white children is 10% to 25% higher than for African-American children.[30] This is ac-

TABLE 2–3. *Annual Incidence per Million of Cancer Among White Children Under 15 Years of Age in the United States: SEER Program, 1973–1982*

	RATE PER MILLION					
	0–4 YR		**5–9 YR**		**10–14 YR**	
SITES	**MALE**	**FEMALE**	**MALE**	**FEMALE**	**MALE**	**FEMALE**
Leukemia	72.5	61.3	35.6	32.5	27.9	16.8
CNS tumors	27.3	25.0	28.1	22.5	23.3	21.4
Lymphoma	10.1	5.2	22.5	6.4	28.3	22.1
Sympathetic nervous system tumors	28.3	28.5	4.3	2.9	1.3	1.8
Soft tissue sarcoma	8.6	9.0	8.2	6.7	7.4	7.9
Kidney tumors	16.1	19.8	4.7	6.7	1.1	1.1
Bone tumors	1.4	1.7	3.8	4.5	12.2	12.0
Retinoblastoma	9.1	10.9	0.6	0.5	—	—
Other	16.8	10.7	6.7	7.6	12.9	21.5
All sites	190.3	172.2	114.6	90.1	114.4	104.6

Modified from Miller RW. Frequency and environmental epidemiology of childhood cancer. In Pizzo PA, Poplack DG (eds): Priniciples and Practice of Pediatric Oncology. Philadelphia: JB Lippincott, 1989, p 6.

TABLE 2–4. *Annual Cancer Incidence by Type for Children Under 15 Years of Age: SEER data*

HISTOLOGIC CATEGORY	RATE PER MILLION	
	WHITE	AFRICAN-AMERICAN
Leukemia	43.7	25.2
CNS tumors	24.9	22.0
Lymphoma	16.0	10.2
Sympathetic nervous system tumors	12.7	10.4
Soft tissue tumors	8.6	8.3
Kidney tumors	9.0	12.4
Bone tumors	5.5	4.3
Retinoblastoma	4.0	5.1
ALL CANCERS	135.6	107.6

Modified from Robison L. General principles of the epidemiology of childhood cancer. In Pizzo PA, Poplack DG (eds): Principles and Practice of Pediatric Onocology, 2nd ed. Philadelphia: JB Lippincott, 1993, p 8.

counted for by lower rates in African-American children of ALL (53% of whites), lymphomas (41% of whites), and Ewing's sarcoma (89% of whites). There are slightly lower rates of CNS tumors, neuroblastoma, rhabdomyosarcoma, and bone tumors for African-American children but higher rates of Wilms' tumor and retinoblastoma. The reasons for these differences are not understood. Although African-American children have a lower rate of ALL, the prognosis is less favorable for African-Americans than whites.

The incidence of childhood cancers varies markedly throughout the world and by race within geographic locations.[4,74a] The highest rates are found in Israel and Nigeria and the lowest in India and Japan.[4] Table 2–5 lists the geographic areas with particularly high rates of specific cancers. The reason for geographic variations is not known and could be attributed to numerous influences, including racial, genetic, and environmental factors.

Cancer Clusters

Unusually high concentrations of childhood cancers (cancer clusters) have been identified in specific areas of the United States over the past 30 years. The most common clusters usually involve high incidences of childhood leukemia. The first such cluster occurred in a small area of Niles, Illinois, during 1963. An initial explanation focused on a viral cause, but this theory was eventually discredited. Several clusters have been associated with chemical pollution, but the cause was never proved. One reported cluster, identified in Woburn, Massachusetts, in 1979, continued to show a sustained increase in childhood leukemia for the next 6 years.[47] Disagreement continues about the cause or significance of this cluster. Some researchers have suggested a link to factory-caused water pollution, but other researchers dispute these findings.[19] This disagreement underscores the reality that cancer clusters are difficult to study and either to confirm or to attribute to chance. However, the parents in the Woburn case pressed and won a legal battle in 1988, linking the well-water pollution to chemical use at the W.R. Grace Company. This case reinforces the importance of clinicians' facilitating con-

TABLE 2–5. *Geographic Variations in Childhood Cancer*

TYPE	AREAS OF HIGH INCIDENCE
Acute lymphocytic leukemia	Israel, Denmark, Japan, United States (white children)
Acute myelomonocytic leukemia	Turkey, Uganda
Burkitt's lymphoma	West Nile District of Uganda
Hepatic tumors	Far East countries
Hodgkin's disease	Columbia
Intestinal lymphoma	Israel
Nasopharyngeal carcinoma	Southern China
Pineal tumors (germ-cell brain tumor)	Japan
Retinoblastoma	India
Skin cancer	North Africa

tinued epidemiologic investigation when they encounter unexpectedly high rates of specific childhood cancers.

Risk Factors

Through clinical observation and both descriptive and analytic epidemiologic studies, it has been known for many years that certain children are at higher-than-average risk for the development of cancer during childhood. Only relatively recently, as more has been learned in the laboratory about cancer at the cellular level, are the reasons why some children are at higher risk becoming evident. Risk factors are both genetic and environmental; current research interest focuses on their interaction, particularly how environmental factors in the presence of specific genetic alterations promote cancer. This interaction is called *ecogenetics* and probably will continue as an intensive area of study in the coming decade.[66] In the following section an overview of genetic and environmental risk factors for childhood cancer is presented. Chapters 8 and 9 provide a more detailed presentation of risk factors for each specific type of childhood cancer.

Although some genetic and environmental risk factors are known, the majority of children with cancer do not have a history of any of these factors, and for most children the specific causes of each child's cancer cannot be pinpointed. It is likely that a complex interaction of ecogenetic factors rather than any single cause or event will ultimately be accepted as the cause of childhood cancer. Besides the need for health professionals to continue to update their knowledge base in this changing field, children and their families must be helped to understand the complexity of cancer development and to appreciate the differences between causes of childhood cancer and what is known about causes of adult cancer. An example of this confusion is found in an Australian study of parents of children with cancer who were asked what caused their child's illness.[60] Researchers found that, first, parents had a specific explanation about the cause of their child's cancer (only 4.7% said they had no idea) and that, second, the explanations were most likely related to en-

vironmental causes, including life-style factors.

Genetic Factors. Several hundred genetic and congenital disorders are associated with increased risk for cancer. These disorders encompass chromosome alterations, congenital malformations, and immunodeficiency syndromes. Many chromosome abnormalities are associated with childhood cancer.[73,81] Chromosomal changes include aneuploidy, deletions, translocations, and fragility. Table 2–6 describes these changes in relation to childhood cancer. However, examining the cells of individual tumors does not always reveal the expected chromosomal alteration. Some tumors demonstrate the defect in nearly all tumor cells examined, whereas other cancers have a much lower rate of detection of the specific defect. It has been suggested that tumors may have chromosomal defects that are so small that current technologies to examine them are inadequate.[39] Finding similar chromosomal alterations in histologically different cancers (e.g., the deletion of the long arm of chromosome 13 in both retinoblastoma and the bone tumor osteosarcoma) has led to the speculation that they may have a common genetic origin. This speculation has led to the suggestion that tumors could be categorized better by genetic descriptors rather than the traditional histologic classification.[95] Cancer would no longer be viewed as several hundred different diseases but as several groups of cancer based on genetic similarities.

Several congenital malformations demonstrate greater susceptibility for childhood solid tumors. The most well documented is the syndrome of aniridia, hemihypertrophy, and genitourinary tract abnormalities associated with Wilms' tumor. Beckwith-Wiedemann syndrome, characterized by gigantism, large tongue, umbilical hernia, visceromegaly, and mental retardation, also predisposes affected children to Wilms' tumor. Neurofibromatosis is associated with tumors of neural or neural crest origin. Children with known congenital disorders, malformations, or syndromes associated with subsequent cancer development must be screened regularly so diagnosis and treatment can begin promptly if tumors develop.[73]

TABLE 2–6. *Selected Chromosomal Alterations Associated With Childhood Cancers*

TYPE	DEFINITION	ABNORMALITY	CHILDHOOD CANCER
Aneuploidy	More or less than the expected two sets of similar chromosomes	Trisomy 21 (Down syndrome)	Acute leukemia
Deletions	Loss of some genetic material from the chromosome	Deletion of long arm of chromosome 13	Retinoblastoma
		Deletion of short arm of chromosome 11	Wilms' tumor with aniridia and mental retardation
		Deletion of short arm of chromosome 1	Neuroblastoma
		Deletion of long arm of chromosome 13	Osteogenic sarcoma
Translocation	Shifting of a fragment of one chromosome to another chromosome	Translocation between chromosomes 2 and 8 and chromosomes 8 and 14 or 22	Burkitt's lymphoma
		Translocation between chromosomes 11 and 22	Ewing's sarcoma
		Translocation between chromosomes 3 and 8	Renal cell carcinoma
		Translocation between chromosomes 11 and 14	Acute T-cell lymphocytic leukemia
		Translocation between chromosomes 8 and 21	Acute myelogenous leukemia (M2)
Fragility	Breaking of chromosomes	Bloom syndrome	Acute leukemia
		Fanconi's aplastic anemia	Acute leukemia (usually myelomonocytic type)
		Ataxia-telangiectasia	Lymphoma

Some genetic disorders (e.g., ataxia-telangiectasia syndrome and Wiskott-Aldrich syndrome) known to alter the immune system also predispose children to subsequent cancer. The majority of the associated malignancies are lymphomas and leukemias.[74a]

Certain childhood cancers such as retinoblastoma and Wilms' tumor exhibit an inherited pattern and an acquired (noninherited) form. This transmission pattern is described in more detail later in this chapter. There is also a rare cancer family syndrome that includes both childhood and adult cancers, the Li-Fraumeni cancer family syndrome.[50] With this familial syndrome is an excess of certain cancers in the affected family as a group and multiple tumors in individually affected family members. Tumor types include a wide variety of cancers such as sarcomas and bone, brain, and breast cancer. A specific gene on chromosomes 17, p53, has been identified as the site of the predisposing defect. The p53 gene is implicated in other cancers separate from the Li-Fraumeni syndrome, notably colon cancer.[49,91]

Besides direct inheritance and family cancer syndromes, there apparently is an increased risk of childhood cancer in families that have another child with cancer, even when families with inherited genetic defects are removed from the analysis. Environmental factors may be implicated as well. Siblings of an affected child are estimated to be at twice the risk for subsequent childhood cancer compared to the risk for children without siblings with cancer.[4] There have been more specific studies of sibling risk of leukemic children, particularly of twins. Miller[61] found that a twin of a child 5 years of age or less when diagnosed with leukemia had a 10% to 20% chance of also being diagnosed with ALL within weeks to a few months of the initial twin's diagnosis. This heightened risk decreases over time so that by 6 to 7 years of age the twin has the same risk as other non-twin siblings.

Finally, it is known that long-term survivors of childhood cancer have an increased risk of new cancers that peaks for most cancers approximately 15 to 19 years after the initial childhood cancer.[4] Many of these new cancers have been linked to prior radiation therapy, representing either an external or environmental cause or an environmental component with a genetically predisposed child rather than solely a genetic predisposition. However, almost one third are not related to prior radiation therapy and may be related to specific prior chemotherapy agents or demonstrate a genetic predisposition to cancer formation.

Environmental Factors. The role and significance of environmental factors in causing childhood cancer are controversial. Although some environmental factors are associated with certain childhood cancers, how often and to what degree these factors account for childhood cancer are unknown. Part of the controversy lies in the observation that environmental carcinogens generally need repeated exposure and a long latency period before the cancer develops. Children simply have not lived long enough to allow this process to occur. Thus the environmental exposures that do lead to childhood cancer are rare instances associated with an extremely short latent period. The exposure may occur either prenatally or during childhood. The rapid biologic development during both the prenatal and childhood periods may increase the child's vulnerability also.

Prenatal exposures include exposure to drugs or substances that freely pass through the placenta to the fetus from the mother. Fetal alcohol or fetal hydantoin syndrome, which is associated with an increased risk for neuroblastoma, and maternal ingestion of di-ethylstilbestrol (DES), which is linked to clear-cell adenocarcinoma of the vagina in the daughter during early adulthood, are examples of prenatal drug exposures with subsequent childhood cancers. The effect of intrauterine exposure to ionizing radiation has been studied. However, a direct causal link is missing and may never be established. Some studies have shown an excessive rate of all types of childhood malignancy after maternal diagnostic x-ray studies.[58,83] However, there is no link between radiation exposure and subsequent childhood cancer in children who were in utero when their mothers were exposed to radiation from atomic bombs during World War II in Japan.[40] In addition to maternal drugs and radiation exposure, maternal factors, particularly advanced maternal age, maternal smoking, previous miscarriages, and an episode of maternal flu during pregnancy, and infant birth weight of greater than 4000 g may be associated with increased risk for leukemia.[29,75] These factors need further study.

Other potentially important prenatal factors for certain childhood cancers include parental exposures, particularly occupational exposures, advanced maternal age, maternal multiple miscarriages, and maternal use of marijuana.[75,77] Parental occupational exposures that may increase risk for offspring include maternal chemical, agriculture, and metal refining occupations; paternal occupations that involve paper and pulp processing, solvents, plastics, and petroleum products; and either maternal or paternal exposure to pesticides. Parental exposure can be harmful both before conception and during the pregnancy.[75,77]

Childhood environmental exposures associated with childhood cancer include radiation, electromagnetic fields, radon, drugs, and viruses. Although a causal link between prenatal radiation exposure and childhood cancer may be controversial, children exposed to fallout from atomic bombs during World War II did show an increased rate of the acute leukemias, chronic myelogenous leukemias, and thyroid tumors. The latent period was approximately 5 years from exposure to diagnosis.[14] However, in most cases of childhood radiation exposure there is a long latent period of up to 20 years before any cancer is evident.[66]

During the last decade attention has turned to the possible link of electromagnetic field exposure from residential power lines, substations, and operation of small household appliances to childhood cancer, particularly leukemia and brain tumors. Results of some epidemiologic studies have suggested a relationship, and laboratory studies confirm that biologic alterations occur in response to low-level electromagnetic field exposure.[2,92] However, a causal link has not been established, and the epidemiologic studies have methodological and measurement difficulties. In a recent study London et al.[55] reported an association between exposure to a specific household wiring configuration and childhood leukemia but not with direct measurement of the magnitude of electromagnetic fields. Further study will explore this possible environmental risk, including large-scale studies to measure electromagnetic field exposure.

There also is recent interest in the role of radon gas as a cause of cancer. Previously a link between some lung cancers and radon exposure was established. Radon is a colorless, odorless gas that is naturally emitted from rock and soil. Increased radon exposure can be found in some homes built on ground with high radon levels. Several investigators have reported a link between radon exposure and increased risk of acute myelogenous leukemia, brain tumors, and osteosarcoma. However, further study is required to establish radon exposure firmly as a risk factor for these childhood cancers.

Childhood exposure to some drugs is associated with cancer, but because of a long latency period, resulting cancers usually occur during adult years. Drug exposures can occur through direct ingestion by the child or during infancy as a lactational carcinogen in breast milk from the mother. Children receiving immunosuppressive therapy, generally after transplantation, have a higher incidence of lymphoma and other cancers. This is similar to the increased risk for children born with immunodeficiency diseases.

Viral exposure also has been an area of intense study. Evidence is sufficient to link only four viruses confidently with human cancer, and some evidence probably links another four. However, there is no strong association with any childhood cancer, with the exception of the Epstein-Barr virus (EBV), which is a risk factor for the African variety of Burkitt's lymphoma, although not Burkitt's lymphoma in the United States.[22] Certain viral exposures in childhood are related to subsequent adult cancers such as hepatitis B virus and later hepatocellular carcinoma, although these cancers are rare.

Childhood Exposure and Subsequent Adult Cancer Risk. Children are exposed to environmental carcinogens, but because of the long latency period, exposures during childhood are more likely to contribute to cancers in later life. The implications of this include the need for risk reduction actions during childhood aimed at decreasing exposure. Pediatric oncology nurses, along with general pediatric nurses, can play an important role in working with their community and with parents and children to understand how childhood exposure can result in cancer during adult years. Appropriate risk-reduction strategies must be encouraged. Two prominent examples include encouraging the use of sunblock products during sun exposure in childhood to reduce the risk of melanoma and encouraging children and adolescents not to begin smoking or chewing tobacco, activities that increase the risk for a variety of cancers. Tobacco use is the single carcinogen most responsible for human cancer and accounts for almost one of every three cancers diagnosed in the United States.[25] At the same time, it is a carcinogen that can be avoided. An emphasis on children is central to reducing risk because it is much easier to resist beginning tobacco use than to break the habit and dependence once started.

MECHANISMS OF CARCINOGENESIS

In recent years geneticists and cellular biologists have made significant progress in describing some of the mechanisms involved in cancer development. These findings help explain the observations of epidemiologists and the laboratory findings related to chromosomal alterations described in the previous section. New insights into the mechanisms of cancer are occurring at a rapid pace, requiring continual scanning of the literature to remain up-to-date. An overview of the current state of understanding of these mechanisms is provided in the next sections. To understand this area, it helps to have a basic knowledge of genetics and cellular physiology. A glossary of selected basic terms is provided in Table 2–7. In reading the literature, those working in pediatric oncology are challenged to separate

mechanisms of carcinogenesis that are most applicable to adult cancers (e.g., those that require repeated carcinogenic exposure and long latency) from those that explain the development of childhood cancers—information often not made explicit in the particular article being read. Luckily, although childhood cancer represents less than 1% of all cancers, many of the advances in understanding carcinogenesis come from progress in understanding specific childhood cancers.

At the cellular level, most scientists believe

TABLE 2–7. *Glossary of Terms*

Carcinogenesis—process of cancer formation

Proto-oncogene—gene that is the normal, nonactivated counterpart of oncogenes; produces proteins necessary for normal growth and development

Oncogene—a gene, originally a normal proto-oncogene, whose activation, either through increased expression or by alteration of the biologic properties of its protein products, promotes the malignant transformation of the cell

Tumor-suppressor gene—gene whose inactivation by mutation, rearrangement, or deletion leads to malignant transformation of the cell; normally involved with constraining cellular growth; also called *cancer susceptibility gene, antioncogene,* or *recessive cancer gene*

Initiation—first stage of carcinogenesis when initial genetic mutation of a cell occurs

Promotion—second stage of carcinogenesis when cell proliferation and tumor development occur

Progression—third stage of carcinogenesis characterized by cell proliferation, invasion into adjacent tissue, and distant metastasis

Allele—one of two copies of a gene situated at the corresponding positions on homologous chromosomes

Blocked ontogeny—inability of a cell to differentiate fully or mature into specialized function

Mutation—permanent change in the genetic material (DNA); this alteration is transmitted to all subsequent daughter cells

Epigenetic change—abnormal pattern of gene expression with no mutation in the DNA sequence

Stem cell—common ancestor cell or parent cell for a particular tissue or cell type

Differentiation—process of cell maturation and specialization

Differentiation inducers—therapeutic agents that cause immature cells to differentiate fully

Germ cell—primitive gametes (original sperm and egg cells) or progenitor cell; mutation of a germ cell would cause transmission of that defect to every cell in the body

Social control genes—genes whose protein products regulate cellular growth and activity within the context of adjacent cells and surrounding tissue

Gene amplification—increase in the number of copies of a particular DNA sequence

Insertional mutation—addition of a new or altered genetic material into a chromosome

Chromosome translocation—shifting of a fragment of one chromosome to another chromosome

Paracrine growth regulation—growth regulation in which growth factor is produced by one cell and then transported through diffusion to nearby cells for their use

Autocrine growth regulation—growth factors produced and used by the same cell

Contact inhibition—cessation of continued cell division when the cell runs out of room to divide further and is in contact with surrounding cells

Down regulation—inhibition of cell growth

Gap junction—clusters of protein channels that allow biochemical transmission from the inside of one cell to the inside of another cell

Gene therapy—correction of genetic defects or loss by replacement with normal genes

Tumor marker—biochemical indicator for the presence of a tumor

Up regulation—promotion of cell growth

that cancer is a genetic disease. This means that cancer develops because of a permanent alteration in the cell's DNA sequence, the genetic material of the cell. These alterations can be either inherited or acquired and are themselves transmitted to every daughter cell, beginning a cell line that perpetuates the mutation. Some evidence suggests that an alternate process may also occur.[9] Rather than a genetic change, cancer may be due to epigenetic change, which means that the DNA sequence is not altered but the pattern of gene expression is abnormal. The epigenetic change is stable and also transmitted to every daughter cell. Some of the evidence for epigenetic changes include the observations that (1) cancer is associated with altered or blocked differentiation (cellular maturation and specialization) and epigenetic changes are related to this process and involve alteration in normal growth control mechanisms; and (2) some cancers are known to reverse their cancerous state occasionally, as in the spontaneous regression of neuroblastoma. If DNA had been altered (as in genetic change), the regression or reversal of the cancer process would be less likely. Teratocarcinoma, which is an embryonic tumor containing a variety of tissue, including skin, bone, and epithelium, is thought to demonstrate epigenetic origins. However, the current focus is on explanations of genetic change rather than possible epigenetic change. As more is learned about carcinogenesis, it is likely that both mechanisms will be better understood and the relative contribution of each will become clearer.[16]

Carcinogenesis: A Multistage Process

Many studies of tumors in animals and humans have led to the conclusion that a cancer develops in a process involving a number of independent stages.[34] It is further believed that cancers are clonal in origin, that is, the cells of the tumor descend from a single cell.[70] Some evidence suggests that the originating cell is a stem cell.[86] Stem cells are characterized by their ability to have both an extensive potential for self-renewal or proliferation and to evolve into specialized cells in a process known as *terminal differentiation*. This multi-step process of tumor development is commonly described by a three-stage model called *initiation/promotion/progression*.

Initiation usually represents the initial genetic mutation of the cell. It has been hypothesized that initiation stops a once-normal stem cell from terminally differentiating into a mature cell. The inability of the cells to differentiate fully has been called *blocked ontogeny*.[86] Further events, however, are required to result in a tumor.

Promotion requires a secondary factor or influence that does not necessarily genetically change the cell but, in combination with the initiated genes, moves the cell forward to a cancerous clone of cells. Promotion is thought to involve stimulation of cellular proliferation. There is evidence that the normal rapid growth periods associated with fetal development, infancy, and puberty may create an environment conducive to tumor promotion and hence explain the associated observations of peak pediatric tumor incidence in early childhood and adolescence.[34] The theory of blocked ontogeny has also been linked to tumor promotion. Whether a factor in initiation or promotion, the role of blocked differentiation as a component of cancer has led to the intriguing possibility of differentiation therapy. Although only in its infancy, this avenue for treatment has been fueled for many years by the observation that, occasionally, neuroblastoma spontaneously regresses by overcoming blocked ontogeny and terminally differentiating into benign ganglioneuromas. The object of the therapy is to induce differentiation and maturation of malignant cells, leading to a return to normal growth control mechanisms and, eventually, natural cell death without further proliferation. Agents used for this purpose are often called *differentiation inducers*. An example is retinoic acid, which reduces development of second primary head and neck cancers and induces initial remissions in children with acute promyelocytic leukemia, although these remissions have been of short duration.[21,36] Differentiation therapy has application in (1) chemoprevention (prevention of primary tumors in at-risk individuals and prevention of secondary cancers once cancer has occurred), (2) reversing recognized precancerous lesions, and (3) treatment of established cancer. This approach should be an intensive area of study in the future.

Progression, in which the malignant behavior of the tumor is enhanced, fosters further invasiveness, distant spread by metastases, and the ability of the tumor cells to resist lethal damage from chemotherapy. The process of progression includes the accumulation of additional genetic alterations.[34]

In reality, initiation, promotion, and progression are not distinct stages or easily identifiable in human cancers. In fact, genetic events involved in initiation in one tumor are associated with promotion or progression in other cancers. However, all three stages contribute to the understanding of the cascade of events necessary to transform a single cell into a cancerous mass large enough to detect at diagnosis.

Cancer development is a multistage process; the length of time and the number of specific events necessary to form cancer vary. Adult tumors generally demonstrate a long latency period after initiation until promotion and progression are completed. Promotion involves chronic exposure to the promoting agents. There is speculation that several mutations and events are involved in normal cell transformation to cancer. The latency period is much shorter in childhood cancer. Chronic, prolonged exposure is not a feature.

It is also believed that the number of events necessary to transform the normal cell in children is less, perhaps as low as two. In 1971 Knudson[46] proposed the "two-hit" hypothesis of cancer development based on a statistical analysis of age and events surrounding the development of retinoblastoma. Further study has allowed validation and further understanding of this model. Retinoblastoma has two observed patterns. Sixty percent of cases are unilateral disease, and 40% of cases are bilateral disease. Unilateral disease occurs during childhood, involves one tumor in one eye, and is seen in children with no family history of retinoblastoma. In contrast, bilateral disease occurs in infancy, includes multifocal retinal tumors in both eyes, and involves a family history of the disease. The two-hit hypothesis predicts that in the inherited form of retinoblastoma, the first mutation occurs in the germ cell; thus every cell in the child's body inherits the defective gene, and only a second mutation in a retinoblast cell is sufficient for the tumor to develop. Multiple tumors are seen because second mutations are likely to occur in several of the approximately 1 to 2 million retinoblast cells.[91] In noninherited unilateral cases, also referred to as the *acquired* or *sporadic form*, both mutations occur independently in the same cell, a very rare event to occur in one cell, let alone several cells simultaneously. Although occurring less frequently, approximately 8% of the time Wilms' tumor also has a bilateral presentation that suggests a similar germ cell mutation. A familial pattern is less common for Wilms' tumor than for retinoblastoma, making the study of Wilms' tumor more difficult.

NATURE OF CANCER GENES

Cellular repair, growth, and differentiation are carefully regulated in living organisms, assuring the survival of the organism in addition to individual cell survival. Growth is controlled so that there is an optimal balance between the cell birth rate and the cell death rate. As new cells are required (e.g., during childhood growth spurts or to replace damaged or dying cells), previously nondividing cells that have been in a quiescent state are signaled into the cell cycle so that they may replicate. The mechanism by which this balanced growth process occurs is called *social control*. It is regulated by social control genes that specify proteins involved in signaling cellular growth and development.[46] There are two classes of these normal growth regulation genes: proto-oncogenes that promote cell growth and tumor suppressor genes that provide a counterbalance by suppressing cell growth. If these normal genes are altered, the result can be abnormal cellular proliferation and disregard for social control mechanisms—this is what happens in cancer.[93]

During the multistage process of cancer initiation, promotion, and progression, the cell mutations that occur cause disruption of the social control function, and in this context these once-normal genes become cancer genes. The proto-oncogenes in the cancer-activated form are called *oncogenes,* and the normal growth-suppressing genes (that are actually lost in the process of cancer transformation) are called *tumor-suppressor genes.*

Genes and Chromosomes

It is useful to review some basic genetic terminology and concepts. Each normal person has 46 chromosomes that are composed of 23 pairs. Chromosome pairs, called *homologous chromosomes,* have matching genetic information. Chromosomes are composed of complex proteins and deoxyribonucleic acid (DNA). Genes, which are discrete units of genetic information, are located in linear order along the chromosomes. Each gene has a specific position along the chromosome that is called a *locus.* Because there are paired chromosomes, there are double sets of genes called *alleles.*[85] For each species this "map" of gene locations is the same. The Human Genome Project is a major current research project aimed at mapping the complete human DNA sequence by the year 2005. This is a massive project since it requires the sequencing of 50,000 to 100,000 genes. However, if it can be done, it will provide rich dividends for genetic diagnosis, understanding the genetic basis of disease, and knowing where to target genetic engineering to repair genetic defects responsible for disease, including cancer.

The study of chromosomes is known as *cytogenetics.* A specific nomenclature is used when describing chromosomes and sites of abnormalities. In the dividing state, chromosomes look like a rod consisting of two U shapes, one inverted under the other, and joined together at their curved bases. The two sides of each U are called *chromatids* and are composed of a double helix of DNA. The base that joins the two Us together is called the *centromere.* The centromere is important in the process of cell division. Generally the Us are different lengths, each called an *arm.* The shorter arm is designated by the notation *p,* for *petit,* and the longer arm has the notation *q.* Thus a specific chromosome site, gene location, or defect is described by referring to the number and arm, p or q, of the chromosome—for example, the short arm of chromosome 1 is 1p or the long arm of chromo-

some 13 is 13q.[85] See Table 2–7 for an explanation of other genetic terms relevant to cancer genes.

Oncogenes

The involvement of oncogenes in cancer formation was first identified through study of RNA tumor viruses in animals. The importance of these findings for understanding human cancers was not appreciated at first because few human cancers had been associated with viruses. However, in the early 1980s links were made to human cancers when genes homologous to viral oncogenes but without viral involvement were identified in some human tumors.[34] At the cellular level, oncogenes have a dominant expression, that is, only one gene copy (an allele) of the normal proto-oncogene must be altered and activated for the cancer transformation to begin. However, activation of the gene may be necessary but not sufficient to cause the cancer. Other requirements may include activation of additional oncogenes, loss of tumor-suppressor genes, and the cell's being in a state of cell differentiation.[16,45]

The proto-oncogenes are activated into oncogenes by a variety of mechanisms, including mutation, overexpression of the normal nonmutated gene, and genetic rearrangement. Overexpression of the normal proto-oncogene can occur through increases in the number of gene copies in the cell. This process, called *gene amplification,* was described in the neuroblastoma oncogene (N-*myc*) during the early to mid-1980s.[78] Amplification of N-*myc* results in anywhere from a few additional copies to as many as 300 copies present in a tumor cell. Besides increasing the understanding of oncogene activation methods, the neuroblastoma studies have established an association between an increased number of gene copies in tumor cells with advanced stage disease at diagnosis and poor prognosis.[17,18,79] In addition, the expression of N-*myc* can increase after treatment for recurrent neuroblastoma and may serve as a still-unexplained mechanism of drug resistance.[76]

A final example of oncogene activation is the process of gene rearrangement and insertional mutation. Gene expression increases when genetic material that acts as a promoter is incorrectly located adjacent to a proto-oncogene. This mechanism has been demonstrated in tumor viruses but remains controversial in human cancer. However, as described previously in this chapter, a number of chromosome translocations are associated with childhood cancer, and these translocations may promote cancer through this mechanism.[13] An example of insertional mutation relevant to pediatrics is found in Burkitt's lymphoma. In children with Burkitt's lymphoma there is a high frequency of chromosome translocation of the eighth chromosome near the c-*myc* proto-oncogene. This arrangement positions c-*myc* closely to an active immunoglobulin promoter, and the result is overexpression of the c-*myc* oncogene. Clinically, the overexpression of the c-*myc* oncogene may contribute to Burkitt's lymphoma by enhancing the aggressiveness of the disease.[54,84]

Once activated, oncogenes code for proteins that alter or prevent the cell from receiving and/or responding to normal regulatory signals. The protein products of oncogenes require further characterization and remain an active area of study. Proteins identified thus far are normally involved with the transfer of extracellular messages necessary to reach the cell nucleus to regulate cell division, and most of these oncogene-derived proteins serve as growth factor receptors. When the oncogene alters the protein product from the normal proto-oncogene, signals to continue growth are sensed, even when there is no extracellular message. Unregulated growth is the result.[80]

Oncogenes also may alter the cell's interpretation of growth factor messages. This occurs when the activated proto-oncogene originally produced a protein that served as a growth factor. Cells that contain proteins that synthesize growth factors are susceptible not only to proliferation from growth factors produced by other cells (called *paracrine growth*) but can proliferate through self-stimulation by growth factors produced in the cell itself (called *autocrine growth*).[1] The cell must both produce the growth factor and have receptors to bind the factor and receive the growth message. This permits an ominous self-contained

proliferation autonomy in the cell and is an important feature of cancer formation.[82] In studies thus far, autocrine growth mechanisms have been identified through laboratory studies in the childhood cancers osteosarcoma, neuroblastoma, and Wilms' tumor. It is speculated that the growth factor implicated in osteosarcoma may be platelet-derived growth factor. Insulin-like growth factor II may be associated with neuroblastoma and Wilms' tumor.[12,28,74] The identification of these autocrine growth pathways provides another new direction to explore for possible treatment strategies. Research has begun to identify methods to interfere with these pathways.

More than 40 proto-oncogenes have been identified and are believed present in every human cell. The resulting oncogenes have very unusual names. Because the identification of viral oncogenes found in animals preceded human oncogene identification, the naming of an oncogene is tied to the abbreviation of the similar virus-associated oncogene identified in the particular animal. For example, the *sis* oncogene is named after the simian sarcoma virus in monkeys, the *src* oncogene comes from the Rous sarcoma virus in chickens, and the *abl* oncogene is named after the Abelson murine leukemia virus identified in mice. Table 2–8 lists some of the childhood cancers in which oncogenes have been detected. This list should grow and become more detailed as more is learned about mechanisms of oncogene activation, the products of these activated genes, and their role in tumor initiation, promotion, and progression.

Tumor-Suppressor Genes

Tumor-suppressor genes, also sometimes called *cancer-susceptibility genes, antioncogenes,* or *recessive cancer genes,* are normal genes that limit or turn off cellular growth. These genes' role in cancer formation occurs when they become inactivated or deleted, allowing cells the unconstrained growth that is the hallmark of cancer. Because tumor-suppressor genes are lost in the process of tumor formation, making study difficult, the identification of specific tumor-suppressor genes and their pro-

TABLE 2—8. *Selected Oncogenes Identified in Childhood Cancer*

HUMAN ONCOGENE	LOCATION IN CELL	DESCRIPTION	CHILDHOOD CANCER
sis	Cytoplasm (secreted)	Platelet-derived growth factor (PDGF)-like growth stimulation	Glioblastoma
src	Plasma membrane	Protein kinases, specifically tyrosine kinase	Rhabdomyosarcoma, Ewing's sarcoma, osteosarcoma, leukemia, neural tumors
abl	Plasma membrane	Protein kinases, specifically tyrosine kinase	Chronic myelocytic leukemia, acute lymphocytic leukemia
erb B	Plasma membrane	Protein kinases, specifically tyrosine kinase and epidermal growth factor receptor	Glioblastoma
N-*ras*	Plasma membrane	Binds quanine nucleotides	Neuroblastoma, leukemia
H/K-*ras*	Plasma membrane	Binds quanine nucleotides	Neuroblastoma, rhabdomyosarcoma, leukemia
c-myb	Nucleus	DNA-binding protein	Neural tumors, leukemia, lymphoma, neuroblastoma, rhabdomyosarcoma, astrocytoma, Wilms' tumor
N-*myc*	Nucleus	DNA-binding protein	Neuroblastoma
c-myc	Nucleus	DNA-binding protein	Burkitt's lymphoma

Modified from Israel M. Cancer cell biology. In Pizzo PA, Poplack DG (eds): Principles and Practice of Pediatric Oncology, 2nd ed. Philadelphia: JB Lippincott, 1993, p 63.

tein gene products has lagged behind oncogene identification. However, new methods have been developed to identify these genes, and their identification is an area of intensive investigation that should yield important information in understanding mechanisms of carcinogenesis.[90]

Tumor-suppressor genes are termed *recessive genes* because both copies of the gene must be deleted from the paired chromosomes to permit cancer growth. If only one of the gene pairs (one allele) is affected, the normal tumor suppression (growth control) continues, which is in contrast to oncogene expression in which only one allele is required to affect tumor formation.

The mechanisms of tumor-suppressor gene action are connected with growth-regulating signals discussed in the previous section. Besides the growth-promoting activity of proto-oncogene–produced proteins, cells exert counter growth-controlling properties between neighboring cells. Tumor-suppressor gene products are involved in the intracellular signaling pathways that allow the cell to inhibit its growth based on signals from surrounding neighbors. Exactly how growth inhibition occurs is still under study. Thus far three important components are described: (1) the process of contact inhibition in which cell-surface molecules somehow sense the presence of neighbor cells and shut down growth in response (called *down regulation*); (2) gap junction communication that allows growth-inhibiting signals to pass between cells; and (3) specific hormones and growth inhibitors such as tumor growth factor B that inhibits the growth of cells or induces end-stage cell differentiation that takes the cell out of cell-cycle proliferation.[31] The end result of growth inhibition by these mechanisms for the cell is a hold on a phase of the cell replication cycle, particularly the phase of replication before DNA synthesis, called G_1, preventing the progression to the phase of DNA synthesis. Growth inhibition also may result in cell differentiation; a commitment to phase out through the aging process, called *senescence;* or the more active process of cell death, called *apoptosis,* which is programmed cellular self-destruction resulting in cell death. When a tumor-suppressor gene is lost, the cell loses the growth-inhibiting signal network; as a consequence, the cell no longer responds to extracellular growth-inhibiting signals, even though these signals are present in the surrounding tissue. Instead, the cell continues to proliferate to the detriment of the organism.

Initial study of tumor-suppressor genes and cancer has focused on hereditary cancers, many of which are relevant to childhood cancer. Hereditary forms of the childhood cancers such as retinoblastoma and Wilms' tumor demonstrate the deletion of portions of a chromosome in all the child's cells since the deletion was transmitted through the germ line. The genetic defect therefore is the loss of a tumor-suppressor gene. In the case of retinoblastoma, this tumor-suppressor gene is called the Rb gene, and it is deleted from the 13q14 chromosome. Wilms' tumor is still under scrutiny, but a candidate gene, WT1, lost from the short end of chromosome 11, has been identified.[3]

In recent years geneticists have found that genes from parents do not always make equal contribution to a child as Mendel's law of 1865 predicts. It is now believed that certain genes are marked so that they are expressed differently, depending on whether they were inherited from the mother or the father. The mechanism for marking genes in this manner is unknown, but the concept is referred to as *genomic imprinting.*[7] The relevance of this concept for childhood cancer and tumor-suppressor genes is that the loss of tumor-suppressor genes, resulting in subsequent tumor development, may be dependent on which parent contributed the chromosome containing the lost tumor-suppressor genes. Although the evidence is preliminary at this point, an example of the importance of genetic imprinting can be found in the observation that the loss of chromosome 11 in the nonherited form of Wilms' tumor almost exclusively involves the maternally contributed chromosome.[7] Genomic imprinting also may

be a factor in familial cancers and retinoblastoma.

Other childhood cancers suspected of having tumor-suppressor gene connections and exhibiting a loss of genetic material include neuroblastoma, osteosarcoma, and rhabdomyosarcoma. The identification of specific tumor-suppressor genes in these cases is still under investigation.[34] However, a tumor-suppressor gene has been identified for neurofibromatosis, the NF1 gene that is deleted from chromosome 17q11.2. Von Recklinghausen neurofibromatosis arises from cells originating in the embryonic neural crest. It is a genetically transmitted disease associated with benign growths and malignant tumors, particularly malignant peripheral nerve sheath tumors and neurofibrosarcomas. A tumor-suppressor gene is also believed lost, perhaps from chromosome 5, in familial cases of adenocarcinoma of the colon. In addition, the p53 gene, associated with Li-Fraumeni syndrome and once thought to function as an oncogene, is now thought to function normally as a tumor-suppressor gene. This gene and its protein products appear particularly complex.[90]

The identification of tumor-suppressor genes for retinoblastoma has provided support for Knudson's two-hit hypothesis that postulated the loss of both alleles, at that time, of an unknown gene. In the case of familial retinoblastoma, all cells have one allele of the Rb gene lost (first hit) and only require a subsequent loss (second hit) of the other allele of the Rb gene in any retinoblast cell for retinoblastoma to occur. In the acquired or sporadic form, only the tumor has the deletion of the Rb gene, and the normal noncancerous cell retains a functional Rb gene. The Rb gene was first identified in retinoblastoma and was named after the disease; however, it has now been associated with other cancers, including breast cancer, small-cell lung carcinoma, and bladder cancer, making the name of the gene somewhat confusing.[34]

Clinical Implication

New understanding of the nature of cancer genes can be exploited to develop diagnostic and therapeutic strategies.[41] As mentioned previously, it is possible that someday cancers will be renamed or grouped according to genetic similarities rather than by histology or organ site. By characterizing genetic alterations that contribute to cancer formation, it will be possible to identify infants and children at high risk for certain cancers. Combining ecogenetics and risk identification is the focus of molecular epidemiology. This approach will couple laboratory methods with analytic epidemiologic methods to identify markers that precede cancer formation. The ability to identify high-risk children will carry with it certain ethical concerns, particularly the heightened vulnerability and fear on the part of families with at-risk children, and potential difficulties in securing or maintaining health insurance.

The ability to detect cancer-causing genes and their gene products also will aid in cancer diagnosis, prognosis, and progression. For example, since the presence of many copies of the N-*myc* oncogene in neuroblastoma tumor cells is associated with more advanced disease and a poorer prognosis, treatment protocols based on the number of N-*myc* copies are designed to respond to these varying levels of tumor aggressiveness. In addition, since many oncogenes code for growth factors, new therapies will focus on blocking growth factors and receptor coupling.

Another potential new approach is the use of a class of agents called *recombinant toxins*. These agents target cell-surface receptors and antigens on tumor cells. They are composed of an agent that will specifically target a cancer cell such as a growth factor or antigen-binding protein and a toxin, usually a bacterial or plant toxin, that, once delivered to the cell, will kill it.[71]

Gene therapy is probably the most dramatic new treatment on the horizon. The ultimate intent will be to correct the genetic defect or loss through genetic engineering.[5,44] Many technical difficulties are associated with implementing such treatment approaches, but they remain areas of great interest.

CHARACTERISTICS OF CANCER CELLS

Given the significance of the genetic alterations and loss of normal social control and function, it is not surprising that cancer cells look different from normal cells and exhibit abnormal biologic activity. Table 2–9 lists some of the unique characteristics common to cancer cells. However, every cancer cell does not have all these altered characteristics. There is variability among tumors, with some closely resembling normal tissue and retaining some normal function and others so disorganized it is difficult to determine the normal tissue of origin.[59]

The cell-surface changes in cancer are particularly significant for understanding the invasiveness and initial metastatic potential of cancer and the mechanism of immune system defense against cancer,[51] both of which are discussed in further detail in the next two sections of this chapter. In addition, cell-surface and cytoplasm abnormalities foster or produce substances that are found on tumor cells or in blood, spinal fluid, or urine and are therefore identified as markers of specific

TABLE 2–9. *Characteristics of Malignant Cancer Cells*

Intracellular Characteristics

Atypical cell structure
Irregular and increased nuclear size and total DNA
Decreased number of mitochondria
Irregular shape and size of cytoplasm
Decreased or increased number of Golgi complexes
Simplified cell membrane
Increased mitotic activity

Cell-Surface Changes

Loss of cell-to-cell adhesion and contact inhibition
Altered anchoring junctions and gap junctions
Lost or altered surface enzymes, glycolipids, and glycoproteins
Increased lectin agglutination
Presence of new antigens and loss of normal antigens

Growth and Spread

Local increase in cell numbers and loss of normal cell arrangement
Rapid rate of growth
Increased vascularity
Growth by infiltration
Propensity to metastasize
Infinite proliferative life span resulting in death of organism if left untreated or if treatment is unsuccessful in stopping proliferation

tumors. Ideally these tumor markers can be detected and measured and therefore aid in cancer detection, provide estimates of tumor burden, and indicate tumor regression or progression.[88] However, even with known tumor markers, there is considerable inaccuracy in measurement and interpretation of findings. For example, nonmalignant disease can also be associated with the presence of a tumor marker, or a tumor marker may also become detectable relatively late in the disease. Often marker levels are not proportionate to actual tumor burden. Identification of tumor markers is more developed with adult cancer but is a continuing area of study in pediatrics.[56] Thus further work is necessary before tumor markers are developed to their full clinical usefulness.[59]

Tumor markers may be organized into several different categories. Categories relevant to childhood cancers are hormones, enzymes, and antigens. Hormones may be inappropriately produced by tumor tissue. Since the tumor is nonendocrine tissue, the hormones are referred to as *ectopic*. Inappropriate hormonal secretion with pediatric tumors includes increased urinary catecholamines and their metabolites associated with neuroblastoma and β-human chorionic gonadotropin elevations in children with rare hepatomas and nongestational trophoblastic tumors.

Enzymes may be abnormally expressed as an immature, fetal form of an enzyme or as the ectopic production of a normal enzyme. Isoenzymes that have a variable form but function similarly to normal enzymes also are potential pediatric tumor markers. Neuron-specific enolase (NSE) is markedly elevated in children, particularly infants with extensive neuroblastoma. Terminal deoxynucleotidyl transferase (TdT) is elevated with T-cell and B-cell leukemias and in some children with acute myeloblastic leukemia. Thus far TdT usefulness is limited to measuring treatment responsiveness. It also may be elevated during febrile episodes or viral infection. Lactate dehydrogenase (LDH) may be elevated with a number of pediatric cancers, including ALL, non-Hodgkin's lymphoma, osteosarcoma, Ewing's sarcoma, and neuroblastoma.[56]

Antigen markers are measured in the serum after being shed by tumor cells. Three antigens that serve as pediatric tumor markers are α-fetoprotein (AFP) and T-cell and B-cell antigens. AFP is elevated in nonseminoma germ-cell testicular tumors and hepatomas. Clinically, AFP is useful in making initial treatment decisions and for follow-up after treatment when increased levels are associated with increased tumor burden. T-cell and B-cell antigens are useful in differentiating between the various forms of leukemia and lymphoma.[56]

TUMOR INVASIVENESS AND METASTASIS

As described previously, oncogenes and tumor-suppressor genes circumvent normal social control. An important component of this is the loss of normal cell-to-cell communication in patients with cancer. Four alterations seen with cancer cells include the loss of (1) density-dependent inhibition of growth, (2) anchorage dependence, (3) contact inhibition, and (4) adhesiveness. Cells normally cease proliferating when they conform to a given space in a single layer, which is called *density-dependent inhibition*. However, cancer cells continue to proliferate, producing multiple, disorganized layers of cells. Normal cells also attach to substratum in the extracellular tissue to maintain cohesive movement known as *anchorage dependence*. Anchorage dependence is not found in cancer cells, and this loss facilitates increased independent movement. Contact inhibition is exhibited by normal cells when they come into contact with each other, preventing cell-on-cell overlap and maintaining single layer growth. The loss of this inhibition is well known in cancer and accounts for the characteristic of cell clumping. A final cancer cell characteristic is the loss of cell-to-cell adhesiveness that is seen in normal cells. When adhesiveness is lost, the cancer cell has increased freedom of movement.

These characteristics occur because of biochemical changes in cancer cells such as the decrease in normal fibronectin secretion and the concurrent increase in proteases, the cellular proteolytic enzymes. Loss of the glycoprotein fibronectin, which is necessary for anchorage dependence and cellular adhesiveness, contributes to cellular disorganization and increased ease in movement of the cancer cell. Proteases such as plasminogen activators, lysosomal enzymes, and collagenases are released from cancer cells and contribute to the destruction of extracellular material, thereby facilitating local invasiveness.[27]

For many years mechanical pressure by the growing tumor mass on surrounding tissue was seen as key to eventual local invasion. However, it is possible to demonstrate tumor invasiveness when pressure is not a factor, and in some large benign tumors in which there is significant pressure on adjacent normal tissue, there is no invasiveness.[37] It is likely that for any given tumor, a variety of biochemical mechanisms and perhaps mechanical pressure in combination contribute to local spread of the tumor.

Local invasiveness begins the dynamic multistep process of metastasis, referred to as the *metastatic cascade*. It is an essential first step in a process that is now seen as arduous and inefficient (less than 1 in 10,000 cancer cells survive the dissemination process) but is directly responsible for most cancer deaths. Table 2–10 outlines the steps of the metastatic cascade.

Angiogenesis

Angiogenesis, meaning new blood vessel growth, is necessary to provide oxygen and essential nutrients to the tumor at both primary and distant sites. Angiogenesis also occurs in normal processes such as placental nourishment of the fetus and wound healing. In these normal processes, however, the neovascularization follows an orderly path, eventually regressing or ceasing further growth, in contrast to the continued proliferation of blood vessels around the tumor.

The mechanism of angiogenesis is very interesting. Rather than tumor cells' directly forming the new blood vessels, the tumor produces a substance known as either *angiogenin* or *tumor angiogenesis factor (TAF)* that causes surrounding normal tissue to make blood vessels for the tumor.[53] Vascularization of the tumor is essential for the tumor to spread to a distant site as a metastasis.

Tumor Spread

Once vascularization has occurred, the metastatic cascade continues with three basic patterns of spread: (1) local invasion and invasion of tumor cells through (2) blood vessels and (3) lymphatics. It again should be emphasized that this is an extremely inefficient process—it is estimated that less than 0.01% of cancer cells that separate and spread from the primary tumor ever become a metastasis.[27] More recent research also suggests that those cells that do survive and carry out the metastatic mission have unique characteristics unlike other cells within the tumor.[43]

The newly formed blood vessels in tumors are loosely structured; therefore it is quite easy for cancer cells to penetrate them. Once inside the blood vessel, the cancer cells are transported into the general circulation. The lymphatic system also provides an avenue for metastatic transport of cancer cells. Lymphatic vessels are not found in tumors themselves but are accessed in naturally occurring lymphatics next to the primary tumor. From entry into lymphatics at the tumor periphery, cancer cells are transported to regional lymph nodes. These regional nodes can actually serve as a barrier and delay the continued spread of the cancer cells, but this protection eventually becomes ineffective. Because of frequent lymphatic–blood vessel intercon-

TABLE 2–10. *Metastatic Cascade*

Primary tumor
↓
Tumor angiogenesis
↓
Local invasion
↓
Invasion into blood vessels and lymphatics
↓
Movement through blood vessels and lymphatics
↓
Lodging in capillary bed of organ site
↓
Escape from vessel
↓
Invasion and growth at new metastatic site
(represents less than 0.01% of cells
that separate from primary tumor)

nections, many tumor cells that enter the lymphatics end up in the venous circulation.[52]

The sites for metastatic spread generally follow the natural downstream circulatory anatomy. In 1873 Paget suggested a "seed and soil" theory to explain site-specific metastasis. This theory underscored the importance of conducive characteristics of the metastatic site (the soil) for the particular tumor cells (the seed) to grow. Elements of this theory are still considered valid. Specific factors thought to contribute to the eventual site of metastasis for particular tumors include hormones, growth-promoting factors, genetics, age, tumor angiogenesis at the metastatic site, immune status, and blood flow.[27] Again, this is a perilous journey during which most cells die in the capillaries because they cannot tolerate the turbulence created by the circulating blood or they are destroyed by immune system defenses.[52] Table 2–11 lists frequent metastatic sites of childhood cancers. Early metastasis is a prominent feature of most childhood cancers, with approximately 80% having metastasized at diagnosis.[30] Once the metastatic site is established, additional new metastases can be initiated from both this secondary site and the primary tumor.

The invasiveness of cancer cells is seen at several points along the metastatic cascade and has been studied extensively. An example of this process is the steps necessary for tumor cells to escape the capillary circulation to create a metastatic site in tissue. The tumor cells first must penetrate the layer of endothelial cells that line the inside of the capillary. Tumor cells are known to attach preferentially to endothelial surfaces. This attachment stimulates the endothelial layer actually to retract, exposing underlying tissue called the *extracellular matrix*. There are several compartments in the matrix that are separated by special membranes. One of these membranes, the basement membrane, covers the blood vessels and muscle cells and nerves. Another matrix, located next to the basement membrane, is the interstitial stroma that compartmentalizes other tissues and the lymphatic vessels. The complex extracellular matrix serves as an important barrier for the tumor cells to breach. Liotta[52] has identified a three-step process used by tumors to penetrate the basement membrane: (1) attachment of the tumor cells to the membrane by tumor cell-surface receptors' binding with elements of the membrane; (2) secretion of enzymes that destroy basement membrane molecules, creating an opening; and (3) movement of the tumor cells through the opening into the tissue.

The discovery of oncogenes and tumor-suppressor genes as a primary mechanism of carcinogenesis has led to the exploration of genes that are involved with metastatic expression. Researchers have found that tumor-suppressor genes also may be involved in blocking metastatic mechanisms. Liotta[52] has proposed the existence of metastasis-suppressor genes in normal cells and cancer cells that can inhibit the invasive behavior of cells. Loss of metastasis-suppressor genes would stop the production of proteins that block cells from expressing metastatic behavior. As established tumors begin the process of invasion, oncogenic-produced proteins may increase and stimulate the cell migration and enzyme production necessary to penetrate the extracellular matrix. Further research is needed to verify this mechanism.

Clinical Significance and Treatment Strategies

The challenge of curing cancer is achieving the ability to prevent or successfully eradicate

TABLE 2–11. *Common Metastatic Sites for Selected Childhood Cancers*

PRIMARY TUMOR	METASTATIC SITES
Ewing's sarcoma	Lung, other bones
Neuroblastoma	Lymph node, liver, spleen, bone, bone marrow, skin
Osteosarcoma	Lungs, brain, occasionally other bone
Retinoblastoma	Brain, spinal cord, bone marrow, long bones, lymph nodes, liver
Rhabdomyosarcoma	Regional lymph nodes, lung, liver, bone marrow, bones, brain
Wilms' tumor	Lung, liver, bone, brain, lymph nodes

metastases. Unfortunately, most children have metastatic disease at diagnosis, and even with those children who do not demonstrate metastases at diagnosis, it is not possible to predict whose disease will eventually spread. Thus understanding the detailed process of metastasis is critical to developing effective treatment strategies. Several approaches to prevention of metastasis have been proposed that address the unique mechanisms of the metastatic cascade. Examples of these approaches include (1) protease enzyme inhibitors that decrease the production of protease; (2) antiadhesive therapy using a peptide inhibitor that blocks the adhesive properties of fibronectin and laminin; (3) anticoagulation therapy using warfarin and other agents that alter coagulation and presumably hematogenous spread (although this remains controversial); (4) antiangiogenesis therapy using agents known to interfere with neovascularization; and (5) biologic response modifiers that increase the immune system's defense against tumor cells.[27]

Effective treatment strategies for children with metastatic disease also are under investigation. Generally, the use of multiple-agent therapy is aimed at the diversity of cells found in advanced tumors and metastatic sites. A class of synthetic compounds called *carboxyamide aminoimidazoles* has been identified that may block the continued growth of metastatic tumor sites, perhaps by altering the flow of calcium ions into the cell and preventing growth signaling messages. The usefulness of these compounds and their applicability to childhood cancers await further exploration.[52]

Additional research has focused on the reasons for eventual drug resistance to many of the chemotherapeutic agents. A gene has been identified as the multidrug resistance (MDR) gene that produces a glycoprotein called *P-glycoprotein*. This protein is thought to act as a efflux pump that decreases drug concentration in the cell.[24] Most childhood cancer cells have not shown this protein at diagnosis but can be found in some childhood cancers relapsing after chemotherapy, particularly neuroblastoma.[24] Once more is understood about the mechanisms of multidrug resistance, treatment strategies to overcome multidrug resistance gene expression will be forthcoming.

IMMUNE SYSTEM AND CANCER

The immune system is the body's defense system against anything identified as foreign or nonself. It is complicated, not yet fully understood, and composed of many different physiologic mechanisms. Although a cancer cell originates from a once-normal cell, transformation to cancer results in sufficient genetic change to permit elements of the immune system to recognize the cell as nonself and destroy it. However, the differences are relatively small, and tumor cells frequently circumvent the protection against cancer offered by the immune system.[35]

Immune System Overview

The immune system has three primary functions: (1) defense against foreign microorganisms; (2) homeostasis through the orderly removal of damaged or dead cells; and (3) surveillance to identify and destroy abnormal or mutated cells.[6] These functions are carried out through two mechanisms that comprise the immune system: innate immunity and adaptive immunity.[6] The innate mechanisms are those with which the individual is born, including all the physical (e.g., skin, mucous membranes) and chemical (e.g., cytolytic components in the respiratory, genitourinary, and gastrointestinal systems) barriers and the specific cellular components (i.e., monocytes and macrophages, eosinophils, neutrophils, and natural killer cells). The cellular components of the innate system do not have the capacity for immunology memory and therefore do not increase potency with repeated exposure to the invading microorganism.[6] The adaptive component of the immune system provides antigen-specific protection and can be strengthened by repeated exposure. It is composed of the following cellular elements: monocytes and macrophages, thymus-derived lymphocytes (T cells), and bone marrow-derived lymphocytes (B cells).

The cells that comprise the immune system are distributed throughout the body, with particular concentration in the lymphatic system. This system includes the lymph nodes, lymphatic vessels and fluid, mucosal-associated lymphoid tissue, spleen, thymus gland, tonsils and adenoids, and components of the bone marrow and liver. Immune system cells originate from the bone marrow stem cell that provides red blood cells, platelets, and leukocytes. The immune elements are derived from the leukocyte line that also differentiates to granulocytes (neutrophils, basophils, and eosinophils), lymphocytes (B lymphocytes; T lymphocytes; and non-T, non-B lymphocytes), and mononuclear phagocytes.

The immune system has two important subsystems that orchestrate the destruction of foreign or nonself cells: humoral immunity and cell-mediated immunity.

Humoral immunity involves B lymphocytes that in the mature form are also called *plasma cells* and produce serum glycoprotein immunoglobulins (antibodies). Immunoglobulins bind to antigens that become targeted cells because they have nonself antigens and, in binding, form antigen-antibody complexes. These complexes neutralize antibodies and also are important in neutralizing bacterial toxins and viruses, opsonizing bacteria (promoting phagocytosis), and activating the inflammatory response. There are five classes of immunoglobulins: IgA, IgD, IgE, IgG, and IgM. IgG is an important component in the development of memory cells that are responsible for the subsequent secondary response to a similar antigen exposure in the future. In addition to immunoglobulins, humoral immunity also involves the complement system. Complement involves at least 10 proteins that are activated in a cascade response when there is antigen-antibody interaction. Most effective against bacterial infection, the complement system is involved with the inflammatory response, cell lysis, and phagocytosis.

T cells are the primary component of cell-mediated immunity. They are capable of becoming sensitized to and directly attacking specific antigens. T cells can be further subdivided by function and surface proteins into killer T cells (cytotoxic cells), lymphokine-producing cells, helper T cells, suppressor T cells, and memory T cells. After macrophage presentation of the antigen, killer T cells attack the nonself antigens; lymphokine-producing cells transfer delayed hypersensitivity; and helper cells and suppressor cells control the activation and down regulation (stopping the action) of both cell-mediated and humoral responses. Helper cells enhance the production and function of other immune system cells. Memory cells induce the subsequent secondary response to an identical antigen. Figure 2–1 summarizes the original and specialized cell lines of both T and B lymphocytes.

Granulocytes, monocytes, and natural killer cells comprise the nonspecific components of cell-mediated immunity. Granulocytes destroy targeted cells through ingestion. Monocytes are phagocytes that are the precursors of tissue macrophages. They also destroy targeted cells through ingestion. In addition, macrophages get the antigens on targeted cells ready for recognition by the immune system; this is called *antigen processing*. This is a specific rather than nonspecific immune response. The natural killer cells are large granular lymphocytes that lack T-cell or B-cell markers and primarily kill abnormal cells, particularly cancer cells and cells invaded by viruses.

For a successful immune response, there must be interaction between the humoral and cell-mediated elements. Cytokines are immune system proteins that provide this interplay and in the process augment the immune response. Cytokines are also known as biologic response modifiers and are the primary immune system components currently used in treatment strategies for cancer. Cytokines are divided into two subtypes: monokines and lymphokines. Produced by macrophages, monokines include (1) interferons (alpha and beta) that bind to target cell antigens; (2) interleukin-1 that stimulates T cells, macrophages, and monocytes; (3) tumor necrosis factor, also called *cachectin*, that is either directly cytotoxic to cancer cells or damages tumor capillaries; and (4) several colony-stimulating factors that regulate growth of bone marrow stem cells. Lymphokines are produced by various activated interleukins that stimulate and enhance other immune cell function and include (1) interferon-γ, which enhances other interferons, interleukins, and tumor necrosis factor; (2) granulocyte-mac-

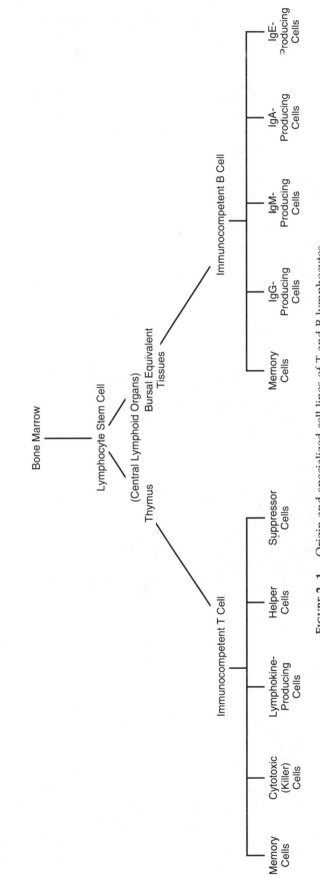

FIGURE 2–1. Origin and specialized cell lines of T and B lymphocytes.

rophage colony stimulating factor, which regulates differentiation of granulocytes and macrophages; and (3) lymphotoxin, which is cytotoxic to viruses.

The lymphocytes respond to foreign or nonself challenges in two phases: (1) afferent response and (2) efferent response. The afferent response involves recognition of the antigen by the lymphocyte, resulting in activation of the lymphocytes as an effector cell.

The efferent phase involves mature lymphocyte response in eliminating the antigen. Both afferent and efferent phases are very complicated events controlled by immune response genes, also called the *human leukocyte antigen (HLA)* genes, that are part of the major histocompatibility complex. An example of the complexity of these phases is the process by which the helper T cell is activated in the afferent phase. First, an antigen is picked up by a macrophage and presented to the helper T cell. Surface receptors on the helper T cell allow it to bind with the antigen and macrophage. The macrophage, in turn, produces the cytokine, interleukin-1, that signals between components of the immune system; this, in combination with the surface receptor-binding, activates the helper T cell as either an effector cell or a memory cell. The activated effector helper T cell then produces lymphokines, including α-interferon, which enhance proliferation and differentiation of T cells. All this activity is in preparation for the efferent phase, which includes antibody production, lymphokine release, cytoxicity, and immunoregulation, that results in the elimination of the antigen. Memory cells are stored and are not used for response to the initiating antigen but are reactivated in a subsequent exposure to the same type of antigen.[6,33]

Development of Immunity in Children

The immune system begins development in the fetus early in gestation. At birth it resembles the adult system but is relatively immature and lacks experience in responding to antigens.[10] However, the immune system develops rather rapidly after birth and is nearly mature by 6 months of age. The antigen-specific adaptive component is last to mature

fully because of the need for repeated exposure to develop sufficient memory cells. For example, the child is generally 5 to 6 years old before there is enough antigen-specific immunity to result in a decrease in episodes of infection.[57] The significance of the developing immune system to childhood cancer during fetal and early life remains open to speculation. Overall, cancer is associated with advancing age when the immune system loses significant function as a part of the aging process rather than with youth, so the primary influence of the immature immune system in the young may not be strong.[96] On the other hand, the relative immaturity of the immune system during fetal development may facilitate the escape of mutated cells from identification and disposal by immune elements and helps to explain the occurrence of embryonal tumors in childhood.

Influence of Immune System on Cancer Development and Progression

Since the early 1900s a role for the immune system in preventing or restraining cancer growth has been postulated.[35] But it was not until the late 1950s when T cells were found to be cytoxic that the modern immune surveillance theory was hypothesized as the key to antitumor resistance. There still is considerable controversy about the validity of this hypothesis. The primary clinical support for the role of the immune system in cancer control is the observation that cancer is more common in individuals who have either congenital or acquired immune defects.[32] However, the majority of cancers seen in children with the immunodeficiency diseases are limited to those with the acute leukemias, Hodgkin's disease, and non-Hodgkin's lymphoma rather than the wide variety of cancers that actually occur. Other evidence for the role of the immune system in cancer resistance is the identification of tumor antigens on the cell surface of cancer cells called *tumor-associated antigens (TAAs)*. Once called *tumor-specific antigens*, TAAs are now known to express themselves on normal cells; thus TAA is a more accurate term.[35] There are a number of known TAAs. One is tumor-associated transplantation antigen (TATA). This antigen can cause immunologic-specific resistance to tumor growth by a mechanism similar to that found in rejection of foreign tissue transplants. Other TAAs may prove valuable as tumor markers for diagnosis and disease monitoring.

The immune surveillance theory has been extended to include the possibility that immune resistance to cancer may be more than a T cell–mediated mechanism. Broadening the theory, cancer cells are now believed to express cell-surface antigens, and they may have other structures that allow a number of components of the immune system to recognize them as nonself. In response, both innate and adaptive effector mechanisms can eliminate or slow the spread of the cancer. In addition to T cells and their products as components of tumor resistance, macrophages, natural killer cells, and antibodies may play significant roles.[35] Natural killer cells have spontaneous cytotoxic activity against cancer cells. They also secrete cytokines and are augmented by exposure to other cytokines, primarily interferon and interleukin-2. Natural killer cells may be especially important in resistance to metastases.[32] Initial studies suggest that natural killer cells are particularly effective in removing tumor cells from the capillary circulation, thus discouraging blood-borne spread.[8]

Unfortunately, the immune system's cancer protection mechanisms can be circumvented by tumor cells, possibly as a combination of both changes in the child's immunologic potential and the evasive characteristic of the tumor cells. Six different mechanisms are proposed, including antigenic modulation, tumor secretion of immunosuppressive substances, escape and sneaking by tumor mechanisms, blocking factor, immunostimulation, and tumor-associated–antigen-suppressor T lymphocytes.

Clinical Implications of Cancer–Immune System Interaction

Adequate knowledge of the complex interaction involving the immune system and cancer resistance requires further study. However, current information provides insight into harnessing elements of the immune system for diagnosis, monitoring, and actual treatment of cancer. Although most of the clinical trials have involved adult cancers, pediatric trials are increasing. Chapter 7 on biologic response modifiers provides a detailed description of the strategies now used to control cancer through use of the body's own natural defenses in the immune system.

CLINICAL MANIFESTATIONS OF CHILDHOOD CANCER

Because childhood cancer is a group of different diseases involving a variety of organ and tissue sites, the manifestations of these cancers are numerous. Generally, a critical mass of cells or, in the case of leukemia, the systemic presence of many cells is needed before clinical manifestations are evident. The clinical manifestations are caused by one or more of the following mechanisms: (1) compression, infiltration, and obstruction caused by space-occupying tumors; (2) disease-related changes in blood cell production, including cytopenias due to disease replacement of the bone marrow and overproduction of lymphocytes and their immature elements; and (3) metabolic, electrolyte, hormonal, or immunologic alterations in response to or as a consequence of tumor metabolism by-products and cell death. Table 2–12 lists some specific manifestations associated with childhood cancer.

A complicating factor in isolating clinical manifestations of cancer is that most treatment approaches also contribute to or accelerate the problem. For example, cancer-related immunosuppression is compounded by immunosuppressive treatment such as chemotherapy. Chapters 11 through 14 discuss many of these clinical manifestations along with the appropriate medical treatment and nursing interventions. The pathophysiology of cancer-related cachexia, fatigue, and pain is explained in more detail in the next sections.

Cachexia

Cancer cachexia is a syndrome composed of a number of nutritional abnormalities, includ-

TABLE 2–12. *Disease Manifestations and Complications of Childhood Cancer*

MANIFESTATIONS AND COMPLICATIONS	CANCER-RELATED CAUSE
Anemia	Replacement of bone marrow with tumor cells or leukemic cells
Bruising, bleeding, hemorrhage	Thrombocytopenia due to replacement of bone marrow with tumor cells or leukemic cells
Cachexia	Hypothesized as a combination of factors: increased energy expenditure, decreased food intake, altered metabolism, by-products of tumor metabolism
Cardiac tamponade	Tumor involving cardiac muscle or pericardium, resulting in accumulation of fluid in pericardial space
Disseminated intravascular coagulation (DIC)	In children with acute leukemias release of enzymes from leukemic cells that activate coagulation system (rare) or consequences of sepsis, particularly with gram-negative organisms
Effusions (pleural, pericardial, abdominal)	Local invasion or metastatic spread to chest or abdomen
Fatigue	Hypothesized as a combination of factors: altered metabolism, increased energy expenditure, decreased food intake, anemia, by-products of tumor metabolism
Fever	Infection from cancer-related neutropenia and immunosuppression or noninfection-related fever from tumor stimulation of cells that produce interleukin-1, a pyrogen (hypothesized)
Hyperleukocytosis or hyperviscosity of blood	Leukemia with peripheral white blood count >100,000
Immunosuppression	Release of immunosuppressive factors by cancer cells
Increased intracranial pressure	Pressure from primary or metastatic brain tumors, resulting in headache, visual disturbances, nausea and vomiting, and/or behavioral changes
Infection or sepsis	Cancer-related neutropenia and immunosuppression and local tumor growth that disrupts normal pathogen barriers
Pain	Tumor infiltration and stretching or compression of pain-sensitive structures
Respiratory distress	Mediastinal tumors
Spinal cord compression	Tumor-related compression of the spinal cord, resulting in edema and ischemia of the cord and possible destruction from direct tumor infiltration
Superior vena cava syndrome	Mediastinal tumor compression of the superior vena cava, resulting in airway obstruction, respiratory distress, and edema
Tumor lysis syndrome	Cancers with high growth fractions and rapid cell lysis, resulting in hyperuricemia, hyperkalemia, hyperphosphatemia, hypercalcemia, and possible renal failure

ing weight loss, anorexia, weakness, taste alterations, decreased food intake, anemia, and altered protein, lipid, and carbohydrate metabolism.[42] It is the most severe form of malnutrition associated with cancer and results in wasting, emaciation, and decreased quality of life. Progressive cachexia often leads to death, especially with advanced-stage cancer.

Elements of cachexia are present in approximately one half of adults newly diagnosed with cancer.[48] However, cachexia at diagnosis is infrequent in childhood cancer.[87] In those instances in which it is found at diagnosis, the child is most likely to have neuroblastoma. Cachexia in childhood cancer is more common with progressive and metastatic disease; the incidence is estimated at 40% in this population.[3a] In addition, some childhood cancers are not associated with cachexia, whereas other tumors such as neuroblastoma and Ewing's sarcoma have strong associations. As a general rule, if children experience significant weight loss during the course of their disease, a poorer prognosis and shortened survival are suggested.[3a]

Although cancer cachexia has been studied for many years, much remains to be learned about the cause of this syndrome. An unanswered question is whether tissue wasting results from decreased food intake or from increased energy expenditure. In noncancer states, during pregnancy for example, an increase in metabolic rate is followed by an increase in food intake. But this does not happen with cancer, and for children this problem is compounded because they have increased nutrient demands simply as a part of normal childhood growth.

Anorexia with resulting decreased food intake is a fundamental component of cachexia. Anorexia in children is attributed more to cancer treatment than the disease itself.[48] Decreased interest in food is also attributed to altered taste perceptions. Of particular interest is a lower threshold for bitter foods such as high-protein products (e.g., meat). In addition, there is evidence that children can develop food aversions associated with cancer treatment.[11] Animal studies suggest that food aversion also may develop in response to some unknown biochemical consequence of tumor growth that is unrelated to treatment.[11]

Significant protein, carbohydrate, and lipid abnormalities occur with tumor growth. Loss of body protein through skeletal muscle wasting and hypoalbuminemia is seen with cancer cachexia. As skeletal muscle is depleted, the freed amino acids are incorporated by the tumor.[26] Altered carbohydrate metabolism includes increased gluconeogenesis, glucose intolerance secondary to insulin resistance, and lactic acidosis. In particular, sarcomas have been shown to use excessive amounts of glucose.[68] Hyperlipidemia and loss of fat stores are common features of altered lipid metabolism with cancer cachexia. This may represent increased mobilization and decreased deposition of fat.[3a]

For a number of years researchers have investigated tumor metabolites that could be responsible for the cachectic state. Several factors have been identified (e.g., serotonin, lipolytic factors), but they only have been measured in a limited number of cancers that are associated with paraneoplastic syndromes.[48] Of more importance in inducing cancer cachexia is a group of cytokines produced by the body in response to the presence of cancer. Predominant in this model is the macrophage-produced tumor necrosis factor (called *cachetin* because of its role in the cachexia syndrome). Other components include interleukin-1, interleukin-6, and interferon-γ. The research is still preliminary and shows some contradictions. Further study is necessary to clarify this intriguing finding—that the body's own defensive response to the presence of cancer may actually promote the cachexia syndrome.[48]

Fatigue

Research of any kind on the experience of fatigue associated with cancer is limited. However, fatigue is a feature of several childhood cancers at diagnosis and of most childhood cancers during treatment and advanced disease. Fatigue directly interferes with quality of life. Cancer fatigue is usually chronic and does not improve with a "good night's sleep." The cause of fatigue with cancer is unknown. Several explanations from general research on fatigue have been proposed, including (1) the accumulation hypothesis that attributes fatigue to the buildup of waste products in the body; (2) the depletion hypothesis that attributes fatigue to inadequate nutrient resources; (3) the biochemical imbalance hypothesis that attributes fatigue to altered nutrient and hormonal balance; and (4) the CNS hypothesis that attributes fatigue to understimulation of the brainstem reticular-activating system or, conversely, the overstimulation of the normal inhibitory system that depresses activity of the reticular-activating system.[67] Each of these explanations of fatigue may have some merit in explaining cancer fatigue. It is most likely a multifactorial cause and may be tied to mechanisms similar to those involved with cachexia, including the cytokine, cachetin. Further research is needed before the mechanisms and, more importantly, treatment approaches to fatigue are understood.

Pain

Pain is a much-feared component of the cancer experience. Multiple sources contribute to pain development during cancer, including pain from the disease itself, treatment-associated complications, and invasive procedures. Although studies have documented a high incidence of disease-related pain in adults with cancer, the most common cause of pain in childhood cancer is procedure related.[65] However, disease-related pain can occur in children. In one study of children at the time of cancer diagnosis, 78% were experiencing disease-related pain.[64] In a second study of children receiving treatment for cancer in which procedure-related pain was excluded, pain was still prevalent in one half of hospitalized children and one quarter of children in ambulatory settings.[65] The difference in pain sources between adults and children may relate to increased treatment-related pain in children caused by more aggressive protocols, more rapid response of children to treatment that would decrease disease-related pain, and shorter period of end-stage disease for those children who do not survive cancer.[65]

Depending on the location and structures involved, cancer pain involves three different types: (1) somatic pain, (2) visceral pain, and (3) neuropathic pain. Somatic pain involves activation of pain receptors in cutaneous and deep-seated tissues. It causes gnawing and aching that is usually constant and well localized. Pain from bone metastasis or tumor infiltration in musculoskeletal structures provides examples of somatic pain. Visceral pain involves activation of pain receptors in major organ systems, including the cardiovascular, respiratory, gastrointestinal, and genitourinary systems. It is poorly localized, and the pain sensation can be referred and therefore felt at a distant cutaneous site. It causes deep pressure and squeezing or knotting sensations and is described as vague and dull. Tumor irritation of mucosal surfaces, torsion and traction of the mesentery, and obstruction of hollow organs are examples of cancer-caused visceral pain. Neuropathic pain is caused by peripheral or CNS damage. The pain is usually described as burning or stabbing.

The pathophysiology of pain is complex. When stimulated by painful input, primary afferent fibers, called *nociceptors*, become activated. Biochemical mediators are released. These mediators, also called *neurotransmitters*, include potassium, bradykinin, prostaglandin, and a peptide that causes vasodilation and edema known as *substance P*. The primary afferent fibers become depolarized, opening sodium channels that cause an influx of potassium and a change in charge that transmits painful stimuli to the dorsal horn of the spinal cord. At this site there is further release of neuropeptides, particularly substance P, which binds on secondary neurons called *spinothalamic tract neurons*. This tract ascends to the thalamus, with a few fibers terminating in the midbrain. At the thalamus, the nociceptive message is transmitted to several areas of the brain. It is here that perception of pain is felt by the child.[71]

Concurrently, a modulatory system exists that permits a natural inhibitory mechanism for pain often called the *descending pain system*. This system involves those fibers that end in the midbrain and act by stimulating the descending transmissions back to the dorsal horn of the spinal cord. Substances, including serotonin and norepinephrine, inhibit the transmission of painful stimuli within the dorsal horn. In addition, noradrenergic neurons located in the pons have descending transmission to the spinal cord and also are known to inhibit nociceptive transmission in the dorsal horn.[71]

However, pain cannot be simply reduced to a biochemical, neurotransmitted phenomenon. Once the child experiences the pain, a psychologic response becomes an integrated component of the pain experience.[71] This psychologic response is individualized and involves many factors, including developmental level, past experience, family support, anxiety, depression, fatigue, and suffering. Pain therefore is a complicated personal experience. As defined by the International Association for the Study of Pain,[38] "Pain is an unpleasant sensory and emotional experience associated with actual or potential tissue damage, or described in terms of such damage. Pain is always subjective." Children of any age feel pain. Although newborns and infants have maturing CNS, they still can experience pain and require prompt and thorough pain relief interventions.[65]

CONCLUSION

Unraveling the causes and mechanisms of cancer has been a slow and arduous process. Historically, a chapter on the pathophysiology of childhood cancer would have focused heavily on descriptive epidemiology. It has only been in the last 10 to 15 years that description of the actual pathophysiology and genetic basis of cancer has begun. Much more awaits discovery. Understanding cancer remains a dynamic process. It is an exciting area because important new knowledge literally is reported on a monthly basis. At the same time, the dynamic nature of the field makes it difficult to stay current.

Understanding the nature of cancer provides the basis for effective prevention and treatment strategies. The treatment of childhood cancer has enjoyed remarkable progress, even without a solid understanding of the mechanisms involved. New knowledge in the future should translate into treatment that ultimately will remove childhood cancer from the list of diseases considered life-threatening. What will be even more exciting is the application of preventive strategies so that the incidence of childhood cancer will be a truly rare event.

REFERENCES

1. Aaronson SA. Growth factors and cancer. Science 1991; 254:1146–1152.
2. Ahlbom A. A review of the epidemiologic literature on magnetic fields and cancer. Scand J Work Environ Health 1988; 14:337–343.
3. Alberts B, Bray D, Lewis J, et al. Cell growth and division. In Molecular Biology of the Cell, 2nd ed. New York: Garland Publishing, 1989.
3a. Alexander HR, Norton JA. Nutritional supportive care. In Pizzo PA, Poplack DG (eds): Principles and Practice of Pediatric Oncology, 2nd ed. Philadelphia: JB Lippincott, 1993, pp 1021–1038.
4. Altman AJ, Schwartz AD. The cancer problem in pediatrics: Epidemiologic aspects. In Altman AJ, Schwartz AD (eds): Malignant Disease of Infancy, Childhood, and Adolescence, 2nd ed. Philadelphia: WB Saunders, 1983.
5. Anderson WF. Human gene therapy—Scientific and ethical considerations. Recomb DNA Tech Bull 1991; 8:55–63.
6. Appelbaum JW. The role of the immune system in the pathogenesis of cancer. Semin Oncol Nurs 1992; 8:51–62.
7. Austin KD, Hall JG. Nontraditional inheritance. Pediatr Clin North Am 1992; 39:335–348.
8. Barlozzari T, Reynolds CW, Herberman RB. In vivo role of natural killer cells. J Immunol 1983; 131:1024–1027.
9. Barrett JC. Genetic and epigenetic mechanisms of carcinogenesis. In Barrett JC (ed): Mechanisms of Environmental Carcinogenesis, vol 1. Boca Raton, Fla.: CRC Press, 1987, pp 129–142.
10. Bellanti JA, Boner AL, Valletta E. Immunology of the fetus and newborn. In Avery GB (ed): Neonatology—Pathophysiology and Management of the Newborn. Philadelphia: JB Lippincott, 1987, pp 850–873.
11. Bernstein I. Etiology of anorexia in cancer. Cancer 1986; 58:1881–1866.
12. Betsholtz C, Westermark B, Elk B, et al. Co-expression of a PDGF-like growth factor and PDGF receptors in a human osteosarcoma cell line: Implications for autocrine receptor activation. Cell 1984; 39:447–457.
13. Bishop JM. The molecular genetics of cancer. Science 1987; 235:305–311.
14. Bizzozero OJ Jr, Johnson KG, Ciocco A. Radiation-related leukemia in Hiroshima and Nagasaki 1946–1964. N Engl J Med 1966; 274:1095.
15. Bleyer WA. The impact of childhood cancer on the United States and the world. CA 1990; 40:355–367.
16. Boyd JA, Barrett JC. Genetic and cellular basis of multistep carcinogen. Pharm Ther 1990; 47:469–486.
17. Brodeur GM, Seeger RL, Schwab M, et al. Amplification of N-*myc* in untreated human neuroblastoma correlates with advanced disease stage. Science 1984; 224:1121.
18. Brodeur GM, Seeger RL, Schwab M, et al. Clinical implications of oncogene activation in human neuroblastomas. Cancer 1986; 58:541–545.
19. Caldwell GG, Heath CW Jr. Case clustering in cancer. South Med J 1976; 69:1598–1602.
20. Cancer Facts and Figures 1993. Atlanta: American Cancer Society, 1993.
21. Castaigne S, Chomienne C, Daniel MT, et al. All-trans-retinoic acid as a differentiation therapy for acute promyelocytic leukemia. Blood 1990; 76:1704.
22. De-Thè G. The epidemiology of Burkitt's lymphoma: Evidence for a causal association with Epstein-Barr virus. Epidemiol Rev 1979; 1:32–54.
23. Developmental genetics and childhood cancer—Meeting report. Cancer Res 1991; 51:5435–5439.
24. DeVita VT. The problem of resistance. Principles Pract Oncol—Update 1990; 4:1–12.
25. Doll R, Peto R. The causes of cancers: Quantitative estimate of avoidable risks of cancer in the United States today. J Natl Cancer Inst 1981; 66:1226–1237.
26. Douglas R, Shaw J. Metabolic effects of cancer. Br J Surg 1990; 77:246–254.
27. Dudjak LA. Cancer metastasis. Semin Oncol Nurs 1992; 8:40–50.
28. El-Badry OM, Romanus JA, Helman LI, et al. Autonomous growth of a human neuroblastoma cell line is mediated by insulin-like growth factor II. J Clin Invest 1989; 84:829.

29. Everson RB. Individuals transplacentally exposed to maternal smoking may be at increased risk in adult life. Lancet 1980; 2:123.

30. Fernbach DJ, Vietti TJ. General aspects of childhood cancer. In Fernbach DJ, Vietti TJ (eds): Clinical Pediatric Oncology, 4th ed. St. Louis: Mosby–Year Book, 1991.

31. Friend SH, Dryja TP, Weinberg RA. Oncogenes and tumor-suppressing genes. N Engl J Med 1988; 318:618–622.

32. Gorelik E, Herberman RB. Role of natural killer (NK) cells in the control of tumor growth and metastatic spread. In Herberman RB (ed): Cancer Immunology: Innovative Approaches to Therapy. Boston: Martinus Nijhoff, 1986, pp 151–176.

33. Grady C. Host defense mechanisms: An overview. Semin Oncol Nurs 1988; 4:86–94.

34. Helman LJ, Thiele CJ. New insights into the causes of cancer. Pediatr Clin North Am 1991; 38:201–221.

35. Herberman RB. Principles of tumor immunology. In Holleb A, Fink D, Murphy G (eds): Textbook of Clinical Oncology. Atlanta: American Cancer Society, 1991, p 69.

36. Honig WK, Lippman SM, Itri LM, et al. Prevention of secondary primary tumors with isotretinoin in squamous-cell carcinoma of the head and neck. N Engl J Med 1990; 323:795.

37. Hubbard SM, Liotta LA. The biology of metastases. In Baird S, McCorkle R, Grant M (eds): Cancer Nursing: A Comprehensive Textbook. Philadelphia: WB Saunders, 1991, pp 130–142.

38. International Association for the Study of Pain, Subcommittee on Taxonomy. Pain terms: A list with definitions and notes on usage. Pain 1979; 6:249–252.

39. Israel M. Cancer cell biology. In Pizzo PA, Poplack DG (eds): Principles and Practice of Pediatric Oncology, 2nd ed. Philadelphia: JB Lippincott, 1993, pp 57–80.

40. Jablon S, Kato H. Childhood cancer in relation to prenatal exposure to atomic-bomb radiation. Lancet 1970; 2:1000–1003.

41. Jenkins J. Biology of cancer: Current issues and future prospects. Semin Oncol Nurs 1992; 8:63–69.

42. Kern K, Norton J. Cancer cachexia. J Parenter Enteral Nutr 1988; 2:286–298.

43. Killion JJ, Fidler IJ. The biology of tumor metastasis. Semin Oncol 1989; 16:106–115.

44. Kinnon C, Levinsky RJ. Gene therapy for cancer. Eur J Cancer 1990; 26:638–640.

45. Klein G, Klein E. Oncogene activation and tumor progression. Carcinogenesis 1984; 5:429–435.

46. Knudson AG. Mutation and cancer: Statistical study of retinoblastoma. Proc Natl Acad Sci U S A 1971; 68:820–823.

47. Lagakos SW, Wessen BJ, Zelen M. An analysis of contaminated well water and health effects in Woburn, Massachusetts. J Am Stat Assoc 1986; 81:583–596.

48. Langstein H, Norton J. Mechanisms of cancer cachexia. Hematol Oncol Clin North Am 1991; 5:103–123.

49. Li FP. Cancer family syndrome: The nurse's role in identifying patients at risk. Fifteenth annual APON conference. Boston, Mass., 1991.

50. Li FP, Fraumeni JF Jr. Prospective study of a family cancer syndrome. JAMA 1982; 247:2692–2694.

51. Lind J. Tumor cell growth and cell kinetics. Semin Oncol Nurs 1992; 8:3–9.

52. Liotta LA. Cancer cell invasion and metastasis. Sci Am 1992; 226:63–65.

53. Liotta LA, Steeg PS, Stetler-Stevenson WG. Cancer metastasis and angiogenesis: An imbalance of positive and negative regulation. Cell 1991; 64:327–336.

54. Lombardi L., Newcomb EW, Dalla-Favera R. Pathogenesis of Burkitt lymphoma: Expression of an activated c-*myc* oncogene causes the tumorigenic conversion of EBV-infected human B lymphoblasts. Cell 1987; 49:161–170.

55. London SJ, Thomas DC, Bowman JD, et al. Exposure to residential electric and magnetic fields and risk of childhood leukemia. Am J Epidemiol 1991; 134:923–937.

56. Lovejoy NC, Halliburton P. Pediatric tumor markers. J Pediatr Nurs 1989; 4:357–369.

57. Lowery GH. Growth and Development of Children. Chicago: Year Book Medical Publishers, 1986, pp 259–266.

58. MacMahon B. Prenatal x-ray exposure and childhood cancer. J Natl Cancer Inst 1962; 28:1173–1191.

59. McCance KL, Mooney KH, Roberts KK. Tumor biology. In McCance KL, Huether SE (eds): Pathophysiology: The Biologic Basis for Disease in Adults and Children. St. Louis: CV Mosby, 1990.

60. McWhirter WR, Kirk D. What causes childhood leukemia? Some beliefs of parents of affected children. Med J Aust 1986; 145:314–316.

61. Miller RW. Deaths from childhood leukemia and solid tumors among twins and other sibs in the United States 1960–1967. J Natl Cancer Inst 1971; 46:203–209.

62. Miller RW. Frequency and environmental epidemiology of childhood cancer. In Pizzo PA, Poplack DG (eds): Principles and Practices of Pediatric Oncology. Philadelphia: JB Lippincott, 1989.

63. Miller RW, Myers MH. Age distribution of epithelial cancers. Lancet 1983; 2:1250.

64. Miser AW, McCalla J, Dothage JA, et al. Pain as a presenting symptom in children and young adults with newly diagnosed malignancy. Pain 1987; 29:85–90.

65. Miser AW, Miser JS. Management of childhood cancer pain. In Pizzo PA, Poplack DG (eds): Principles and Practice of Pediatric Oncology, 2nd ed. New York: JB Lippincott, 1993, pp 1039–1050.

66. Mulvihill JJ. Childhood cancer, the environment and heredity. In Pizzo PA, Poplack DG (eds): Principles and Practice of Pediatric Oncology, 2nd ed. Philadelphia: JB Lippincott, 1993, pp 11–27.

67. Nail LM. Fatigue. In Groenwald SL, Frogge HM, Goodman M, et al. (eds): Cancer Nursing: Principles and Practice, 2nd ed. Boston: Jones & Bartlett Publishers, 1990, pp 485–494.

68. Norton JA, Peacock JL, Morrison SD. Cancer cachexia. Crit Rev Oncol Hematol 1987; 7:289–293.

69. Deleted.

70. Nowell P. The clonal evolution of tumor cell populations. Science 1976; 194:23–28.

71. Paice JA. Unraveling the mystery of pain. Oncol Nurs Forum 1991; 18:843–849.

72. Pastan I, FitzGerald D. Recombinant toxins for cancer treatment. Science 1991; 254:1173–1177.

73. Pizzo PA, Horowitz M, Poplack D, et al. Solid tumors of childhood. In DeVita VT, Hellman S, Rosenberg SA (eds): Cancer Principles and Practice of Oncology, 3rd ed. Philadelphia: JB Lippincott, 1989.

74. Reeve AE, Eccles MR, Wilkens RJ, et al. Expression of insulin-like growth factor II transcripts on Wilms' tumor. Nature 1985; 317:258.

74a. Robison L. General principles of the epidemiology of childhood cancer. In Pizzo PA, Poplack DG (eds):

Principles and Practice of Pediatric Oncology, 2nd ed. Philadelphia: JB Lippincott, 1993, pp 3–10.

75. Robison L, Mertens A, Neglia J. Epidemiology and etiology of childhood cancer. In Fernbach D, Vietti T (eds): Clinical Pediatric Oncology, 4th ed. St. Louis: Mosby–Year Book, 1991.

76. Rosen N, Reynolds CP, Thiele CJ, et al. Increased N-*myc* expression following progressive growth of human neuroblastoma. Cancer Res 1986; 46:4139–4142.

77. Savitz DA, Chen JH. Parental occupation and childhood cancer: Review of epidemiological studies. Environ Health Perspect 1990; 88:325–337.

78. Schwab M, Alitalo D, Kleinpnauer KH, et al. Amplified DNA with limited homology to *myc* cellular oncogene is shared by human neuroblastoma cell lines and a neuroblastoma tumor. Nature 1983; 305:245.

79. Seeger RC, Brodeur GM, Sather H, et al. Association of multiple copies of the N-*myc* oncogene with rapid progression of neuroblastoma. N Engl J Med 1985; 313:1111.

80. Skinner MA, Iglehart JD. The emerging genetics of cancer. Surg Gynecol Obstet 1989; 168:371–379.

81. Solomon E, Borrow J, Goddard A. Chromosome aberrations and cancer. Science 1991; 254:1153–1160.

82. Sport MB, Roberts AB. Autocrine growth factors and cancer. Nature 1985; 313:745.

83. Stewart A, Webb J, Giles D, et al. Malignant disease in childhood and diagnostic radiation in utero. Lancet 1956; 2:447.

84. Taub R, Moulding C, Battey J, et al. Activation and somatic mutation of the translocated c-*myc* gene in Burkitt lymphoma cells. Cell 1984; 36:339–348.

85. Thompson MW, McInnes RR, Willard HF. In Thompson & Thompson Genetics in Medicine, 5th ed. Philadelphia: WB Saunders, 1991.

86. Trosko JE, Chang CC. Stem cell theory of carcinogenesis. Toxicol Lett 1989; 49:283–295.

87. vanEys J. The pathophysiology of undernutrition in the child with cancer. Cancer 1986; 58:1874–1880.

88. Virji MA, Mercer DW, Herberman RB. Tumor markers in cancer diagnosis and prognosis. CA 1988; 38:104–126.

89. Vital Statistics of the United States. Washington, D.C.: U.S. Government Printing Office, 1986.

90. Weinberg RA. Tumor suppressor genes. Science 1991; 254:1138–1146.

91. White R. Cancer genetics. In Jorde L, Carey J, White R (eds): Human Genetics. In press.

92. Wilson BW, Stevens RG, Anderson LE (eds). Extremely Low-Frequency Electromagnetic Fields: The Question of Cancer. Columbus, Ohio: Battella Press, 1990.

93. Yarbro JW. Oncogenes and cancer suppressor genes. Semin Oncol Nurs 1992; 8:30–39.

94. Young JL Jr, Reis LG, Silverberg E. Cancer incidence survival and mortality for children younger than age 15 years. Cancer 1986; 8:598–602.

95. Yunis JJ. Chromosomes and cancer: New nomenclature and future directions. Hum Pathol 1981; 12:494–503.

96. Ziegler JL. Cancer in the immunosuppressed host. In Stites DP, Terr AI (eds): Basic and Clinical Immunology. Norwalk, Conn.: Appleton & Lange, 1991, pp 588–598.

Nursing Implications of Diagnostic and Staging Procedures

Marcia Leonard

The nurse caring for the child suspected of having a malignancy is in a unique position to offer support and guidance to a family experiencing extraordinary stress. The nurse should possess a thorough understanding of the various diagnostic measures used for pediatric malignancies and the usual sequence in which they are obtained. Preparing the child and family for tests and procedures and facilitating patient safety are key nursing responsibilities.

ESTABLISHING THE DIAGNOSIS

Although cancer is the second leading cause of death in children greater than 1 year of age, it is still an uncommon disease in children. The diagnosis of childhood cancer is often delayed, even though the family has brought the child to the family doctor or pediatrician. The greatest aid in diagnosing malignant disease in children is a high index of suspicion,[35] for there is no classic, universal symptom of cancer in children. Signs and symptoms are influenced by the age of the patient, the type of tumor, and the extent of the disease. Rather than focusing on any particular symptom or group of symptoms, the practitioner should be alert to children with *persistent* symptoms.

The goals of diagnostic and staging pro-

cedures are to determine the presence of a cancer, to identify the kind and type of cancer, and to localize the cancer. These procedures should be carried out expeditiously to allow appropriate therapy to begin as quickly as possible. It is essential to blend general knowledge of the disease and treatment with as much information as possible about the histology and biology of the individual child's tumor so the appropriate amount and type of therapy can be delivered.[27]

Basic noninvasive imaging procedures that confirm the presence of a mass and basic laboratory work that suggests organ dysfunction such as an abnormal blood count can be performed by the local health care provider, and in light of the results, prompt referral should be made to a pediatric oncologist. Further community-based diagnostic testing usually cannot be as extensive as the disease warrants and subjects the child and family to unnecessary delay, expense, and trauma.

New and sophisticated tests that provide detailed information and prognostic data are available only at established pediatric cancer centers. As the pediatric oncologists' understanding of the disease process increases, treatment has become precisely tailored and often more complex. The child deserves state-of-the-art therapy and psychosocial support provided by a team of professionals experienced in the care of children with cancer. In a study published by Meadows et al.,[23] childhood cancer survival rate was positively influenced by place of treatment and the use of cancer protocols.

History

Diagnosis begins with obtaining a detailed medical history. Special attention is given to factors that suggest the possibility of malignancy. The interview is conducted in private, with consideration for the comfort of both the parents and child and without interruptions. The parents will be more relaxed if adequate provision has been made for the child's needs. An ill child is assigned to the care of a staff member. A more active child may be provided with toys or other activities. The parent may prefer to hold an infant or an older child, or the child may be placed on the examination table close to the parent.

Begin the interview process by greeting both parent and child. Include a friendly comment to the child (e.g., a remark about his or her appearance, clothing, or toy). During the interview make frequent eye contact with the child. Engage the child verbally during anxiety-producing moments.[8]

The older child and adolescent actively participate in the initial history taking and throughout their course of care. Comments that directly address the patient help pull the older child into the interview. The adolescent is given the opportunity to provide information without parents in the room, usually after the initial interview with the parents and before the physical examination. The parents can be reassured that the pertinent findings of the physical examination will be shared with them. Respecting the teen's independence and establishing a sense of confidentiality with the teen are best achieved if begun at the onset of treatment. Of course, if the teen is frightened and prefers parental presence, this wish is respected.

To collect relevant information, the examiner phrases questions in language that the parent and adolescent understand, listens carefully to the responses, and encourages the family to express ideas and concerns freely. If the parents are not fluent in English, an interpreter with some degree of medical knowledge should be obtained as soon as possible.

The examiner elicits the information by following a specific pattern. First, determine the chief complaint. Many health professionals ask the parents, "Why did you come to see us today?" Record the duration of the illness or complaint that brought the child to the attention of a physician. The examiner then develops the sequence of the present illness by inquiring about the date symptoms appeared, the order of occurrence, the diagnosis made by the referring health care provider who examined the patient, and response to any treatment prescribed. Listen intently to the parent's description of the child's illness or complaint. Parents describe a child's problem as they perceive it, and their story frequently includes a theory of the cause of the problem. Understanding such theories may be helpful later in counseling parents.[8]

The examiner next reviews the child's past history. The child's prenatal, neonatal, and subsequent growth and development are essential information. Record all immunizations and past illnesses and obtain a thorough social history. Included in a routine pediatric social history are age, marital status, and occupation of the parents, including stepparents or those with whom the child lives, and the age of siblings. The parent or the older child is asked to discuss school performance and adjustment.

Pertinent family medical history also is documented. Any history of cancer in family members, including the health status of grandparents, parents, and siblings, is noted, with special attention given to any pediatric cancers.

Finally, the patient history concludes with a review of body systems. The examiner attempts to elicit any symptoms that the parent has not recognized or considered relevant. Questions are asked about each body system. Before concluding the interview, the examiner asks the parent if all questions and concerns have been discussed. No concern should be minimized or automatically dismissed.

Physical Examination

Physical examination generally begins as the examiner observes the child while obtaining the medical history. Initial impressions about parent-child interactions, the child's general appearance, and whether the child behaves in an age-appropriate manner are made. A developmental assessment is an integral part of a pediatric physical examination. During the physical examination there must be regard for privacy and comfort. The child is treated with respect and consideration. An infant or toddler can be examined almost completely while on the parent's lap.

During the physical examination adolescents may raise concerns about their health or their bodies that were not mentioned in the initial interview. Many teens have misguided ideas about the cause of their illness, the extent of their symptoms, and the prognosis of childhood cancer. With skill and sensitivity, the examiner elicits this information from the adolescent and corrects any misconceptions. The skilled practitioner conveys to the adolescent that he or she is the primary concern of the medical team. The teen should be the primary source of information and is encouraged to be active and involved throughout treatment and decision making.[25]

Vital signs are obtained and recorded during the initial examination. Height and weight are measured and plotted on the appropriate growth chart, and the head circumference of infants and young children is measured also. Care is taken to assure accurate height and weight. Metric measurements are taken because they will be used to calculate the patient's body surface area. The surface area is measured in square meters, "m^2," and is computed with the use of a slide rule nomogram or by using the following formula:

$$\sqrt{\frac{Height \times Weight}{3600}}$$

The growth chart is an important tool for evaluating growth failure or dysfunction secondary to cancer treatment. Such dysfunction may be recognized sooner if baseline and incremental height and weight measurements are obtained and recorded regularly.

The four methods of examination are incorporated: inspection, auscultation, palpation, and percussion. Each body system is assessed for abnormality. Careful physical examination may indicate the site of a primary tumor, spread to lymph nodes or other organs, or both. In addition, detailed thorough documentation of physical findings is made.

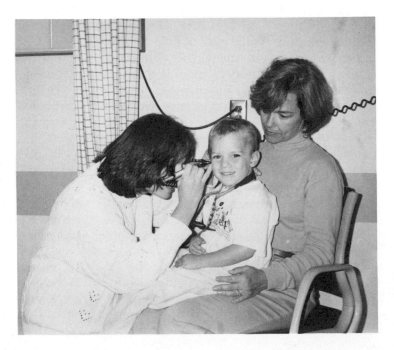

FIGURE 3–1. Young children may prefer to sit on their parent's lap during examination.

Enlarged or abnormal areas discovered during the physical examination are recorded in concise, descriptive, and quantitative terms whenever possible. For example, "shotty" or "pea-sized" lymph nodes may have entirely different meanings to different examiners, whereas "1.5 cm × 1 cm" can mean only one size. Likewise, organ span, testicular size, abdominal girth, lymphadenopathy and tumors, if present, are measured and their actual dimensions recorded.

After the initial history and physical examination the health care provider orders a battery of tests to aid in confirming the diagnosis of a malignancy. These tests help define the source and the extent of the tumor and its effect on other organ systems in the body. The required tests fall into three broad categories: (1) blood or laboratory work; (2) imaging studies; and (3) direct examination of tumor for pathologic confirmation of diagnosis.

The nurse expedites the child's initial diagnostic phase by knowing and assuring that the proper preparative regimens are maintained. Educate the family to understand why nothing by mouth (NPO) status is necessary before some scans, and make sure that meals are not inadvertently delivered at those times. Facilitate the sequencing of various tests, making sure that certain preparative procedures do not conflict with each other and that enough time is allowed to travel physically from one department to another. Timely scheduling of tests and scans can also permit a more judicious use of sedatives for the young child.

Parents may become frustrated by the length of time needed to establish the diagnosis, frustration that can be exacerbated further by the unavailability of some scans and laboratory tests over the weekends. Often parents had their child in for examination and blood work for weeks or even longer before the initial hospitalization. Most parents are anxious for a definitive diagnosis and the start of treatment. The nurse helps the family by emphasizing the vital importance of making an accurate diagnosis and fully defining the extent and histology of the malignancy. The nurse who can sit patiently with the family, acknowledge their frustration, and provide information and support will do much to help them through a very anxious, difficult time.

BLOOD WORK AND LABORATORY STUDIES

In most medical centers the child routinely has a complete blood count (CBC), serum blood chemistries, and urinalysis at the time of admission. Depending on the location of the tumor, additional blood and urine studies are required.

Complete Blood Count

The CBC measures the formed elements that are suspended in plasma: erythrocytes (RBCs), leukocytes (WBCs), and platelets. Hemoglobin (main physiologic component of RBCs) and hematocrit (percentage of RBCs per volume of whole blood) levels are also included. In addition, RBC indices provide both qualitative and quantitative information about erythrocytes. The RBC indices reflect the size, weight, and hemoglobin content of an individual RBC. They consist of mean corpuscular volume (MCV), mean corpuscular hemoglobin concentration (MCHC), and mean corpuscular hemoglobin (MCH). MCV is the average or mean volume of each RBC. MCH is a measure of the weight of hemoglobin in each RBC, and MCHC is the average amount of hemoglobin in each RBC but expressed as a percentage of the volume of the RBC.

Determining the WBC differential is standard for the hematology-oncology patient. The differential identifies the relative proportions of the different WBCs that comprise the total white count. Five types of WBCs normally are present in blood: lymphocytes, monocytes, eosinophils, basophils, and neutrophils. There are two types of neutrophils: segmented neutrophils, referred to as *segs* or *polys*, and banded neutrophils, commonly called *bands* or *stabs*. To determine exactly what percentage of each type of WBC is present, 100 WBCs are counted, and each cell is identified individually. The total of each type is reported as a percentage of the total number of WBCs.

A normal CBC does not guarantee that the bone marrow is free of tumor. Children with leukemia invariably have some degree of abnormality of the CBC at diagnosis. Typically the normal bone marrow is replaced by malignant cells. However, a child with a solid tumor may also have malignant cells present in the bone marrow but in significantly less numbers and have no alteration of the hemogram.

Serum Chemistry

Biochemical evaluation of the blood serum is a routine screening procedure performed on admission. The biochemical studies of the child suspected of having cancer will measure and reflect ongoing metabolic processes and the status of specific organs.[4] Most hospitals have panels or combinations of serum chemistry tests that allow multiple assays from a single blood sample. These panels typically include "routine" electrolytes (sodium, potassium, chloride, carbon dioxide) and tests that measure renal function (blood urea nitrogen, creatinine) and liver function (serum aspartate aminotransferase [SGOT or AST], serum alanine aminotransferase [SGPT or ALT], bilirubin). Some panels may measure various proteins (total protein, albumin), enzymes (amylase, lipase), and additional electrolytes (calcium, phosphorus, and magnesium).

Serum lactate dehydrogenase (LDH) is typically part of the panel. LDH is a cellular enzyme that contributes to carbohydrate metabolism. Specifically it catalyzes the conversion of lactic acid to pyruvic acid within cells. It is present in many cells of the body, including the liver, heart, kidney, and skeletal muscles. LDH often is elevated at the time of diagnosis in children with several types of malignancies, particularly lymphomas, leukemias, and bone tumors. LDH may be elevated for reasons other than malignancy; thus it cannot be considered a specific tumor marker. However, levels are obtained at diagnosis, and elevations that recur after remission is induced may be significant.[20]

Alkaline phosphatase is an isoenzyme associated with bone, liver, and gastrointestinal (GI) metabolism. Levels are increased when cells such as osteoblasts, the cells that make bone, are active. Children with bone tumors usually have very high levels of this enzyme. However, healthy bone growth in children also causes elevated values.[7]

Uric acid is routinely measured at diagnosis. It is a by-product of cell destruction and is released as cells lyse. Malignant cells, particularly in children with leukemia and non-Hodgkin's lymphoma, have a rapid doubling time and turnover rate. Consequently, uric acid levels may be elevated at diagnosis in these children. Uric acid levels are monitored closely in children with cancer after therapy has begun because levels often rise as the malignant cells are killed in response to chemotherapy, enhancing the possibility of tumor lysis syndrome.

Urinalysis

A urinalysis is obtained routinely on most children as a general screening test. The kidneys provide a semipermeable membrane that reabsorbs some substances from plasma and excretes others via urine. Urinalysis results reflect plasma homeostasis in a normally functioning kidney, or they may indicate pathology directly related to the genitourinary tract. The microscopic urinalysis measures the presence of WBCs, RBCs, casts, and epithelial cells. The macroscopic examination measures specific gravity, pH, protein, glucose, and ketones. Children with renal or bladder tumors occasionally have hematuria as an initial presenting sign.[10]

Tumor Markers

Tumor-associated substances or tumor markers detected in body tissues, blood, urine, or cerebrospinal fluid (CSF) would ideally enable the clinician to screen patients for neoplastic development.[37] Markers would also enable the physician to stage patients with a malignant disease more effectively. The concentration of tumor marker could allow for detection of minimal residual disease or early recurrence.[11] Unfortunately, in the pediatric population the technology required to achieve these objectives is just beginning to develop, and there are few reliable tumor markers. The best-documented and most sensitive are those associated with neuroblastoma, hepatoblastoma, and germ cell tumors.

Occasionally large abdominal tumors are difficult to categorize preoperatively, even with sensitive scans. Tumor markers can help differentiate neuroblastoma, Wilms' tumor, or hepatoblastoma. They often clarify the diagnosis, and their presence becomes an important component for follow-up of therapy. Elevated marker values may also have a role in determining prognosis. Elevated levels of serum ferritin and neuron-specific enolase (NSE), a neuronal glycolytic enzyme, occur frequently with neuroblastoma. Abnormal levels of alpha-fetoprotein (AFP) and β-human chorionic gonadotropin (β-hCG), both normally occurring only in fetal cells, are often found in patients with liver tumors. AFP and β-hCG are also elevated in germ cell tumors of both gonadal and central nervous system (CNS) origin.

Urine collection for catecholamine measurement is obtained if the child has an abdominal tumor. This may be one aliquot of urine, but more often a 24-hour collection is requested. Vanillylmandelic acid (VMA), the main metabolite of epinephrine and norepinephrine, and homovanillic acid (HVA), the main metabolite of dopamine, metanephrine, and normetanephrine, are the catecholamines secreted by the adrenal medulla and sympathetic nervous tissue. Seventy percent to 95% of patients with neuroblastoma have elevated catecholamine levels at diagnosis either because of overproduction by individual cells or because of rapid release caused by defective storage within tumor cells.[18] In fact, elevations of these levels in the urine are so pathognomonic for neuroblastoma that, combined with a positive bone marrow test result, the diagnosis of neuroblastoma is confirmed on that basis, precluding the need for a surgical biopsy.

Timed urine collections pose particular difficulties for the pediatric population, especially the young patient. Babies and children still in diapers or with only daytime bladder control usually require an indwelling catheter to obtain acceptable collections. Older children need frequent reminders to save all urine and to use only one commode

or urinal during the collection period. The stress and anxiety of hospitalization, combined with intravenous hydration, may cause enuresis in previously toilet-trained children. Diurnal variations occur in the excretion of catecholamines, and the loss of even one aliquot of urine may be crucial.[22] The physician should be notified if urine loss occurs so he or she can decide whether to restart the 24-hour period or continue with the present collection. The container for urinary catecholamine studies contains concentrated hydrochloric acid to maintain a pH of 2 to 3 throughout the collection period. Boys should be instructed not to urinate directly into the jug.

Serum copper, a trace mineral found in plasma, may be elevated in patients with Hodgkin's disease. Carcinoembryonic antigen (CEA), normally produced during rapid multiplication of epithelial cells, may be elevated with a number of malignancies, including retinoblastoma, neuroblastoma, and germ cell tumors.

Polyamines, specifically putrescine and spermine, are small molecules involved in nucleic acid metabolism and thus in cellular proliferation.[28] They may be elevated in the spinal fluid and serum of patients with brain tumors, most notably in children with medulloblastoma. Elevations of polyamines have predicted tumor regrowth several weeks in advance of cytology or radiologic scans.[13]

During the initial workup numerous other blood and laboratory tests may be ordered. It is crucial to evaluate organ systems other than those of tumor origin for any dysfunction caused by the disease and to evaluate specific baseline organ function before the initiation of therapy. The natural history of the cancer and its known pattern of spread influence the selection of tests. Table 3–1 lists normal ranges of various tumor-associated markers.

Every attempt should be made to coordinate all aspects of the child's care and obtain all blood specimens from a single venipuncture. The child should have no more than one or two venipunctures per day during acute phases of illness, with decreasing frequency as the child's condition improves. The nurse serves as the child's advocate, coordinating tests and intervening if excessive invasive procedures are requested.

TABLE 3–1. *Tumor-Associated Laboratory Studies*

LABORATORY TEST	NORMAL RANGE	ASSOCIATED MALIGNANCIES
Alpha-fetoprotein (AFP)	<20 ng/ml	↑ Hepatomas ↑ Germ cell tumors (teratocarcinomas) ↑ Retinoblastoma
Alkaline phosphatase	20–150 U/L	Nonspecific elevations can occur in normal settings ↑ Bone tumors
β-Human chorionic gonadotro-pin (β-hCG)	5 mIu/ml	↑ Hepatoblastoma ↑ Germ cell tumors
Carcinoembryonic antigen (CEA)	2.5 ng/ml	↑ Gastrointestinal cancers
Catecholamines (urine):		↑ Neuroblastoma (elevations may occur in one or all)
Epinephrine	0–5 µg/24 hr	
Norepinephrine	0–20 µg/24 hr	
Metanephrine	0–300 µg/24 hr	
Normetanephrine	50–800 µg/24 hr	
Vanillylmandelic acid (VMA)	2–10 mg/24 hr	
Homovanillic acid (HVA)	0–10 mg/24 hr	
Copper	80–160 µg/dl	↑ Hodgkin's disease
Ferritin	7–150 µg/L	↑ Neuroblastoma
Lactate dehydrogenase (LDH)	60–170 U/L	Nonspecific ↑ Non-Hodgkin's lymphomas ↑ Acute lymphocytic leukemia (ALL), osteo-sarcoma, neuroblastoma ↑ Germ cell tumors, Ewing's sarcoma
Neuron-specific enolase (NSE)	15 ng/ml	↑ Neuroblastoma
Polyamines	58–278 pmol/nol	↑ Medulloblastoma

Data from references 19 and 27.

The child with cancer will be subjected to hundreds of blood tests during the course of therapy. The routine placement of a venous access device for most newly diagnosed patients eliminates much of the pain and trauma involved with repeated venipuncture. However, before its insertion or for those children without a catheter, venipuncture is frequently required. Everyone *must* be honest and open with the child from the beginning. Venipunctures are performed in the treatment room, which makes the child's bed and room a "safe place." The parents are allowed to stay with the child, if they wish, to provide support. At least initially, consider placing the child on the examination table with his or her arm or hand firmly held in place by someone other than the parents before performing veni-puncture. It may be advisable to allow the child to sit up for the procedure once it has been determined that he or she can truly hold still. A second person is mandatory for maintaining proper positioning of the arm or hand, even with older children. Simple age-appropriate explanations for the blood work are given, reminding the child that the venipuncture is not a consequence of or punishment for his or her behavior. Praise is given once the "poke" is over, and a small reward in the form of a special bandage, sticker, or small toy may be given.

DIAGNOSTIC IMAGING STUDIES

Diagnostic imaging helps define and delineate the primary tumor and examine regional and distant sites for spread from the organ of origin. These studies are also crucial for follow-up to determine response to therapy. Once again, tests are ordered in a logical sequence, with the biology and known metastatic pattern of the suspected disease in mind. Imagining falls into four general categories: (1) radiologic studies, (2) magnetic resonance studies, (3) nuclear medicine studies, and (4) ultrasonography.

Radiologic Studies

Initial radiology studies include x-ray examinations, which use small amounts of x-radiation to visualize organs and structures within the body. The four densities in the human body (air, water, fat, and bone) absorb radiation in varying degrees. Air has the least density, causing dark images on film, and bone has the highest density, resulting in light images.[15] The varying degrees of radiation absorption cause darker or lighter structures to appear on the film.

A chest x-ray study is obtained on every patient, either as a baseline or for diagnosis. X-ray studies are ordered as *anteroposterior* (A-P), indicating that the beam will be directed from the patient's front to back; *lateral*, indicating side-to-side beam direction, and/or *decubitus*, indicating the films are obtained while the patient is lying down. X-ray studies of affected areas may also be ordered (e.g., leg studies if the child has a limp). These x-ray studies or "plain films" of specific areas are usually used for screening purposes and are followed by more extensive tests if indicated.

A skeletal survey is a collection of plain x-ray films of the entire skeletal system. This study is useful in detecting bony lesions in diseases that metastasize to the bone. Further corroborating studies may be ordered if the skeletal survey results are positive.

No pain is involved in obtaining x-ray films. However, the child must hold very still, and parents are not routinely allowed in the room. The nurse helps minimize radiation exposure through patient education. Even young children understand the basic concept of a camera, film, and the taking of a picture. Simple statements explaining the x-ray cam-era takes a picture of "your insides" may help a child cooperate. Reassurance that parents are waiting outside the door (e.g., in the hall) will also provide comfort. Very young children and babies may require assistance with positioning and restraints.[17] This should be explained in a simple factual manner and never implied as a punishment for noncompliance. Restraints and straps must be applied gently with respect and consideration for the child.

Computerized Tomography. In children with a known or suspected solid tumor, extensive computerized tomography (CT) scans will be obtained. CT was developed in 1972 and has greatly diminished the need for many previously routine scans and tests. CT scan may also be referred to as *computerized axial tomography (CAT)* scan. The terms are interchangeable.

The conventional x-ray image is formed by the casting of shadows of internal structures when a large x-ray beam is projected through the area. In contrast, the CT image is formed in a two-step process. In the first step the CT scanner produces a narrow x-ray beam, which examines only one layer or slice of the body. As previously stated, this x-ray beam is absorbed differently by body structures of different densities. Receptors, which are located directly across from the x-ray beam source, detect the number of x-rays remaining after the beams have passed through the body. This information is relayed to a computer and stored there. The x-ray beam source rotates 360 degrees around the body. Thousands of readings are taken by the receptors and are recorded in the computer. The computer analyzes the receptor's readings and calculations at thousands of different points. In the second step the calculations are converted into an image on a videoscreen, which may be photographed or stored on videotape.[33]

Radioiodinated contrast material highlights blood vessels and can be used to enhance the image of particular organs.[17] Intravenous (IV) contrast is often used during brain CT scans if a tumor is present or suspected. The IV contrast may cause a temporary flush and a sensation of warmth, waves of nausea, and a metallic or bitter taste. The

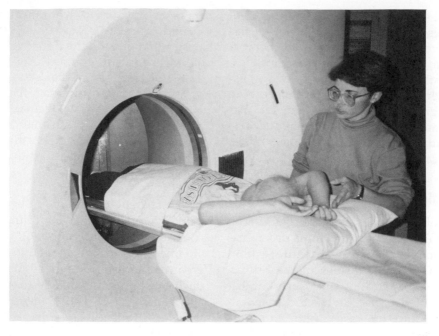

FIGURE 3–2. Technician positioning child for abdominal CT scan.

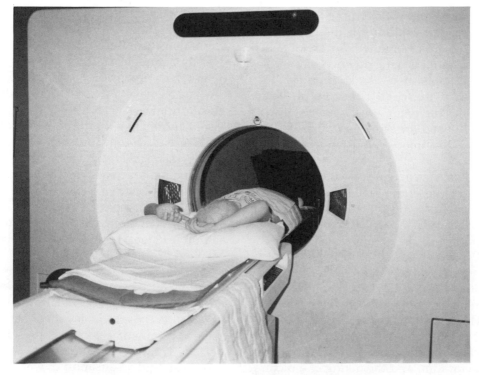

FIGURE 3–3. Child in place for a chest CT scan.

duration of these symptoms is usually only 1 to 3 minutes, but they can be very frightening. The child should be told of this possibility before the scan and again just before the injection. Most radiology departments prefer that the child is NPO for 3 to 6 hours before the test to decrease the risk of aspiration should vomiting occur. IV contrast can be safely administered through permanent right atrial catheters, including implanted venous ports.

CT scanning of the abdomen and pelvis is enhanced by oral contrast material. The family should be instructed in the proper mixing and administration of the oral contrast medium if the child is an outpatient. For the medium to work effectively, the child must drink the entire volume within 45 to 60 minutes. The parents may mix the material in a palatable drink such as fruit juice, Hawaiian Punch, or 7-Up. Several varieties of oral contrast are available. Specific instructions vary slightly with each brand. Most brands, however, require oral ingestion 10 to 12 hours before the scan and again 2 hours before the scan to allow peristalsis to move the contrast material to all aspects of the GI tract. The volume of contrast depends on the child's age. Most children can be coaxed into drinking the contrast orally; however, some children refuse to drink the solution or may vomit the entire volume shortly after ingestion. In these cases the oral contrast should be administered through a nasogastric tube.

The child undergoing a CT scan must remain very still for approximately 30 to 90 minutes, the typical duration of the scan. In addition, IV access is usually required in the event that the radiologist believes IV contrast is indicated. Very young children typically require some form of sedation. Most children respond well to chloral hydrate (50 to 100 mg/kg administered by mouth 20 to 30 minutes before the scan).[6] Chloral hydrate is also available in rectal suppository form. In general, rectal medications are not used for the pediatric oncology patient because of the potential to cause trauma or infection in the rectal mucosa; however, chloral hydrate can be judiciously administered per rectum to patients who require sedation and cannot or will not swallow the drug. Most newly diagnosed pa-

tients with solid tumors do not have compromised bone marrow function. The nurse should ascertain, however, that the child is neither thrombocytopenic nor neutropenic before administering the drug by this route. If either condition is present, the nurse alerts the physician and recommends another drug. For the occasional child who does not respond to chloral hydrate, stronger sedation is needed. Most pediatric radiology departments have protocols in place for pharmacologic sedation of children. Nurses should become familiar with their own institution's preferences. Care must be taken not to overmedicate the child and depress respiration. A heavily sedated child is monitored by a nurse or physician throughout the entire length of the scan.[1]

Older children can cooperate quite satisfactorily during the CT scan if they have been adequately prepared ahead of time. The nurse can show the child pictures of the CT scanner and explain positions expected during the scan. Children should practice holding their breath because this is sometimes required during the scan. Reassure the child that the loud noises the machine makes will not hurt in any way. Let the child know where his or her parents will be waiting during the scan. It is helpful if parents are on hand immediately after the completion of the study to praise and hug their child.

Intravenous Pyelogram. In the past intravenous pyelogram (IVP) was routinely used in the evaluation of a child with an abdominal mass. Today its use as a diagnostic tool has largely been supplanted by CT scans. During an IVP a radiopaque dye is injected intravenously, and during its elimination through the kidney via glomerular filtration, normal renal tissue is opacified. Cysts, tumors, and other tissue defects remain free of contrast. Obtaining satisfactory IVP results requires that all intestinal contents be evacuated before the examination because the kidneys are located behind the intestines. Laxatives or bisacodyl suppositories are administered the night before and the morning of the test.

As stated previously, an IVP is rarely obtained for primary evaluation of an abdominal mass. However, if the tumor probably is of renal origin (e.g., Wilms' tumor), an IVP is obtained in addition to the CT scan to delineate the tumor further before surgery. An IVP also can assess the function of the remaining kidney after nephrectomy and therapy for Wilms' tumor.[29]

Gastrointestinal Tract Studies. The entire GI tract can be visualized by using barium sulfate as the contrast material and fluoroscopy. Barium studies ("upper and lower GI") may be ordered when neoplastic involvement of the GI tract is suspected. These studies, however, like the IVP, largely have been replaced by CT scans.

Preparation for an upper GI tract evaluation (upper GI series) requires that the child receive nothing by mouth after midnight before the test. This fasting state continues until the child receives the oral barium suspension. The esophagus, stomach, and small intestine are then visualized under direct fluoroscopic examination. Fluoroscopy enables continuous visualization on a monitor of the movement of body parts. A blockage or abnormality becomes evident as the barium travels through the GI tract. A disturbance in flow often points to the location of an early anatomic change.

Nursing intervention can facilitate this procedure. Upper GI tract procedures customarily are performed early in the morning. Nursing staff members, however, must assess the child's hydration and obtain orders for appropriate IV support. During fluoroscopy x-ray films are taken for permanent records. The procedure may last from 30 minutes to 3 hours, depending on the speed of peristalsis. The child must remain fasting until the last film is taken. A follow-up film customarily is taken 24 hours later. Parents and child are informed that the child's bowel movements will be chalky for the next few days as the barium travels through the GI tract. A laxative is usually prescribed to eliminate the barium.

A barium enema (lower GI series) requires careful preparation for adequate visualization of organ contour and motility. For 2 days before the examination the child receives a low-residue diet. A clear liquid diet is required the day before examination. No milk or dairy products are given without prior arrange-

ments with the radiologist. After the evening meal on the day before the examination, a cathartic such as mineral oil or bisacodyl or a rectal suppository is administered. On the day of the examination children may receive clear liquids until 3 hours before the examination, and cleansing enemas are administered until clear results are obtained. Children are informed that no pajama bottoms or undergarments may be worn during the procedure because of the necessity to instill and expel the barium.

Lymphangiogram. A lymphangiogram (LAG) permits direct radiologic visualization of the lymphatic system. This is achieved by introducing radiopaque contrast material into a lymph vessel. Since the lymphatics are not palpable, an intradermal injection of a blue dye is given into the first interdigital space of each foot. The dye is taken up by the lymphatic vessels, allowing their visualization. X-ray films are taken of the chest and abdomen, visualizing the lymphatic tissue and lymph nodes in the field. The contrast dye remains in the lymph system for 6 months or longer, thus allowing long-term evaluation of disease progression.

LAG was routinely obtained for suspected diagnosis of Hodgkin's disease and non-Hodgkin's lymphoma in the past. Its use today remains somewhat controversial, and many centers forego LAG in favor of CT scans. The cannulation procedure is technically difficult, invasive, and painful. Heavy sedation is usually required for young children. It is, however, the only imaging procedure that allows thorough evaluation of intrinsic lymph node architecture. CT can identify nodes that are even minimally enlarged; however, LAG gives more information about lymph node architecture and has the potential to differentiate nodes enlarged because of tumor from nodes enlarged for benign reasons.[29]

The parents and child must be informed that the dorsal surface of the child's feet will be swollen and stained blue after the test. Patients may be unable to wear their usual shoes for several days because of the swelling. The cannula insertion is closed with a single stitch or Steri-strips skin closures. Generally a small-bandage dressing is placed over the site. Urine may contain the blue dye for several days after the test. The feet retain diminishing amounts of the blue color for a week or less.

Myelogram. Myelograms allow fluoroscopic and radiologic examination of the spinal canal. They are used to detect obstruction and tumors within the spinal canal and to detect spinal nerve root injury and arachnoiditis.[15] During the myelogram a lumbar puncture is performed, and a radiopaque contrast agent is instilled into the spinal canal. The child is strapped to the examination table in several places. After the injection of the dye the table is tilted until the entire canal or problem area can be visualized. Care is taken to prevent the dye from entering the cranial space. Most often a water-soluble dye (e.g., mitrizamide) is used.

Children are generally heavily sedated for a myelogram. Often general anesthesia is used. The child must be NPO for 4 to 8 hours (depending on age) before the test. Some hospitals require inpatient overnight admission after completion of the study. Others discharge patients after several hours of observation. Vital signs are monitored frequently to check for hemodynamic changes. The head of the bed is elevated to prevent meningeal irritation from the dye. Infrequently, the contrast material can precipitate seizures because of the meningeal irritation; thus phenytoin (Dilantin) may be ordered prophylactically before the scan.

Magnetic Resonance Imaging

The use of magnetic resonance imaging (MRI) has expanded greatly over the last several years. MRI has become the scan of choice for certain malignancies, most notably brainstem tumors and bone tumors. MRI scans use strong, steady magnetic fields created by a large round magnet. Under normal conditions the protons inside the atoms that comprise the human body spin in random directions. The magnetic field causes the protons to align and spin in the same direction. Throughout the scan a radio-frequency signal is intermittently beamed into the magnetic field, causing the protons to move out of alignment. When the signal is stopped, the protons move back to their aligned positions and release energy. A receiver coil measures the energy released by the disturbed protons and the time it takes for the protons to return to the aligned positions. These measurements provide information about the type of tissue in which the protons lie and its condition. A computer then uses this information to create an image on a television monitor. This image can be recorded on film or magnetic tape to retain a permanent copy.[5]

The MRI scan lasts approximately 60 minutes, and for most of that time the child must lie very still. Children who cannot do so or who may become frightened by the loud noises made by the machine or become claustrophobic because of the close quarters are sedated before the scan. Because no x-rays are used during the scan, many MRI departments allow a parent to stay with the child during the entire procedure. There have been no short-term deleterious effects of magnetic field exposure described, but long-term side effects are as yet unknown.

The strong magnetic field precludes entry to persons who have any implanted metallic objects in their body.[9] These objects may include orthodontic braces, metal (dental) bridgework, surgical plates or clips, implanted orthopedic rods, and certain implanted venous ports.[3] Jewelry and other metallic objects must be removed. In addition, IV poles, infusion controllers, and cardiac monitors are not permitted in the MRI suite. Personnel working in MRI are familiar with the restrictions and can help the nurse adapt the patient's equipment appropriately.

MRI pictures are extremely precise, and often as much information can be obtained from MRI as from direct visualization of the tissue. MRI can target specific atoms, so it "sees" right through bone and clearly defines soft tissue.

Gadolinium IV contrast media is used as an enhancing agent during MRI at the discretion of the radiologist. When assessing the spinal canal for metastatic brain tumors or paraspinal masses, gadolinium is usually used.

MRI may not be a suitable test for all pa-

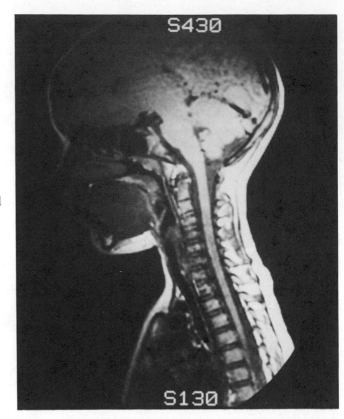

FIGURE 3–4. Sagittal view of cervical and thoracic spinal cord.

tients. Scanning time is slow, and patient movement affects scan quality. Most monitoring and ventilatory support equipment cannot be brought into the MRI suite. Patients who are having their upper body scanned must be enclosed deep within the machine and are difficult to see or evaluate during the scan. Hence an unstable patient may not be a good candidate for MRI. Additionally, because of the magnetic fields generated during the scan, MRI suites are usually isolated at an imposing distance from patient care areas, which further decreases accessibility.

Lastly, MRI is costly, generally 25% to 30% higher than CT scanning.[2] Third-party payers are demanding increasing accountability for hospital costs and may insist that less costly imaging studies are adequate for good patient care.

Nuclear Medicine Scans

Nuclear medicine scans use radioactive material, isotopes, for diagnostic and therapeutic purposes. Various radioisotopes or radionu-

clides such as technetium, xenon, and iodine can be used for nuclear medicine scans. A mandatory precaution before all nuclear medicine procedures, as is the case with x-ray studies and CT scans, is to assure that the patient is not pregnant since even small amounts of radioactivity or radiation can damage the fetus.

The radionuclide or radiopharmaceutical selected is used as a simple salt compound or is chemically bound to another element. Once the radiopharmaceutical enters the body, it functions like the chemical the organ normally metabolizes so that the organ tissue "takes up" the radionuclide. For example, radioactive iodine concentrates in the thyroid just as stable iodine does. Radionuclides delineate cancer in one of two ways: (1) the tumor concentrates the radionuclide from the rest of the organ in a "hot" spot; or (2) the rest of the organ concentrates the radionuclide, and the tumor shows up as a "cold" spot.

The gamma scintillation camera is the most common imaging device. The camera

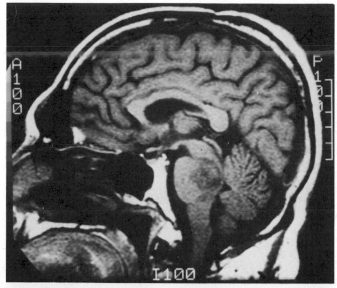

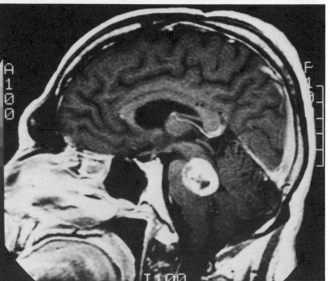

FIGURE 3–5.   MRI scan, **A,** without and, **B,** with gadolinium enhancement of patient with a brain stem glioma.

detects, not unlike a Geiger counter, the gamma rays emitted after the IV administration of radionuclide and projects the image on a screen. The results are transferred to x-ray film.[36] Timing of the scan after administration of the radionuclide is dependent on its uptake in the targeted organ.

Various organs can be studied by means of nuclear medicine scans. Bone scans are the most commonly ordered nuclear medicine study in pediatric oncology. Thyroid scans are used to detect masses or tumors in the thyroid gland; however, this is a rare site of pediatric cancer. Kidney, liver or spleen, and brain

scans are no longer routinely obtained because these organs can be more easily and better assessed by CT scan or MRI scan. Gallium scans were standard for metastatic workup for lymphoma patients in the past. Generally replaced by CT scan for malignancy detection, gallium scans are still used to detect occult infections and inflammation. Gallium is particularly useful in detecting pelvic and abdominal abscesses. Metaiodobenzylguanidine (MIBG), radio-labeled monoclonals, positron emission tomography (PET), and single photon emission computed tomography (SPECT) scans are new and exciting applications of nuclear medicine and are described in further detail.

Bone Scan.   Technetium 99m (TC 99m)–labeled compounds, the radio-pharmaceuticals used for bone scan, have a relatively low radiation exposure.[17] The uptake of bone-seeking agents by the skeleton is nearly complete within 30 minutes after the IV injection. In practice, images are generally obtained after a 2- to 4-hour delay to permit additional renal clearance of the radiopharmaceutical from extracellular fluid.

The bone scan is a highly sensitive method for detecting malignant lesions. However, increased focal accumulation of tracer elements may indicate a number of abnormalities in addition to malignant lesions. Bone scanning is based on the uptake of a nuclide by the crystal lattice of bone. The degree of nuclide uptake by a particular bone is related to bone blood flow. Primary skeletal disease (e.g., osteosarcoma), secondary skeletal disease (e.g., metastases), inflammatory bone disease (e.g., osteomyelitis), and bone trauma are all associated with increased bone blood flow. Therefore the existence of any of these disease processes will be seen on a bone scan as increased nuclide uptake.[17] Because of the non-

specificity of the bone scan, scan results are correlated with clinical findings and conventional radiographs such as a skeletal survey. The actual scan takes 30 to 60 minutes. No pain is involved with the scanning procedures, but the child must lie still during the procedure. Sedatives such as chloral hydrate are often used for young children.

Tc 99m is completely excreted by the kidneys in 24 hours or less. The dose of radiation from radionuclide imaging is usually less than the amount of radiation received from diagnostic x-ray studies.[15] The injected radionuclide should not affect parents or hospital staff.

MIBG   Scans.   I-metaiodobenzylguanidine (MIBG) is a specific radioisotope marker that was synthesized for the detection of pheochromocytoma, a benign vascular tumor of the adrenal gland. MIBG is taken up and stored in tissues in a manner similar to that for norepinephrine; thus it accumulates in adrenergic tissues. MIBG is extremely useful in the diagnosis and follow-up of neuroblastoma, a tumor of the sympathetic nervous system.[16] MIBG apparently is superior to bone scan in detecting metastatic neuroblastoma.[29,31] In clinical practice the two nuclear

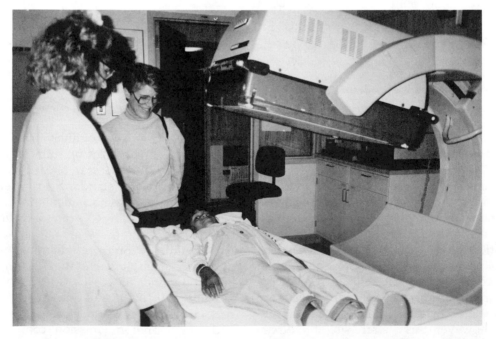

FIGURE 3–6.   Child in proper position to begin bone scan.

studies are often used in a corroborative fashion. As previously stated, bone scan uptake occurs in areas with any bone activity, including bone growth. Bone scans may continue to read an area as positive with malignancy when in fact the lesions have responded to therapy and active bone repair is occurring. MIBG, on the other hand, is picked up only by active tumor; therefore an area of bone regrowth would not take up the radioisotope. The major disadvantage of MIBG is that a small but significant percentage of biopsy-proven neuroblastomas do not take up MIBG.

The MIBG study requires imaging on 3 consecutive days after the tracer dose is given. After injection of MIBG on day 1 the patient is seen 24, 48, and 72 hours later for imaging. Drugs such as hydroxyzine (Vistaril), phenothiazines, and sympathomimetics (e.g., pseudoephedrine [Sudafed]), block the uptake of norepinephrine and thus MIBG. They should be avoided for 4 to 6 weeks before the scan.

MIBG is bound to radioactive iodide and is taken up by the thyroid without adequate prophylaxis. Administration of saturated solution of potassium iodide (SSKI) drops or Lugol's solution (1 drop three times per day) must begin 1 day before the scan and continue for 6 days after the administration of MIBG. Parents must be aware of the need for strict compliance with SSKI administration and the potential for damage to the thyroid if radioactive iodine is absorbed.

As is true with most imaging studies, the child must hold very still during the nuclear medicine scans. Young children may require sedation. Older children should be informed about the scan and be allowed to see the machine before the test. The radioisotopes are usually injected through a small-gauge butterfly needle. Some institutions may not permit the use of permanent right atrial catheters for radioisotope injection because of the radioisotope's propensity to adhere to the catheter lining and thus obscure the image in the area of the catheter.

Positron Emission Tomography. PET is one of the newer scans added to the nuclear medicine arsenal. PET scan combines conventional nuclear medicine techniques with transaxial tomography (e.g., CT scans) and adds double photon imaging (produced by the radiopharmaceutical), which images metabolic activity.[36] Substances normally used by the body such as glucose, water, or fatty acids are made radioactive and administered intravenously before the PET scan. The most commonly used PET radiopharmaceutical is fluorine 18 (F-18-FDG), a labeled glucose analogue. It is one of the few known molecules with the ability to pass through the normal blood-brain barrier.[34] Glucose is the only source of energy used by brain cells. By measuring the location and quantity of F-18-FDG, detailed information about the biochemical activity within cells and precise organ function can be determined. Brain metabolism is a reliable indicator of brain tissue viability and helps determine the degree of malignancy present. PET scan can also help distinguish recurrent or residual (i.e, active) tumor from necrotic tissues in the tumor area. To date, PET is used mainly for evaluation of brain and cardiac function. The positron-emitting radioisotopes used in PET typically have a very short half-life; thus local production of the radioisotopes in an in-house or regional cyclotron is required. Use of PET scanners thus most likely will be limited to major centers with a cyclotron available. Use in the pediatric population is limited in 1993, but the next decade will no doubt bring clinical applications of PET to the pediatric brain tumor population.

Single Photon Emission Computed Tomography. SPECT is likewise a new computer-aided nuclear medicine scan similar in concept to PET scan. The SPECT scan technology combines the technique of conventional nuclear medicine imaging with that of CT. Rather than using x-rays as in CT, the SPECT relies on gamma-emitting radioactive isotopes. Unlike PET scan, conventional isotopes such as technetium 99m and iodine 131 are used, greatly reducing its cost and increasing the scan's accessibility. The image produced in SPECT is not merely in one plane; instead the gamma camera rotates 360 degrees around the patient, just as the PET scanner does. Therefore the targeted organ is reconstructed and displayed in axial, para-sagittal, and coronal sections.[24] SPECT scan looks at only one photon (or gamma ray) instead of the double photons generated in PET and provides approximately half the information that a PET scan provides. The SPECT process is analogous to drawing the floor plan of a house by looking through the windows of the house. The viewer is confined to the outside of the house, but by walking around the house and looking into each window, he or she can see the details of the house.[34]

Radiolabeled Monoclonal Antibodies. Monoclonal antibodies that bind to specific types of cancer cells have been produced since the mid-1970s. It is possible to tag these monoclonal antibodies with radionuclides. The injected radionuclide-monoclonal antibody will bind to cancer cells in areas of tumor involvement and be clearly detectable on scan.

Radiolabeled monoclonals also show promise for therapeutic use. Studies of bonded radionuclides have begun. These substances engage in high-linear energy transfers, enabling delivery of therapeutic doses of radiation to the targeted cancer cells, often without needlessly irradiating the surrounding normal tissues.[34]

Ultrasound

Ultrasound is a noninvasive procedure used to visualize body structures. The ultrasound probe is called a *transducer* and contains a crystal that vibrates when subjected to a small electric current. The vibrations produce sound waves. The transducer is held against the patient's skin, and the sound waves are intermittently transmitted to the tissues; this step is followed by periods of time during which the transducer listens for sound waves or echos reflected back from the body tissues. These waves are then recorded on film, videotape, oscilloscope, or recorder and read by the ultrasonographer. No radiation is involved.

An ultrasound is most often ordered as an initial screening test for the child with a palpable mass. It is a fast and relatively inexpensive test with no known potential side effects. The ultrasound beam cannot penetrate air, so its usefulness is limited in the lung or in the GI tract if it is filled with gas.

The parent should be allowed to stay with the child during the ultrasound examination. The child must hold still, but often a skilled technician, along with the parent's presence, can get even the younger child to cooperate. A jelly substance is applied to the skin to allow the transducer to move freely. Many children feel that the transducer "tickles" and may have a harder time holding still because of sensitive skin rather than fear. It is essential to keep excessive gas or air from the abdomen. When a baby cries, air is swallowed, and the ultrasound quality may suffer. Giving the baby a bottle with juice may help alleviate crying during the scan. Occasionally a full bladder is required to help differentiate various organs. Achieving this is very difficult for some children. Compliance may be improved with abundant verbal encouragement and praise, but the child is not scolded if he or she urinates before the scan.

Miscellaneous Studies

Several other tests or procedures are performed on the child with cancer once the diagnosis is suspected or confirmed but before initiating therapy. Baseline evaluations of certain organs are performed to ascertain normal function and as a means of evaluating drug toxicity during the course of therapy. For children with a solid tumor, it is not unusual for some of these tests to be ordered even before the definitive surgical procedure. There is often a strong suspicion of the tumor type, and using free time to evaluate normal organs during the metastatic workup allows therapy to begin promptly after surgical recovery. Additionally, tests that require the child's full cooperation and participation are best obtained before surgery when postoperative pain and discomfort will not interfere with performance.

A hearing evaluation is indicated before and during therapy with cisplatin. The older, cooperative child can be monitored with an audiogram, but the younger child, baby, or older child who is unable to cooperate will require brain stem auditory evoked response testing (BAER). Auditory neural activity is recorded as it passes from the peripheral or cochlear end organ through the brain stem to the cortex. Both acoustic nerve response and upper brain stem response are measured.[26]

Normal cardiac function should be documented before anthracycline use. This is most commonly done with an echocardiogram and an electrocardiogram (ECG). An echocardiogram examines the sizes, shape, and motion of cardiac structures with high frequency sound waves, and an ECG records the electric current generated by the heart. Some centers routinely perform a multiple gated acquisition (MUGA) scan, a nuclear medicine study that evaluates cardiac function. The MUGA scan is more precise in evaluating cardiac function but is also more expensive and time-consuming. A sample of blood is tagged with the radioactive isotope technetium (Tc 99m). A scintillation camera measures the radioactivity emitted by the isotope as it passes through the left ventricle. The percentage of isotope ejected during each heartbeat can then be calculated to determine the ejection fraction, a reliable measure of ventricular function. The choice of MUGA versus echocardiogram is generally up to individual institutions or physicians. However, the same study should be used consistently to monitor the child throughout therapy.

Pulmonary function tests are used to diagnose and quantify the degree of restrictive lung disease. They may be performed before, during, and after bleomycin therapy, which is known to cause severe restrictive lung disease. Pulmonary function tests require full cooperation of the patient. During the test the patient must inhale and exhale and hold his or her breath on demand. Pulmonary function tests therefore cannot be administered to young children, generally ones less than age 5 years, or to an uncooperative older child. Currently there is no reliable substitute for the pulmonary function tests in these children; however, transcutaneous oxygen saturation monitoring measures the oxygen tension (PO_2) of blood and provides general information about lung function. Table 3–2 lists the various diagnostic imaging studies used for specific tumors, which may vary among institutions and study groups.

PATHOLOGIC CONFIRMATION OF DIAGNOSIS

Once the entire metastatic workup is complete and laboratory and imaging studies indicate the likelihood of cancer, direct examination of the tumor is performed. The safest and most reliable method of obtaining tissue samples should be used.

Bone Marrow Aspiration and Biopsy

When a child presents with an abnormal CBC suggesting malignancy, an examination of the bone marrow is warranted. The bone marrow is a potential site of metastasis for many solid tumors as well. Under normal conditions an adequate specimen of bone marrow can be obtained through the aspiration method. Although various sites may be used to obtain a specimen of bone marrow, the most common sites in children are the anterior or posterior iliac crests. The tibia is sometimes used in infants. The spinous processes are used by some clinicians when both bone marrow aspiration and lumbar puncture must be performed. The patient is positioned for a lumbar puncture, and a local anesthetic is injected. The lumbar puncture is usually done first. The bone marrow aspiration is then performed in the spinous process through the same locally anesthetized site.

In the child marrow is easily and safely obtained from the pelvic bone from either the anterior or posterior iliac crest. The child should be permitted to climb onto the procedure table with minimal assistance and should be instructed to lie in a prone position if the posterior iliac crest is selected or supine if the anterior aspect of the bone will be used. If the child is chubby, a pillow or folded blanket can be placed under the abdomen to elevate the hips and facilitate access to the posterior site. Parents should be allowed to stay during the procedure if they wish. The supporting parent may sit on a stool adjacent to the child's head. In this position the parent is able to offer physical and verbal support by talking to the child and holding his or her hand.

In several published studies most parents report that they would like to stay with their

TABLE 3–2. *Diagnostic Imaging Studies for Various Malignancies*

DISEASE	PRIMARY TUMOR	METASTATIC SEARCH
Leukemia	Bone marrow aspirate and biopsy*	Spinal tap* Chest x-ray examination
Neuroblastoma	Computed tomography (CT) scan (abdomen, chest)	Bone marrow biopsy* Magnetic resonance imaging (MRI) for paraspinal lesion Bone scan Metaiodobenzylguanidine (MIBG) scan Skeletal survey Pelvic CT scan
Wilms' tumor	Abdominal CT scan	Chest x-ray examination Chest CT scan Intravenous pyelogram (IVP)† Head CT scan (unfavorable histology) Skeletal survey (unfavorable histology)
Non-Hodgkin's lymphoma	CT scan of primary tumor area (abdomen, chest, pelvis)	Bone marrow aspirate or biopsy and spinal tap* Chest x-ray examination Chest CT scan Bone scan Skeletal survey Gallium scan† Lymphangiogram† Head CT scan† (if clinically indicated)
Hodgkin's disease	CT scan of primary tumor area (chest, abdomen)	Chest x-ray examination Chest CT scan Bone marrow aspirate or biopsy* Lymphangiogram†
Rhabdomyosarcoma	Involved region or extremity CT scan	Chest x-ray examination Chest CT scan Abdominal CT scan Bone scan Head MRI or CT scan and spinal tap (for parameningeal tumors) Bone marrow aspirate or biopsy*

Bone tumors
  Osteosarcoma
  Ewing's sarcoma
	Extremity or involved bone MRI (preferred) or CT scan
	Bone x-ray examination
		Chest x-ray examination
		Bone scan
		Bone marrow aspirate or biopsy for Ewing's sarcoma*

Hepatoblastoma	Abdominal or pelvic CT scan	Chest x-ray examination Chest CT scan Liver-spleen scan† Hepatic angiography†
Germ cell tumors	Abdominal or pelvic CT scan	Chest x-ray examination Chest CT scan Bone scan Brain CT scan or MRI if clinically indicated
Brain tumors	Brain CT scan with or without enhancement or MRI Dependent on tumor location	Bone scan (medulloblastoma) MRI of spine with gadolinium if indicated or myelogram Spinal tap* Bone marrow aspirate or biopsy* (medulloblastoma) Chest x-ray examination

*Not an imaging study; included for completeness.
†Optional studies.

child during painful procedures, but many are unsure about their role and have received little communication from the hospital staff in this area.[21,39] The nurse should briefly inform the parents of the positive effects of their presence during painful procedures and, in effect, grant "permission" for the parent or parents to remain.

The parent, however, should not be placed in the position of having to restrain the child physically. Parents have very little experience in proper restraining techniques, and more importantly, to do so may cause considerable distress to both parent and child. Parents are not forced to stay during the procedure against their wishes, nor should they feel guilty about their decision to leave.

Many pediatric centers are using various forms of sedation or anesthesia for children undergoing bone marrow examination. Short-acting, quick-onset methods of achieving general anesthesia are widely available, and many cancer centers use the anesthesiology department to anesthetize the child during these procedures. Occasionally the care of a child with a solid tumor can be coordinated so that the marrow for completion of the metastatic workup is obtained while the child is in the operating room under general anesthesia for biopsy, debulking, or insertion of a central venous catheter. The judicious use of such timing spares the child the pain of the procedure and should not hamper or delay making the diagnosis. Coordination is required among the oncology, anesthesia, and surgery staffs.

Some centers rely on short-acting medications that produce sedation, relaxation, or an amnesic effect. Midazolam (Versed) has become increasingly popular because of its rapid onset, short duration, and potent sedative and amnesic effect. Profound slumber is rarely obtained with midazolam, however, and the child may still require personnel to assist and restrain him or her during the procedure. The child is monitored by nursing personnel; in addition, a pulse and oxygen saturation monitor is used during the short procedure and recovery period. Midazolam has no analgesic effect, so it is often used in combination with an opioid. Morphine sulfate, fentanyl (Sublimaze), or meperidine

(Demerol) has been used. The addition of one of these drugs can potentiate respiratory depression. Numerous studies have reported apnea as a frequent side effect, and respiratory arrest has been reported secondary to anoxia.[40] Newer studies, however, have documented the safety and effectiveness of midazolam, with or without opiate analgesia.[32] In 1990 the American Academy of Pediatrics Subcommittee on the Management of Pain in Childhood Cancer published age-specific recommendations and guidelines for managing pain associated with bone marrow and lumbar puncture.[42]

Many centers use local anesthesia with no systemic sedation. Non-pharmacologic methods of helping the child cope are used. Age-appropriate descriptions of the procedure before its use, guided imagery, and distraction can all enhance the child's coping skills. Older children need help to hold still, and young children may require firm restraint. Once again, the parent should be there to offer love and support but should not be expected to provide restraint. See Chapter 12 for an in-depth review of pain and pain management in children.

When the desired site for bone marrow aspiration is identified, the area is prepared with a povidone-iodine solution. Surface anesthetic is most commonly injected through a small-gauge needle and syringe or by means of a pressurized dispenser. The pressurized dispenser (often referred to as the "zinger" or "pop-gun" by children and staff alike) provides superficial surface anesthesia. Children may be reassured by the absence of a needle and the speed of injection and many object far less than with conventional methods. A deeper injection of anesthetic may be given once the skin is numb. If a biopsy is required, the anesthetic is delivered directly into the periosteum of the bone. In some pediatric centers topical anesthetics such as EMLA and ethyl chloride are used in place of injected agents.[14,38,41]

After anesthesia has been achieved, the aspiration needle with stylet in place is inserted through the cortex of the bone with a slight twisting motion. The stylet is then removed and a syringe is attached to the needle hub. Manual suction is applied until marrow appears in the syringe. If awake, the child will feel pain as the needle goes through the periosteum of the bone and a second sharp transient pain as the marrow is withdrawn into the syringe. Both pain sensations last only a few seconds. Many patients request that the nurse press firmly on the posterior aspect of both knees during aspiration. The firm pressure behind the knees reassures the patient that the correct position will be maintained and the needle will not be inadvertently dislodged.

When marrow appears in the syringe, the syringe is removed and the bone marrow expressed onto a glass slide. Bone marrow spicules will appear as whitish, granular particles throughout the bloody aspirate. Their presence indicates that the specimen is satisfactory. Bone marrow cell morphology is determined by examining the cells on the slide under a microscope. In addition, a child with newly diagnosed or suspected leukemia will require additional bone marrow samples for cytogenetic analysis, karyotype, and flow cytometry (immunophenotyping). Individual institutional studies may require additional specimens of the child's bone marrow.

The initial bone marrow aspirate on a newly diagnosed leukemic patient may be extremely difficult to withdraw because, in part, of the marrow's being very hypercellular and packed with leukemic cells. Often several sites and attempts are needed to obtain the proper specimens, and at times marrow can be obtained only through bone marrow biopsy. These diagnostic marrow specimens and marrow specimens obtained during periods of extreme hypocellularity may not contain the characteristic spicules. Although not ideal, these specimens still may be adequate for diagnosis.

Many oncologists require a bone marrow biopsy in which an actual core of bone and marrow are obtained in addition to aspiration, especially for evaluation of children with solid tumors. A Jamshidi biopsy needle is used for a bone marrow biopsy. The needle is manufactured in infant, pediatric, and adult sizes. The usual bone marrow sites are customarily used, but deeper local anesthesia is administered. A local anesthetic should be administered into tissue and bone periosteum in ad-

dition to the skin surface. While obtaining the specimen, the practitioner must grasp the needle firmly with both a rotating and rocking motion to cut a sliver of bone. The bone sliver remains in the core of the needle as it is removed from the patient. The biopsy material is ejected from the needle core with a metal probe and is placed on a glass slide for immediate examination or is placed in a tube containing formalin for later study. It is not uncommon for solid tumor protocols to require two separate sites for bone marrow aspiration and biopsy. Sampling marrow from more than one site helps lessen the chance of completely missing tumor clumps that may be few in number.

A pressure bandage customarily is applied at the site of a bone marrow aspiration or biopsy if the child's platelet count is 50,000 or less. If the platelet count is adequate, a simple adhesive bandage is the only dressing necessary. The child or parent is instructed to remove the original dressing no earlier than 8 hours and no later than 24 hours after the procedure. Leaving the bandage in place for longer periods predisposes the compromised child to infection. Many children are reluctant to have the dressing removed, especially the larger pressure bandage. In such a case the parent is advised to remove the bandage during the child's next bath because a wet bandage can be removed more easily.

Lumbar Puncture

Children with leukemia, lymphoma, parameningeal rhabdomyosarcoma, and medulloblastoma require a spinal tap or lumbar puncture as part of the diagnostic or staging workup.

Lumbar puncture is a sterile procedure that provides information about the pressure and dynamics of the CSF circulation and, more importantly, the composition of the fluid. The procedure is explained to the child and parents in advance. The importance of correct positioning *must be emphasized*. The nurse can demonstrate the improved access obtained with proper positioning by bending and permitting the child to palpate between the nurse's vertebrae. Before the procedure, the child is requested to void to ensure an

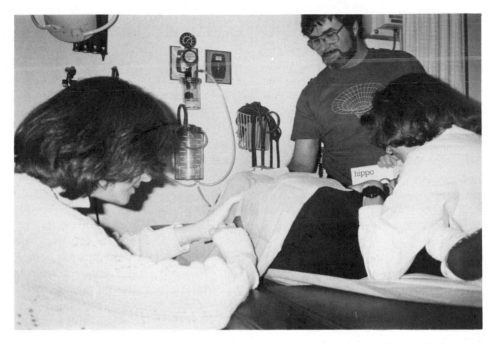

Figure 3–7. During a spinal tap both parent and nurse help comfort and distract a school-age child.

empty bladder. Parents are informed that they are welcome to accompany the child, observe the procedure, and assist and support the child.

During the procedure the child is positioned on the table with knees drawn up under the chin and head bent over the chest. This position arches the lumbar section of the back, offers maximal widening of the interspinous spaces, and provides easy entry into the subarachnoid space. A nurse usually assists the child to maintain this position by using locked hands to provide support behind the child's knees and neck. The child's back *must not rotate* forward or backward, for this can make access to the lumbar spaces very difficult. The entire back in its curved position should be completely perpendicular to the table. The assisting nurse constantly provides verbal reassurance and continuously assesses the child's status. Physical support prevents sudden movements that could dislodge the needle placement, causing tissue injury and bleeding, thus obscuring the correct diagnosis.

The parent is encouraged to sit on a stool close to the child's head and to hold the child's hand. The parent is thus able to offer both physical and verbal support during the procedure. The child may be offered objects that will provide distraction once the needle is in place and the fluid is being collected. A helpful object for use with young children is "pop-up" storybooks. They seem to delight children and help them relax. The parent or restraining nurse can hold the book and read the story out loud while turning pages that pop out at the child.

The American Academy of Pediatrics Subcommittee on Cancer Pain in Children recommends some type of sedation during the initial lumbar puncture.[42] As is true for bone marrow procedures, many pediatric medical centers offer short-acting general anesthesia or sedation for lumbar punctures as well. The administration and doses needed for spinal taps are similar to those necessary for bone marrow aspiration.

The lumbar puncture site is prepared with povidone-iodine. The pressurized dispenser, intradermal and subcutaneous injection, or the topical anesthetic agent is used to anesthetize the skin surface. The child's body is then positioned correctly, and the spinal needle is inserted between the third and fourth or fourth and fifth lumbar vertebrae into the interspace. When the needle is in place, the nurse reassures the child that there will be no further pain. Children usually relax when they know the needle is in position. The practitioner then requests that the child slowly straighten his or her legs. This change in position prevents a false increase in interspinal pressure caused by body curvature.

An elevated spinal fluid pressure is indicative of disease or abnormality. However, the nurse must remember that muscle tension and compression of the abdomen can give a falsely elevated spinal fluid pressure. The child is encouraged to lie quietly and breathe normally while the spinal fluid pressure is measured. Hyperventilation can lower a truly elevated pressure. CSF pressure is measured by attaching a manometer to the spinal needle. Specimens of fluid are obtained through a stopcock on the manometer. The fluid is examined to determine if WBCs are present and to ascertain the numbers and differential of those cells. RBC levels are also noted. Biochemical evaluation of spinal fluid includes glucose and protein measurements. Abnormal amounts of glucose and protein obtained in the initial lumbar puncture may indicate disease. Specimens of fluid sometimes are sent for bacteriologic culture and for cytologic examination for cancer cells if indicated.

At the completion of the lumbar puncture, the stylet is replaced, the needle is withdrawn, and an adhesive bandage is placed over the site. The child and parents are informed that it may be helpful for the older child to remain flat for 30 minutes to prevent a headache, although unlike in adults, this is not a common occurrence in children. The nurse may suggest that the child pass the time in quiet play.

Biopsy

With only a few exceptions, the child with a solid tumor must undergo a surgical procedure to obtain tissue for direct pathologic visualization. Pathologic confirmation is paramount in diagnosing pediatric malignancy and must precede any decision about choice and timing of treatment. Precise biologic classification is performed by the pathologist using light microscopy (standard microscopic

evaluation) and electron microscopy. An electron microscope uses an electron beam rather than light for illumination and allows greater magnification and resolution. The tumor sections can be stained with various dyes to define further the cells' appearance.

The surgeon, along with the oncologist, must decide if biopsy alone is sufficient for the child with a solid tumor or if complete surgical resection should be attempted. Because pediatric cancers encompass such a diverse group of diseases, no single surgical procedure has universal applications. Obviously, the primary goal is cure, which entails total eradication of the malignant cells. However, eradication may be achieved best with chemotherapy alone or chemotherapy and radiation combined rather than with surgery.

STAGING

The imaging studies obtained before the pathologic confirmation, along with direct surgical examination, assist the oncologist in determining the stage of the tumor. Staging is the accurate definition of the extent of disease locally, regionally, and systematically and in most solid tumors is the cornerstone of appropriate, specific therapy.[30] A system of staging has been designed for each tumor and depends on the experience gained, relating the extent of disease at diagnosis to the subsequent clinical course.[19] It is based on the premise that cancers of similar histologic features and site of origin will extend and metastasize in a predictable manner. Staging helps determine prognosis and treatment.

The prognosis of most childhood cancers is dependent on the stage and/or the histology of the disease. Assessment of prognosis is therefore integral to determining appropriate therapy and improving the child's chance of achieving cure. Most large institutions discuss new patients with solid tumors at a multispecialty conference commonly called the *Tumor Board.* Pediatric cancer specialists, including medical oncologists, surgeons, radiation therapists, radiologists, and pathologists, convene to share their findings and to determine a strategy for treating the pediatric solid tumor patient. All of the data compiled during the staging and diagnostic workup are discussed and considered. Chemotherapy, radiation therapy, and surgery are all integral parts of a combined program of care, and each plays a role at a specific point, the timing of which is highly dependent on the effects of the other(s).[12] During the tumor board meeting a medical plan of care is established, using the expertise of the various represented disciplines.

CONCLUSION

The diagnostic phase of cancer treatment is emotionally shattering to most families. Many parents are devastated, and the diagnosis will cause irrevocable change in their lives. Nurses caring for a child at this time often become deeply involved in the child's long-term therapy. A sound knowledge of the tests involved, the general sequence and timing of the diagnostic evaluation, and the disease itself permits nurses to respond realistically to the families. The diagnostic phase begins the long-term education, guidance, and support these families need and deserve.

REFERENCES

1. American Academy of Pediatrics. Guidelines for the elective use of conscious sedation, deep sedation and general anesthesia in pediatric patients. Pediatrics 1985; 76:317–321.
2. Bragg DG. State of the art assessment: Diagnostic oncologic imaging. Cancer 1989; 64(suppl):261–265.
3. Camp-Sorrell D. Magnetic resonance imaging and the implantable port. Oncol Nurs Forum 1990; 17:197–199.
4. Cella JH, Watson J. Nurse's Manual of Laboratory Tests. Philadelphia: FA Davis, 1989.
5. Channing Bete Co. What you should know about magnetic resonance imaging. South Deerfield, Mass.: The Company, 1990.
6. Cole CH. Harriet Lane Handbook. Chicago: Year Book Medical Publishers, 1989.
7. Corbitt JV. Laboratory Tests in Nursing Practice. Norwalk, Conn.: Appleton-Century-Crofts, 1982.
8. DeAngelis C. Interviewing to obtain a medical history. In DeAngelis C (ed): Pediatric Primary Care, 3rd ed. Boston: Little Brown & Co., 1984.
9. Elster AD. Magnetic Resonance Imaging: A Reference Guide and Atlas. Philadelphia: JB Lippincott, 1986.
10. Fletcher BD, Pratt CG. Evaluation of the child with a suspected malignant solid tumor. Pediatr Clin North Am 1991; 38:223–247.
11. Given CJ, Vogel V, Strauss L. Tumor markers and their significance in adolescent oncology. In Tibbs C (ed): Major Topics in Adolescent Oncology. New York: Futura Publishing, 1987.

12. Hays DM, Atkinson JB. General principles of surgery. In Pizzo P, Poplack D (eds): Principles and Practice of Pediatric Oncology, 2nd ed. Philadelphia: JB Lippincott, 1993, pp 247–272.
13. Heideman RL, Packer RJ, Albright LA, et al. Tumors of the central nervous system. In Pizzo P, Poplack D (eds): Principles and Practice of Pediatric Oncology, 2nd ed. Philadelphia: JB Lippincott, 1993, pp 633–682.
14. Kapelushnik J, Koren G, Solh H, et al. Evaluating the efficacy of EMLA in alleviating pain associated with lumbar puncture; Comparison of open and double-blinded protocols in children. Pain 1990; 42:31–34.
15. Kee JL. Handbook of Laboratory and Diagnostic Tests With Nursing Implications. Norwalk, Conn.: Appleton & Lange, 1990.
16. Kelly JU. The use of an investigational radiopharmaceutical in neuroblastoma: A nursing perspective. J Pediatr Oncol Nurs 1989;6:133–138.
17. Kirks DR, Hedlund GL, Gelfand MJ. Techniques. In Kirks DR (ed): Practical Pediatric Imaging, 2nd ed. Boston: Little, Brown & Co, 1991, pp 1–55.
18. Krishner BH, Cheung NK. Neuroblastoma. Pediatr Ann 1988; 17:269–283.
19. Leventhal BG. Neoplasms and neoplasm-like structures. In Behrman RE, Kliegman RM, et al. (eds): Nelson Textbook of Pediatrics, 14th ed. Philadelphia: WB Saunders, 1992, pp 1291–1322.
20. Lovejoy NC, Halliburton P. Pediatric tumor markers. J Pediatr Nurs 1989; 4:357–369.
21. Lutz WJ. Helping hospitalized children and their parents cope with painful procedures. J Pediatr Nurs 1986; 1:24–31.
22. MacFarland MB, Grant MM. Nursing Implications of Laboratory Tests, 2nd ed. New York: John Wiley & Sons, 1988.
23. Meadows AT, Kramer S, Hapson R, et al. Survival in childhood A.L.L.—The influence of protocol and place of treatment. Cancer Invest 1983;1:49–55.
24. Miller JH, Reed BS. Nuclear imaging. In Miller J (ed): Imaging in Pediatric Oncology. Baltimore: Williams & Wilkins, 1985.
25. Nunstein LS. Adolescent Health Care: A Practical Guide, 2nd ed. Baltimore: Urban & Schwargnburg, 1990.
26. Nurse's Reference Library. Diagnostics, 2nd ed. Springhouse, Penn.: Intermed Communications, 1986.
27. O'Mary SS. Diagnostic evaluation, classification and staging. In Groenwald SL, Frogge MH, et al. (eds): Cancer Nursing Principles and Practice, 2nd ed. Boston: Jones & Bartlett, 1990.
28. Ortega J, Siegel S. Biological markers in pediatric solid tumors. In Pizzo P, Poplack D (eds): Principles and Practice of Pediatric Oncology, 2nd ed. Philadelphia: JB Lippincott, 1993, pp 179–194.
29. Parker BR, Moore SG. Imaging studies in the diagnosis of pediatric malignancies. In Pizzo P, Poplack D (eds): Principles and Practice of Pediatric Oncology, 2nd ed. Philadelphia: JB Lippincott, 1993, pp 153–178.
30. Segel S, White L. The importance of imaging in the current practice of pediatric oncology. In Miller J (ed): Imaging in Pediatric Oncology. Baltimore: Williams & Wilkins, 1985.
31. Shulkin BL, Shapiro B, et al. Neuroblastoma: Detection of extraskeletal and skeletal deposits by Tc99M-MDP and I-131 MIBG. Society of Nuclear Medicine, June 1991. (Abstract.)

32. Sievers TD, Yee JD, et al. Midazolam for conscious sedation during pediatric oncology procedures— Safety and recovery parameters. Pediatrics 1991; 99:1172–1179.

33. Sprawls P. The principles of computed tomography image formation and quality. In Gedgaudas-McClees RK, Torres W (eds): Essentials of Body Computed Tomography. Philadelphia: WB Saunders, 1990.

34. Stubbs JB, Wilson LA. Nuclear medicine: A state-of-the-art review. Nuclear News 1991; 50–54.

35. Sumer Timii. Neoplastic disease in pediatrics. In Ziai M, Janeway CA, Cooke RE (eds): Pediatrics, 4th ed. Boston: Little, Brown & Co, 1990.

36. Tressler KM. Clinical Laboratory and Diagnostic Tests: Significance and Nursing Implications, 2nd ed. Norwalk, Conn.: Appleton & Lange, 1989.

37. Tuchman M, Woods W. Introduction: Neuroblastoma screening laboratory, clinical and epidemiological aspects. Am J Pediatr Hematol Oncol 1992; 14:95–96.

38. Waters L. Pharmacologic strategies for managing pain in children. Orthop Nurs 1992; 11:34–40.

39. Watt-Watson JH, Evernden C. Parent's perception of their child's acute pain experience. J Pediatr Nurs 1990; 5:344–349.

40. Yaster M, Nichols DG, et al. Midazolam-fentanyl intravenous sedation in children: Case report of respiratory arrest. Pediatrics 1990; 86:463–466.

41. Zappa SC, Nabors SB. Use of ethyl chloride topical anesthetics to reduce procedure pain in pediatric oncology patients. Cancer Nurs 1992; 15:130–136.

42. Zeltzer LK, Altman A. Report of the Subcommittee on the Management of Pain Associated with Procedures in Children With Cancer. Pediatrics 1990; 86:826–831.

CHEMOTHERAPY

Alice Renick-Ettinger

CELL CYCLE

To understand how chemotherapy works, it is necessary to review normal cellular proliferation. There are four phases in the cellular growth cycle (Fig. 4–1). Mitosis *(M)* represents actual cell division. Between mitotic events, the cell is in an interphase period distinguished by two gaps (G_1 and G_2) on either side of DNA synthesis *(S)*. There is also a period during which the cell is "out of cycle" or in a resting phase *(G_0)*. During this phase cells are not actively dividing.[35]

G_1, the first gap, is the postmitotic phase in which synthesis of ribonucleic acid (RNA) and protein occurs. G_1 has the most variable time span (8 to 48 hours) and is the phase in which cells spend the greatest portion of their active lives. The length of time that a cell spends in this phase influences the rate of cell proliferation. Rapidly growing cell populations have very few cells in this phase, whereas slow-growing populations have many cells in the G_1 phase.

The S phase is the synthesis phase in which the cell replicates its DNA in preparation for cellular division. This phase lasts 10 to 20 hours.

After the S phase is a resting period called G_2 in which a second gap occurs. This premitotic phase lasts 2 to 10 hours and is when RNA synthesis occurs.

Mitosis, the actual cell division, takes approximately 1 hour to complete and is accomplished in a four-step sequence (Fig. 4–1).

During *prophase* the nuclear membrane breaks down and disintegrates, and the chromosomes begin to clump. The chromosomes align in the middle of the cell during *metaphase*. Then the chromosomes segregate to the centrioles during *anaphase*. The final step is *telophase* in which actual cell division results in the production of two identical daughter cells.

G_0 represents a "resting" phase when cells are not dividing. Normal cells are in this phase for the majority of the time; cancer cells in this phase are extremely difficult to treat.[8]

Under ordinary conditions cells move from G_0 and G_1 when stimulated by growth factors or specific hormones. These growth factors, or hormones, present on the surface membrane of a cell, bind to specific receptors on the target cell and trigger it into the cell cycle.[35]

Cells proceed through the other phases until there is no longer a need for additional cells; then they reenter G_0. Although normal cells and cancer cells have similar cell cycles, normal cells reproduce in response to the body's feedback mechanism, but cancer cells ignore this system and replicate uncontrollably.[34,35]

Cell proliferation is also influenced by age and developmental status. In adults, many cell populations are inactive. For example, muscle cells and neurons are irreversibly differentiated and do not replicate. Some cells replicate only under special circumstances. Normally quiescent hepatocytes of children

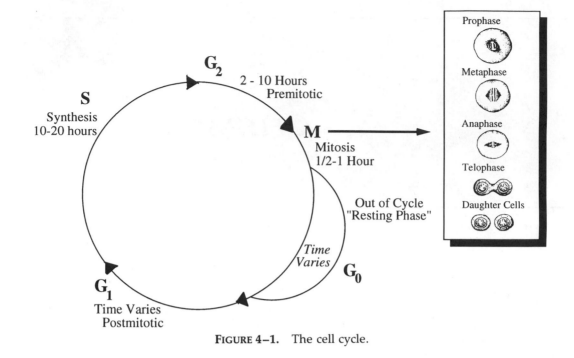

FIGURE 4–1. The cell cycle.

and adults can proliferate after hepatic injury.[34,53] Other cells such as hematopoietic cells and the mucosal cells lining the gastrointestinal tract replicate constantly in adults and children. Children and adolescents, unlike adults, have dividing cell populations because of developing or changing body systems and structures. Both cerebral and somatic growth and development may be susceptible to the acute and long-term adverse effects of chemotherapy.

TUMOR CELLULAR KINETICS

The development of a therapeutic plan (called a *protocol*) for the treatment of a patient with a malignancy incorporates cellular dynamics and tenets of the Gompertzian model. Originally derived by the eighteenth century mathematician, Gompertz, this mathematic model theorizes that tumors grow exponentially at first, with a high growth fraction and a very short doubling time. The *growth fraction* is the percentage of cells undergoing division at any one time. The *doubling time* is the time for any given number of cells to double. The growth fraction decreases and the doubling time slows as the tumor size increases.[43] In

part, this may be related to the tumor mass' outgrowing the blood supply. Cells situated more deeply may be relatively hypoxic, have a low growth fraction, and be less sensitive to the tumorcidal effects of chemotherapy.[22]

Another theory important for protocol development is the *fractional cell kill hypothesis*, which states that if a given drug concentration is applied for a specific time period, a constant percentage of the cell population will be killed, regardless of the number of cells present.[9] Most antineoplastic agents are more effective against malignancies with high rates of cellular proliferation and microscopic amounts of tumor cells rather than against ones with a larger tumor burden. Many pediatric cancers have a high growth fraction,[2] and it is theorized that this is one of the reasons that childhood malignancies are so susceptible to treatment.

PHARMACOKINETICS AND PHARMACODYNAMICS

Pharmacokinetics is the study of drug absorption, distribution, metabolism, and excretion, or what the body does to the drug. *Pharmacodynamics* is the study of relationships between drug concentrations and effect, or what the drug does to the body.[11,48] Principles of pharmacokinetics and pharmacodynamics are used in therapeutic protocols to optimize drug dosage and schedule, giving the greatest cell kill while minimizing toxicities.[12]

The following definitions help in understanding the principles of pharmacokinetics:

- The *area under the concentration-time curve (AUC)* represents the actual exposure over time of the drug in the body.
- *Bioavailability* is the rate and extent of absorption of a drug.
- *Biotransformation* is the enzymatic metabolism of a drug.
- *Clearance* is the rate of drug elimination calculated in terms of volume of plasma cleared of drug per unit of time.
- The *half-life* of a drug is the time needed to reduce the concentration of the drug by 50% within the body.

Although these principles help determine the optimal route, schedule, and dose of a drug, both physiologic and cellular factors are involved in the failure of chemotherapy to induce a response. Physiologic factors include absorption, distribution, metabolism, and elimination of the drug in the individual (Table 4–1).

Pharmacodynamics is concerned with dose-response relationships. For example, the same total dose of an agent given by rapid versus prolonged intravenous (IV) infusion may result in significantly different efficacy and toxicity. The use of biochemical modulators such as leucovorin rescue may allow the safe use of potentially lethal doses of high-dose methotrexate, with greater killing of malignant cells.

Pharmacodynamics and pharmacokinetics of drugs are intertwined within each individual. It is necessary to assess the patient each time chemotherapy will be administered. Variability within the same patient may account for differences in pharmacokinetics. For instance, many agents produce myelosuppression after repetitive doses. Although this may represent the continuous exposure of the bone marrow to the drug, slowing the production of new cells, it may also represent

TABLE 4–1. *Potential Abnormalities in Cancer Patients Altering Pharmacokinetics of Anticancer Agents*

ABNORMALITY	CAUSE
Abnormalities of absorption	Nausea/vomiting
	Prior surgery, radiotherapy, or chemotherapy
	Concurrent antiemetics affecting gut motility
	Patient adherence to treatment
Abnormalities of distribution	Weight loss
	Obesity
	Decreased body fat (lipophilic drugs)
	Pleural effusions or ascites (methotrexate)
Abnormalities of elimination	Hepatic dysfunction due to tumor replacement or prior (or concurrent) therapy
	Renal dysfunction due to malignant involvement of prior (or concurrent) therapy
Abnormalities in protein-binding	Hypoalbuminemia
	Concomitant medications

From Ratain MJ, Schilsky, RL: Principles of pharmacology and pharmacokinetics. In Perry MC (ed): The Chemotherapy Source Book. Baltimore: Williams & Wilkins, 1992, p 30. © 1992, the Williams & Wilkins Co., Baltimore.

decreased clearance of the drug, resulting in increased drug exposure.[11,49]

Careful monitoring of the patient through patient history, physical examination, and blood work is necessary before each course of chemotherapy begins. It may be necessary to recalculate doses based on changes in weight and renal and hepatic status.

CHEMOTHERAPEUTIC PROTOCOLS
Definitions

Some definitions help with understanding how chemotherapy is used in the treatment of patients with malignancies. *Multimodal therapy* is the use of chemotherapeutic agents with other forms of treatment such as surgery and/or radiation. The treatment of Wilms' tumor uses multimodal therapy.

Adjuvant chemotherapy is used in patients who are at high risk for recurrence but without clinical evidence of residual disease after receiving local therapy with surgery or radiation. Many treatment protocols for pediatric solid tumors use this approach.

Combination chemotherapy is the use of several active agents (each of which is active against a particular cancer) together in multidrug regimens. For example, regimens designed to treat leukemia use combination chemotherapy.

Neoadjuvant chemotherapy is used preoperatively in an effort to reduce bulk disease before a definitive surgical procedure is performed. This type of chemotherapeutic approach currently is used in the treatment of osteosarcoma.

Sanctuary therapy is administered into an area where malignant cells are sequestered and concentrations of systemic chemotherapy may not be sufficient to eradicate them. The central nervous system (CNS), which is protected by the blood-brain barrier, is such an area. Chemotherapy is administered intrathecally, through lumbar puncture, or through an Ommaya reservoir, described later in this chapter, to eliminate malignant cells.

In certain types of pediatric cancers such as the leukemias, therapy is given in regimens with several phases of treatment. The initial *induction phase* consists of extremely intensive therapy with the goal of killing enough cells to induce a remission. It is followed by a *consolidation phase* in which subclinical disease remains and continued intensive therapy is given to destroy remaining cancer cells. *Maintenance* is the next phase, which continues for a specified period of time or the remainder of therapy. The object of this phase is to destroy any residual cancer cells. The *observation phase* is the period of time when therapy has ended and the child is followed for recurrent or late effects of the disease or its treatment.

Resistance

Some malignant cells are sensitive to the chemotherapy used, and remission and cure may be achieved. Other cells demonstrate either an intrinsic or acquired resistance.[3,16] Resistant cells contain a gene known as the *multidrug resistant (MDR) gene*. In intrinsic, or de novo, resistance the MDR gene is present from the onset of the disease, even before exposure to any chemotherapeutic agents. In the acquired form the presence of the MDR gene is the result of genetic mutation after exposure to antineoplastic drugs.

In either case the resistant cells express a protein on the cell's membrane, P-glycoprotein. This protein acts as a pump to eliminate certain chemotherapeutic agents rapidly from the cell. Chemotherapeutic agents particularly sensitive to this glycoprotein are the antitumor antibiotics, vinca alkaloids, and the epipodophyllotoxins.[3,18,26]

Two main hypotheses are used to develop chemotherapeutic protocols that try to avoid this problem of drug resistance. The Goldie-Coldman hypothesis[27] suggests that early use of effective drugs given at maximal dosage as frequently as possible will achieve the best tumor cell kill and prevent multiple drug resistance.

Norton and Simon's[44] treatment model describes "spikes" of intensity or a late intensification phase of therapy. Intense induction and consolidation therapy are given to reduce the gross total volume of cancer cells. A recovery phase follows in which there is either a "waiting period" with no treatment or a low-dose maintenance phase. The waiting period is followed by a second, or "late," intensification phase, which could consist of "rapidly alternating, high-dose, sequenced therapy." Theoretically, there are smaller numbers of cancer cells that then would respond to high-dose therapy.

Principles of Combination Chemotherapy

Therapeutic protocols use a combination of drugs that individually are active against a specific disease entity. (See the section "Clinical Trials" in this chapter.)

Drugs used in combination may show synergy. It is not completely understood how agents work synergistically to provide maximal cell kill, but it is known that certain agents display a greater antitumor effect when used together than when used as single agents. Since tumor cells do not all progress through the cell cycle at the same time, it is important to use agents that exert effects at different stages of the cell cycle.

Using agents that have toxicities that do not overlap by organ system or timing minimizes the risk of severe or lethal effects. Since myelosuppression usually is the dose-limiting toxicity for many chemotherapeutic agents, scheduling and dosage of drugs become essential when combining agents.[37] It is possible to give higher doses of all agents if the nadir, or low point, of the myelosuppressive agents comes at different times. Drugs should be used at the highest possible dosage and be given as frequently as possible. However, there must be adequate time between cycles to allow for healthy tissues to recover.

CLASSIFICATION OF CHEMOTHERAPEUTIC AGENTS

Chemotherapeutic agents are classified according to their chemical structure and their cell cycle activity, either *cell cycle (phase) specific* or *cell cycle (phase) nonspecific*, depending on their mode of action:

1. Cell cycle specific agents have their effect during a specific phase of the cell cycle, exerting maximal effect on rapidly dividing cells.
2. Cell cycle nonspecific agents act on cells regardless of their phase. They are dose dependent, whereby the degree of cell kill is directly proportional to the dose administered. These agents can be effective on neoplasms that grow more slowly because they are cytotoxic even to resting cells.[8]

Table 4–2 classifies chemotherapeutic agents by their mechanism of action.

In classifying agents by chemical structure, they are divided into six major categories: alkylating agents, antimetabolites, antitumor antibiotics, plant alkaloids, hormonal agents (corticosteroids are used for pediatric malignancies), and miscellaneous agents.[23]

Alkylating Agents

During alkylation the hydrogen atoms of some molecules within the cell are replaced by an alkyl group. Replacement by this alkyl group causes breaks in the DNA molecule and the cross-linking of its twin strands; this process interferes with DNA replication and RNA transcription, resulting in an inability of the cell to carry on its metabolic activities and to replicate. Alkylating agents are cell cycle nonspecific and can exert their effects on either slow-growing tumors or rapidly proliferating ones. They vary considerably in speed and duration of their action. For example, nitrogen mustard acts directly and almost instantly, but cyclophosphamide, which must be activated metabolically, is slower and has relatively long lasting effects.

Antimetabolites

Antimetabolites are agents that are structurally similar (analogues) to the normal cellular metabolites that are required for cell function and replication. They interfere with normal cell metabolism, interacting directly with the specific enzyme, either to inhibit the enzyme or to produce a nonfunctional end product. Cell processes dependent on the enzyme or the end product thus are blocked, causing interruption in the synthesis of protein, RNA, or DNA within the cell. For example, methotrexate competes with folic acid to bind the enzyme dihydrofolate reductase. When methotrexate binds with this enzyme, folic acid cannot be metabolized further, thus interfering with DNA synthesis.

Antitumor Antibiotics

Antineoplastic antibiotics are synthesized naturally by various bacterial and fungal species. They interfere with cellular metabolism in widely differing ways by forming relatively stable complexes with DNA, thereby inhibiting DNA or RNA synthesis or both. An example is dactinomycin, which forms a complex with DNA. This complex interferes with the transcription of DNA and the synthesis of RNA. Doxorubicin also binds to DNA but exerts its effect primarily by inhibiting DNA replication. Since the antibiotics are active at many stages within the cell replication cycle, they apparently are cell cycle phase nonspecific agents.

TABLE 4–2. *Classification of Chemotherapeutic Agents*

CLASSIFICATION	MECHANISM OF ACTION	AGENTS
Cell Cycle Nonspecific		
Alkylating agents	Substitute an alkyl group for the hydrogen atom, causing the two strands of DNA to become cross-linked, usually bonding the two guanine pairs; this leads to an inability of DNA to replicate	Busulfan Chlorambucil Cyclophosphamide Ifosfamide Mechlorethamine Melphalan Thiotepa
Nitrosoureas	Cause cross-linking and breakage in DNA strands Lipid soluble and cross blood-brain barrier	Carmustine Lomustine
Antitumor antibiotics	Interfere with nucleic acid synthesis by binding or reacting with the DNA molecule, blocking DNA-directed RNA and DNA transcription	Bleomycin Dactinomycin Daunorubicin Doxorubicin Mitomycin
Hormonal agents	Interfere with protein synthesis and alter cell metabolism	Corticosteroids
Cell Cycle Specific		
Antimetabolites (S phase specific)	Interfere with normal cellular metabolism by substitution for natural metabolite	5-Azacytidine 5-Fluorouracil 6-Mercaptopurine 6-Thioguanine Cytosine arabinoside Methotrexate
Plant alkaloids (M phase specific)	Bind to and crystalize the microtubular proteins in the cell, causing metaphase arrest; in high concentrations there is inhibition of nucleic acid and protein synthesis	Etoposide Teniposide Vinblastine Vincristine
Miscellaneous Agents		
Hydroxyurea (cell cycle specific [S phase])	Inhibits ribonucleotide reductase enzyme system, inhibiting DNA synthesis Functions as antimetabolite	
Procarbazine (cell cycle nonspecific)	Inhibits DNA, RNA, and protein synthesis Functions as alkylating agent	
Asparaginase (cell cycle nonspecific)	Inhibits DNA, RNA, and protein synthesis by hydrolyzing serum asparagine to nonfunctional aspartic acid and ammonia	
Cisplatin Carboplatin (cell cycle nonspecific)	Probably function as alkylating agents by binding to DNA	

Data from references 7, 18, 20, and 22.

Plant Alkaloids

Alkaloids used in anticancer therapy are agents derived from plants that interfere with mitosis and other cellular processes. This group includes the vinca alkaloids (vincristine, vinblastine, and vindesine) and the epidophyllotoxins (etoposide and teniposide). The vinca alkaloids, by binding to critical proteins within the cell, inhibit the passage of cells through metaphase and thus block cell division. They also may interfere with normal DNA and RNA metabolism. Although they differ structurally by only a single oxygen atom, vincristine and vinblastine have widely different clinical applications. The epidophyllotoxins are semisynthetic derivatives of plant extracts that also produce mitotic arrest at metaphase. In addition, they may inhibit DNA synthesis. The alkaloids apparently are cell cycle phase M–specific agents.

Corticosteroids

Steroids appear to enter the cell passively and bind with macromolecules in the cytoplasm of the cell. This complex then enters the cell nucleus, binds with DNA, and modifies the transcription process.

Miscellaneous Agents

Several chemotherapeutic agents do not fit into the above classifications. They have various mechanisms of action and are described in Table 4–2.

ACUTE SIDE EFFECTS OF CHEMOTHERAPEUTIC AGENTS

Most of the side effects commonly associated with chemotherapy occur because these agents are relatively nonselective. They are cytotoxic to both rapidly dividing normal cells and cancer cells. The hematopoietic system, the GI tract, and the integumentary system are composed of rapidly dividing cells; therefore they are highly susceptible to acute adverse effects.

Hematopoietic System

The hematopoietic system is responsible for the proliferation, differentiation, and maturation of the various blood-forming cells. Since blood cells have a relatively short life span, requiring constant regeneration, hematopoiesis is a continuous process (Table 4–3).

The blood-forming cells in humans are found in the microenvironment of the bone marrow. In infants and young children hematopoiesis occurs in nearly every bone; by adulthood it occurs mainly in flat bones such as the sternum, ribs, skull, and proximal ends of long bones.[19]

Bone marrow suppression is the most significant dose-limiting toxicity of many chemotherapeutic regimens. With a few exceptions (e.g., classic alkylating agents such as nitrogen mustard and the nitrosoureas), chemotherapeutic agents affect actively dividing cells. A significant number of cells in the bone marrow are not actively dividing, and they are spared the toxic effects of chemotherapy.[53]

The time of the most profound bone marrow suppression is known as the *nadir*. The time to recovery depends on the agent or agents used and the patient's past treatment history. For example, a patient who has had considerable prior chemotherapy or radiation therapy may have a prolonged nadir.

Phase-specific agents produce the most rapid decrease of the white blood cell (WBC) count. Ultimately, these cells will have a rapid recovery. Agents that are cell cycle specific but not phase specific cause a slightly more delayed nadir and recovery. Cell cycle–nonspecific agents produce late nadirs and prolonged depression.[20,37]

TABLE 4–3. *Life Span and Function of Hematopoietic Cells*

CELL TYPE	LIFE SPAN	FUNCTION
Mature RBCs	120 days	Carry oxygen to cells
Neutrophils	6–8 hr	Phagocytosis
Eosinophils	5–24 hr	Allergic reactions
Lymphocytes	100–300+ days	Antibody production (B) Cellular immunity (T)
Monocytes	8 hr	Phagocytosis
Platelets	10 days	Prevent or stop bleeding

Since WBCs divide at an extremely rapid rate, they are most susceptible to the effects of chemotherapy. A decrease in WBCs is termed *leukopenia.*

WBCs are divided into several types. Granulocytes are the neutrophils, eosinophils, and basophils. Neutrophils help the body fight bacterial and fungal infection. They are produced in the bone marrow and are divided into bands, which are slightly immature, and polymorphonuclear cells, or "polys," which are the mature cells. Severe neutropenia increases the risk for serious infection.

Monocytes are the body's scavengers. Eosinophils are minimally phagocytic and are involved in allergic responses. Basophils are not phagocytic; they release histamine and heparin into the bloodstream.

Lymphocytes are responsible for cell-mediated (T-cell) and humoral (B-cell) immunity. Severe lymphopenia places the host at risk for serious viral infection. In patients with varicella, a lymphocyte count of less than 500/mm^3 presents a greater risk for viral dissemination.[23a]

Platelets are also adversely affected by chemotherapy, resulting in thrombocytopenia, which can occur within 7 days or as late as 21 days after administration of the agents. A platelet count less than 20,000/mm^3 is associated with an increased risk of spontaneous hemorrhage. If bleeding occurs, platelet transfusions are indicated. The use of platelet transfusions when there is no bleeding, even with a low platelet count, is controversial because of the risk of antibody formation and therefore destruction of platelets with subsequent transfusions.[17]

The red blood cell (RBC) line is also affected by chemotherapeutic agents. Because the life span of the RBC is approximately 120 days, it is usually the least affected. However, some agents can cause a decrease in the RBC count as early as 10 days after their administration and may result in a lengthy recovery time. Reticulocytes are the precursors to mature RBCs in the peripheral blood smear (normal level, 0.5% to 1%). A rising reticulocyte count suggests recovery of the bone marrow from the effects of chemotherapy.

Table 4–4 depicts standard toxicity criteria as used by the National Cancer Institute (NCI). These criteria are used in determining the toxic effects of chemotherapy and provide a mechanism for uniform reporting for therapeutic protocols. Toxicities rated grades 3 and 4 are considered significant.

Gastrointestinal Tract

Many chemotherapeutic agents cause anorexia, nausea, or vomiting by a direct effect of the agent on the vomiting center. The use of high-dose chemotherapy and combinations of drugs increases the risk and severity of nausea and vomiting.[55] Vomiting occurs when the true vomiting center, located on the floor of the medulla, is stimulated by emetic neurotransmitters. Chemotherapeutic agents stimulate the vomiting center through afferent pathways resulting from changing chemical levels of neurotransmitters in the brain and cerebrospinal fluid (CSF).[21,54]

There is also a strong psychologic component to chemotherapy-induced nausea and vomiting that suggests it is a conditioned response resulting in anticipatory vomiting that can develop before any agents are administered.[32,33]

Table 4–5 reviews the emetogenic potential and the expected time frame after administration of chemotherapeutic agents.[6] When known emetogenic drugs are used, it is always best to try to prevent nausea and/or vomiting rather than try to treat it once it begins. To do so may prevent anticipatory vomiting in the future because the child does not become conditioned to expect nausea and vomiting with chemotherapy. Antiemetic agents are administered approximately ½ hour before therapy is to begin and may be continued on a scheduled, around-the-clock basis, depending on the antiemetics used.

Many children are also able to use relaxation techniques to decrease their feelings of nausea. The use of hypnosis, visual imagery, or supportive counseling, which can be used by the child at home and before visits to the clinic to receive chemotherapy, allows the child to gain control of the situation. These techniques can decrease symptoms of distress

TABLE 4–4. *Common Toxicity Criteria of National Cancer Institute*

TOXICITY	GRADE				
	0	**1**	**2**	**3**	**4**
White blood count	≥4	3–3.9	2–2.9	1–1.9	<1
Platelets	Within normal limits (WNL)	75–normal	50–74.9	25–49.9	<25
Hemoglobin	WNL	10–normal	8–10	6.5–7.9	<6.5
Granulocytes/bands	≥2	1.5–1.9	1–1.4	0.5–0.9	<0.5
Lymphocytes	≥2	1.5–1.9	1–1.4	0.5–0.9	<0.5
Hemorrhage (clinical)	None	Mild, no transfusion	Gross, 1–2 units transfusion per episode	Gross, 3–4 units transfusion per episode	Massive, >4 units transfusion per episode
Infection	None	Mild	Moderate	Severe	Life-threatening
Nausea	None	Able to eat reasonable intake	Intake significantly decreased but can eat	No significant intake	—
Vomiting	None	One episode in 24 hr	Two to five episodes in 24 hr	Six to 10 episodes in 24 hr	>10 episodes in 24 hr or need for parenteral support
Diarrhea	None	Increase of two to three stools/day over pretreatment period	Increase of four to six stools/day or nocturnal stools or moderate cramping	Increase of seven to nine stools/day or incontinence or severe cramping	Increase of ≥10 stools/day or grossly bloody diarrhea or need for parenteral support
Stomatitis	None	Painless ulcers, erythema, or mild soreness	Painful erythema, edema, or ulcers but can eat	Painful erythema, edema, or ulcers and cannot eat	Requires parenteral or enteral support
Bilirubin	WNL	—	<1.5 × N	1.5–3 × N	>3 × N
Transaminase SGOT (AST) SGPT (ALT)	WNL	≤2.5 × N	2.6–5 × N	5.1–20 × N	>20 × N
Alkaline phosphatase *or* 5′ nucleotidase	WNL	≤2.5 × N	2.6–5 × N	5.1–20 × N	>20 × N
Liver—clinical	No change from baseline	—	—	Pre-coma	Hepatic coma
BUN*	<20	20–39	40–59	60–79	>80
Creatinine clearance*	100%	75%–99%	50%–74%	25%–49%	<25%
Creatinine	WNL	<1.5 × N	1.5–3 × N	3.1–6 × N	>6 × N
Proteinuria	No change	1+ or <0.3 g% or <3 g/L	2–3+ or 0.3–1 g% or 3–10 g/L	4+ or >1 g% or >10 g/L	Nephrotic syndrome
Hematuria	Negative	Microscopic only	Gross, no clots	Gross and clots	Requires transfusion
Alopecia	No loss	Mild hair loss	Pronounced or total hair loss	—	—

*Taken from Childrens Cancer Group Toxicity Criteria.
N = normal.

Table continued on following page.

TABLE 4–4. *Common Toxicity Criteria of National Cancer Institute* Continued

TOXICITY	GRADE				
	0	1	2	3	4
Pulmonary	None or no change	Asymptomatic, with abnormality in pulmonary function tests	Dyspnea on significant exertion	Dyspnea at normal level of activity	Dyspnea at rest
Cardiac arrhythmias	None	Asymptomatic, transient, requiring no therapy	Recurrent or persistent; no therapy required	Requires treatment	Requires monitoring; or hypotension or ventricular tachycardia or fibrillation
Cardiac function	None	Asymptomatic; decline of resting ejection fraction by <20% of baseline value	Asymptomatic; decline of resting ejection fraction by >20% of baseline value	Mild congestive heart failure (CHF); responsive to therapy	Severe or refractory CHF
Cardiac Ischemia	None	Nonspecific T-wave flattening	Asymptomatic, ST and T wave changes suggesting ischemia	Angina without evidence for infarction	Acute myocardial infarction
Pericardial	None	Asymptomatic effusion; no intervention required	Pericarditis (rub, chest pain, ECG changes)	Symptomatic effusion; drainage required	Tamponade; drainage urgently required
Hypertension	None or no change	Asymptomatic; transient increase by >20 mm Hg (D) or to >150/100 if previously WNL; no treatment required	Recurrent or persistent increase by >20 mm Hg (D) or to >150/100 if previously WNL; no treatment required	Requires therapy	Hypertensive crisis
Hypotension	None or no change	Changes requiring no therapy (including transient orthostatic hypotension)	Requires fluid replacement or other therapy but no hospitalization	Requires therapy and hospitalization; resolves within 48 hr of stopping the agent	Requires therapy and hospitalization for >48 hr after stopping the agent
Neurologic Sensory	None or no changes	Mild paresthesias; loss of deep tendon reflexes	Mild or moderate objective sensory loss; moderate paresthesias	Severe objective sensory loss or paresthesias that interfere with function	—
Motor	None or no changes	Subjective weakness; no objective findings	Mild objective weakness without significant impairment of function	Objective weakness with impairment of function	Paralysis

TABLE 4–4. *Common Toxicity Criteria of National Cancer Institute* Continued

TOXICITY	GRADE				
	0	1	2	3	4
Cortical	None	Mild somnolence or agitation	Moderate somnolence or agitation	Severe somnolence, agitation, confusion, disorientation, or hallucinations	Coma, seizures, toxic psychosis
Cerebellar	None	Slight incoordination, dysdiadochokinesia	Intention tremor, dysmetria, slurred speech, nystagmus	Locomotor ataxia	Cerebellar necrosis
Mood	No change	Mild anxiety or depression	Moderate anxiety or depression	Severe anxiety or depression	Suicidal ideation
Headache	None	Mild	Moderate or severe but transient	Unrelenting and severe	—
Constipation	None or no change	Mild	Moderate	Severe	Ileus for >96 hr
Hearing	None or no change	Asymptomatic; hearing loss on audiometry only	Tinnitus	Hearing loss interfering with function but correctable with hearing aid	Deafness not correctable
Vision	None or no change	—	—	Symptomatic subtotal loss of vision	Blindness
Skin	None or no change	Scattered macular or papular eruption or erythema that is asymptomatic	Scattered macular or papular eruption or erythema with pruritus or other associated symptoms	Generalized symptomatic macular, papular, or vesicular eruption	Exfoliative dermatitis or ulcerating dermatitis
Allergy	None	Transient rash, drug fever <38° C (100.4° F)	Urticaria; drug fever of 38° C (100.4° F), mild bronchospasm	Serum sickness, bronchospasm requiring parenteral medications	Anaphylaxis
Fever in absence of infection	None	37°–38° C (98.7°–100.4° F)	38.1°–40° C (100.5°–104° F)	>40° C (>104° F) for <24 hr	>40° C (104° F) for >24 hr or fever accompanied by hypotension
Local	None	Pain	Pain and swelling with inflammation or phlebitis	Ulceration	Plastic surgery indicated
Weight gain or loss	<5%	5%–9.9%	10%–19.9%	≥20%	—

Table continued on following page.

TABLE 4–4. *Common Toxicity Criteria of National Cancer Institute* Continued

TOXICITY	GRADE				
	0	**1**	**2**	**3**	**4**
Hyperglycemia	<115	115–160	161–250	251–500	>500 or ketoacidosis
Hypoglycemia	>64	55–64	40–54	30–39	<30
Amylase	WNL	<1.5 × N	1.5–2 × N	2.1–5 × N	>5.1 × N
Hypernatremia*	135–145	146–149	150–155	156–164	>165
Hyponatremia*	135–145	130–134	125–129	116–124	<115
Hyperkalemia*	3.5–5.4	5.5–5.9	6–6.4	6.5–6.9	>7
Hypokalemia*	3.5–5.4	3.1–3.4	2.6–3.0	2.1–2.5	<2
Hypercalcemia*	8.5–10.5	10.6–11.5	11.6–12.5	12.6–13.5	>13.5
Hypocalcemia*	8.5–10.5	7.8–8.4	7–7.7	6.1–6.9	<6.1
Hypomagnesemia	>1.4	1.4–1.2	1.1–0.9	0.8–0.6	≤0.5
Fibrinogen	WNL	0.99–0.75 × N	0.74–0.5 × N	0.49–0.25 × N	≤0.24 × N
Prothrombin time	WNL	1.01–1.25 × N	1.26–1.5 × N	1.51–2 × N	>2 × N
Partial thromboplastin time	WNL	1.01–1.66 × N	1.67–2.33 × N	2.34–3 × N	>3 × N

*Taken from Childrens Cancer Group Toxicity Criteria.

and eliminate anticipatory stress, nausea, or vomiting.[13,14,32,56]

Chemotherapy-induced stomatitis is a painful tissue injury to the basal layers of the oral mucosa that occurs within a few days to a week after treatment. It is caused by the cytotoxic effects of the agent on the rapidly dividing oral mucosa, which has a life span of 10 to 14 days.[51] There is an actual loss of cells that results in mucosal ulcerations, which can result in infection with organisms such as *Staphylococcus*, *Candida*, and herpes simplex virus.

Antimetabolites, particularly methotrexate and 5-fluorouracil, and antibiotics such as bleomycin, dactinomycin, daunorubicin, and doxorubicin are more likely to cause stomatitis than other drugs.

The other tissues of the GI tract also are greatly affected by these agents. The generation time of the cells in the stomach, intestines, colon, and rectum ranges from 1 to 6 days,[42] making the cells extremely susceptible to the effects of chemotherapy. These effects can result in anorexia, ulcerations from the mouth to the anus, malabsorption, and diarrhea.

Integumentary System

The tissues of the skin and hair follicles are affected by many chemotherapeutic agents. Skin problems can include a mild maculopapular rash, erythema, pruritus, or discoloration of skin or nailbeds.[4] (See Tables 4–6 and 4–7 for specific agents associated with skin lesions.) Local skin reactions can occur when vesicant agents leak outside of the vein (*extravasate*), which can cause a burn or sloughing of the surrounding tissue. (For further discussion, refer to section, "Extravasation.")

The human scalp has hairs in different phases of growth. Approximately 10% to 15% are in the resting phase (telogen), which lasts approximately 3 months, and the rest are in the growing phase (anagen), lasting 2 to 6 years. The hairs in the anagen phase are most susceptible to the effects of chemotherapy and account for the major hair loss, termed *alopecia*, with some drugs.[8] Hair regrowth may take place, even though the drugs are still being given. However, the new hair may be a different texture and shade. When therapy is completed, hair usually returns to normal.

Text continued on p. 108.

TABLE 4—5. *Emetogenic Potential of Chemotherapeutic Agents in Children*

DRUG	INCIDENCE	TIME FROM ADMINISTRATION (HOURS)
Acridinyl anisidide (AMSA)	Low	—
Asparaginase	Very low	1–3
5–Azacytidine	Moderate to severe	1–4
Bleomycin	Low	3–6 Rarely given as a single agent
Busulfan	Very low	—
Carboplatin	Moderate	1–4
Carmustine (BCNU)	High	2–4
Cisplatin	Severe	1–6
Corticosteroids	Very low	—
Cyclophosphamide (Cytoxan)	High to very high	4–12
Cytarabine (ARA-C)	Low to high (dose dependent)	4–12
Dacarbazine (DTIC)	Very high	Immediate to 3
Dactinomycin (Actinomycin-D)	High (variable) Younger children have less vomiting	Immediate to 6
Daunorubicin (Daunomycin)	Moderate	2–6
Doxorubicin (Adriamycin)	Moderate	4–6
Etoposide (VP-16)	Low	3–8
Fazarabine	Moderate	—
Fludarabine	Low	—
5-Fluorouracil (5-FU)	Moderate	3–6
Homoharringtonine	Low	—
Hydroxyurea	Low (nausea more common)	6–12
Idarubicin	Moderate	2–6
Ifosfamide	Moderate	1–2
Lomustine (CCNU)	High	2–6
Mechlorethamine (nitrogen mustard)	Very high to severe	Immediate to 2
Melphalan	Low	6–12
Mercaptopurine (6-MP, Purinethol)	Very low	—
Methotrexate	Very low: oral dose	—
	Low to moderate: intermediate dose	4–12
	Moderate to severe: high dose	2–4
Mitoxantrone	Low to moderate	—
Paclitoxel (Taxol)	Low	Nausea during infusion
Piritrexim	Mild to moderate	—
Procarbazine	Moderate (nausea)	24
Retinoic acid	Very low	—
Teniposide (VM-26)	Low	3–8
Thioguanine (6-TG)	Very low	—
Thiotepa	Low to moderate	6–12
Vinblastine	Low	4–12
Vincristine	Very low	—

Data from author's experience and reference 6.

TABLE 4—6. *Table of Chemotherapeutic Agents*

DRUG	CLASSIFICATION	ROUTE
Acridinyl anisidide (AMSA, Amsacrine) Investigational	Acridine dye derivative	Intravenous (IV) Diluted solution is stable for 48 hr but should be discarded in 8 hr because no bacteriostatic agent is included
Asparaginase (L-asparaginase, Elspar) Erwinia and PEG-L-asparaginase (long-acting form of *E. coli* L-asparaginase with less risk for serious hypersensitivity reactions) are investigational	Enzyme from *Escherichia coli* or *Erwinia carotovora* Inhibits protein synthesis by hydrolyzing serum asparagine to nonfunctional aspartic acid and ammonia Cell cycle nonspecific	Intramuscular (IM) IV May be reconstituted with 1 cc for 10,000 U/ml or 2 cc for 5000 U/ml Use within 8 hr Refrigerate
5-Azacytidine (5-AC, 5-AZA)	Antimetabolite	IV infusion Refrigerate Dilution in nonbuffered, highly acidic; basic media degrades drug, therefore dilution is in Ringer's lactate only
Bleomycin sulfate (Blenoxane)	Antibiotic	IV IM SQ Intracavitary Intra-tumor Refrigerate May be diluted with as little as 0.5 ml of sterile water, sodium chloride, 5% dextrose, or bacteriostatic water
Busulfan (Myleran)	Alkylating agent	By mouth (PO) 2 mg tablets

A = anorexia, N = nausea, V = vomiting, D = diarrhea.

SIDE EFFECTS	SPECIAL CONSIDERATIONS
Leukopenia with nadir at 10 days; recovery by 25 days N, V Hepatic toxicity Cardiac arrhythmias Phlebitis is a serious problem unless a central line is used Alopecia	**Vesicant** — severe tissue damage if extravasation occurs Solution is red-orange color and will cause colored urine Not compatible with chloride-containing solutions (precipitation may occur) Use glass syringes for reconstitution Do not give unless potassium, calcium, and magnesium levels are normal
Coagulation abnormalities A, N — mild Pancreatitis, hyperglycemia, transient diabetes mellitus Convulsions Abnormal liver function test (LFT) results Somnolence, lethargy Allergic reactions ranging from mild urticaria to anaphylaxis	IV administration associated with increased risk of anaphylaxis Have emergency equipment and drugs available Observe patient for at least ½ hr after dose Dipstick urine for glucose before each dose (treat with insulin if ordered for hyperglycemia)
Myelosuppression Neutropenia — dose dependent, with nadir from 2–3 wk N, V, D — severe with IV or subcutaneous (SQ) pulse dosing; less severe with continuous infusion Skin rash Liver damage rare but severe Rare and dose-dependent muscle pain, weakness, lethargy Fever during and for 24 hr after administration	Careful administration to patients with liver disease or decreased serum albumin level (<3.8 g/dl) Continuous infusions should be changed every 3 hr
N, V, A Pneumonitis with dry cough, dyspnea, rales, progressive pulmonary fibrosis — total cumulative lifetime dose of 400 U Fever with or without chills Skin rash, cutaneous hyperpigmentation, discolorations — dose related Mild stomatitis	Rare, lethal anaphylactoid reactions with severe fever and hypotension — have emergency equipment available Administer test dose of 1–2 U IM; wait 1 hr and give remaining dose Lower dose may be given when pulmonary radiotherapy is used Pulmonary function tests are done as baseline, throughout course of therapy, and for a period of time after therapy; pneumonitis can progress to fatal fibrosis
Myelosuppression, pancytopenia with nadir from 11–30 days and recovery at 24–54 days Hyperpigmentation Gynecomastia — rare GI disturbances — mild	Interstitial pulmonary fibrosis within a year of starting therapy is rare and can occur after long-term therapy

Table continued on following page.

TABLE 4–6. *Table of Chemotherapeutic Agents* Continued

DRUG	CLASSIFICATION	ROUTE
Carboplatin (Paraplatin)	Heavy metal	Vials contain equal parts by weight of carboplatin and mannitol IV infusion Room temperature Discard after 8 hr Protect from light Dilution yields concentration of 10 mg/ml
Carmustine (BCNU, BiCNU)	Nitrosourea Lipid-soluble alkylating agent that crosses blood-brain barrier	IV infusion Refrigerate Reconstitute with absolute alcohol diluent
Cisplatin (Cis-Platinum, Platinol)	Heavy metal	IV infusion Do not refrigerate reconstituted solution Protect from light Diluted solutions must contain at least 0.45% sodium chloride (NaCl)
Corticosteroids Prednisone (Deltasone, Liquid Pred Syrup) Dexamethasone (Decadron) Hydrocortisone (Solu-Cortef) Methylprednisolone (Solu-Medrol)	Lympholytic (effective in the treatment of acute lymphoblastic leukemia [ALL], non-Hodgkin's lymphoma [NHL], and certain other malignancies) Decreases edema produced by tumor or caused by tumor necrosis	PO IV Intrathecal (IT) For IT use, mix with saline, lactated Ringer's, or Elliott's B solution

SIDE EFFECTS	SPECIAL CONSIDERATIONS
Myelosuppression N, V Renal impairment, electrolyte wasting Peripheral neuropathies Ototoxicity Liver function abnormalities	IV infusion over 15 to 60 min or longer Aluminum reacts with carboplatin, causing precipitate formation and loss of potency; therefore do not allow needles or IV sets containing aluminum parts to come in contact with the drug
Delayed myelosuppression — leukopenia, thrombocytopenia (nadir 3–4 wk and resolving slowly) N, V appearing within 2 hr of administration and lasting up to 6 hr Liver and renal dysfunction Alopecia Pulmonary fibrosis with long-term use Hypotension	**Irritant** — may cause pain and phlebitis at injection site and facial flushing, hypotension from alcohol diluent, especially with rapid infusion; solution may be further diluted, IV rate slowed, ice or warm pack applied to extremity to decrease pain May cause pain and brown staining of skin
Severe and often protracted N, V Myelosuppression Nephrotoxicity during second week after dose, becoming more severe with repeated courses of drug Ototoxicity, especially high-frequency hearing loss and tinnitus Electrolyte wasting, especially calcium and magnesium Hypomagnesemia may be protracted, requiring magnesium replacement therapy Allergic reactions — rare Hyperuricemia Peripheral neuropathy	Aluminum reacts with cisplatin, causing precipitate formation and loss of potency; therefore do not allow needles or IV sets containing aluminum parts to come in contact with drug Premedicate with antiemetics; continue throughout course of therapy It may be necessary to replace emesis "ml for ml" Monitor creatinine clearance, blood urea nitrogen (BUN) and creatinine levels before each dose During course of therapy carefully monitor input and output Maintain urinary output at least at 1–2 ml/kg/hr Administer furosemide (Lasix) or mannitol as ordered to assure adequate urinary output Intensifies aminoglycoside toxicity and should be used with caution when administered concurrently
Salt or fluid retention, electrolyte depletion, hypertension, cushingoid appearance, increased appetite, obesity Hyperglycemia, diabetes Muscle weakness, osteoporosis Gastritis, gastric and peptic ulcers, gastrointestinal (GI) bleeding Immunosuppression, impaired wound healing Personality and mood changes Acne Growth retardation with long-term high dose use IT — sterile arachnoiditis	Decrease salt intake; protect from infection; observe for hyperglycemia To decrease or prevent GI upset, take with meals or snacks; may need to take with histamine H_2-receptor antagonist such as cimetidine, ranitidine May mask infection

Table continued on following page.

TABLE 4–6. *Table of Chemotherapeutic Agents* Continued

DRUG	CLASSIFICATION	ROUTE
Cyclophosphamide (Cytoxan, CTX)	Alkylating agent	IV push or infusion PO tablets May be difficult to dissolve when diluted Observe for any particulate matter Store at room temperature once reconstituted and discard in 24 hr Reconstitute with paraben-preserved diluent, not benzyl alcohol Oral liquid preparation may be made from parenteral solution mixed in aromatic elixir
Cytarabine (ARA-C, Cytosine Arabinoside, Cytosar-U)	Antimetabolite	IV, SQ, IM, IT Reconstituted solution is stable at room temperature for 48 hr May be diluted with 1–2 ml for SQ or IM use Do not use diluent that is packaged with drug for IT use because it contains benzyl alcohol
Dacarbazine (DTIC-Dome)	Alkylating agent	IV push, infusion
Dactinomycin (Actinomycin D, ACT-D, Cosmegen)	Antibiotic	IV push Golden colored Protect vial from light Vial contains 0.5 mg of drug; reconstitute with 1.1 ml sterile water without preservative to equal a concentration of 0.5 mg/ml; dose is usually ordered in micrograms
Daunomycin (daunorubicin, Cerubidine, Rubidomycin) *and* Doxorubicin (Adriamycin)	Anthracycline antibiotic	IV push or infusion Continuous infusion Red color

SIDE EFFECTS	SPECIAL CONSIDERATIONS
Hemorrhagic cystitis resulting from chemical irritation of bladder by metabolites of CTX N, V — may be severe, beginning 4–8 hr after administration and lasting 8–10 hr Leukopenia is dose-limiting, toxicity reaching nadir at 7–10 days; recovery in 14–24 days Syndrome of inappropriate antidiuretic hormone (SIADH; water intoxication) with seizures Alopecia Sterility related to dose and pubertal status Cardiac toxicity and pulmonary fibrosis — rare May be carcinogenic (second malignant neoplasms)	Maintain adequate hydration, urinary output, urinary specific gravity <1.010 before giving high dose; administer drug in morning or early afternoon Check urine for blood before, during, and after giving drug Encourage patient to urinate before going to bed for the night to empty bladder completely With high dose, maintain urinary output at 1500 ml/m^2/12 hr and measure q2h × 12 hr Furosemide may be given to maintain urinary output (0.5 mg/kg; maximum 40 mg IV)
A, N, V — may be severe at high doses or IT Myelosuppression with nadir of 7–14 days ARA-C syndrome — flulike symptoms, conjunctivitis, fever, maculopapular rash occurring 6–12 hr after administration Alopecia IT — headache, vomiting, pleocytosis; rare convulsions and paresis High-dose ARA-C regimens may result in severe myelosuppression lasting at least 28 days	Anticipate vomiting immediately or within 2 hr after IT dose Administer steroid eye drops to prevent conjunctivitis with high dose
Myelosuppression with nadir of 21–25 days N, V can be severe Diarrhea — rare Alopecia Flulike syndrome Facial flushing Facial paresthesias Erythematous and urticarial rashes — rare	**Irritant** — severe local pain and burning at injection site and along vein; thought caused by degradation of drug by light Slow infusion; apply cold pack to arm Drug extremely light sensitive Can cause tissue necrosis if drug is extravasated
Myelosuppression — nadir in 2–3 wk N, V — severe Diarrhea Alopecia Skin eruptions, acne Radiosensitizer causing recall phenomenon at prior radiation site Flare-up of erythema or increased pigmentation of previously irradiated skin	**Vesicant** — severe tissue damage if extravasation occurs Do not use with 0.2 μm filters Toxicity may be enhanced if liver damage is present, especially with concomitant radiation to or near liver
Myelosuppression with nadir of 10–14 days; recovery in approximately 1 wk after nadir N, V Alopecia Cardiomyopathy — total lifetime dose of 550 mg/m^2, less if cardiac radiation was given Hyperpigmentation of nailbeds	**Vesicant** — severe tissue damage if extravasation occurs Continuous infusions should be done through patent central line Erythematous streak up the vein of injection or hives at or near injection site

Table continued on following page.

TABLE 4–6. *Table of Chemotherapeutic Agents* Continued

DRUG	CLASSIFICATION	ROUTE
Etoposide (VP-16, VP-16–213, VePesid)	Plant alkaloid — semisynthetic derivative of podophyllotoxin	IV infusion to run over 30–60 min Do not refrigerate reconstituted solution PO — 50 mg capsules Capsules must be refrigerated
Fazarabine (ara-AC) Investigational	Antimetabolite	IV infusion
Fludarabine (Fludara)	Antimetabolite	IV infusion
5-Fluorouracil (5-FU, Fluorouracil, Adrucil)	Antimetabolite	IV push IV infusion PO (parenteral form may be given orally) Intrahepatic artery Protect from light Store at room temperature Clear, light yellow
Homoharringtonine (Cephalotaxine) Investigational	Plant alkaloid	IV — vial contains mannitol and hydrochloric acid to adjust pH Store intact vials in refrigerator (4°–8° C)
Hydroxyurea (Hydrea, HU, HUR)	Antimetabolite	PO 500 mg capsules Keep bottle tightly closed — moisture causes degradation of drug

SIDE EFFECTS	SPECIAL CONSIDERATIONS
Radiosensitizer — recall phenomenon at prior radiation or infiltration site Increased sensitivity to sunlight Stomatitis — may be severe	Cardiac studies with echocardiogram or multiple-gated arteriography (MUGA) scan should be done periodically to monitor cardiac function — must have acceptable cardiac ejection fraction Cardiac toxicity may be less with continuous infusions Urine may have red-orange tinge
Myelosuppression with nadir of 7–14 days and recovery by 10–16 days Hypersensitivity reactions, including bronchospasm, fever, erythema, pruritus N, V — mild Headache Neurotoxicity Alopecia Hypotension	**Irritant** — severe hypotension can occur with rapid infusion Look for precipitates in dextrose solutions
With 24-hr infusions, granulocytopenia and thrombocytopenia with nadirs between 12–19 days With 72-hr infusions, neutropenia with nadir in 3 wk N, V Headache, malaise Stomatitis	Unstable in aqueous solutions, so infusions of 3 hr or less can be diluted in Ringer's lactate solution; for >24-hr infusion, dilute in DMSO with slow injection through a side port into a 5% dextrose solution (DMSO has a pungent, garliclike smell, which will cause the breath and skin to exude this odor) Must be given through polyolefin-lined IV tubing
Leukopenia with nadir at day 8; thrombocytopenia with nadir at day 15 Neurotoxicity Pulmonary toxicity with interstitial pneumonitis	Must have adequate pulmonary function Monitor pulmonary function tests (PFTs)
Myelosuppression — leukopenia with nadir of 9–14 days; thrombocytopenia with nadir of 7–14 days N, V, D Stomatitis beginning in 5–8 days; can be severe Esophagitis Alopecia Dermatitis Hyperpigmentation of nail beds	For oral administration mix parenteral solution of 5-FU with flavored water or carbonated beverage; avoid acidic fruit juices Take on empty stomach (at least 2 hr before or after food)
Myelosuppression Severe lassitude N, V, D Alopecia Stomatitis Skin rash Hypotension Tachycardia or arrhythmias Hyperglycemia Increased liver enzymes, serum creatinine level	When given IV bolus, severe hypotension, often with tachycardia and cardiac arrhythmias, may occur May cause changes in mentation (e.g., confusion, agitation, depression) Data not available for compatibility with other agents
Myelosuppression with rapid drop in WBC N, V, D — mild Stomatitis Rash and/or facial erythema	Renal impairment enhances toxicity

Table continued on following page.

TABLE 4–6. *Table of Chemotherapeutic Agents* Continued

DRUG	CLASSIFICATION	ROUTE
Idarubicin, Idamycin	Anthracycline	IV slow push or infusion
Ifosfamide (isophospha-mide, IFEX)	Alkylating agent Analogue of cyclophospha-mide	IV infusion
Lomustine (CCNU) (CeeNU)	Nitrosourea	PO — 10, 40, 100 mg capsules
Mechlorethamine hydro-chloride (nitrogen mus-tard, Mustargen, HN$_2$)	Alkylating agent	IV push Diluted to concentration of 1 mg/ml Intracavitary use in presence of pleural, peritoneal, or pericardial effusion due to metastatic tumors
Melphalan (Alkeran, L-PAM) L-Sarcolysin Investigational in parenteral form	Alkylating agent	PO — 2 mg tablets IV agent available with diluent
Mercaptopurine (Purinethol, 6-MP)	Antimetabolite	PO — 50 mg tablets IV (investigational) IT (investigational)
Methotrexate (Amethop-terin, MTX)	Antimetabolite	PO — 2.5 mg tablets IV push or infusion IM IT (mix with preservative-free diluent)

SIDE EFFECTS	SPECIAL CONSIDERATIONS
See doxorubicin	**Vesicant** — severe tissue damage if extravasation occurs See doxorubicin Perhaps less cardiotoxicity than doxorubicin and daunorubicin
Myelosuppression with nadir in 7–10 days and recovery in 16–21 days Renal tubular damage (Fanconi's syndrome) Alopecia N, V — mild Mild, transient abnormal liver and renal function Encephalopathy Peripheral neuropathy	Risk of hemorrhagic cystitis if given without uroprotection from mesna (see Table 4–7) Can be mixed with mesna More severe symptoms may occur at higher doses and after rapid injection Must receive PO or IV hydration for 24 hr after dose Must monitor I&O and urinary specific gravity
Myelosuppression — delayed and persistent N, V 3–6 hr or longer after administration Alopecia Pulmonary fibrosis — rare Confusion, lethargy, ataxia	Take on empty stomach
Myelosuppression with nadir in 10–14 days Leukopenia can occur within 24 hr and thrombocytopenia at 6–8 days N, V — severe Sterility, infertility Hyperuricemia Rash Alopecia May cause second malignant neoplasm	**Vesicant** — can also cause skin irritation with local contact Use within 1 hr after reconstitution May cause thrombosis, phlebitis, and discoloration of vein
Severe myelosuppression with nadir in 14–21 days, lasting 5–6 wk Anorexia Alopecia Profuse diarrhea Dermatitis Stomatitis, mucositis IV — serious hypersensitivity reactions Pulmonary fibrosis	Infusion over 15–30 min Administer within 1 hr after reconstitution Take daily dose at one time Take on empty stomach Good hydration for 24 hr after dose Furosemide may be given to maintain urinary output
Hepatic dysfunction Atopic dermatitis Myelosuppression A, N, V — rare Stomatitis, mucositis Fever — rare	Reduce dose if given with allopurinol Take daily dose at one time, preferably at bedtime Avoid extravasation of IV form Hematuria and crystalluria may occur with high IV doses
Ulcerative stomatitis, glossitis, gingivitis N, V, A, D Myelosuppression Hepatic toxicity Malaise Rash Alopecia Arachnoiditis or leukoencephalopathy after IT use Renal failure (with high-dose administration)	Renal impairment will enhance toxicity Advise patients to use sun screen; severe sunburn can occur even with low weekly doses When intermediate or high-dose methotrexate is given, leucovorin is administered as ordered as a rescue agent (see Table 4–7) Take oral dose at one time

Table continued on following page.

TABLE 4–6. *Table of Chemotherapeutic Agents* Continued

DRUG	CLASSIFICATION	ROUTE
Mitoxantrone (Novantrone)	Anthracycline analogue	IV infusion Dark blue solution
Paclitaxel (Taxol)	Plant product isolated from the stem bark of the western yew, *Taxus brevifolia;* it enhances both the rate and the yield of microtubule assembly, inhibiting interphase and mitotic cellular functions	Supplied as a concentrated sterile solution, 6 mg/ml in 5 ml ampules, in 50% polyoxyethylated castor oil and 50% dehydrated alcohol; contents must be diluted as directed before use Intact ampules are kept dry and refrigerated until reconstituted Dilute paclitaxel to final concentration of 0.3 mg/ml–1.2 mg/ml, which is stable for 12 hr in D5W or normal saline solution All solutions exhibit a slight haze A small number of fibers (within acceptable levels of the USP Particulate Matter Test) have been observed after dilution
Piritrexim (PTX) Investigational	Antimetabolite	IV infusion PO
Procarbazine (Matulane) Investigational in parenteral form	Alkylating agent	PO — 50 mg capsules Keep bottle tightly closed; moisture causes decomposition IV — use immediately after reconstitution

SIDE EFFECTS	SPECIAL CONSIDERATIONS
Photosensitivity	Avoid vitamins containing folic acid in order not to bypass the metabolic block caused by methotrexate Many agents adversely interact with methotrexate (consult *Physicians' Desk Reference*)
N, V Cardiomyopathy Mucositis, stomatitis Myelosuppression with nadir in 7–14 days Transient elevations in liver enzymes Alopecia Radiation recall dermatitis	**Vesicant** — severe tissue damage if extravasation occurs Not recommended for patients who have received full doses of anthracyclines Monitor cardiac status Urine, serum, and sclera may appear green; bluish discoloration of veins and nails Phlebitis at injection site Do not give IV push
Acute hypersensitivity reactions characterized by cutaneous flushing, bronchospasm, tachypnea, bradycardia, hypotension within minutes of administration secondary to dilution vehicles Myelosuppression with white blood count nadir at 10 days and normalization within 18 days Sensory neuropathy Mucositis and ulcerations occurring on day 3–7 and resolving within 5–7 days Joint discomforts and myalgias occurring 2–3 days after administration and resolving within 4–7 days Alopecia Bradycardia N, V during infusion Diarrhea occurring within 1 week after infusion	Premedicate with corticosteroids, H_1 and H_2 antagonists, diphenhydramine, ranitidine Monitor patient frequently — may need cardiac monitor, pulse oximetry Slow continuous IV infusion decreases risk of serious anaphylactic reactions 0.2 μm inline filters must be used Solutions exhibiting excessive particulate formation should not be used PVC bags and sets should be avoided
Leukopenia and thrombocytopenia with nadir at day 8 Mucositis Skin rashes Phlebitis N, V, D with oral dosing Liver function abnormalities with oral dosing	**Irritant** — must have central venous access for continuous infusions to decrease phlebitis Oral doses may be given on a divided-dose schedule to decrease GI toxicity
Myelosuppression — protracted nadir for thrombocytopenia at 4 wk Stomatitis A, N, V, D Alopecia Rash, pruritus Azoospermia; cessation of menses Myalgia, flulike syndrome CNS reactions — headache, paralysis, nervousness, nightmares, dizziness, hallucinations, confusion, coma, or convulsions May induce second malignant neoplasms	Hypertension and/or central nervous system (CNS) depression may occur in the presence of alcohol, monoamine oxidase (MAO) inhibitors, phenothiazines, phenytoin (Dilantin), tricyclic antidepressants, barbiturates, and tyramine-rich foods such as aged cheese, wine, bananas, yogurt, chocolate

Table continued on following page.

TABLE 4–6. *Table of Chemotherapeutic Agents* Continued

DRUG	CLASSIFICATION	ROUTE
Retinoic acid (13-cis-retinoic acid, Isotretinoin, Accutane) All-trans retinoic acid are investigational	Vitamin A and its derivatives Stimulate clonal proliferation of erythroid and myeloid progenitor cells and play a role in growth, reproduction, epithelial cell differentiation, and immune function; functions as a maturation agent in diseases such as neuroblastoma, rhabdomyosarcoma, acute promyelocytic leukemia (APL), and osteosarcoma	Accutane commercially available as soft gelatin capsules in 10 mg, 20 mg, 40 mg sizes Store at room temperature in light-resistant container
Teniposide (VM-26)	Plant alkaloid Epipodophyllotoxin	IV infusion over 60 min
Thioguanine (6-thioguanine, 6-TG)	Antimetabolite	PO — 40 mg tablets IV — investigational in parenteral form
Thiotepa (Triethylene thiophosphoramide, TESPA)	Alkylating agent	IV infusion IT IM SQ Intracavitary Intratumor
Vinblastine (Velban, VBL)	Plant alkaloid	IV push Reconstituted to concentration of 1 mg/ml Stable for 4 wk in refrigerator
Vincristine (Oncovin)	Plant alkaloid	IV push 1 mg/ml

A = anorexia, N = nausea, V = vomiting, D = diarrhea.

SIDE EFFECTS	SPECIAL CONSIDERATIONS
Adverse mucocutaneous effects, primarily cheilitis, xerosis, and conjunctivitis Hypertriglyceridemia Transient increase in gamma-glutamyl transferase (GGT), serum glutamic oxaloacetic transaminase (SGOT), serum glutamic pyruvac transaminase (SGPT) May produce birth malformations and **should not** be administered during pregnancy or to women who may become pregnant while undergoing treatment	Capsules can be swallowed directly or opened with a large needle and contents mixed with food
Allergic reactions Myelosuppression with nadir in 3–14 days Hypotension with rapid infusions Chemical phlebitis Fever, chills Alopecia	**Irritant** — avoid extravasation Anaphylaxis with rapid infusions May appear "oily" or foamy when mixed, but this effect disappears quickly
Myelosuppression A, N, V, D — mild Hepatic toxicity Atopic dermatitis Stomatitis	Take oral dose at one time Refrigerate after IV reconstitution; precipitate will form if stored at room temperature
Myelosuppression N, V Dizziness, headache Stomatitis Pain at injection site Alopecia Rash	Reconstitute to hypertonic or isotonic solution; avoid acidic diluents Solution must be clear — discard otherwise Do not use with succinylcholine
Myelosuppression Stomatitis Alopecia A, N, D or constipation Neurotoxicity — loss of deep tendon reflexes, paresthesias, peripheral neuropathy, hoarseness, ptosis, double vision	**Vesicant** — severe tissue damage if extravasation occurs Administer stool softeners; increase bulk and fiber in diet
Minimal myelosuppression Alopecia SIADH Peripheral neuropathies such as numbness and tingling of distal extremities, myalgias, cramping, foot drop, jaw pain, seizures, constipation, paralytic ileus, ptosis, vocal cord paralysis, cranial nerve palsies, absent deep tendon reflexes	**Vesicant** — severe tissue damage if extravasation occurs Stool softeners may be given prophylactically or for constipation Liver dysfunction may enhance toxicity Infants may have difficulty sucking because of jaw pain Maximal single dose: 2 mg regardless of body surface area (BSA)

TABLE 4–7. *Miscellaneous Agents**

DRUG	USE	ROUTE	SIDE EFFECTS	NURSING CONSIDERATIONS
Allopurinol (Zyloprim)	Enzyme inhibitor; blocks uric acid production by inhibiting xanthine oxidase	PO—100 mg and 300 mg tablets IV—500 mg vials Parental use investigational	Liver function abnormalities, pruritic maculopapular rash, anorexia; nausea Fever	Dose may need alteration when administered with 6-MP, azathioprine, cyclophosphamide, warfarin, oral antidiabetic drugs, ampicillin, amoxicillin, thiazide diuretics Adequate hydration Physically incompatible with methotrexate—do not give in same IV fluid
Trimethoprim (TMP) and sulfamethoxazole (SMZ) (Bactrim, Septra)	Antibiotic used prophylactically to prevent *Pneumocystis carinii* pneumonia	PO—80 or 160 mg tablets TMP or 400 or 800 mg tablets SMZ 40 mg TMP/ 200 mg SMZ in 5 ml suspension IV	Myelosuppression Anorexia, nausea, vomiting, diarrhea GI upset Hepatic dysfunction Rash, Stevens-Johnson syndrome	May be given as prophylaxis for *P. carinii* on a schedule of 3 consecutive days weekly Must be diluted in D5W solution for IV administration; infuse parenteral solution over 60–90 min; monitor for hyponatremia Not compatible with other drugs in IV solution
Leucovorin calcium (Citrovorum Factor, Folinic Acid)	Vitamin Bypasses the inhibitor action of folic acid antagonist (methotrexate)	PO IV IM	Rash, pruritus, erythema Nausea, vomiting Allergic sensitization	Used as cellular rescue when intermediate or high-dose methotrexate is given May be given as a single dose after IT methotrexate, especially if patient is neutropenic Must be given exactly at the times ordered
Mesna (Mesnex)	Uroprotecting agent Prevents hemorrhagic cystitis	IV push IV infusion IV form may be given PO	Nausea, vomiting, diarrhea Skin hypersensitivity Abdominal pain Headache Limb and joint pain Lethargy Transient hypotension	False positive test for urinary ketones Not compatible with cisplatin May be mixed with cyclophosphamide or ifosfamide Must be given exactly at the times ordered

*These drugs are not chemotherapeutic agents but are commonly used as an adjunct in the management of the child with cancer.

Hair elsewhere on the body is not as long and hence has a shorter growth phase. Body hair may not be affected as greatly by chemotherapy as scalp hair, although loss of eyebrows, eyelashes, pubic hair, and other body hair is not uncommon.

There are various methods to decrease hair loss such as applying scalp tourniquets or ice bags during the administration of chemotherapy. These methods cause vasoconstriction to the scalp and thereby prevent the drugs' reaching hair follicles. These practices are controversial because some clinicians believe the methods provide a sanctuary site for cancer cells if the drugs are prevented from reaching all parts of the head.[8]

CLINICAL TRIALS

In 1955 the NCI undertook a national effort to develop new, effective, and less toxic anticancer drugs.[2] The process for developing new drugs can take 10 to 12 years, beginning with the acquisition of the agent, testing in animals and then in humans, and the final marketing of the drug by pharmaceutical companies.

Initially drugs are screened for in vitro activity against tumor cell lines. Once a compound is judged as active in the tumor panel, toxicology studies are performed in several animal species to ascertain its toxic effects and to help determine a safe dose for humans.[24] Only one or two agents out of 15,000 per year complete the testing procedures and are released for use in humans.

The initial stage of human testing is called a phase I trial. It is designed to determine the maximal tolerated dose (MTD) of the drug in humans, to determine qualitatively the types of toxicities that may occur, and to study the clinical pharmacology of the agent. Phase I testing is performed in a small group of patients (15 to 30) with refractory cancer and is not intended to determine the therapeutic effect of the agent. There are separate phase I trials in adult and pediatric populations.[2]

A phase II trial is undertaken after the optimal dose and scheduling have been determined. Phase II trials define the spectrum of activity and response rate in various cancers. Patients who have been heavily treated for cancer usually are not candidates for phase II trials because they are likely to have resistant tumors.

Once efficacy has been established for a drug, it is moved into frontline therapeutic protocols for use in newly diagnosed patients. These phase III trials compare new therapy to standard therapeutic designs. This comparison usually is done in a random fashion.

In pediatrics the majority of testing of new therapeutic protocols has been performed in national collaborative groups—the Pediatric Oncology Group (POG) and the Childrens Cancer Group (CCG). These groups provide organized research efforts to advance the body of knowledge about childhood cancer and its treatment. It is through these efforts that many childhood cancers potentially are curable.[30,39] The collaboration within pediatrics provides the foundation for cancer research and clinical trial development for adults with cancer.

It is mandatory when entering a patient on a clinical trial that informed consent be obtained. The process of obtaining informed consent varies, depending on institutional policy.

DRUG ADMINISTRATION

Chemotherapeutic agents most commonly are administered by nurses, although recently the use of central lines in children has made it possible for parents to administer chemotherapy at home.

Dosage Calculation

Chemotherapy doses usually are computed according to body surface area (BSA), which is calculated using the child's height (in centimeters) and weight (in kilograms), as plotted on a nomogram. This calculation determines the surface area (SA) or square meters (m^2) of the child. The dose is calculated using a "mg/m^2" formula.

The dose can be calculated for children under the age of 12 months or who weigh 10 kg or less by using a milligrams per kilogram formula rather than a SA formula. Some protocols decrease doses for these infants by 50% of the regular dose.

Dosage for intrathecal and intraommaya therapy is based on age because the volume of CSF is a known quantity according to the age of the individual. Spinal fluid volume is proportionally much larger in infants and young children, reaching adult volume by the age of 3 years. Therefore a dose based on BSA might underdose a young child and overdose an adolescent.[5]

If there has been a severe toxicity from prior treatment, the dose of the offending agent may be adjusted to prevent or minimize recurrence of the toxicity.

Some agents are radiosensitizers such as dactinomycin and doxorubicin and require dose reductions during concomitant radiotherapy. Agents that have cumulative toxicities such as bleomycin and doxorubicin have maximal lifetime dose restrictions (see Table 4–6).

To assure accuracy when determining the dose of chemotherapy, two persons should calculate the SA and the dose. These values should be recalculated before every phase or course of therapy since significant changes in weight may occur during the course of treatment.

EXTRAVASATION

Some chemotherapeutic agents are vesicants and can cause tissue damage if not administered directly into the vein (Table 4–8). The degree of tissue damage apparently is related to the concentration and quantity of the drug extravasated. There is no apparent relationship between degree of damage and dose of the drug. The symptoms and appearance of an area in which a vesicant or irritant has been extravasated can range from hyperpigmentation, burning, erythema, or inflammation to ulceration, necrosis, prolonged pain, tissue sloughing, infection, or loss of mobility.[8]

There is no general consensus about the management of local tissue toxicity after extravasation.[50] Table 4–9 summarizes some of the antidotes and methods used. Below are some guidelines for treatment.

1. Prevention is the best way to avoid toxicity from extravasation of drugs. Careful administration by persons skilled in IV therapy helps to prevent serious complications.

2. Some chemotherapeutic agents have an antidote identified that can be infused through the needle and infiltrated into the surrounding tissues. If an extravasation antidote will be given, as much residual drug as possible must be aspirated from the needle and tubing before administering the antidote.

3. Notify the physician immediately if there is a definite or suspected extravasation. It may be necessary for a plastic surgeon to consult for a serious extravasation.

4. An extravasation kit, which contains agents used as antidotes, may be available on the unit where chemotherapeutic agents are administered.

Agents that can cause less severe reactions if infiltrated are known as *irritants*. Their reactions can range from redness to burning or inflammation at the injection site.

DRUG DELIVERY SYSTEMS

There are several new methods for the delivery of chemotherapeutic agents. They have been developed to maximize the effectiveness of the agents while minimizing toxicity. The

TABLE 4–8. *Vesicant and Irritant Chemotherapeutic Agents*

VESICANT AGENTS	IRRITANT AGENTS
Acridinyl anisidide (AMSA)	Carmustine (BCNU)
Dactinomycin (Actinomycin D)	Dacarbazine (DTIC)
Daunorubicin (daunomycin)	Etoposide (VP-16)
Doxorubicin (Adriamycin)	Piritrexim
Idarubicin (Idamycin)	Teniposide (VM-26)
Mechlorethamine (nitrogen mustard)	
Mitoxantrone (Novantrone)	
Vinblastine (Velban)	
Vincristine (Oncovin)	

TABLE 4–9. *Local Antidotes for Chemotherapy Extravasation*

CATEGORY OF AGENT	ANTIDOTE	COMMENTS
Anthracyclines	Dimethyl sulfoxide (DMSO)	Elevate extremity and apply ice for 15 min Rest extremity for 24–48 hr Apply DMSO topically to large area around site q6h for 14 days
Vinca alkaloids	Hyaluronidase	Apply heat Administer local, liberal injection of hyaluronidase into extravasation site
Nitrogen mustard	Thiosulfate	Inject into extravasation site in excess of amount of nitrogen mustard extravasated

Data from references 4 and 50.

following discussion is an overview of the existing drug delivery systems in use today.

Ommaya Reservoir

The Ommaya reservoir was developed in the early 1960s by a neurosurgeon, A.K. Ommaya.[46] It is a hollow-domed, self-sealing silicone reservoir with a catheter attached, which allows access to the CSF. Figure 4–2 depicts the placement of the Ommaya reservoir in the lateral ventricle.

Before accessing the reservoir, the patient's head is shaved over the reservoir, the skin is cleaned with povidone-iodine, and aseptic technique is maintained. A small-gauged needle is inserted into the reservoir, and a quantity of CSF is removed equal to the amount of chemotherapy to be instilled. Then the reservoir is pumped with the fingertip to distribute the drug directly into the ventricles. The reservoir is easy to access, eliminates the need for repeated lumbar punctures, and affords a much better distribution of drug.[15,29]

Potential complications of the Ommaya reservoir are infection and failure of the device to function. Postoperatively the site must be monitored closely for signs of infection. Once the incision has healed, the child's hair can be shampooed on a regular basis to decrease the chance of infection. Inability to withdraw CSF or insert medication indicates failure of the reservoir.

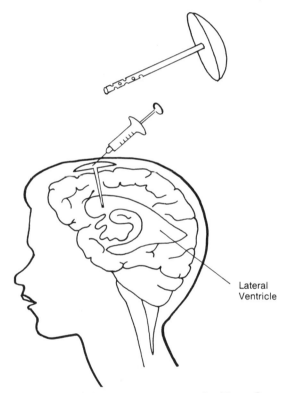

Lateral Ventricle

FIGURE 4–2. The Ommaya reservoir. (*From Cornwell CM. The Ommaya reservoir: Implications for pediatric oncology. Pediatr Nurs 1990; 16:249. Used with permission of publisher, Anthony J. Jannetti, Inc.*)

Implantable Pump

Implantable pumps are designed to provide continuous or bolus chemotherapy infusions, maximal portability, and protection against infection. They are used for intraperitoneal, intracavitary, or intra-arterial infusions. These pumps have a power source, which operates either by an equilibrium between an internal fluorocarbon liquid and the agent for delivery or by a battery with an expected life of approximately 2 years. They can be programmed to deliver a drug by continuous or bolus infusion and can be refilled easily.

The pump consists of a drug-filled chamber, an outlet catheter, a power source, and a rubber septum for access. The pump is placed in a subcutaneous pocket in either the lower abdominal wall or the upper chest. It is sutured into the pocket and situated so that the incision is not directly over the septum. The catheter is sutured in place to prevent migration or displacement.

To access the device, the septum is palpated and the area prepared using aseptic technique. Depending on the device, either a Huber needle or a straight needle is used to access the pump and to refill it.

There is a risk of extravasation of vesicant agents. The nurse must educate the patient and family to notify the health care provider if there are signs of infection, fever, pain, and/or leakage at the incision site.

These pumps allow the patient to continue with daily activities with minimal limitations. The patient should avoid both situations that raise the body temperature and contact sports or activities that involve a change in atmospheric pressure.[7] The implantable pump provides comfort for the patient and because it is not visible, allows the patient to continue with a normal life-style.

Ambulatory Infusion Pumps

Several small, portable infusion pumps are available to deliver continuous infusions with or without bolus therapy to the ambulatory patient. They are easy for patients and family members to use, lightweight, portable, and concealable, thus enabling the patient to continue with normal activities and remain an outpatient.[41,47]

The method of venous access, the drug, the patient and family's ability to participate, and third-party reimbursement are considered in deciding if a patient is a candidate for home infusions.[25]

If the agent is a vesicant, central venous access is mandatory for home infusion therapy. However, nonvesicant drugs such as cytosine arabinoside may be given through a peripheral IV site. If infiltration occurs, the infusion can be stopped, and there will be relatively little harm to the tissue from the infiltrate.

NURSING CARE OF THE CHILD RECEIVING CHEMOTHERAPY

Many other people are involved in the care of the child with cancer. Among them are siblings, grandparents, extended family members, teachers, school nurses, and primary care physicians. They may need education about the treatment and associated side effects.

Many chemotherapeutic agents are available only for oral administration. It may be necessary for the nurse and family to find creative methods for giving oral medications to children. Table 4–10 describes problems and approaches in oral administration of chemotherapeutic agents.[38]

When liquids are given, the dose should be measured in a liquid medication measuring device available from local pharmacies. Also available are crushing devices and pill "scissors" to divide scored tablets accurately.

It may be necessary to watch older children take their medications. Nonadherence to treatment among older children and adolescents is a complex issue. These are the years when it is important for the child to develop independence and to be like peers. They may find the side effects so unpleasant that they do not take their medications.[10,45] Blood assays can be performed to determine if certain medications are being taken, but open discussion with the child and family of the child with suspected nonadherence may produce the same result.

Caution is necessary with all medications, supplies, and equipment at home. Medications, needles, and syringes must be stored in a locked box and kept out of reach. Children must never be told that their medication is candy.

TABLE 4–10. *Guidelines for Administration of Oral Chemotherapy to Children*

PROBLEM	APPROACH
Administering oral drug to a child who cannot swallow	Do not use a medication that has an unpleasant taste (e.g., prednisone) to teach child to swallow a tablet.
Tablets	Some tablets may be chewed—consult pharmacist.
	Enteric-coated tablets should not be chewed, broken, or crushed.
	Crush tablet into fine powder and dissolve in warm water; mix solution with small amount of juice or food acceptable to child (e.g., ice cream, applesauce); child must take all to receive total dose.
Capsules	Open capsule (e.g., CCNU, hydroxyurea) and sprinkle contents into food.
	Not all capsules should be opened—consult pharmacist.
Administering liquid chemotherapy to an infant or very young child	Place liquid in empty nipple; place nipple in infant's mouth, and allow child to suck.
	Draw medication up into syringe, place along inside of cheek, and administer slowly.
	Raise child's head slightly during administration to avoid aspiration.
Administering medication with an unpleasant taste (e.g., prednisone)	Discourage chewing of tablets.
	Mix crushed tablet in small amount of juice or food with strong or sweet taste or in sticky food (e.g., peanut butter, maple syrup, fruit roll); child must take all to receive total dose.
	Do not mix with essential food items (e.g., milk, cereal).
Administering partial doses	Crush pills and place in gelatin capsule.
	Break scored tablets only (refer to text).
	Pharmacy will crush tablets and dispense in unit-dose packages.
Administering oral medications to promote drug absorption	Notify physician if child vomits after oral administration of medication; may be necessary to repeat drug.
	Control vomiting with antiemetics.
	With single doses, administer all tablets at one time to achieve maximal blood levels.
	Some medications should be given between meals on an empty stomach—consult pharmacist.

Modified from Meeske K, Ruccione KS. Cancer chemotherapy in children: Nursing issues and approaches. Semin Oncol Nurs 1987; 3:118–127.

When administering chemotherapy, explain the procedures, the agents, and the expected potential side effects. Present all of the information to the child at an age-appropriate level and repeat as necessary. Children cooperate more fully if they are included in the discussions about their care. It may be necessary to provide a strategy involving rewards for appropriate behaviors.

SAFE DRUG HANDLING[1]

Concern has been growing about the safe handling of chemotherapeutic agents. Research has shown that many agents are capable of causing carcinogenic, mutagenic, and teratogenic effects in animals and humans.[40] Mutagenic activity can be detected in urine for 2 days after administration of single agents and for at least 5 days after multiagent chemotherapy.[36] Further research is necessary to determine the implications of administration of these agents.

The Occupational Safety and Health Administration (OSHA) has developed guidelines to protect workers from undue exposures to cytotoxic agents.[52] The main concern is to decrease exposure through inhalation, absorption, and ingestion of these agents. It is also inherent in the guidelines that all persons at risk for contact be educated in the safe handling of these agents.[28,40]

Preparation

The first recommendation is the use of a class II, type A, vertical air flow biologic safety cabinet (BSC) when reconstituting, mixing, or drawing up chemotherapeutic agents. The person preparing the drug wears nonpowdered, surgical latex gloves and a back-closing or closed-front protective gown with long sleeves and elastic or cuffed wristbands. The gloves are pulled over the cuffs.

If mixing must be performed without a BSC, it must be done in a vented room away from drafts and ceiling fans to prevent aerosolization. A plastic face shield or splash goggles are worn, and hydrophobic filter needles should be used to prevent solution from back-spraying. Ampules are broken with a sterile gauze or alcohol pad covering the neck.

The preparation area should be away from traffic and distractions. Eating, drinking, and smoking in the area are prohibited. Plastic-backed absorbent pads are used to cover the work surface.

All preparation is done using aseptic technique. It is necessary to label the prepared agents as chemotherapy so that proper handling and disposal will be followed.

Individuals who administer the drugs should wear gowns and gloves as noted above. If tubing is not primed within the BSC, the end of the tubing should be placed in a sealable plastic bag with a sterile gauze to catch any fluid. The end of the tubing is wiped with alcohol to remove any drug. All tubing and syringes must have Luer-lok connections to prevent accidental disconnection. A plastic-backed absorbent pad is placed under the tubing during administration to catch any leakage.

Disposal

Everything that comes in contact with cytotoxic agents is considered hazardous waste and must be disposed of in the recommended manner. Included are containers, tubing, syringes, needles, bottles, bags, gloves, gowns, masks, protective pads, and body excretions (urine, feces, emesis) from the individual receiving the drugs. Syringes, needles, IV tubing, bottles, and bags should be discarded intact; they should not be disconnected from each other. Maximal protection should be given to all personnel, parents, family members, and the environment.

Sealable plastic- or wire-tie bags are used for all disposable materials and are labeled "Cytotoxic Waste" or "Hazardous Waste." Needles, syringes, ampules, and other breakable items are disposed of in a puncture-proof, labeled box. Never clip or recap needles because of the risk of aerosolization into the environment or accidental needle puncture.

Linens and clothing contaminated with chemotherapy or body excreta from a patient who has received chemotherapy are handled with gloves and disposable gown and disposed of as hazardous waste. If they are wet, they are placed in impenetrable, waterproof bags to protect all other personnel who come in contact with dirty linen.

Gloves should be worn when changing diapers or assisting with urinals, bedpans, and emesis basins for up to 48 hours after the patient has received chemotherapy. The excreta is flushed in the toilet. The containers are placed in sealable plastic bags and labeled properly.

Spills

Cytotoxic spills and breaks must be cleaned up immediately. The area of the spill is identified to protect others from exposure. For a large spill, absorbent sheets or pads are placed on the spill to cover and contain it completely. Powder spills are covered with moist towels. Protective apparel should be worn by personnel handling the spill. The area must be thoroughly cleaned, and all contaminated materials must be disposed of as hazardous waste.

Family Teaching

Parents must be taught safety procedures for administering chemotherapy at home and for disposal of contaminated equipment, supplies, and excreta. Precautions must be taken for 48 hours after single-agent administration and 5 days after multiagent chemotherapy. Arrangements must be made for the disposal of waste containers. This information must be incorporated into family teaching to avoid unnecessary cytotoxic exposures.

Reproductive Issues in Handling Chemotherapy

There is no general agreement regarding the handling of cytotoxic agents by the pregnant or lactating woman or by females and males of childbearing years. OSHA believes it is reasonable to assume that if appropriate procedures are followed, risks are minimized. They also suggest that if a staff member requests no involvement in handling these agents, the nurse can negotiate with the institution for transfer to another area. This action must be consistent with the policies and procedures of individual institutions.

REFERENCES

1. Association of Pediatric Oncology Nurses. Cancer Chemotherapy. Richmond, Va.: Association of Pediatric Oncology Nurses, 1990.
2. Balis FM, Holcenberg JS, Poplack DG. General principles of chemotherapy. In Pizzo PA, Poplack DG (eds): Principles and Practice of Pediatric Oncology, 2nd ed. Philadelphia: JB Lippincott, 1993, pp 197–245.
3. Bertino JR, O'Keefe P. Barriers and strategies for effective chemotherapy. Semin Oncol Nurs 1992; 8: 77–82.
4. Betcher D. Local toxicities of chemotherapy. J Assoc Pediatr Oncol Nurs 1987, 4.56–60.
5. Bleyer WA, Dedrick RL. The clinical pharmacology of intrathecal methotrexate. 1. Distribution kinetics in nontoxic patients after lumbar injection. Cancer Treat Rep 1977; 61:703–708.
6. Borison HL, McCarthy LE. Neuropharmacology of chemotherapy-induced emesis. Drugs 1983; 25(suppl 1):8–17.
7. Brown JK, Hogan CM. Chemotherapy. In Groenwald SL, Frogge MH, Goodman M, et al. (eds): Cancer Nursing. Principles and Practice, 2nd ed. Boston: Jones & Bartlett Publishers, 1990, pp 230–283.
8. Burke MB, Wilkes GM, Berg D, et al. Cancer Chemotherapy: A Nursing Process Approach. Boston: Jones & Bartlett Publishers, 1991.
9. Chabner BA. Clinical strategies for cancer treatment: The role of drugs. In Chabner BA, Collins JM (eds): Cancer Chemotherapy: Principles and Practice. Philadelphia: JB Lippincott, 1990, pp 1–15.
10. Cohen DG. Treatment refusal in adolescents. Semin Oncol Nurs 1986; 2:112–116.
11. Collins JM. The principles of pharmacokinetics in cancer patients. In American Society of Clinical Oncology Educational Book. 28th Annual Meeting, San Diego, Calif. May 1992, pp 88–91.
12. Collins JM. Pharmacokinetics and clinical monitoring. In Chabner BA, Collins JM (eds): Cancer Chemotherapy: Principles and Practice. Philadelphia: JB Lippincott, 1990.
13. Cotanch P. Relaxation training for control of nausea and vomiting in patients receiving chemotherapy. Cancer Nurs 1983; 277–283.
14. Cotanch P, Hockenberry M, Herman S. Self-hypnosis as antiemetic therapy in children receiving chemotherapy. Oncol Nurs Forum 1985; 12:41–46.
15. Cornwell CM. The Ommaya reservoir: Implication for pediatric oncology. Pediatr Nurs 1990; 16:249–251.
16. Dalton WS, Miller TP. Multidrug resistance. Principles Pract Oncol Updates 1991; 5:1–13.
17. Deisseroth A, Wallerstein R. Use of blood and blood products. In DeVita VT, Hellman S, Rosenberg SA (eds): Cancer. Principles & Practice of Oncology, 3rd ed. Philadelphia: JB Lippincott, 1989, p 2045–2059.
18. DeVita VT. Principles of chemotherapy. In DeVita VT, Hellman S, Rosenburg SA (eds): Cancer. Principles & Practice of Oncology, 3rd ed. Philadelphia: JB Lippincott, 1989, pp 276–300.
19. DiJulio J. Hematopoiesis: An overview. Oncol Nurs Forum 1991; Suppl 18:3–6.
20. Dorr RT, Fritz WL. Cancer Chemotherapy Handbook. New York: Elsevier, 1980.
21. Egan AP, Taggart JR, Bender CM. Management of chemotherapy-related nausea and vomiting using a serotonin antagonist. Oncol Nurs Forum 1992; 19:791–795.
22. Fischer DS, Knobf MT. The Cancer Chemotherapy Handbook, 3rd ed. Littleton, Mass.: Year Book Medical Publishers, 1989.
23. Fochtman D, Foley G. Nursing Care of the Child With Cancer. Boston: Little Brown & Co, 1982.
23a. Fresfeld AG, Hawthorne JW, Pizzo PA: Infectious complications in the pediatric cancer patient. In Pizzo PA, Poplack DG (eds): Principles and Practice of Pediatric Oncology, 2nd ed. Philadelphia: JB Lippincott, 1993, pp 987–1019.

24. Galassi A. The next generation: New chemotherapy agents for the 1990s. Semin Oncol Nurs 1992; 8: 83–94.

25. Garvey EC. Current and future nursing issues in the home administration of chemotherapy. Semin Oncol Nurs 1987; 3:142–147.

26. Goldie JH. Drug resistance. In Perry MC (ed): The Chemotherapy Source Book. Baltimore: Williams & Wilkins, 1992, pp 54–66.

27. Goldie JH, Coldman AJ. A mathematic model for relating the drug sensitivity of tumors to their spontaneous mutation rate. Cancer Treatment Rep 1979; 63:1727–1731.

28. Gullo SM. Safe handling of antineoplastic drugs: Translating the recommendations into practice. Oncol Nurs Forum 1988; 15:595–601.

29. Hagle ME. Implantable devices for chemotherapy: Access and delivery. Semin Oncol Nurs 1987; 3: 96–105.

30. Hammond GD. Keynote address: The cure of childhood cancers. Cancer 1986; 58(suppl):407–413.

31. Deleted.

32. Hockenberry MJ. Relaxation techniques in children with cancer: The nurse's role. J Assoc Pediatr Oncol Nurs 1988; 5:7–11.

33. Hockenberry-Eaton M, Benner A. Patterns of nausea and vomiting in children: Nursing assessment and intervention. Oncol Nurs Forum 1990; 17:575–584.

34. Israel MA. Cancer cell biology. In Pizzo PA, Poplack DG (eds): Principles and Practice of Pediatric Oncology, 2nd ed. Philadelphia: JB Lippincott, 1993, pp 57–80.

35. Lind J. Tumor cell growth and cell kinetics. Semin Oncol Nurs 1992; 8:3–9.

36. Maniar AC, Williams TW, Hammond GW, et al. Excretion of mutagens following chemotherapy. Am J Pediatr Hematol Oncol 1991; 13:160–163.

37. Maxwell MB, Maher KE. Chemotherapy-induced myelosuppression. Semin Oncol Nurs 1992; 8: 113–123.

38. Meeske K, Ruccione KS. Cancer chemotherapy in children: Nursing issues and approaches. Semin Oncol Nurs 1987; 3:118–127.

39. Miller RW, McKay FW. Decline in US childhood cancer mortality. JAMA 1984; 251:1567–1570.

40. Miller SA. Issues in cytotoxic drug handling safety. Semin Oncol Nurs 1987; 3:133–141.

41. Mioduszewski J, Zarbo AG. Ambulatory infusion pumps: A practical view at an alternative approach. Semin Oncol Nurs 1987; 3:106–111.

42. Mitchell EP, Schein PS. Gastrointestinal toxicity of chemotherapeutic agents. In Perry MC (ed): The Chemotherapy Source Book. Baltimore: Williams & Wilkins, 1992, pp 620–634.

43. Norton L. The Norton-Simon hypothesis. In Perry MC (ed): The Chemotherapy Source Book. Baltimore: Williams & Wilkins, 1992, pp 36–53.

44. Norton L, Simon R. New thoughts on the relationship of tumor growth characteristics to sensitivity to treatment. Methods Cancer Res 1979; 17:53–90.

45. Olson R, Kaufman D, Ware L, et al. Compliance with treatment regimens. Semin Oncol Nurs 1986; 2: 104–111.

46. Ommaya AK. Subcutaneous reservoir and pump for sterile access to ventricular cerebrospinal fluid. Lancet 1963; 2:983–984.

47. Pasut B. Home administration of medications in pediatric oncology patients: Use of the Travenol infusor. J Pediatr Oncol Nurs 1989; 6:139–142.

48. Ratain MJ. Important aspects of pharmacodynamics and pharmacogenetics: Considerations for use of cytotoxics. In American Society of Clinical Oncology Educational Book. 28th Annual Meeting, San Diego, Calif. May 1992, pp 92–95.

49. Ratain MJ, Schilsky RL. Principles of pharmacology and pharmacokinetics. In Perry MC (ed): The Chemotherapy Source Book. Baltimore: Williams & Wilkins, 1992, pp 22–35.

50. Rudolph R, Larson DL. Etiology and treatment of chemotherapeutic agent extravasation injuries: A review. J Clin Oncol 1987; 5:1116–1126.

51. Sonis ST. Oral complications of cancer therapy. In DeVita VT, Hellman S, Rosenburg SA (eds): Cancer. Principles & Practice of Oncology, 3rd ed. Philadelphia: JB Lippincott, 1989, pp 2144–2152.

52. U.S. Department of Labor, Office of Occupational Medicine: Occupational Safety and Health Administration. Work practice guidelines for personnel dealing with cytotoxic (antineoplastic) drugs. Publication No. 8-1.1. U.S. Printing Office, 1986.

53. Vietti TJ. Cellular kinetics and cancer chemotherapy. In Fernbach DJ, Vietti TJ (eds): Clinical Pediatric Oncology, 4th ed. St. Louis: Mosby–Year Book, 1991, pp 173–212.

54. Wickham R. Managing chemotherapy-related nausea and vomiting: The state of the art. Oncol Nurs Forum 1989; 16:563–574.

55. Wujcik D. Current research in side effects of high-dose chemotherapy. Semin Oncol Nurs 1992; 8: 102–112.

56. Zeltzer L, LeBaron S, Zeltzer PM. The effectiveness of behavioral intervention for reduction of nausea and vomiting in children and adolescents receiving chemotherapy. J Clin Oncol 1984; 2:683–690.

RADIATION THERAPY

Patsy McGuire

Radiation as a therapeutic modality originated with the discovery of x-rays by Roentgen, a German physicist, in 1895. Shortly thereafter, Becquerel, a French physician, produced dermatitis on himself by carrying radium in his pocket. The element radium was subsequently successfully isolated by Marie and Pierre Curie in 1898. Interest in the area of radiation sparked many early, somewhat uncontrolled experiments. Emil Grubbe, a medical student in Chicago, for example, persisted in exposing his hand to x-ray cathode tubes until he developed a skin reaction similar to that experienced by Becquerel. In the early decades of the twentieth century, radiation was used in the treatment of benign conditions such as thyrotoxicosis, rheumatism, herpes, and gout.[25] The first successful use of radiation as a therapeutic modality for cancer was reported in 1898 in the treatment of a patient with basal cell carcinoma.[16,22,28]

Initially the therapeutic benefit of radiation was hindered by many scientific and technical factors. For several decades treatments were administered in a single large fraction that delivered the entire dose to the surface of the skin, often producing severe and life-threatening reactions. Superficial tumors such as skin lesions responded to this treatment. The technology of the day, however, was limited in the therapeutic usefulness of radiation for the treatment of deepseated tumors to avoid unacceptable and often irreversible toxicity.

The practice of giving radiation treatments over a period of days or weeks was developed by Régaud in 1922. *Fractionation*, or the division of the total desired radiation dose into equal portions administered on a set schedule, was developed approximately 10 years later by Coutard.[28,66] Application of the modality of radiation to the full spectrum of susceptible malignancies was hampered, however, until increasingly sophisticated equipment became available. After the development of the atomic bomb during World War II, technology became available that facilitated the production of more sophisticated teletherapy equipment using high-energy gamma radiation from cobalt 60. Subsequent development of the linear accelerator, using photon or electron therapy, further advanced and refined treatment capabilities.[25] Increased electronic sophistication and the advent of computer-assisted equipment have allowed the administration of radiation therapy in a more precise fashion, with minimal "scatter" or diffusion of radiation out of the planned treatment field to surrounding, uninvolved tissues.

Although radiation therapy has been used

for almost a century, knowledge about the most effective use of this modality in the treatment of pediatric cancer continues to develop. Equipment is regularly upgraded and refined to ensure accuracy. Acute clinical outcomes and late effects of treatment are being managed better as research findings are integrated into practice applications. This has become particularly important in the care of the pediatric oncology patient receiving radiation therapy. The unique needs of the pediatric patient require particular attention to the details of treatment and the management of side effects, both acute and chronic. Children and adolescents, unlike adult patients, have incompletely developed or changing body systems and structures. Both cerebral and somatic growth are incomplete and susceptible to the effects of radiation. Developmentally and psychologically, the radiation experience may be a frightening one for the child and family. Proper preparation and instruction are necessary to minimize anxiety. The pediatric oncology nurse must be cognizant of the physical and biologic basis of radiation therapy to realize the primary goal of comprehensive care of the child and family.

BIOLOGY OF RADIATION THERAPY

The goal of radiation therapy is delivery of a therapeutic dose of radiation to tumor cells while sparing healthy tissue. Radiation affects single-strand or double-strand breaks in the DNA molecule, which results in future inability of tumor cells to divide, division with subsequent inability to function, or death during cellular division. The specific process that causes this cellular damage is called *ionization*. Ionization is a complex process whereby a source of radiation emits energy sufficient to cause the atoms of cells it encounters to lose orbiting electrons. Liberated electrons attach themselves to other nearby atoms, converting these atom fragments to a negative state. A chain reaction is set up as electrons continue to displace other orbiting electrons, generating a release of energy. This energy has the capacity to cause both physical and chemical changes in living cells, which further result in modifications in cell structure and function.[16,18,22,32,44]

Therapeutic radiation is classified as either electromagnetic (x-rays, gamma rays) or particulate (alpha particles, beta particles, neutrons). Electromagnetic radiation is character-

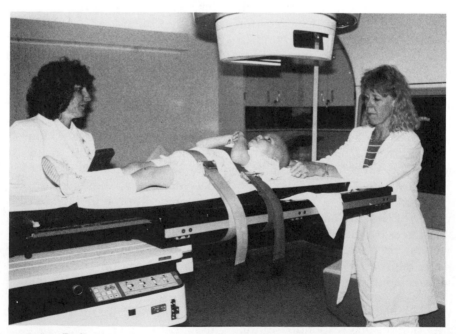

FIGURE 5–1. Pediatric patient positioned for administration of daily radiation treatment to the brain by linear accelerator.

ized by high energy and absence of mass[25] and may be machine generated (x-rays, gamma rays) or produced spontaneously through emission by radioactive substances undergoing transition. Radioactive cesium and cobalt are examples of such substances. Both x-rays and gamma rays are best described as *photons*, discrete packets of energy. They have no charge, but their energy is transferred to the absorbing medium when they collide with orbiting electrons of an atom.[16]

Three different types of electromagnetic radiation are currently used in clinical practice. *Superficial radiation* (also called *roentgen rays*) encompass the 10 to 125 keV (a unit of electric force equals 10^3 volts) spectrum; *orthovoltage radiation* involves the midrange of 125 to 500 keV; and *supervoltage radiation* (also called *megavoltage*) spans the range above 500 keV. An important concept regarding radiation is that as the voltage level increases, so does the level of penetration. In addition, supervoltage radiation, unlike orthovoltage, achieves its maximal dose in the tissues rather than on the skin surface. When orthovoltage therapy was in use, skin reactions were often the dose-limiting toxicity. Since this form of therapy is in very limited use today, such problems are not the norm.[16,20]

Three methods of ionization of electromagnetic radiation have been identified.[22] In *photoelectric absorption* photon interaction results in the ejection of a tightly bound electron. The empty space is subsequently filled by another electron from the atom's outer shell or from outside in domino-like fashion. All, or at least the majority, of the photon's energy is lost in this process. Photoelectric absorption varies with the cube of the atomic number (Z^3); thus the higher the atomic number, the less is the absorption. This explains why lead (high atomic number) is such an effective shielding agent. It also means that bones will absorb more radiation than muscle or soft tissues at lower photon energies, a concept also important in the field of diagnostic radiology. In *Comptontype absorption* interaction with distant, rather than proximal, electrons is involved. In this case the photon gives up part, but not all, of its energy to a single interaction. A portion is reformulated

as a secondary photon capable of undergoing subsequent ionization processes. Finally, high-energy photons are also capable of interacting with the atom's nucleus; when this occurs, the resultant energy is converted to matter.[56] Two charged particles (positive and negative electrons) result from this interchange. Ionization that occurs in this manner is referred to as the *pair production process* and is possible only at energies higher than 1.02 meV (i.e., million electron volts). Electrons produced by the pair production process are also capable of further ionization reactions.

Lysis of the cell membrane or a break in both strands of DNA causes prompt cellular death. These processes are responsible for the immediate tumoricidal effects seen and the acute toxicities associated with radiation therapy. Conversely, cellular death is delayed when only a single DNA strand has been damaged. Such cells may not die until they attempt to divide. Normal and malignant cells that divide frequently are most susceptible to the effects of radiation. Highly mitotic normal cells such as those of the skin, gastrointestinal (GI) mucosa, hair follicles, and bone marrow are particularly susceptible to radiation effects. Tumors with rapid generation times such as leukemias and lymphomas often respond quickly to radiation therapy, whereas tumors that grow more slowly such as tumors of soft tissue and muscle (rhabdomyosarcoma, synovial cell sarcoma, spindle cell sarcoma) are affected more slowly and respond over a more prolonged period of time. Molecular oxygen is considered the most important modifier of the biologic effect of radiation.[40] Studies have shown consistently that greater doses of radiation are required under hypoxic conditions to achieve optimal cell destruction.[41] Thus tumors with necrotic or poorly oxygenated regions respond poorly to radiation therapy.

Malignant cells have less ability to recover from the acute effects of radiation therapy than do normal cells. Both normal and malignant cells, however, will attempt to repair themselves within 3 to 4 hours after exposure to radiation. This repair process is responsible for the fibrosis and atrophy of normal tissue in the treatment field often observed in patients who have received this treatment modality.[7,17,25,32,36,45,54] Repair is further inhibited by a variety of related factors such as exposure to cold, radiation-enhancing chemotherapeutic agents such as actinomycin-D, anthracyclines, bleomycin, cisplatin, and methotrexate, and tissue hypoxia, which may inhibit cellular abilities at self-repair.[4,6,7,12,40,41,64]

IMPLEMENTATION OF THE RADIATION PLAN

Before implementing a plan for radiation therapy, the overall goal of treatment must be defined. For most children radiation therapy is used with *curative* intent; for some children, however, with recurrent or metastatic disease, radiation therapy provides *palliation* of troublesome symptoms. Data that must be assembled before initiating therapy include (1) the goal of therapy; (2) pertinent facts about the tumor such as size, location, and histologic grade; (3) relative volume of necrotic or poorly vascularized tissue in the treatment field (may be assessed by, for example, angiography or computed tomography [CT]); (4) other complicating medical conditions; and (5) the age and physiologic and psychologic condition of the child. The radiation oncologist then determines the dose, volume of tissue to treat, number of treatments to deliver, and frequency of treatment.[18,22,32,48]

The *therapeutic ratio*, the relationship between the amount of radiation required to kill the tumor and the amount of radiation that normal adjacent tissue can safely tolerate, must be established before the initiation of therapy. The radiation field must be designed to exclude as much surrounding normal tissue as possible. As the tumor decreases in volume, the radiation field also is decreased in size. This technique, known as the *shrinking field method*, also spares tissue adjacent to the tumor from unnecessary toxic effects.[22,32] Radiation therapy is *fractionated* (divided into multiple separate treatments) and *protracted* (delivered over a specified period of days or weeks). The usual range of time for radiation therapy is dependent on the total dose that will be delivered. For example, radiation therapy to the central nervous system (CNS) for acute leukemia may be accomplished in 10 days, whereas the usual plan for whole-brain radiation for malignant astrocytoma takes approximately 6 weeks because of the higher total dose of radiation required to complete the therapy.[66]

The majority of radiation prescriptions (treatment plans) used today require sophisticated three-dimensional analyses to establish the correct treatment field. This is accomplished by interfacing planning computers with CT or magnetic resonance imaging (MRI) scans. The *radiation absorbed dose* (rad) describes the interaction between radiation and matter. In 1984 the term *gray* was officially designated as the unit of absorbed dose, measured in joules per kilogram. One gray (Gy) equals 100 rads, and 1 centigray (cGy) equals 1 rad. Both terms (*rad* and *cGy*) are currently used interchangeably as the newer designation becomes the norm.[17]

Once the specific radiation prescription for a given patient has been established, diagnostic x-ray films of the designated treatment area are obtained by using a *simulator machine*, which uses diagnostic, rather than therapeutic, doses of radiation to simulate the treatment field in terms of size, shape, angle, and volume. The radiographs obtained during this procedure are used to demonstrate adequate coverage of the tumor volume and the reproducibility of the treatment field. These films are kept as a permanent record of the patient's treatment and are also used for quality-control purposes.

The treatment field is defined in a variety of ways using skin marks or tatoos. The inked lines are usually replaced during treatment by tiny permanent tatoos that assist with reconstruction of the treatment field.[25] Although not extremely painful, the procedure may be viewed as intrusive by children, and careful attention to patient and family preparation is essential. Plaster casts and molds constructed of plastic materials such as Aquaplast are used to immobilize the pediatric patient for purposes of treatment reproducibility. Shielding devices, usually constructed of lead and individually designed for each patient, protect healthy surrounding tissues and organs from unnecessary radiation exposure. Additionally, in certain situations surgical procedures such as moving the ovaries in a young female child who is to receive pelvic radiation are used to prevent irreversible damage to these organs.

The accurate planning, organization, and implementation of the radiation program is a true team effort that requires the input, involvement, and expertise of a variety of involved professionals. The *radiation oncologist* is a physician who clinically supervises and directs the therapy, manages the patient's care during treatment, delineates the area for treatment, and prescribes the appropriate radiation dose and plan of care. The *radiation physicist* is instrumental in the planning of the specific treatment field. Trained *radiation therapists* deliver the ordered therapy on a daily basis. *Registered nurses, clinical nurse specialists,* and *nurse practitioners* specializing in radiation oncology provide physical assessment, education, and longitudinal follow-up for patients undergoing treatment.[24,26,67]

Once the radiation planning has been accomplished, the actual treatment sessions may begin. Radiation therapy treatments are generally scheduled daily on a Monday to Friday basis. In emergency situations, such as airway compromise, daily treatments may be administered, although the more common practice is to increase the dose per fraction in such situations. With certain resistant tumors such as brainstem glioma, hyperfractionated schedules, which use multiple treatments at specific intervals during the same day, are being studied. Theoretically, such schedules allow an increase in the total delivered dose without a concomitant increase in toxicity.[5,11,35] Treatment verification films are obtained at various points during therapy to assess the reproducibility of the treatment fields. These *portal films* can be used to compare the proper positioning of the patient and appropriate shielding of sensitive organs.

PSYCHOSOCIAL CONSIDERATIONS

The entire radiation experience is a stressful one for the pediatric oncology patient and his or her family. Fears and misinformation associated with radiation add to the level of stress experienced by both child and family. Concrete explanations of the mechanisms of radiation and printed information about the procedures are useful. The child and family should be informed that, even though radiation is a brief and silent treatment, the machinery involved in the delivery of the therapy makes a variety of noises. The child is alone during the treatment but is observed constantly on a video monitor. The child can communicate verbally with staff, and it is often helpful to allow a parent to communicate with the child throughout the short period

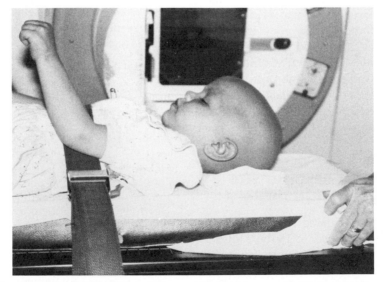

FIGURE 5–2. Patient positioned for delivery of lateral beam of radiation by linear accelerator.

that he or she is actually alone in the treatment room.[1,26,27,29,52]

Children and adolescents may become uncomfortable when required to lie still on a hard flat surface. Simulation procedures at the beginning of therapy often take an hour or more to complete. Thereafter total treatment time may be as little as 5 to 10 minutes. Agitation may develop and interfere with efficient administration of the treatments. Parents can help their child learn to cope with the imposed immobility by having the child practice lying still on a table at home. Immobilization appliances can produce a sense of claustrophobia in young children, leading to refusal to cooperate with the procedure. A mild sedative such as chloral hydrate or oral diazepam (Valium) administered 1 hour before the scheduled treatment time can help correct this problem. Occasionally individual age and temperament necessitate the daily administration of a short-term general anesthetic to deliver therapy effectively.[34,39] In such rare circumstances a pediatric anesthesiologist should be consulted to prescribe and administer an anesthetic that is appropriate to the situation and has the lowest cumulative toxicity.

Parents may be concerned that their child will be "radioactive" after leaving the radiation department and fear that their child's skin, clothing, urine, and stool will be contaminated and dangerous to others. Information should be provided to reinforce the fact that no radiation safety precautions are required for those undergoing external beam radiation therapy. Since many children receiving radiation treatments also attend school or day-care centers, at least on a part-time basis, school personnel and other students should also be provided with this basic information.[19]

MANAGEMENT OF SPECIFIC SIDE EFFECTS OF RADIATION THERAPY

The majority of anticipated side effects of radiation begin to develop 7 to 10 days after the initiation of treatment.[60] These toxicities usually continue throughout the course of treatment and may last for several weeks to months after therapy has been completed.

Since most children receiving radiation therapy are treated on an outpatient basis, it is extremely important to give parents and caregivers adequate information about anticipated side effects and their management[9,24,26,60,61] (Table 5–1).

The generalized effect of radiation therapy to the *skin* ranges from a mild erythema progressing to dry desquamation, wet desquamation, and, rarely, necrosis.[20,23] It is advisable to instruct parents to observe the skin daily for areas of breakdown and to avoid friction, unnecessary scrubbing, and use of hot water and abrasive soaps. Children will be more comfortable if clothing is loose rather than constrictive. Exposure of treated skin to the sun should be avoided since radiated skin may burn more easily. Creams, deodorants, and lotions can also promote skin reactions, and it is recommended that parents discuss

TABLE 5–1. *Acute Responses to Radiation Therapy*

SITE	RESPONSE
Skin	Loss of epidermal layer
	Erythema, dryness
	Wet desquamation
Gastrointestinal tract	Mucositis
	Pain
	Dysphagia
	Ulceration
	Nausea, vomiting
	Diarrhea
Salivary glands	Decreased formation of saliva
	Dryness of mucous membranes
	Taste distortion
Kidney or bladder	Cystitis
	Ulceration
Bone marrow	Myelosuppression
	Anemia
	Thrombocytopenia
Hair follicle	Hair loss (temporary or permanent)
Lungs	Pneumonitis
Heart	Myocarditis or pericarditis
Brain or spinal cord	Edema
Ovary	Permanent sterility possible
Testes	Mature sperm: radioresistant
	Immature sperm: permanent sterility

their use with radiation therapy staff. Recent research has shown that a moisture vapor permeable dressing (Tegaderm) is particularly useful in hastening healing of denuded skin.[57]

Radiation to the scalp produces *alopecia*, which often has already begun after the administration of chemotherapy. Generally speaking, radiation doses of less than 3000 cGy will produce reversible alopecia, whereas doses greater than 4500 cGy generally produce permanent loss of hair in the treated area. Doses in the intermediate range of 3000 to 4500 cGy result in variable amounts of permanent hair loss.[60] Children and their families need factual information about the possible permanent nature of hair loss and should be encouraged to obtain appropriate head covering suitable to the child's age, gender, and developmental level. Adequate head covering is very important during the winter months when excessive body heat loss can occur and during periods of intense summer sun.

Radiation to the head and neck, often administered to children with orbital, parameningeal, or facial tumors such as rhabdomyosarcoma, produces *dryness of the oral mucosa, alterations in taste sensation*, and *mucositis*. Care should be taken to maintain moisture of the mucous membranes by frequent intake of fluids and meticulous mouth care.[59] A complete baseline dental evaluation by a pedodontist with knowledge and interest in the area of pediatric oncology is recommended before the initiation of radiation therapy. Use of fluoride carriers (appliances similar to orthodontic retainers that are filled with topical fluoride solution) may be indicated to prevent *radiation caries*, which develop as a result of a decrease in saliva production, with subsequent disruption of tooth enamel. Special attention should be paid to the care of the gums in an effort to prevent the development of gingivitis. Recent research has shown that children who receive head and neck radiation have missing or blunted tooth roots and may be candidates for early permanent tooth loss if ongoing consistent dental care is not given.[42,43] In addition, artificial saliva products such as Oralube are helpful in maintaining a more normal, moist mucosal surface.

An adequate nutritional status must be maintained in spite of the development of alterations in taste secondary to altered composition of saliva and disruption in normal taste bud function. Some children develop food aversions, and special care must be taken to provide adequate intake for them. Taste acuity can be heightened by serving foods hot or cold rather than warm and by seasoning foods adequately. If mucositis is present, however, foods of a more bland nature may be more acceptable.[59,60]

It is recommended that the extent and severity of mucositis be assessed on a daily basis. Care should be taken to prevent infection of the oral mucosa. The child's weight should be monitored frequently, ideally twice per week, and on the same scale if at all possible. Weight loss greater than 10% of "ideal" body weight for age is an indication for the institution of home parenteral nutrition.

Radiation to the chest or upper back can cause *esophagitis, indigestion*, and *nausea*. Less commonly, *pneumonitis* occurs in approximately 10% of patients who receive full-dose radiation to this area and usually occurs 6 weeks to 3 months after completion of treatment. Parents should be taught to assess daily for the presence of esophageal pain, regurgitation, or excessive burping. Milk and milk products can help ease discomfort. Sucralfate (Carafate), an agent commonly used in ulcer regimens, often helps relieve symptoms and is usually well tolerated by children.[65]

Nausea and vomiting, generally seen only with radiation to the abdomen, pelvis, or lower back, can be alleviated by standard antiemetic agents. The use of phenothiazide category agents such as chlorpromazine (Thorazine) and prochlorperazine (Compazine) is not recommended, however, because of the possibility of the development of extrapyramidal side effects. Currently, minimal data are available on the relative efficacy of the new serotonin-antagonist antiemetic agent ondansetron (Zofran) in the radiation therapy setting; however, it has shown considerable efficacy in pediatric patients receiving emetogenic chemotherapy.

Radiation-induced *pneumonitis* may be a serious condition necessitating hospitalization and occasionally mechanical ventilation before recovery occurs. Prompt attention should be sought for respiratory symptoms such as tachypnea, orthopnea, dyspnea, dry cough, or increased respiratory effort. Influenza vaccine should be administered annually to all pediatric cancer patients receiving chemotherapy or radiation therapy since these children are particularly vulnerable to the consequences of influenza.[12,36] Patients deemed at risk for *Pneumocystis carinii* pneumonia should take trimethoprim-sulfamethoxazole in prophylactic doses (e.g., 5 mg/kg/day divided BID for 2 to 3 days per week) on a consistent basis.[51,53] In the event of allergy to sulfa drugs, inhaled pentamidine may be substituted for oral trimethoprim-sulfamethoxazole prophylaxis.

Radiation therapy delivered to the abdomen, pelvis, and lower back can cause *nausea, vomiting, diarrhea,* and *cystitis*. A low-residue diet, elimination or restriction of milk and milk products, and optimal fluid intake are helpful interventions parents may use. The anal mucosa should be inspected daily for evidence of ulceration, especially if myelosuppression and resultant neutropenia have developed. Daily sitz baths may provide comfort and cleanliness. Parents should be instructed not to take the child's temperature via the rectal route. Likewise rectal suppositories and enemas are contraindicated. Antidiarrheal agents may be used in accordance with a physician's recommendations.

The development of cystitis is hastened by inadequate fluid intake and an alkaline urinary pH. Encouraging a high fluid intake and maintaining an acidic (< 7.0) urinary pH by increasing the child's intake of citrus juices, for example, is helpful in this regard. If symptoms persist or worsen, a urinalysis and urine culture should be obtained, urinary tract analgesics used, and appropriate antibiotic therapy instituted if bacterial infection is proved.[60]

Many patients receiving radiation therapy report vague symptoms of *fatigue* and *malaise* that develop after the initiation of treatment. *Headache* is a common complaint of children receiving cranial radiation. Many children will feel energetic in the early portion of the day and may want to attend school in the morning. They may, however, display decreased energy reserve and require more sleep and a daily nap during the time that they are receiving radiation.[21,31] The postra-

diation "somnolence syndrome" that may persist for several months after completion of radiation therapy to the head may be worrisome for staff and families alike since they may perceive it as a worsening of CNS symptoms related to the child's underlying disease. After radiographic confirmation that tumor progression or regrowth has not occurred, care revolves primarily around supporting patient and family until symptoms abate.

The effect of radiation therapy on the *hematopoietic system* should not be overlooked. Areas of bone marrow within the radiation field are affected in a manner similar to the general effects of chemotherapy on the blood-forming organ. Neutropenia, anemia, and thrombocytopenia may all result and contribute to the cumulative toxicities the child experiences. For example, the child receiving radiation to the spinal axis may experience prolonged neutropenia and anemia. Since ionizing radiation depends on the availability of oxygen to produce free radicals, a minimum of 10 g/dl of hemoglobin is needed for effective treatment (the "oxygen effect"). Hemoglobin levels below this level can compromise the efficacy of therapy. Children receiving radiation therapy should have weekly complete blood counts (CBCs) performed, and these results should be communicated to the radiation oncology department promptly. Packed red blood cell (RBC) transfusions are indicated in the event that the child's hemoglobin level is below acceptable limits.[51,53]

Although the acute effects of radiation have been addressed in this chapter, long-term effects of this treatment modality such as growth retardation, body asymmetry, endocrine dysfunction, cataracts, and cognitive problems are identified elsewhere in this text (see Chapter 17 for further discussion).

INNOVATIVE TREATMENT APPROACHES
Hyperfractionated Radiation Therapy

Hyperfractionation refers to the delivery of more than one radiation treatment per day. In the pediatric arena hyperfractionated radiation therapy has been used in bone marrow conditioning regimens before transplantation, in the treatment of aggressive CNS tumors (specifically those in the brainstem), and in recalcitrant muscle and soft tissue tumors such as advanced rhabdomyosarcoma.[49] The rationale underlying this modality is that treating cells with a high mitotic index twice in one day, rather than once, may prevent tumor healing and repair between doses. Although each treatment uses a lower dose, the total dose delivered over the entire period is actually higher. Although preliminary data in brain tumor patients do not indicate a higher incidence of toxicities with this method, the need for more longitudinal analyses is indicated.[11] The potential of serious or possibly irreversible GI toxicity in patients receiving hyperfractionated radiation therapy to the abdomen and/or pelvis should be considered, and meticulous attention and assessment must be paid to symptom development in all children receiving this treatment modality.[50] Scheduling multiple treatments a day may be problematic for patients and families, especially if sedation is required. Coordination between family schedules and radiation department timetables is essential.

Intraoperative Radiation Therapy

Intraoperative radiation therapy involves delivery of a large-dose (1000 to 1500 cGy) single treatment administered while the patient is undergoing surgery. Theoretic advantages of this treatment plan are that the tumor bed is directly visualized, the treatment field is precisely defined, and normal adjacent structures are physically moved out of the radiation field.[8]

The usual pediatric intraoperative radiation dose to solid tumors is 1000 cGy, although higher doses are possible. At the time of surgery, the tumor bed is measured to accommodate introduction of a Lucite cone, which in turn is attached to the radiation machine for delivery of the therapy. After resection of as much of the tumor as possible, the radiation dose is delivered, and the operative procedure is completed. Although the theoretic benefit of intraoperative radiation would seem maximal with microscopic or minimal residual disease, benefit also may still be gained from radiating inoperable masses. In the pediatric setting intraoperative radiation therapy has been used in patients with large,

initially unresectable abdominal and pelvic tumors such as rhabdomyosarcoma, neuroblastoma, and Ewing's sarcoma and with thoracic and chest wall tumors such as primitive neuroepithelioma. Small sample results indicate that local control is improved by addition of this method of therapy.[8,15,30]

Initial concerns regarding increased infection rates and delayed wound healing have not been borne out in published research.[62,63] A primary limiting factor of this modality is the logistic dilemma of orchestrating a true multidisciplinary, and often multi-institutional, effort. Many institutions do not have operating suites adjacent to a radiation therapy department. Transportation to a different facility can cause stress to both patient and family. If possible, a preoperative tour is advisable so that staff, patient, and family will all feel more comfortable when the day of surgery arrives. Families must be informed that institutional procedures must be followed with regard to admission, discharge, blood-banking requirements, and visitation in the postanesthesia recovery unit, to name a few. Safety concerns exist regarding the fact that an anesthetized patient must be left alone, albeit briefly, in the radiation suite. Parents must be given adequate reassurance that extensive audiovisual monitoring will be used during this period of time. Metabolic and renal abnormalities as a result of tumor lysis in unresectable tumors treated with intraoperative radiation, while possible, have not been reported to any great degree in the literature.[2]

Interstitial Radiation Therapy

Interstitial radiation therapy, also known as *implant therapy* or *brachytherapy*, has not been used extensively in the pediatric population to date but may be incorporated to a greater degree in the future. This modality differs from external beam radiation therapy in that the radioactive material is implanted directly into the tumor bed. The radiation sources used (radium, iridium, radioactive iodine, gold seeds, cesium) are nonpenetrating so that large local doses of radiation can be administered with minimal delivery to adjacent tissues. Such implants provide an additional "boost" to recalcitrant tumors without damaging normal tissues.[13,14,58]

Interstitial implants provide improved local control for pediatric patients with retinoblastoma, soft tissue tumors, and certain malignant brain tumors since many of these tumors tend to recur locally rather than metastasize distantly. Interstitial implants have been used in adult patients with brain tumors who have received prior radiation.[3,46] The catheters are placed with CT guidance and are loaded with the radioactive isotope when the patient is neurologically stable. They are left in place for 50 hours and deliver a dose of 5000 cGy. To date, minimal problems have been reported, although experience with this technique in children has been limited.[33,55]

Safety precautions should be followed stringently for nurses and other personnel caring for children receiving brachytherapy. A distinction, however, must be made between *sealed* and *unsealed* sources of radiation. *Iodine 131*, used in the treatment of thyroid diseases such as hyperthyroidism and thyroid cancer, is administered systemically and is an example of an unsealed source. Excretion occurs via the feces, urine, emesis, saliva, sweat, and other body fluids. Fifty percent of such radioactive iodine is excreted in the first 48 hours after administration; thus rubber gloves should be worn while providing direct care to the patient. Patients and parents should be instructed to flush the toilet twice after each use. Linen and gowns used in these situations must be kept in properly labeled separate isolation bags. Permanent room fixtures (e.g., telephone, television) should be covered with plastic, and disposable food trays and utensils should be used.[1]

Sealed sources of radiation such as radium or cesium tubes, iridium ribbon, and gold or iodine 125 seeds are enclosed in sealed sources. The radioactivity from these sources is not absorbed by the body, nor is it excreted. General guidelines for care of a child receiving implant radiation using sealed sources include assigning the child to a private room with a private bath, placing a caution sign on the door, and if feasible, grouping such patients at the end of a hall to avoid contact with other patients. Nursing personnel should wear a dosimeter film badge at all times while caring for such patients. Additionally, nurses who are pregnant should not care for such patients, nor should pregnant women or children under 18 years of age visit. Visits should be limited to 30 minutes per visitor per day. In the unlikely event that the radioactive source dislodges, it should be retrieved by using long-handled forceps and should be deposited in a lead container. Such isolating techniques may prove stressful to the pediatric patient, and appropriate education and orientation of the child and family should be conducted before the initiation of this therapy.[1]

Hyperthermia

Hyperthermia refers to the use of heat to destroy tumor cells. Clinically, the use of hyperthermia has been limited by available technology and an inability to measure the precise distribution of applied heat. Heat augments and enhances the body's response to radiation.[10] Additionally, heat apparently is more damaging to cancer cells than to normal tissues. Presumably, hypoxic cells are more heat sensitive than well-oxygenated tissues, and tumor cells are often more hypoxic than normal surrounding tissues.[37]

The actual mechanism by which heat damages or destroys cells is not completely understood. One hypothesis is that cell membrane damage leads to increased cell permeability and subsequent death. A second theory postulates that lysosomes in the cell cytoplasm are damaged by heat, causing the release of digestive enzymes that destroy the cell.[10] Finally, heat may also stimulate the immune system, thereby contributing to individual host capabilities such as tumor necrosis factor.

Although it may be delivered to the whole body, hyperthermia is more commonly administered locally or regionally, using microwaves or ultrasound heat to the tumor and surrounding tissue. In the adult population hyperthermia has been used as an adjuvant therapy to surgery, chemotherapy, and radiation therapy, especially in patients with hepatic tumors. Although this modality shows promise, its use in the pediatric population has been quite limited to date.[38,47]

Chemical Modifiers

Two categories of compounds are being evaluated as adjuvants to radiation therapy at the present time: (1) radiation sensitizers and (2) radioprotectors.[50] *Radiation sensitizers* theoretically increase oxygenation to hypoxic cells and thereby render them more sensitive to the effects of radiation. The first agent tested in this group, Misonidazole, proved to possess unacceptable neurologic and GI toxicity.[32] Newer compounds currently are under study, including certain chemotherapeutic agents in the alkylating group. *Radiation protectors* theoretically shield normal cells from radiation damage by using substances absorbed by healthy cells but not by tumor cells. Research aimed at the isolation of such compounds that do not possess unacceptable systemic toxicities is ongoing.[50]

DEVELOPMENTAL ISSUES

Infants have a basic need for trust, and this can be facilitated best by providing consistent caregivers in the radiation department and establishing a routine for the treatment schedule each day. Fears of separation can influence both infant and toddler behavior in the radiation department. Since the child must be alone in the treatment suite, allowing and en-

couraging parents to speak or read to their child over the intercom system may help calm an anxious child. Security needs for toddlers and preschoolers may be met by allowing them to take a favorite toy or a "security" blanket into the treatment suite.

Young children have little ability to understand complex explanations of the anticipated procedure. Anxiety also contributes to a poor ability to process the information cognitively. Explanations should be simple and concrete and should be given in close temporal proximity to the actual radiation treatment. Explanations should focus on sensory experiences such as what the child will see, feel, and hear. Children should be allowed to explore the treatment suite with appropriate supervision. Having a wagon in which a small child can ride to the treatment room provides diversion, and providing a "treasure box" with small inexpensive toys can serve as motivation to cooperate with the therapy. Allowing a child to see an adult patient receiving treatment may also help allay fears. Allowing the child to wear his or her own clothes into the treatment suite may be helpful, especially with preschool age children in whom body integrity fears are paramount.

School-age children typically are most interested in the actual workings of the equipment and are able to process more sophisti-

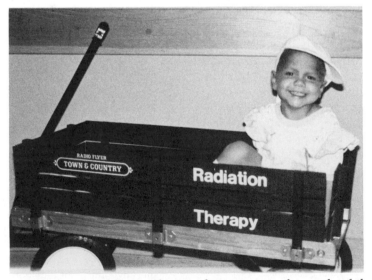

FIGURE 5–3. Adapting the radiation therapy department to the needs of the pediatric patient is important to successful delivery of therapy.

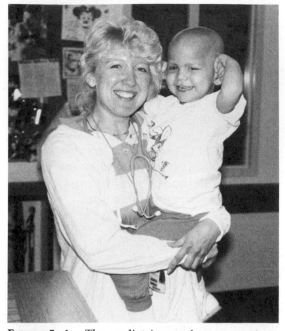

FIGURE 5-4. The pediatric oncology nurse is instrumental in family education for the child undergoing radiation therapy.

cated information. They may enjoy watching the control panels while other patients are receiving treatment and should be encouraged to ask questions and build their fund of knowledge. Adolescents are particularly resistant to the idea of permanent skin tatoos that must be applied to reconstruct the treatment field accurately. Sensitivity to the adolescent patient's need to preserve his or her body image must be maintained and reassurance given that, although they are permanent, these markings are barely noticeable. Close collaboration between radiation department personnel and pediatric oncology nursing staff helps provide a smooth transition for required care.[34]

REFERENCES

1. Anderson BL, Tewfik HH. Psychological reactions to radiation therapy: Reconsideration of the adaptive aspects of anxiety. J Pers Soc Psychol 1985; 48:1024–1032.
2. Bashein G, Russel AH, Mommii ST. Anesthesia and remote monitoring for intraoperative radiation therapy. Anesthesiology 1986; 64:805–807.
3. Bouzaglou A, Dyck P, Solt-Bohman L, et al. Stereotactic interstitial implantation of brain tumors. Endocur Hypertherm Oncol 1985; 1:99–113.
4. Brown JM. Clinical trials of radiosensitizers: What should we expect? Int J Radiat Oncol Biol Phys 1984; 10:425–429.
5. Cox J, Cuse C, Asbell S, et al. Tolerance of normal pelvic tissues to hyperfractionated radiation therapy: Results of protocol 83–08 of the radiation therapy oncology group. Int J Radiat Oncol Biol Phys 1988; 15:1331–1336.
6. D'Angio GJ. Early and delayed complications of therapy. Cancer 1983; 51:2515–2518.
7. D'Angio GJ, Farber S, Maddock CL. Potentiation of x-rays effects of actinomycin-D. Radiology 1959; 73:175–177.
8. Dobelbower RR, Abe M. Intraoperative radiation therapy. Boca Raton, Fla.: CRC Press, 1990.
9. Dodd MJ. Patterns of self-care in cancer patients receiving radiation therapy. Oncol Nurs Forum 1984; 11:23–27.
10. Dritschilo A, Piro A. Therapeutic implications of heat as related to radiation therapy. Semin Oncol 1981; 8:83–92.
11. Freeman CR, Krischer J, Sanford R, et al. Hyperfractionated radiation therapy in brain stem tumors: Results of a pediatric oncology group study. Int J Radiat Oncol Biol Phys 1988; 15:311–318.
12. Fu KK. Biological basis for the interaction of chemotherapeutic agents and radiation therapy. Cancer 1985; 55:2123–2130.
13. Gerbaulet A, Panis X, Flamant F, et al. Iridium afterloading curie–therapy in the treatment of pediatric malignancies. Cancer 1985; 56:1274–1279.
14. Glicksman A. Radiobiologic basis of brachytherapy. Semin Oncol Nurs 1987; 3:3–7.
15. Hailbeck SV. Intraoperative radiation therapy. Oncol Nurs Forum 1988; 15:143–147.
16. Hall EJ. The particles compared. Int J Radiat Oncol Biol Phys 1982; 8:2137–2140.
17. Halperin EC, Kun LE, Constine LS, et al. Pediatric Radiation Oncology. New York: Raven Press, 1989.
18. Halpern J, Maor MH. Radiotherapy in the pediatric oncology patient. In Gottlieb RA, Pinkel D (eds): Handbook of Pediatric Oncology. Boston: Little, Brown & Co, 1989; pp 62–70.
19. Hassey KM. Principles of radiation safety and protection. Semin Oncol Nurs 1987; 3:23–29.
20. Hassey KM, Rose CM. Altered skin integrity in patients receiving radiation therapy. Oncol Nurs Forum 1982; 9:44–50.
21. Haylock PJ, Hart LK. Fatigue in patients receiving localized radiation. Cancer Nurs 1979; 2:461–467.
22. Hellman S. Principles of radiation therapy. In DeVita VT, Hellman S, Rosenberg SA (eds): Cancer: Principles and Practice of Oncology, 3rd ed. Philadelphia: JB Lippincott, 1991, pp 227–255.
23. Hilderley LJ: Skin care in radiation therapy. Oncol Nurs Forum 1983; 10:51–56.
24. Hilderley LJ. The role of the nurse in radiation oncology. Semin Oncol 1980; 7:39–47.
25. Hilderley LJ. Radiation oncology: Historical background and principles of teletherapy. In Hassey Dow K, Hilderley LJ (eds): Nursing Care in Radiation Oncology. Philadelphia: WB Saunders, 1992, pp 3–15.
26. Israel MJ, Mood DW. Three media presentations for patients receiving radiation therapy. Cancer Nurs 1982; 5:57–63.
27. Johnson JE, Nail LM, Lauver D, et al. Reducing the negative impact of radiation therapy on functional status. Cancer 1988; 61:46–51.
28. Kaplan H. Historic milestones in radiobiology and radiation therapy. Semin Oncol 1979; 4:479–490.

29. King K, Nail L, Kraemer K, et al. Patients' descriptions of the experience of receiving radiation therapy. Oncol Nurs Forum 1985; 12:55–61.
30. Kinsella TJ, Glatsein E, Sindelar WF. Intraoperative radiation therapy. Hosp Pract 1985; 20:125–141.
31. Kobashi-Schoot JAM, Hanewald G, Van Dam F. Assessment of malaise in cancer patients treated with radiotherapy. Cancer Nurs 1985; 8:303–313.
32. Kun LE, Moulder JE. General principles of radiation therapy. In Pizzo PA, Poplack DG (eds): Principles and Practice of Pediatric Oncology, 2nd ed. Philadelphia: JB Lippincott, 1993, pp 273–302.
33. Lashford LS, Clarke J, Kemshead JT. Systemic administration of radionuclides in neuroblastoma as planned radiotherapeutic intervention. Med Pediatr Oncol 1990; 18:30–36.
34. Lew CC. Special needs of children. In Hassey Dow K, Hilderley LJ (eds): Nursing Care in Radiation Oncology. Philadelphia: WB Saunders, 1992, pp 177–202.
35. Ludgate C, Douglas B, Dixon P, et al. Superfractionated radiotherapy in grade III and IV intracranial gliomas. Int J Radiat Oncol Biol Phys 1988; 15:1091–1095.
36. Miller RW, Fusner JE, Fink RJ, et al. Pulmonary function abnormalities in long-term survivors of childhood cancer. Med Pediatr Oncol 1986; 14:202–207.
37. Moore C. Hyperthermia: A modern experiment in cancer treatment. Oncol Nurs Forum 1984; 11:31–37.
38. Moore C. Nursing management of the patient receiving local or regional hyperthermia. Oncol Nurs Forum 1984; 11:40–45.
39. Morrison JE, Friesen RH, McGuire P. Serum bromide elevation following multiple anesthetics for cranial irradiation treatment of posterior fossa ependymoma in a child. Proceedings Second Int Neuro-Onc Symp. Philadelphia: 1990.
40. Mottram JC. Factors of importance in radiosensitivity of tumors. Br J Radiol 1936; 9:606–614.
41. Moulder JE, Rockwell S. Tumor hypoxia: Its impact on cancer therapy. Cancer Metastasis Rev 1987; 5:313–341.
42. Mueller WA, Cullen JW, Abrams RB, et al. Late effects of cancer therapy on developing dentition. J Dent Res 1990; 69:250.
43. Mueller WA, Cullen JW, Abrams RB, et al. Effect of cranial radiation on tooth abnormalities in ALL patients. J Dent Res 1991; 70:424.
44. Muzenrider JE, Shipley WU, Verhey LJ. Future prospects of radiation therapy with protons. Semin Oncol 1981; 8:110–114.
45. Newman NM, Donaldson S, DeWit S, et al. Neuro-ocular damage in pediatric oncology patients: Predictor of long-term visual disability or tool for limiting toxicity. Med Pediatr Oncol 1986; 14:262–270.
46. Novaes PE. Interstitial therapy in the management of soft-tissue sarcomas in childhood. Med Pediatr Oncol 1985; 13:221–224.
47. Overgaard J. The current and potential role of hyperthermia in radiotherapy. Int J Radiat Oncol Biol Phys 1989; 16(suppl):S35–S51.
48. Perez CA, Brady LH (eds). Principles and Practice of Radiation Oncology. Philadelphia: JB Lippincott, 1987.
49. Peters LJ et al. Radiobiological considerations in the use of total body irradiation for bone marrow transplantation. Radiology 1979; 131:243.
50. Phillips T. Sensitizers and protectors in clinical oncology. Semin Oncol 1981; 8:65–83.
51. Plowman PN. The effects of conventionally fractionated extended portal radiotherapy on the human peripheral blood count. Int J Radiat Oncol Biol Phys 1983; 9:829–839.
52. Rainey LC. Effects of preparatory patient education for radiation oncology patients. Cancer 1985; 56:1056–1061.
53. Rubin P, Scarantino CW. The bone marrow organ: The critical structure in radiation-drug interaction. Int J Radiat Oncol Biol Phys 1978; 4.3–23.
54. Russo A, Tomarchio S, Pero G, et al. Abnormal visual evoked potentials in leukemic children after cranial radiation. Med Pediatr Oncol 1985; 13:313–317.
55. Saleman M, Sewchand W, Amin P, et al. Technique and preliminary results of interstitial irradiation for primary brain tumors. J Neurooncol 1986; 4:141–149.
56. Sarna LP. Concepts of nursing care for patients receiving radiation therapy. In Vredevoe DL, Derdiarian A, Sarna LP, et al. Concepts in Oncology Nursing. Englewood Cliffs, N.J.: Prentice-Hall, 1981, pp 154–206.
57. Shell JA, Stantz F, Grimm J. Comparison of moisture vapor permeable (MVP) dressings to conventional dressings for management of radiation skin reactions. Oncol Nurs Forum 1986; 13:11–16.
58. Stowe SM, Mittman P, Wara W, et al. The use of implantation in childhood tumors: The experience of the Children's Cancer Study Group member institutions. Am J Clin Oncol 1982; 5:129.
59. Strohl R. Nursing management of the patient with cancer experiencing taste changes. Cancer Nurs 1983; 65:353–359.
60. Strohl R. Nursing role in radiation therapy: Symptom management of acute and chronic reactions. Oncol Nurs Forum 1988; 15:429–439.
61. Strohl RA. Radiation therapy: Recent advances and nursing implications. Nurs Clin North Am 1990; 25:309–329.
62. Tepper JE, Gunderson LL, Goldson AL, et al. Quality control parameters of intraoperative radiation therapy. Int J Radiat Oncol Biol Phys 1986; 12:1687–1695.
63. Tepper JE, Gunderson LL, Orlow E, et al. Complications of intraoperative radiation therapy. Int J Radiat Oncol Biol Phys 1984; 10:1831–1839.
64. Trott KR. Radiation-chemotherapy interactions. Int J Radiat Oncol Biol Phys 1986; 12:1409–1413.
65. Welch D. Radiation-related nausea and vomiting: A review of the literature. Oncol Nurs Forum 1979; 6:8–11.
66. Withers HR. Biologic basis for altered fractionation schemes. Cancer 1985; 55:2086–2095.
67. Yasko JM. Care of the patient receiving radiation therapy. Nurs Clin North Am 1982; 17:631–648.

6

BONE MARROW TRANSPLANTATION

Beth Frederick
Mary Jo Hanigan

HISTORY

The earliest recorded therapeutic use of bone marrow in man ". . . for the treatment of leukemia and other diseases believed to be characterized by defective homogenesis . . . " was attempted in 1891.[134] Small amounts of bone marrow were given by mouth to patients with anemias of varying etiology in hopes the bone marrow would replenish a deficient substance or factor necessary to correct anemia. The first reports of intravenous (IV) and intramedullary (sternal) administration of bone marrow as alternatives to oral administration were recorded in 1939 and 1940, respectively, in two patients suffering from aplastic anemia.[118,123] These initial attempts to use bone marrow therapeutically were unsuccessful.

The discovery of atomic energy in 1945 raised concerns about severe radiation injury and its effects on human bone marrow.[54,150] Initial bone marrow transplantation (BMT) research grew out of efforts to understand and treat bone marrow failure resulting from irradiation injury.[38] The hallmark experiments of BMT were conducted in 1949 and 1951 by Jacobson et al.[84] and Lorenz, Congdon, and Uphoff,[105] respectively. Jacobson et al. established that lethally irradiated mice could be protected from death by shielding the spleen (a hematopoietic organ in the mouse). Lorenz, Congdon, and Uphoff showed that lethally irradiated mice and guinea pigs could be protected from death through an IV infusion of bone marrow. Initially the origin of the effect that protected the lethally irradiated animals against death was thought to be a humoral, noncellular substance produced by the living cells of the shielded spleen or injected bone marrow.[83,105] However, it was shown through the use of genetic markers in donor bone marrow cells that the protective effect against lethal irradiation was from the colonization of the recipient bone marrow donor cells and not through the secretion of a humoral factor.[102]

Several attempts were made in the late 1950s and 1960s to apply BMT to the treatment of human diseases.[38] Early results of human marrow transplantation were not encouraging. Most bone marrow transplants were done on end-stage patients who died either before the status of the graft could be evaluated or as a result of a lethal immunologic reaction between the donor graft and the recipient (now known as *graft-versus-host disease [GVHD]*), in addition to fatal viral and fungal infections.[38,150]

Current advances in BMT have benefited from several significant developments including *identification of the human leukocyte antigen (HLA) system* that controls the genetic identity of human tissues and bone marrow,[150] *identification and characterization of the pathophysiology of GVHD,* and *advances in blood banking.* Progress in microbiology, new treatments for infections, development and use of total parenteral nutrition (TPN), and the development of the Silastic central venous catheter, which provided a reliable mechanism to administer large volumes of TPN, fluids, and blood components safely, have been invaluable in the advancement and application of BMT.[158,176]

OVERVIEW OF BMT

The bone marrow is the soft tissue that fills the cavities of the bone. Its primary functions are to provide and maintain the body's source of blood cells through hematopoiesis and maintain the integrity of the immune system through lymphopoiesis. The pluripotent stem cell, which is capable of self-replication and differentiation, is the key progenitor cell responsible for these functions.[104] A BMT is possible because these stem cells can be removed from one individual, through a process called *harvesting,* and transplanted or infused into a recipient. The transplanted stem cells migrate to the recipient's marrow spaces, engraft, and produce a new hematopoietic and immune system in the recipient.

Bone marrow transplantation is a therapy performed for the treatment of cancer, diseases that affect the immune and hematopoietic systems, and certain metabolic diseases (Table 6–1). The sources of bone marrow that can be used for a transplant are *autologous (auto-BMT),* which uses the patient's own bone marrow, and *allogeneic (allo-BMT),* which uses bone marrow from a donor other than the patient. Usually the donor is a sibling, but in some cases the donor can be a twin (syngeneic BMT), a parent, another relative, or a carefully matched unrelated person (unrelated BMT [UBMT]).

HLA is a protein antigen that is a tissue-type marker located on an individual's nucleated cells. The HLA can be typed by a blood test specifying the individual's tissue typing. The HLA system is responsible for recognizing foreign tissue and activating the immune system to fight foreign tissue. The HLA typing of an individual is inherited from his or her parents. In allo-BMT HLA typing is used to determine the most genetically compatible bone marrow donor for a patient.

All patients must undergo ablative therapy before receiving bone marrow. The ablative therapy, also known as the *conditioning regimen,* is an intensive, very high-dose combination chemotherapy with or without radiotherapy (total body irradiation [TBI]). It is designed to destroy any unwanted cell population (e.g., cancer cells), suppress the body's immune system, and create "space" in the marrow cavity for the stem cells of the new marrow to engraft, or to take root and grow.[149] Effective suppression of the immune system is important to prevent rejection of the donor marrow in patients receiving allogeneic transplants. The greater the incompatibility between the patient's HLA type and the donor marrow, the higher is the risk for rejection. Additional immunosuppression may be necessary in these situations.

Immediately on completion of the ablative therapy, the patient will receive the harvested bone marrow. In auto-BMT the bone marrow is harvested from the patient weeks to months before the ablative therapy is given and is frozen (cryopreserved) until it is needed. In allo-BMT the marrow is harvested from the selected donor when the ablative therapy is completed and is transfused directly into the patient. The process by which the transplanted marrow successfully takes root and grows in the patient's marrow cavities is known as *engraftment* and usually occurs 10 to 21 days after BMT.

Although the precise mechanism by which the intravenously infused marrow cells "home" or migrate to the bone marrow cavities is unknown, it is speculated that the process involves molecules on the infused hematopoietic cells that have preferential binding sites on bone marrow stromal cells. After infusion the stem cells of the marrow probably circulate throughout the blood system until the hematopoietic cells come in contact with the bone marrow tissue in the empty cavities. Once in contact with the stromal tissue, the hematopoietic cells engraft and begin replication and differentiation.[170]

Aggressive supportive care to manage the

TABLE 6-1. *Rationale and Potential Uses of Bone Marrow Transplantation in Children*

FOR MALIGNANCY	FOR BONE MARROW FAILURE OR DYSFUNCTION	FOR SYSTEMIC DEFICIENCY IN ENZYME PRODUCTION
Rationale for BMT		
Rescue myeloablative effects of high dose chemotherapy or radiotherapy	Traditional concept of transplantation; replace diseased non-functioning bone marrow with healthy functioning bone marrow	Replace damaged cells with normal functioning bone marrow that can produce normal enzyme
Treatment Goal		
Erradicate malignancy and restore normal bone marrow function	Restore normal bone marrow function; reconstitute hematologic and immune function	Stabilize and prevent further deterioration from the effects of the genetic disease process
Donor Bone Marrow		
Auto-BMT, Allo-BMT, UBMT	Allo-BMT, UBMT	Allo-BMT, UBMT
Diseases Transplanted		
Leukemias	*Acquired*	*Mucopolysaccharidoses*
ALL, AML, CML, JCML, Myelodysplasia	Severe aplastic anemia	Hurler syndrome
	Congenital	Hunter syndrome
Lymphomas	Fanconi's anemia	Maroteaux-Lamy syndrome
Non-Hodgkin's lymphoma		Others
Hodgkin's disease	*Immune Dysfunction*	*Mucolipidoses*
	SCIDS	Metachromatic leukodystrophy
Solid Tumors	X-linked agammaglobulinemia	Adrenoleukodystrophy
Neuroblastoma		Other lipidoses
Brain tumors	*Monocyte or Granulocyte Dysfunction*	
Ewing's sarcoma	Chronic granulomatous disease	*Other Lysosomal Diseases*
Rhabdomyosarcoma	Infantile agranulocytosis	Lesch-Nyhan syndrome
PNET	Leukocyte adhesion defects	Type IIa glycogen storage disease
Wilms' tumor	Osteopetrosis	
Retinoblastoma		
	Erythrocyte Dysfunction	
	Blackfan-Diamond anemia	
	Thalassemia	
	Sickle cell disease	
	Miscellaneous	
	Glanzmann's thrombasthenia	
	Wiscott-Aldrich syndrome	

Data from references 36, 153, and 161.
ALL = acute lymphocytic leukemia; ANLL = acute nonlymphocytic leukemia; CML = chronic myelogenous leukemia; JCML = juvenile chronic myelogenous leukemia; PNET = primitive neuroectodermal tumor; SCIDS = severe combined immunodeficiency syndrome.

effects of pancytopenia and other toxicities resulting from the ablative therapy is the hallmark of post-transplant medical and nursing care. GVHD is an immune reaction of the engrafted bone marrow (graft) against the patient's (host) tissues. GVHD occurs in patients who have received an allo-BMT. It affects the skin, liver, and gastrointestinal (GI) systems.

Symptoms of GVHD usually become evident within 30 days after transplant as marrow engraftment is evident. Patients receive prophylaxis for GVHD, which may include cyclosporine, methotrexate, glucocorticoid, or antithymocyte globulin (ATG). Discharge from the hospital depends on the resolution of side effects and complications and successful patient and family teaching about post-transplant care. Discharge can occur within the first 30 days after transplant.

The success of any BMT depends on an acceptable source of donor marrow; the effectiveness of the pretransplant conditioning regimen; successful engraftment, which signals the return of hematopoietic functions or production of all blood cell lines and immune reconstitution; and cure or stabilization of the disease state for which the transplant was performed.

Use Against Malignant Disease

Although childhood malignancies are very sensitive to chemotherapy,[13] increasing the dose beyond what is used in conventional treatment plans may be necessary to produce a better tumor response for certain cancers.[135] If a source of bone marrow is available to engraft and "rescue" the patient from the severe myeloablative effects, higher doses of these agents can be used to eliminate enough residual or micrometastatic tumor to achieve a cure.

Use Against Nonmalignant Disease

Nonmalignant diseases for which BMT is considered a viable form of treatment are characterized by a defect in normal bone marrow function. The defect can vary from (1) complete bone marrow failure of hematopoiesis as seen with severe aplastic anemia (SAA)[165]; (2) defects in immunologic functioning, typical of a child diagnosed with severe combined immunodeficiency syndrome (SCIDS)[4,56]; and (3) defects in single blood cell lines such as the erythrocytes in patients with thalassemia major.[28,174] Other types of genetic diseases can be corrected or partially repaired by BMT. For example, children diagnosed with Gaucher's disease can be treated by BMT.[138] Gaucher's disease is a systemic defect in the production of the enzyme glucocerebrosidase, which controls the production and disposition of glucocerebroside in certain hematopoietic cells. In nonmalignant diseases BMT plays the traditional role as in solid organ transplants—the replacement of a diseased organ. The donor

for a transplant in nonmalignant diseases must be allogeneic.

The majority of these diseases are congenital. Some forms of SAA are acquired through unknown causes. Aplastic anemia and SCIDS are life threatening, and BMT is the curative therapy. However, in other diseases of bone marrow function, the risk of morbidity and mortality with BMT must be contrasted with the long-term effects of the disease and the methods of supportive care available. Many illnesses such as sickle cell anemia or thalassemia major could be cured by a bone marrow transplant, yet at the present time, the risks of BMT may outweigh the benefits.[85,137,157,174]

Increasing attention is being given to other genetic diseases in which the defect in enzyme production is systemic and the clinical effects of the genetic disorder are evident in body tissues other than the bone marrow such as the central nervous system (CNS). Included are diseases such as Hurler syndrome, Hunter syndrome, and the leukodystrophies. BMT may be indicated in the treatment of these diseases because the cells from a healthy bone marrow donor could provide the missing enzyme, which could potentially stabilize and reverse the systemic toxic effects of the disease.[80,187]

ALLOGENEIC BONE MARROW TRANSPLANTATION

Allo-BMT relies on the availability of a suitable bone marrow donor. In most cases the donor is a "matched" sibling, although in rare cases a parent whose tissue type by definition is at least half identical to that of the child has been used. Unrelated donors, identified through national bone marrow registries, have been used. The specific science and nursing considerations related to UBMT are discussed later in this chapter.

Donor Identification

Histocompatibility typing is the first step in identifying a potential donor. The "typing" includes HLA and mixed lymphocyte culture (MLC) analyses. The HLAs are protein antigens on the cell surfaces of all nucleated cells that function in immune recognition. They

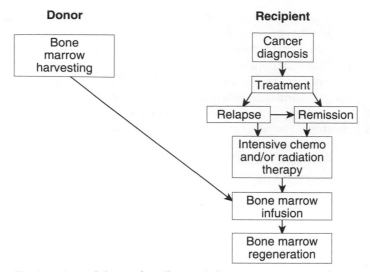

FIGURE 6–1. Schema for allogeneic bone marrow transplant.

recognize foreign tissues and mount an immune response against them. Approximately 100 HLA antigens have been classified. The antigens are expressed in combinations that are the genetic "thumbprints" of an individual, determining self from non-self.

The genes that code the HLAs are situated at the major histocompatibility complexes (MHCs) on the short arm of chromosome 6. An individual inherits half of his or her HLA type from each parent, meaning that the HLA type is "haploidentical" to that of the parent. According to principles of genetics, full siblings have a 1 in 4 (25%) probability of inheriting the same HLA typing. In the current experience of transplantation, however, the probability is actually closer to 35%,[136] for certain HLA genes express gene-linkage disequilibrium, that is, are inherited together as a group. Gene-linkage disequilibrium frequently occurs in ethnic groups, for certain HLA genes can be more prevalent in a specific ethnic group; therefore parents of the same ethnic background may share some common HLA types. When parents share common HLA types, the offspring may have an HLA type that closely resembles that of one parent or the other.[39]

The HLAs that currently play the significant role in matching tissue types for BMT are the HLA-A, HLA-B, HLA-DR, and HLA-D antigens. A child inherits two of each as a group, or *haplotype*. One haplotype is inherited from each parent. The matched set of genes (e.g., A from the mother and A from the father) that code for alternate expressions for the same characteristic are called *alleles*. Individuals can be homozygous (same alleles) or heterozygous (different alleles) for any pair. The inherited HLA combinations are referred to as the individual's *genotype*, and the morphologic or biochemical expression of the inherited genes is called the *phenotype*. Identical twins are genotypically and phenotypically identical. Other siblings can be phenotypically identical for HLA expression despite not being genetically identical. Unrelated donors are genotypically different but may be phenotypically exact or similar, which is why in select cases they can be used as BMT donors.

Current testing methods are neither sophisticated nor precise for other important antigens, the *minor HLA antigens*. Despite their identification as "minor," they actually may play a major role in the immune responses of BMT patients. In fact, the minor antigens may be responsible for adverse immune reactions in transplants in which the recipient and donor are HLA and MLC compatible. The degree to which a donor and the recipient are histocompatible determines the degree of marrow rejection and more importantly, the degree of graft reaction against the immunocompromised host tissue. Ongoing research is directed toward precise identification of additional HLAs.

The HLA-A, HLA-B, and HLA-DR antigens are tested serologically by a process similar to that for the identification of the ABO antigens. This technique, the microlymphocytotoxicity test, mixes the viable lymphocytes of an individual with controlled antisera. Antisera antibodies attach to the cell surfaces of the lymphocytes and combine with the HLAs. After an immune reaction, the cells lyse and are stained. From the staining technique, the HLAs are characterized and identified.

The DR antigen is the most significant match in the HLA series in determining a compatibility between donor and patient. Monoclonal antibody assays are being used more routinely to identify these antigens.

D antigen typing is determined by mixed lymphocyte culture reaction testing, which analyzes lymphocyte proliferation. The D locus is located on the major histocompatibility complex next to the A, B, and DR loci. Viable lymphocytes from the patient are mixed with those of the potential donor and incubated. Blast cell stimulation occurs if the D antigens are discordant or disparate in antigen expression. Blast cell transformation can be controlled (stimulated or blocked) by laboratory measures so that the reactions can be evaluated as donor reactivity against the patient (in the direction of GVHD) or as patient reactivity against the graft (in the direction of graft rejection). A low reactivity response during laboratory analysis suggests compatibility and can be correlated chemically to increased immune tolerance.

The best matches are an identical twin and a full sibling identical at the HLA-A, HLA-B, and HLA-DR loci and MLC compatible or "nonreactive." Since the HLA-A, HLA-B, and HLA-DR loci and the D locus are situated together on the MHC, there is a greater than 95% probability that HLA-A, HLA-B, and HLA-DR matched siblings are also MLC compatible.

Some transplant centers are using mismatched family donors when necessary. If the mismatch is minor, for instance at the A or B loci, or exists between two antigens known to be cross-reactive (complementary), the match is a better choice than if the mismatch involves the DR loci or there is a highly reactive MLC response. The degree of histocompatibility determines the suitability of a particular donor and dictates the amount and intensity of immune suppression required to prevent GVHD and graft rejection.

Allo-BMT can occur across ABO blood groups. It is not necessarily contraindicated when the patient and recipient are ABO incompatible. However, a potential exists for infusion of donor erythrocytes along with the bone marrow cells, called the *marrow inoculum*, causing hemolysis of the graft. Therefore the erythrocytes must be removed before transplant by a variety of laboratory methods. Plasma is also removed from the marrow inoculum by centrifugation if there is an incompatibility against the recipient's erythrocytes by the donor antibodies. In cases in which the recipient and donor ABO blood types are discrepant, the recipient's blood type will change to that of the donor once myeloid (and thus erythroid) engraftment has occurred and residual recipient ABO antigens have been depleted from the circulation. The donor's erythrocytes then repopulate the marrow.

UNRELATED BONE MARROW TRANSPLANTATION

UBMT has had a dramatic impact on the potential for cure in those children who do not have a matched family marrow donor.[69] Unrelated marrow donors are altruistic volunteers whose HLA typing has been done and who are registered in a file of potential marrow donors. Several small privately operated registries exist in this country. The largest registry, however, is the National Marrow Donor Program (NMDP), with its coordinating center in St. Paul, Minnesota. The NMDP, established in 1987 by the federal government, cooperates with several international registries and private registries. Any transplant physician can request a preliminary search of the files on behalf of a patient who might benefit from BMT. There is no cost for a preliminary search. Other aspects carry associated financial costs. There is an approximate 10% to 15% success rate in identifying HLA-matched,

MLC-compatible unrelated donors for patients.[110] Clinical investigation is ongoing to (1) determine the most effective timing of UBMT compared to high-dose, nonablative therapy; (2) determine more sophisticated identification of HLAs; (3) determine more effective methods to prevent GVHD in UBMT; and (4) compare the outcome of UBMT to that of partially matched family donors.

The classic study of chronic myelocytic leukemia (CML) patients undergoing UBMT found that, although there was a higher incidence of acute GVHD in patients undergoing UBMT compared to matched family donor transplants, the median time to engraftment and +100-day survival was not significantly different between the two groups.[114] These findings are scientifically motivating and have been the impetus toward increased research to determine the role of UBMT in childhood cancer treatment.

AUTOLOGOUS BONE MARROW TRANSPLANTATION

Auto-BMT uses the patient's own bone marrow for hematopoietic and immune reconstitution and currently is used only for the treatment of malignant disease. The use of autologous marrow avoids the risk of the GVHD seen in allogeneic transplantation along with its attendant morbidity and mortality. Since

only 20% to 30% of the patients have a genetically matched sibling donor, the use of autologous marrow allows offering high-dose therapy with marrow rescue to a greater number of patients.

Chemotherapy drugs appropriate for use in auto-BMT conditioning regimens demonstrate the following key characteristics: (1) activity for the tumor type, (2) myelosuppression as the primary dose-limiting toxicity, and (3) a steep dose response curve, showing an increasing tumor cell kill response with higher drug dose.[52,153] Based on these criteria, alkylating agents such as cyclosphosphamide and L-phenylalanine mustard have become the primary agents used in auto-BMT-conditioning protocols.[52] The steep dose-response curve of alkylating agents allows dose escalation several times the standard treatment dose so that nonhematopoietic toxicity becomes their dose-limiting factor.[52] Because alkylating agents have different nonmyelosuppressive toxicities and minimal cross-resistance, several of these drugs can be used in combination, which is a highly successful component of conventional chemotherapy regimens.[51,153] This allows a more aggressive treatment approach for malignancies that have not responded well or demonstrate incomplete responses to conventional chemotherapy and radiotherapy.

The first auto-BMT was performed in the

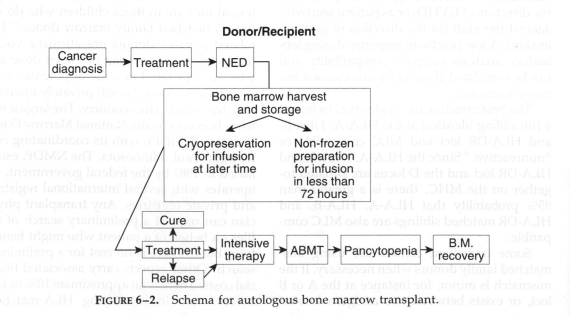

FIGURE 6–2. Schema for autologous bone marrow transplant.

late 1950s[95] and the first in children in 1961.[27] Since 1984 the use of auto-BMT in the treatment of malignancies has expanded rapidly.[82] Early clinical studies from allogeneic transplantation in patients with leukemia[18,147] and autologous transplantation in patients with lymphoma[125] and neuroblastoma[141] demonstrated that the use of BMT is most successful in achieving long-term disease-free survival in patients with malignancies if performed early in the disease course. There is a smaller disease burden with a less resistant cell population, and patients are usually in better physical state clinically to tolerate a transplant procedure. Currently auto-BMT is used as a form of consolidation therapy immediately after completing initial remission-induction therapy or as salvage therapy for patients after early relapse. Auto-BMT is most appropriate for patients identified by clinical staging or other forms of prognostic analysis at diagnosis as high risk for failing conventional chemotherapy, surgery, and/or radiation or for patients who develop progressive disease during or after conventional treatment.[153]

Purging Autologous Bone Marrow

The major limitation in the application of auto-BMT to the treatment of malignancy is tumor contamination of the harvested bone marrow and the subsequent risk of infusing tumor cells that could contribute to disease recurrence in the patient. Indirect evidence from nonrandomized human trials in patients with leukemia and neuroblastoma suggest that tumor cells infiltrating autologous bone marrow can regrow if infused into the patient.[60,62,154] Bone marrow considered in clinical "remission" has also been shown as infiltrated with tumor.[12,86] It is impossible to determine the number of tumor cells that will produce cancer in the patient, which may vary between and within disease states.[153] This is a significant concern in the treatment of leukemias since the bone marrow may be more heavily infiltrated with tumor cells. With solid tumors, the question of bone marrow metastasis varies by tumor type.

In an effort to minimize the risk of bone marrow contamination with tumor, various methods of "purging," or cleaning, harvested

bone marrow of contaminating tumor cells have been developed. All purging techniques are based on the ability to detect and exploit reliably and consistently the different physical, functional, and/or immunologic characteristics between normal bone marrow stem cells and the malignant cells in the bone marrow. Unfortunately, the more a tumor cell resembles a normal stem cell physically, functionally, and immunologically, the more difficult it is to design purging methods that remove only the tumor cells and preserve the normal stem cells necessary for engraftment.

Purging methods vary in degree of specificity and thus efficacy in tumor removal.[128,153] The purging process itself is performed immediately after the bone marrow harvest. The marrow is taken from the operating room to the laboratory for processing. Most purging procedures take several hours to complete. Afterward, the purged marrow is cryopreserved (frozen) for future use in transplantation.

The risks of bone marrow purging are (1) contamination of the bone marrow with infectious organisms during the harvest or processing procedure; (2) incomplete elimination of tumor cells from the harvested marrow; and (3) delayed or nonengraftment of the marrow in the patient.

In spite of sterile conditions in the operating room during the bone marrow harvest and in the laboratory during processing, manipulation of the bone marrow is extensive and can lead to marrow contamination with infectious agents. Cultures of the marrow are taken for bacteria and fungi. Policies and procedures for handling the bone marrow in the operating room and the purging laboratory to prevent contamination are followed closely.

The optimal goal of purging autologous bone marrow is to remove enough contaminating malignant cells so they will not regrow after the processed marrow has been infused.[128] This requires a system sensitive beyond the level of clinical morphologic remission for detecting the presence of tumor cells in the bone marrow. For instance, for neuroblastoma a detection system has been developed that uses monoclonal antibody staining of cell-surface antigens. Depending on the antibodies and methods used, this system can detect the presence of tumor beyond the level of clinical remission from 1 tumor cell in 1000 to 1 tumor cell in 100,000 normal bone marrow cells.[10,119] Using this detection system, autologous marrow is infused only if tumor cells are not detected in a random sampling of the purged marrow.[141]

A variety of factors can impede engraftment of an autologous purged bone marrow. Any purging process results in a degree of nonspecific cell loss. Thus fewer normal stem cells are given back during the transplant process, potentially causing delayed engraftment.[153] In addition to cell loss, manipulation of the bone marrow during purging procedures may damage the normal stem cell population sufficiently to delay engraftment. The amount of therapy the patient has received before bone marrow harvesting can damage stem cells so that their hematopoietic function is diminished.[57,153] Any variable that prolongs the time to engraftment of the bone marrow leaves the patient at risk for prolonged severe pancytopenia.

Frequently an autologous "backup marrow" is obtained. The backup marrow contains enough cells to ensure engraftment and is not processed in any manner that could influence the engraftment process. Backup bone marrow is routinely obtained when a new purging process is being evaluated. Obtaining backup marrow is attempted at the time of initial harvest but sometimes requires a subsequent harvest.

Purging of autologous bone marrow is controversial.[2] Disagreement among investigators is related to the inability to evaluate directly the efficiency of tumor cell removal by any specific purging technique. If a patient relapses after auto-BMT, it is difficult to evaluate whether the relapse is due to recurrence of residual disease in the patient or contaminated marrow infused during transplant.

OUTCOME

Multiple variables affect both event-free survival and long-term disease-free survival after BMT. Patients and family members seeking information about survival statistics are given factual, updated information, with explanations clarifying how the variables affect their outcome. Important variables include patient factors (e.g., age and adherence to therapy), disease factors (e.g., stage of disease at BMT), therapy-related factors (e.g., amount and type of previous cytoreductive treatment), and supportive care factors (e.g., availability of sophisticated blood bank support), to name a few. Table 6–2 summarizes the current research-based survival statistics for a variety of diseases treated by BMT. Outcome statistics are constantly evolving as new treatment modalities evolve and the criteria for transplant candidacy mature.

THE TRANSPLANT PROCESS
Choosing a Transplant Center

Deciding to undergo a BMT and determining where to have it performed are based on many factors. The age, diagnosis, and overall health status of the patient, donor availability, bed availability, family dynamics, and the degree of social and financial support of the family are considered by the family and health care team in the decision-making process.[188] Although an increasing number of beds are becoming available for pediatric BMT across the country, most transplant programs are based in tertiary care centers located in urban areas.[3,185] As a result, many families pursuing transplant face the prospect of traveling to a BMT center some distance from their home to have the procedure performed.[24,185]

A family's decision in favor of BMT must be based on an understanding of the rationale, risks, possible outcomes, and commitment involved in the transplant process.[188] It is the major responsibility of the primary or referring physician, nurses, and social worker to prepare the family for the BMT and transfer of care.[24,185] The referring physician provides the family with current scientific data on BMT, alternative treatment options, and potential appropriate transplant centers with available beds. Helping a family make a well-informed decision about BMT can be a highly influential process, a fact that must be recognized by everyone involved.[24] In making a decision, families should visit a transplant center of their choice, talk with the members of the transplant team, and tour the institution.[3,24,188] Spending time with other families who have

TABLE 6–2. *Selected Indications and Clinical Results of BMT in Children*

DISEASE	INDICATIONS	CLINICAL RESULTS
Malignancies		
Acute lymphoblastic leukemia (ALL)	Second complete remission or higher	30%–40% actuarial 2 yr disease-free survival with HLA-matched sibling donor 2+ complete remission
	First complete remission with poor prognostic factors (e.g., Philadelphia chromosome positive, chromosome translocation [4;11])	
	Extramedullary relapse (e.g., testicular, CNS)	20% actuarial 2-yr disease-free survival; dependent on duration of initial remission
	Auto-BMT for ALL (with purging procedure)	
Acute myelogenous leukemia (AML)	First complete remission	45%–65% actuarial 2-yr disease-free survival with HLA-matched sibling donor in first complete remission
	Early first relapse and second complete remission versus resistant first relapse	34% 3-yr survival rate and 24% 3-yr survival in resistant first relapse with HLA-matched sibling donor
	Auto-BMT with hydroperoxycyclophosphamide-purged bone marrow	40% actuarial disease-free survival in second and third complete remission
Chronic myelogenous leukemia (CML) or juvenile CML	Treatment of choice with suitable donor; improved results with BMT <1 yr from diagnosis	63% 3-yr survival in chronic phase 36% 3-yr survival in accelerated phase 12% 3-yr survival in blast crisis
Myelodysplasia (preleukemia, refractory anemias)	Treatment of choice with suitable donor	60%–70% without excess blasts in bone marrow
Lymphomas: non-Hodgkin's lymphoma and Hodgkin's disease	Chemotherapy-responsive disease	42% 2-yr disease-free survival
Neuroblastoma	6 mo S/P diagnosis with poor prognostic features, N-*myc* amplification, poor histology, stage III and IV, diagnosed over 1 yr of age	20%–40% long-term disease-free survival at 5-yr with auto-BMT
Brain tumors		
Primitive neuroectodermal tumor (PNET)		
Rhabdomyosarcoma	Initial pilot studies confirm potential efficacy of procedure in high-risk subgroups; ongoing studies needed	
Osteosarcoma		
Ewing's sarcoma		
Wilms' tumor		
Bone Marrow Failure		
Severe aplastic anemia	Treatment of choice with suitable donor	80%–90% 2- to 16-yr survival with HLA-matched sibling donor without transfusion; 70% with transfusion
Severe combined immunodeficiency syndrome (SCIDS)	Treatment of choice with suitable donor	90%–100% cured with HLA-matched sibling donor; 70% cured with haploidentical parent donor
Thalassemia major	Identify poor prognostic factors; balance risks of supportive care versus BMT	75% 2-yr disease-free survival when patient is <16 yr of age at BMT
Systemic Enzyme Deficiency Diseases		
Inborn errors of metabolism	Initial studies indicate a potential for BMT in some disease states	

Data from references 44, 65, 99, 136, 155, 161, 175, 191.

gone through the transplant experience and reading the available literature also help prospective families make their decision about BMT.[24,188]

The most critical factor enabling a smooth transition between the referral institution and transplant centers is the communication of information between the different health care teams and the family to maintain consistency and foster the family's trust in the new system.[3,24,185] Information about the BMT process and specific routines of the transplant center should be accurate, and differences in technique or routines between the referring and transplant center should be presented in a way that does not prejudice the family or jeopardize the development of trust in the transplant center.[3] Tables 6–3 and 6–4 list nursing responsibilities in transferring the patient and family to the BMT center.

Pre-BMT Evaluation

Patient Evaluation. Before admission all prospective patients, donors, and their families participate in a comprehensive evalua-

tion process at the transplant center (Table 6–5). The pre-BMT evaluation period allows for a thorough clinical assessment of the child and donor while providing an introduction to the transplant center, transplant team, and the BMT environment. The evaluation is generally performed on an outpatient basis, with the child, donor, and family arriving at the transplant center from weeks before the transplant to days before the tentative admission date. Appropriate baseline tests are performed to confirm the child's overall clinical condition and disease status pre-BMT. The donor undergoes a physical examination and limited clinical testing to ensure he or she is an appropriate candidate for general anesthesia.

A psychosocial assessment of the family is done, and families who could benefit from special ongoing support are identified. The evaluation period is a time of anxiety and uncertainty for the child and family. This anxiety is heightened if test results indicate any reason why the BMT should be delayed or is contraindicated such as relapse or identification of significant organ damage.[67] During the

TABLE 6–3. *Responsibilities of Referring Nurse in Transition, Orientation, and Education of Patient and Family to BMT*

Assist patient and family to make an informed decision about performing BMT by providing information and clarifying misinformation.

Identify a nursing contact at the BMT center who will help the patient and family plan for their stay at the BMT center, and obtain pertinent information to share with the patient and family regarding:

Nursing care delivery system (e.g., primary nursing).

Basic nursing care routines and how they are performed at the BMT center.

Isolation policies and procedures practiced on the BMT unit.

Parent accomodations on the BMT unit (e.g., are parents allowed to stay in the child's room at night).

Restrictions on personal items that may be brought to the BMT unit (e.g., TV, VCR, computers, and video games).

Pre-BMT evaluation: how long does it take; what tests are involved; estimate of the average length of time between completion of pre-BMT evaluation and actual admission.

Average length of stay at BMT center after discharge.

Obtain any written information that could be heplful for the family.

Provide reinforcement and reassurance about daily routines that change from institution to institution.

Encourage patient and family to identify what routines and aspects of care are important to them so they can be discussed with the BMT unit nursing staff.

Facilitate social work contact to help patient and family with issues of lodging, travel, and funding.

Help patient and family, in conjunction with social worker, to plan a strategy to deal with a 2- to 3-month absence from home.

Provide nursing contact at BMT center with pertinent information about patient and family to help facilitate transition of care.

Data from references 32 and 185.

TABLE 6—4. *Responsibilities of the BMT Nurse in Transition, Orientation, and Education of the Patient and Family to BMT*

Outpatient

Provide formal introduction to BMT center and multidisciplinary team.
Provide formal education about BMT and side effects to prepare the patient and family for the consent process.
Facilitate adaptation to the transplant center and geographic locale.
Assist with transition of patient and family to inpatient setting.

Inpatient

Provide orientation and reinforce education about the daily routine and procedures on the BMT unit.
Provide continuing education and information processing about the transplant process and complications.
Provide ongoing patient and family support and facilitate integration into the BMT unit.
Conduct discharge teaching and organize transition of patient and family back to outpatient or referral center.

Data from references 32 and 127.

TABLE 6—5. *Patient Evaluation for BMT*

1. Complete medical history and physical examination
   a. Confirmation of diagnosis
   b. Previous treatment history
   c. Diagnosis or treatment-related problems
   d. Other medical problems
   e. Transfusion history
   f. Allergy and immunization history
   g. Psychosocial assessment and neuropsychologic testing
2. Histocompatibility
   a. Confirmation of HLA and MLC testing and selection of donor
   b. Transfusion support planning; ABO typing of patient
   c. Determination of markers of engraftment for allogeneic patients
3. Major organ and body system screening and assessment
   a. Complete blood count, differential, and platelets
   b. Chemistry panel, electrolytes, creatinine, magnesium
   c. Hepatitis screen (A, B, and C)
   d. Viral assessment (cytomegalovirus, herpes simplex virus, varicella-zoster virus, Epstein-Barr virus, human immunodeficiency virus)
   e. Pulmonary function tests (if <5 yrs old, use another measure of pulmonary function)
   f. Cardiac evaluation: ECG and echocardiogram and/or multiple gated acquisition (MUGA)
   g. Creatinine clearance and/or glomerular filtration rate (GFR) study
   h. Chest x-ray, sinus films
   i. Nutritional evaluation
   j. Dental evaluation
   k. Ophthalmology evaluation
   l. Hearing evaluation
   m. Occupational and physical therapy evaluation
4. Tumor status evaluation
5. Genetic disease status evaluation
6. Central line placement
7. Sperm banking
8. Ancillary support evaluation (education therapy, child life, clergy)
9. Informed consent, discussion with patient and family about BMT
10. Education
11. Blood product donor screening: family and relatives, friends

Data from references 32 and 127.

psychosocial assessment, financial screening for BMT is completed if it has not been investigated before the pretransplant evaluation. Pediatric BMT is an expensive treatment modality. Most transplant centers require a written guarantee or contract of full or partial payment for services before recommending BMT. The recommendation to use it as therapy is subject to intense scrutiny for payment benefits from both insurance companies and medical aid programs. Transplant coordinators and/or financial officers at BMT centers can provide estimated costs analysis for individual patients. Most transplant coordinators assist in securing medical benefits for patients by providing documentation and research-based medical support to insurance companies and other payors. The degree to which transplant centers actively participate in individual fund-raising varies according to institutional policies. The financial prescreening is laborious and anxiety provoking to families.

During the pre-BMT evaluation the child and family become acquainted with the new staff and the transplant setting. The transplant team consists of several physicians, inpatient and outpatient nursing staff, social workers, and possibly a psychologist or psychiatrist.[127,159] Numerous other consulting services may be involved with transplant patients as clinically indicated. Nurses play a key role in coordination of services and education and soon become identified by the family as a resource for questions and for help in processing information.[33,67]

In addition, nurses teach the child and family the basic concepts of BMT, the conditioning regimen, and about subsequent toxicities. Patients and families may be asked to participate in various clinical research protocols underway on the transplant unit. The nurse can provide information to help the child and family understand the research process and the purpose of clinical trials.[67] Various teaching methods, including written materials, videotaped instruction, and play therapy with younger children, may be used.[33,188] Since large volumes of information must be absorbed by the family, written materials (e.g., copies of consent forms and information on BMT routines) are helpful and should be provided in a systematic fashion to allow time for individual review and assimilation.

Patients and families come to the transplant center with varying amounts of information and expectations about BMT. Obtaining consent from the patient and family for the transplant procedure is a thoughtful, deliberate process conducted by the transplant physician with a nurse and possibly a social worker in attendance.[33,127] During the consent conference basic information about the child's disease status and the natural history of the disease are reviewed, and the general rationale for BMT and its specific indication in that child's illness are discussed. The child's prognosis and any other treatment options are presented.

Results of the pre-BMT evaluation are summarized, and acute and chronic toxicities of the transplant are discussed. The impact of long-term side effects of BMT on the child's physical health and quality of life must be given careful consideration in the consent process.[31,127] The child and family often have the misconception BMT is invariably curative.[127] It is crucial to help families understand the role of BMT in the therapeutic outcome for the child. Children 6 years of age and older need developmentally appropriate discussions to obtain assent for the transplant.[45] The nurse's professional knowledge of the transplant experience, combined with an understanding of the patient's and family's needs and comprehension of the pre-BMT teaching, makes him or her a unique advocate for the patient and family during the decision-making process. Additionally, some centers use an objective child advocate to safeguard the rights and needs of minor children involved in decisions about BMT and marrow harvests.

Donor Evaluation. Parental consent is required for a minor child to donate bone marrow for transplantation. Special consents may be required for a very young child or a child with developmental disabilities. Children 6 years of age and older assent to the procedure after receiving developmentally appropriate information. When an appropriate donor has been identified for BMT, the donor undergoes a thorough preharvest evaluation. The information obtained from the evaluation is used as a baseline to monitor the donor throughout the harvest process, to diagnose comorbidity that may preclude the use of a particular donor, and to obtain marrow chromosomes that may be necessary to document engraftment in the recipient.

Included in the routine preharvest workup are a physical examination, complete blood count (CBC) with indices, clotting time, liver and renal function studies, and viral studies (e.g., cytomegalovirus titer, hepatitis screen, herpes simplex screen, Epstein-Barr virus serology, toxoplasmosis titer). A specimen is collected from the donor to crossmatch the donor's blood with that of the recipient on the day of the transplant if the recipient-donor pair is ABO incompatible. If the HLA and MLC analyses are equivocal, the tissue typing is repeated at the transplant center. Many transplant centers repeat these tests routinely, using their own quality control measures to avoid problems associated with inaccurate tissue typing.

Peripheral blood chromosomes may be collected, which, in conjunction with the marrow chromosomes, are used to document donor cell engraftment in the recipient. Other routine evaluation studies may include urinalysis and chest x-ray examinations. Allogeneic donors may undergo a bone marrow aspiration before the bone marrow harvest to document cellularity, normal marrow histology, and chromosomal constitution. In some cases this is done at the time of the harvest. Donors old enough to cooperate and who have adequate venous access are asked to donate a unit of autologous blood 7 to 10 days before the harvest for transfusion during the procedure. Generally autologous blood donation is successful if the child is age 7 or older. For younger donors and in select cases for autologous BMT patients, directed donor blood components are collected for transfusion during the harvest. These measures are done to minimize the possibility of bloodborne diseases.

Bone Marrow Harvest. Emotional preparation and patient teaching for the donor and family are nursing responsibilities. Whether the donor is an allogeneic sibling or is the autologous donor, the harvest experience is new and frightening. The donor is given age-appropriate information that explains how marrow is removed from the bone marrow spaces and emphasizes his or her body will replace the removed bone marrow after the harvest. In the hematologically healthy donor the blood system begins to replenish itself immediately.

Many younger children have the misconception that bones actually will be removed during the harvest procedure. Most BMT centers have patient education tools to explain the transplant process and the bone marrow harvest. When possible, the donor should have an opportunity to view films preoperatively and to tour the surgical area.

Emotional support and encouragement should be provided to the parents at the time of the bone marrow harvest. Although they may have a very sophisticated understanding of the underlying disease and the BMT process, they may still have many misconceptions and concerns about the bone marrow harvest. The parents must sign informed consent for the harvest procedure. Financial and insurance reimbursement issues for the bone marrow harvest are an additional source of stress for them. With allo-BMT, many parents struggle with the ethical conflict of subjecting a healthy child to the risks of surgery and anesthesia to collect marrow that may be the only source of curative therapy for the ill child.

Harvesting is performed in the operating room using sterile technique. A team of bone marrow harvesters (usually two or three individuals) prepare the bilateral posterior iliac crests under sterile conditions. Small scalpel incisions are made over the area of the iliac crest bones. The bone marrow aspiration needles are inserted numerous times, often up to 50 to 100 times, on each side to aspirate the appropriate amount of marrow. The marrow is placed in heparinized culture medium to prevent clotting. It is filtered through several fine and coarse mesh screens to remove bone spicules, fat particles, and blood clots, which can cause emboli formation in the recipient. During the procedure the donor may receive blood transfusions and colloid or crystalloid fluid support. Transfusion is avoided if possible; however, when it becomes nec-

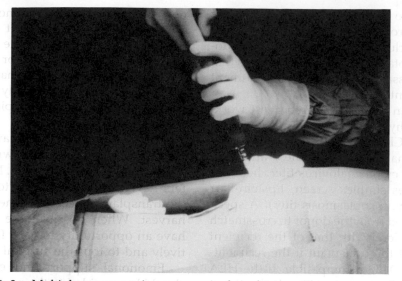

FIGURE 6–3. Multiple puncture sites are required to obtain sufficient marrow from the donor. *(Courtesy Peter F. Coccia, M.D., University of Nebraska Medical Center, Omaha.)*

essary, the irradiated autologous or donor packed red blood cells (RBCs) are transfused.

After the harvest procedure small sutures or tape closures are placed over the incision site and are covered with pressure dressings. The pressure dressings are removed the following day and replaced with bandages, which can be removed the next day. Incisions are monitored for postoperative bleeding, although this complication is rare. The donor and parents are told there is a risk for infection and are instructed to keep the incision sites clean and dry. The donor is likely to experience mild to moderate muscle and bone pain in the hips, which is easily alleviated with nonnarcotic analgesics.[77] Typically the donor is released from the hospital the day after the harvest. Supplemental iron is not usually needed.

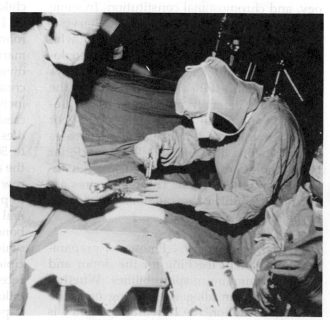

FIGURE 6–4. Bone marrow from the donor is aspirated under the sterile conditions of the operating room. *(Courtesy Peter F. Coccia, M.D., University of Nebraska Medical Center, Omaha.)*

Although the volume of marrow collected provides an estimate of an "adequate" harvest, the actual number of mononuclear cells collected is the essential parameter. The amount harvested is based on the weight of the recipient. Typically a dose of 2 to 6 × 10[8] nucleated cells per kilogram of the recipient's weight is collected.[164] If the marrow will be purged or processed, an additional amount of nucleated cells is required to compensate for cell loss. The usual volume desired is approximately 10 cc per kilogram of the recipient's weight. This volume is most safely and easily obtained when the donor is larger than the recipient or is older than toddler age; however, successful bone marrow harvesting has been reported for donors less than the age of 2 years.[144] When the allogeneic donor is an unrelated HLA-MLC compatible donor identified through a national bone marrow registry, the coordination and implementation of the harvest are complicated. Transplant centers affiliated with the NMDP have trained coordinators responsible for this detailed process.[69]

The harvest procedure is nearly the same for the auto-BMT donor except that the amount of marrow collected is also contingent on the quality of marrow reserve (which may be depleted from previous chemotherapy and/or radiotherapy) and required processing such as purging. It is often necessary to collect an additional amount of marrow to compensate for a potentially inadequate harvest. Auto-BMT donors are also more likely to have comorbid organ system disease (e.g., nephrotoxicity) that may place them at greater risk during general anesthesia.

Autologous marrow is cryopreserved, or frozen, until the patient has completed the preparative regimen. The marrow is frozen in special polyoleifen bags placed in flat metal canisters. Safeguards are taken to label and catalog the marrow accurately. The metal canisters are submerged in liquid nitrogen in specialized freezing tanks at a temperature of −40° to −50° C. A cryopreservative protective agent such as dimethyl sulfoxide (DMSO) or hydroxyethyl starch is added to the marrow before freezing to protect the stem cells from lysis caused by the extreme temperature. Cryopreserved marrow can be thawed and infused up to several years after harvest without appreciable loss in stem cell viability, although there is little research data suggesting how long marrow may be stored without damage to the cells.

Admission and Isolation Technique

Patient Admission. Children are admitted to the transplant unit from 1 to several days before beginning the conditioning regimen. Some patients may also be transferred from another hospital directly to the inpatient unit of the transplant center. Although most major BMT centers have committed BMT intensive care unit beds for BMT patients, some centers admit children to the pediatric or pediatric oncology unit. The extent of isolation precautions varies with the child's clinical condition and institutional policies.

Most patients and families will have toured the transplant unit and possibly gone through some degree of orientation before admission. The outpatient nursing staff communicates with the inpatient nursing staff about the family's level of knowledge and understanding and their assessment of the family's adjustment and coping with the initial aspects of the transplant experience. Nurses work together to determine teaching priorities and communication strategies used with the child and family. The inpatient nursing staff is responsible for assimilating the information received from the outpatient staff and designing an appropriate plan of care to meet the educational and support needs of the child and family.

The immediate nursing concerns when a patient is admitted to the transplant unit are to provide the child and family with (1) a practical orientation to the patient care environment, including the type of isolation room used and isolation techniques; (2) a description of the roles and responsibilities of nursing and other staff of the multidisciplinary team; (3) a list of guidelines governing unit activities; and (4) a discussion of the routine nursing care included in a general patient day. Most BMT units have nursing standards of care for patient education and orientation.[26]

Knowledge of the child's prior medical history, developmental history, and experiences with hospitalization can guide the nurse in assessment, development, and implementation of nursing care strategies designed to integrate the child and family into the BMT environment. For example, a child with a malignancy will be somewhat familiar with basic concepts of BMT care and side effects of chemotherapy and radiation from prior hospitalization experiences. In contrast, a child with a new diagnosis of severe aplastic anemia or SCIDS needs a different, more intensive teaching approach by the nursing staff in orienting and integrating the child and family into the BMT environment.

Isolation. A major risk for patients undergoing BMT is the complication of life-threatening infections that occur during prolonged granulocytopenia after marrow infusion and that can be associated with acute GVHD and its treatment.[19,163] Exposure to exogenous sources of infection is prevented and/or minimized through the control of the physical environment with different types of isolation, with or without concomitant procedures to suppress or eliminate the endogenous microbial flora of the patient through gut decontamination and skin cleansing measures.[19,131]

The most sophisticated and comprehensive type of isolation is the total protected environment. The goal of using the total protected environment is to eliminate the normal microbial flora and to prevent colonization of the patient by new microorganisms from the hospital environment.[131] It includes using a laminar flow isolation room, skin and GI tract decontamination, sterile supplies, and specialized nursing procedures for patient care. Laminar air flow is a complex air filtering and circulation system that makes the air in this type of isolation room essentially germ free or sterile.[131] Gut and skin decontamination measures minimize the role endogenous normal flora can play as a source of infection. Gut decontamination is achieved with a sterile or low-bacteria diet, administration of oral nonabsorbable antibiotics (known as "gut meds"), and an antifungal agent such as nystatin several times daily. Skin-cleansing measures include a daily bath with an antimicrobial soap and application of antibiotic solutions and creams to body surfaces such as the

mouth, nasal passages, anus, vagina, groin, and axilla several times daily.[103,131] The use of sterile supplies and sterile gowning of those entering the laminar air flow room augment strict nursing standards of care to maintain a total protected environment.

A total protected environment can significantly decrease the incidence of serious bacterial and fungal infections in certain patients undergoing BMT (e.g., patients with severe aplastic anemia).[19,163] However, the use of this extreme type of isolation has not improved the overall long-term disease-free survival time of most BMT patients.[19,101,163] Most BMT centers use the total protected environment only for selected groups of patients, based on diagnosis or donor status.

There are no age restrictions for children placed in a total protected environment. Adolescents may have a more difficult time than younger children adjusting to the isolation. Although liberal or unrestricted visitation policies for the immediate family are common in most pediatric transplant units, rooming-in at night is often not permitted for children isolated in the total protected environment to maintain the integrity of the isolation. Parents of younger children initially have difficulty with the physical separation at night. Often it is helpful to introduce parents and patients to other transplant families who have experienced similar fears and frustrations.

The total protected environment requires intensive nursing support and strict adherence to a protocol of care.[103,109] An important nursing goal is to minimize the impact of the isolation setting on an already stressed child and family.[109] Touring the unit before admission is the first step in this process. All types of personal belongings from clothing and toys to stereos, televisions, videocassette recorders (VCRs), and computers are commonly permitted. Particularly for children and families traveling a far distance, personal items and reminders of home, family, friends, and pets take on special importance. Parents of younger children are encouraged to create photo albums of important people, pets, places, and home that can be used in story telling or in creative play therapy with the child. Home videos can be entertaining and therapeutic. Adolescents may prefer a video

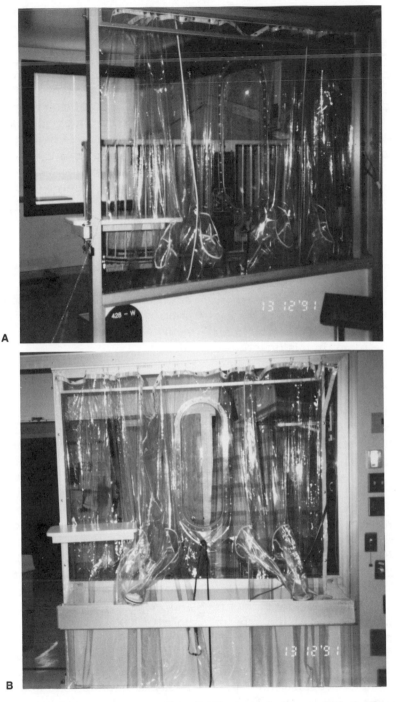

FIGURE 6–5.   Views of laminar air flow (LAF) room: **A,** from outside LAF room looking into the room and, **B,** from inside LAF room looking out. *(Courtesy Children's Hospital, Los Angeles, California.)*

or photographs of special moments with their friends in addition to reminders of home. Classmates from school should be encouraged to write and send cards and other items of interest. Cassette recordings from family and friends are also important to have and help to ease feelings of isolation and separation.

Once the child is admitted, the parents and the child, if old enough, are encouraged to take an active role in the child's care, assisting with bathing, central line and dressing care, and medication administration. Nurses work with the child and family to develop plans for managing care throughout the hospitalization. Children are encouraged to decorate their isolation room. To relieve the tedium and boredom that normally develop with a prolonged hospital stay, parents are encouraged to divide a child's toys into groups that are given back at different intervals. Most personal items brought by the child can be sterilized or cleaned effectively for use in a laminar air flow room.

A more common form of isolation is modified protective (reverse) isolation. The BMT patient is isolated in a single room where good hand washing, with or without the use of gloves, gowns, and masks, is required for those entering the room. In this type of isolation, liberal visitation and parental rooming-in are common practice. A BMT admission and the prolonged period of isolation are demanding for everyone involved. It is important for the nurse, the child, and the family to work together to promote adjustment.

Conditioning

Immediately before the bone marrow infusion, the child receives a course of intensive chemotherapy with or without total body irradiation (TBI). This treatment, known as the *conditioning*, *ablative*, or *preparative regimen*, may last from 4 to 8 days.[50] The specific conditioning regimen selected for the patient is influenced by the disease and the type of BMT.[176] For example, in allogeneic transplants the risk of graft rejection necessitates varying degrees of immunosuppression. In autologous transplants immunosuppression to prevent graft rejection is not necessary. TBI, total lymphoid irradiation (TLI), cyclophosphamide, and ATG may be used to provide effective immunosuppression to prevent graft rejection.[149]

Removal of unwanted cell populations (e.g., with malignant disease and in certain nonmalignant diseases) requires agents with antineoplastic, and thus myeloablative, effects. Cyclophosphamide, busulfan, cytosine arabinoside, and L-phenylalanine mustard have antineoplastic or myeloablative effects and are used most often in conditioning regimens for hematologic malignancies and certain nonmalignant disorders.[29,151,165,173] Against malignant solid tumors, combinations of known tumoricidal agents are used.[25] The majority of conditioning regimens use a combination of drugs that do not have overlapping toxicities, with or without radiation therapy. Rarely is only a single agent used for conditioning a patient for BMT.[165]

Chemotherapy is administered in lethal myeloablative doses, resulting in a dramatic increase in side effects rarely seen outside of the BMT setting.[47] Having astute assessment skills is critical in monitoring and intervening effectively against both anticipated and unanticipated side effects and toxicities in patients receiving transplant conditioning regimens.[47]

Cyclophosphamide (Cytoxan). Cyclophosphamide, an alkylating agent, is the most common drug used in transplant conditioning regimens because of its immunosuppressive and myeloablative or antineoplastic effects. It is used with TBI, is combined with busulfan, or is given as a single agent in certain protocols (e.g., in conditioning for transplantation in a patient with severe aplastic anemia). The BMT conditioning dose of cyclophosphamide varies from 50 to 60 mg/kg to a total dose of 200 mg/kg.[184]

The major dose-limiting toxicity in high-dose regimens is life-threatening myocarditis and/or pericarditis, which can occur at total doses of 200 mg/kg.[184] Clinical manifestations resemble congestive heart failure (CHF), with tachycardia, dyspnea, weight gain, edema, and hepatosplenomegaly, and may occur 3 to 14 days after administration.[17] The electrocardiogram (ECG) shows low-voltage QRS complexes, and the echocardiogram demonstrates decreased left ventricular contractility.[18] Some patients can develop fulminating CHF, with rapid deterioration and death. Those patients who develop a less acute course can be managed successfully with digitalis, diuretics, and fluid restriction until spontaneous resolution of the process occurs.[18] Correct dosing with cyclophosphamide may prevent this toxicity.[184] An important dosing consideration in young children is the significant difference between dose based on body surface area and dose based on body weight. Routine cardiac rhythm strips are assessed for voltage changes before the administration of each cyclophosphamide dose. Nurses must be aware of any prior mediastinal radiation or anthracycline therapy the patient has received and the pre-BMT cardiac evaluation results.

With transplant doses of cyclophosphamide, hemorrhagic cystitis occurs frequently and can be severe. Symptoms range from tea-colored urine to significant blood clots, pain, and urinary retention.[184] Standard therapy includes providing hyperhydration, continuing for 24 to 48 hours after the last cyclophosphamide dose to promote the excretion of toxic metabolites and thus prevent damage to the bladder mucosa. In the BMT unit continuous bladder irrigations are performed, or mesna is administered. Fluid and electrolytes, weight, and intake and output must be monitored closely to assess antidiuretic hormone's effects on the kidneys. Platelet counts must also be monitored because of the risk of bleeding.

Total Body Irradiation. TBI is the single most effective immunosuppressant agent.[173] It lacks cross-resistance to many chemotherapy agents, thus enhancing its antineoplastic effects. It also can reach disease sanctuaries such as the CNS, which is important in the management of hematologic malignancies.[173] However, TBI is associated with numerous toxicities that are dependent on total dose and rate of delivery of the dose.[184] Immediate side effects include nausea and vomiting, diarrhea, hypotension, capillary leak syndrome, and a respiratory distress syndrome. TBI may enhance the toxicities resulting from other agents used in the conditioning regimen.[7] The late effects of TBI include cataracts, restrictive and obstructive lung disease, interstitial pneumonitis, leukoencephalopathy, cognitive impairment leading to poor school achievement, and endocrinopathies such as gonadal failure, hypothyroidism, and growth hormone deficiency.[117,148,180,184] Numerous

protocols avoid using TBI when possible, particularly in children whose developing organ systems are susceptible to the long-term effects of radiation. Organ system toxicity is magnified in infants in whom rapid physical and brain development is occurring.[117]

Busulfan. Busulfan, another alkylating agent, is myeloablative if administered in large doses. The conditioning regimen of busulfan and cyclophosphamide was developed for use in patients with acute myeloblastic leukemia (AML).[151] Busulfan was substituted for TBI to avoid radiation-associated toxicities. Studies have demonstrated similar therapeutic benefit of busulfan combined with cyclophosphamide as compared to TBI and cyclophosphamide in patients with hematologic malignancies with less toxicity.[151]

Busulfan is available only in oral 2 mg tablets. The common transplant dosage is 16 mg/kg divided every 6 hours over 4 days.[151] A major nursing concern is to ensure that patients take and retain each busulfan tablet. If emesis occurs within an hour of administration, the entire dose must be repeated.[143] Antiemetics are used, and occasionally use of a nasogastric (NG) tube is necessary to ensure that the patient receives and absorbs the total dose of busulfan. Patients receiving high doses of busulfan may experience seizures. Prophylactic phenytoin (Dilantin) is given throughout the conditioning regimen to prevent seizure activity.[143] Nurses monitor serum phenytoin levels and assess the child for seizure activity. High doses of busulfan in combination therapy for BMT are associated with the occurrence of veno-occlusive disease (VOD), which is characterized by obstruction of blood flow from the liver.[181]

Cytosine Arabinoside (ARA-C) (Cytarbine). Cytosine arabinoside, a cell cycle–specific antimetabolite, has an excellent antileukemic effect when given in high doses and is effective treatment for meningeal leukemia because it crosses the blood-brain barrier. High-dose cytosine arabinoside and fractionated TBI are highly effective as a preparative regimen in transplant of patients with acute leukemia.[29] Customarily, cytosine arabinoside is administered as 12 doses of 3000 mg/m^2 given twice daily over 1 to 3 hours for 6 days. It is followed by radiation administered twice daily on the subsequent 3 days. In addition to the side effects seen at conventional doses, high-dose cytosine arabinoside causes major skin, ocular, and CNS toxicities.

Patients receiving high-dose cytosine arabinoside may develop an erythematous painful rash localized to the palms of the hands and soles of the feet. Known as *acral erythema*, this rash may be accompanied by swelling, blister formation, and severe desquamation.[20] Additional pain experienced during infusions of cyclosporine is believed caused by the drug's alcohol base.[87] Acral erythema caused by high-dose cytosine arabinoside may mimic the rash associated with acute GVHD.[34] Documentation of other symptoms of acute GVHD helps differentiate the two skin conditions. Other nursing concerns center on pain management, infection prevention, and comfort measures to decrease swelling, to cool the burning sensation, and to soothe the skin.[1] Patients may need assistance with self-care since the tenderness, swelling, and blistering of the hands and feet can limit their use until healing occurs.[1]

Cytosine arabinoside, which can be isolated from the rapidly developing cells of the corneal epithelium, can cause severe chemical conjunctivitis.[97] The route by which the systemic cytosine arabinoside reaches the cornea is unclear. Patients experience intense photophobia, pain, redness, tearing, blurred vision, and a foreign body sensation in their eyes.[97] Administering glucocorticoid eye drops, started 24 hours before treatment and administered every 6 to 8 hours throughout high-dose cytosine arabinoside administration, can prevent or ameliorate the symptoms for the patient.[97]

Toxicity to the CNS is the most severe and dose-limiting side effect with high dose cytosine arabinoside.[76] Patients experience cerebellar dysfunction seen as nystagmus, dysarthria with truncal and gait ataxia, or less commonly, cerebral dysfunction, which can manifest from mild personality changes and difficulties performing calculations to more severe symptoms, including psychoses, seizures, encephalopathy, and coma.[35] Neurotoxicity occurs in 16% to 40% of patients receiving high-dose cytosine arabinoside at doses of 3000 mg/m² and is severe in 7% to 18% of patients.[75,121] It is reversible in 50% to 90% of patients and fatal in the remainder.[75,121] A recent retrospective study found renal insufficiency at the time of receiving high-dose cytosine arabinoside was a significant independent risk factor in the development of neurotoxicity.[35] Nurses should be aware of the renal status of patients receiving high-dose cytosine arabinoside. Other nursing concerns focus on self-care needs, patient safety, and emotional support of the patient and family coping with neurotoxicity.

L-phenylalanine Mustard (Melphalan). L-phenylalanine mustard, another alkylating agent, is a major component of conditioning regimens for neuroblastoma. Most regimens use L-phenylalanine mustard in combination with additional drugs, with or without TBI.[63,74,155] It is administered as a short IV infusion daily over 1 to 3 days. GI and dermatologic side effects can be severe at transplant doses.[155] Altered renal function may increase the toxicity of L-phenylalanine mustard in the transplant setting.[155]

Nausea and vomiting can be severe with the higher dose chemotherapy used in transplant conditioning regimens. Providing aggressive combination antiemetic regimens as premedication and continuing on a scheduled basis are a normal standard of BMT nursing care.

Bone Marrow Infusion

Infusion of the marrow is similar to transfusion of a blood component. Allogeneic, unprocessed marrow may be transported directly from the surgical suite to the patient's room and infused to the recipient through a central venous catheter. If the marrow is plasma depleted, purged, or processed in any other manner, there may be a delay of hours or days before reinfusion. Autologous, cyropreserved marrow is removed from the liquid nitrogen tank and thawed in a warm water bath before infusion. In most institutions the marrow is transported in a plastic blood component transfer pack, whereas others process and preserve marrow in small aliquots that are thawed and pooled for infusion. Strict measures are taken to verify and document that the correct patient's marrow has been infused.

The marrow infusion can be delivered through an IV pump or can be infused by gravity. In some institutions the physicians or transplant coordinators reinfuse the marrow, whereas BMT nurses are responsible for reinfusion in others. Generally the infusion lasts 60 to 90 minutes, depending on the marrow volume and the patient's size. Frequently the patient receives antiemetics and/or diphenhydramine before the infusion to decrease acute toxicities, which usually occur at least in a small degree in most recipients. The nurse is at the bedside throughout the infusion and takes frequent vital signs to assess for fever, hypertension, tachycardia, and/or tachypnea, which may indicate a marrow transfusion reaction or marrow emboli. Large amounts of hydration are given during the infusion to diminish nephrotoxicity secondary to hemolysis. The patient is encouraged to void frequently, and the urine is tested for blood. Patient anxiety is related to the acute care and number of staff present during the infusion and/or may be a symptom of emboli formation. Transplant centers have established protocols for marrow infusion and the management of infusion-related complications. Specific flow sheets are maintained to document and chronicle the marrow infusion.

The marrow infusion is usually anticlimactic for the patient and family. Although it signifies optimism and hope for cure, it is less eventful than most of the procedures and complications of the evaluation process and preparative regimen. At this time of the transplant, many patients and families are consumed with other fears and preoccupations, including fear of complications, fear of disease recurrence, and/or fear that the marrow will fail to engraft.[73] Although patients do not generally experience pain, they may complain of nausea, particularly if DMSO was used as the cryopreservative. DMSO is metabolized and excreted in the lungs and produces a characteristic strong garlic breath odor that may distress the patient and family. Measures should be taken to provide physical comfort to the child, and the entire family is provided emotional support. Some families ask to carry out rituals or celebrations as a way to bring meaning and significance to the infusion procedure.

Acute Side Effects, Engraftment

The period after the transplant can be divided into three chronologic phases for describing expected toxicities and side effects.[32,46,53,193] The immediate post-transplant period covers approximately day 0, the day of transplant, through day +30 after BMT, and the focus is on the management of acute life-threatening toxicities. The intermediate period after transplant extends from day +30 through day +100, and nursing and medical care is focused on the resolution of acute toxicities, patient and family teaching, and discharge planning. The management and control of acute GVHD and its associated effects play a prominent role in allo-BMT during this period. The late or long-term phase begins from day +100. The majority of BMT recipients are outpatients by this time, and the focus of their follow-up care centers on late complications and/or rehabilitation.

Nursing care during the post-BMT period focuses on the prevention and/or treatment of transplant-related complications. Complications are often interrelated and seldom can be considered or managed individually. Clinical symptoms may be similar, and the treatment and management plan for one complication can significantly affect another, which makes nursing care very complex.[32,46,47] Table 6–6 summarizes post-BMT complications and nursing interventions.

IMMEDIATE POST-BMT PERIOD; DAY 0 TO DAY +30
Hematopoietic Complications

Regardless of the source of bone marrow used for the transplant, all patients go through a period of prolonged pancytopenia immediately after BMT while the new bone marrow is engrafting. The period of pancytopenia lasts an average of 2 to 3 weeks but can be longer if various purging methods, T-cell depletion, or acute GVHD prophylaxis exerts an adverse effect on marrow recovery.

TABLE 6–6. *Summary of Nursing Interventions for Post-BMT Complications*

NURSING DIAGNOSIS	NURSING STRATEGIES
Immediate Post-BMT Day 0 to Day +30	
Infection and Bleeding	

Potential for injury
  Infection
  Thrombocytopenia
	Identify risk factors: prior infections, pre-BMT CMV status, extensive use of antibiotics pre-BMT, history of refractory platelet treatment
	Monitor and maintain prophylactic measures: isolation and gut decontamination, prophylactic medications, CMV-negative blood products, and use of WBC depletion filters, routine hygiene, monitor results of weekly surveillance cultures; promote patient safety; administer platelet treatment as ordered

Mucositis	
Impairment of skin integrity Mucositis, enteritis	Assess oral mucosa and skin integrity: provide oral care according to unit policy; maintain skin integrity according to unit protocol
Alteration in comfort	Implement and monitor effectiveness of comfort measures: assess need for IV bolus before oral medications and mouth care

Potential for injury
  Excessive secretions
  Ineffective airway clearance
	Assess for aspiration and respiratory compromise
	Provide Yankauer suction tip for management of secretions
	Elevate head of bed; minimize oral trauma and bleeding

Veno-Occlusive Disease	
Alteration in body fluids Fluid volume excess	Implement oral and IV fluid restriction Administer spironolactone (Aldactone) as ordered Obtain BID weights and abdominal girth Strict intake and output (I and O) assessment; monitor vital signs and electrolytes in blood and urine
Alteration in nutritional status Impaired hepatic function	Assess use of medications extensively metabolized by the liver; monitor coagulation studies, liver functions and bilirubin results Altered protein metabolism; adjust nutritional intake accordingly; maximize calories
Impaired gas exchange Hepatomegaly, ascites	Assess for respiratory difficulty; implement and monitor use of oxygen Elevate head of bed, use pillows for optimal lung inflation
Alteration in comfort	Administer short-acting narcotics, morphine sulfate drug of choice; avoid merperidine Assess effectiveness, monitor respirations, mental status, duration of effect
Potential for injury Encephalopathy	Monitor mental status Keep side rails up, padded if necessary Maintain bed rest, ambulation with assistance only Assess for bleeding and assess skin integrity
Renal Insufficiency	
Alteration in fluid volume, excess or deficit Alteration in body fluid composition	Identify risk factors for renal impairment: use of nephrotoxic agent, prior radiation to kidneys, congenital kidney disease, nephrectomy, liver disease, infection, GVHD Monitor vital signs, daily BID weights, strict I and O, daily abdominal girth, assess level of consciousness Monitor results of serum and urinary laboratory studies Assess for cognitive changes
Acute GVHD	
Impairment of skin integrity	Assess skin q8h; include intertriginous skin folds Administer antihistamines for pruritus

Data from references 30, 32, 94, and 108.

TABLE 6–6. *Summary of Nursing Interventions for Post-BMT Complications* Continued

NURSING DIAGNOSIS	NURSING STRATEGIES
Acute GVHD—cont'd	Give bath or shower daily without soaps; may use medicated emollient Apply antimicrobial ointment to open lesions Apply skin lubricants and emollients prn Trim nails; apply mittens if scratching persistent
Alteration in bowel elimination Diarrhea	Assess amount, color, consistency, guaiac results, and pH of stool Assess perianal area for redness, fissures, or signs of abscess Obtain hemoglobin and hemotocrit values frequently Monitor I and O diligently Cleanse perianal area after diarrhea episodes Perform diligent perianal care; avoid heat lamps Administer anticathartics if ordered
Potential fluid volume deficit	Weigh BID Monitor IVF and PO fluid rates and volumes Monitor I and O Obtain vital signs
Alterations in nutrition Weight loss	Teach child and family causes of weight loss to allay anxiety Obtain dietary consults and calorie counts Perform meticulous oral hygiene; provide artificial saliva if necessary Provide TPN with appropriate monitoring if warranted Teach family appropriate dietary and fluid choices Encourage family to weigh child no more than two or three times per week
Alteration in comfort	Position patient on left side to decrease liver pressure Reposition frequently Administer analgesics as prescribed Provide age-appropriate diversional activities
Potential Compromised or Ineffective Family Coping	
Alterations in patient or family role function, self-concept, and usual mechanisms of coping	Allow child and family to verbalize feelings, concerns, frustrations Promote opportunities for self-care and parent participation Encourage appropriate lighting in room during wakeful periods Arrange a schedule for child to include recreational therapy, Child Life, tutorial, occupational therapy services Obtain psychiatry or psychology consult if warranted Provide familiar, favorite toys or objects in isolation or laminar air flow room Instruct child and family about emotional and metabolic reasons for depression Reinforce teaching about therapy and changes in care Encourage parents to use respite care, maintain adequate nutrition and exercise, maintain communication with support systems Encourage parents to attend appropriate support group meetings for BMT families
Intermediate Post-BMT Day +30 to Day +100	
Interstitial Pneumonia	
Impaired gas exchange Interstitial pneumonia (IP)	Identify risk factors for IP: allo-BMT, acute GVHD grade II-IV, cytomegalovirus (CMV) positive, older age, use of total body irradiation in CMV-seropositive patient Monitor vital signs; assess for respiratory difficulty, oxygenation, and ventilation

Table continued on following page.

TABLE 6—6. *Summary of Nursing Interventions for Post-BMT Complications* Continued

NURSING DIAGNOSIS	NURSING STRATEGIES
Interstitial Pneumonia—cont'd	
	Monitor results of laboratory and diagnostic testing, administer treatments, including oxygen, and monitor effects
Activity level intolerance	Assess activity level intolerance: inpatient by direct observation; outpatient, by patient report
	Promote optimal patient activity; assist with breathing and posturing techniques
Knowledge deficit	Provide patient and family teaching about signs and symptoms of respiratory insufficiency or infection to report to physician
	Describe pathophysiology and rationale for increased risk; note day +60 as a time of increased risk
Potential Knowledge Deficit for Discharge and Home Care	
Increased amount of required learning with potential for anxiety and alteration in parenting role	Assess parent and child readiness to learn
	Initiate discharge teaching as soon as appropriate and use specific unit and institutional protocol and/or discharge manuals
	Deliver information in reasonable amounts or packets that are related and provide consistent instructions in a nonthreatening manner
	Initiate interagency communication with referring center nurses and social workers
	Assure parents and patient of availability of BMT team to problem-solve and offer continued support
	Consider introducing family to another post-BMT family
	At discharge, have conference with parents and child to clarifiy and repeat pertinent instructions
	After discharge, communicate prn with family and referring center nurses about patient and family adaptation at home
	Encourage parent and child to verbalize fears and concerns

While pancytopenic, the patient is at greater risk for infection (particularly bacterial and fungal), thrombocytopenia, anemia, and hemorrhage.[23,179,193] Nursing care focuses on principles and strategies used in the management of the neutropenic or thrombocytopenic child. Transplant patients receive irradiated blood products throughout BMT and for the first 1 to 5 years after BMT. Irradiation, given as a single 1500 to 5000 rad dose to the blood product, attenuates viable allogeneic lymphocytes that may be present in small numbers in homologous blood components. It does not make the product radioactive, nor does it destroy the cell line of the product (i.e., RBCs). Irradiation of the product does, however, inhibit the replication of the transfused nucleated cells, preventing GVHD in immunodeficient patients.[98,183]

The risk of infection increases with the duration and magnitude of the granulocytopenia.[130,193] Disruption of skin and mucosal barriers from the toxic effects of the conditioning regimen can provide a hematologic portal of entry for potentially infectious organisms already colonizing the skin and GI tract. Nurses must continuously assess for signs and symptoms indicating sepsis. Most transplant centers collect weekly surveillance cultures of orifices and overt lesions that can provide valuable information about a potential infectious source. In addition, the nurse should be aware of any prior history of bacterial, fungal, and/or viral infections.[179,193]

Growth factors such as granulocyte-macrophage colony-stimulating factor (GM-CSF) and granulocyte colony-stimulating factor (G-CSF) are being used to promote more rapid marrow recovery after transplantation, especially for those patients experiencing delayed or failed engraftment. GM-CSF and G-CSF are cytokines that accelerate hemato-poiesis. Clinical trials of auto-BMT have shown they decrease the length of neutro-penia and incidence of bacterial infections when administered after the transplant, thereby decreasing the transplant-related morbidity and mortality.[124] Randomized studies are being undertaken to determine the most advantageous dose, timing, and application of growth factors in BMT.

Significant hemorrhage from any body orifice is a persistent risk in the thrombocyto-penic patient. The GI tract, where the effects of mucositis can predispose to significant bleeding episodes, is a common hemorrhagic site. Hemorrhagic cystitis associated with conditioning regimens containing cyclophosphamide or L-phenylalanine mustard can also contribute to complications. Nurses should know if the patient has a past history of platelet refractoriness and should continually assess the patient's response to platelet transfusions.

Nonhematologic Complications

Superimposed on the acute hematologic complications of infection and bleeding are many nonhematologic complications resulting from the effects of the conditioning regimen on multiple organ systems and body tissues. The most common toxicities involve GI, hepatic, and renal function. Cardiac and neurologic complications are less common.[46] Acute GVHD can occur during the immediate post-transplant period in patients receiving allo-geneic, haploidentical, or unrelated donor marrow. The treatment and management of acute GVHD must be balanced with the care of other toxicities occurring simultaneously.[32,46]

Gastrointestinal Complications. The conditioning regimen affects rapidly dividing mucosal epithelial cells lining the GI tract, causing mucositis, a universal complication in BMT patients.[21] Although oral mucositis is most common, the toxic effects of mucositis

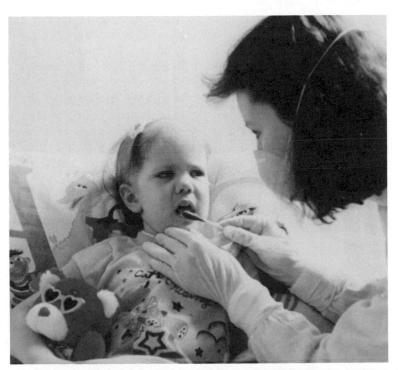

FIGURE 6–6. Meticulous oral hygiene is an integral part of the nursing regimen for bone marrow transplant patients. A trusting relationship between nurse and patient facilitates care. (*Courtesy Peter F. Coccia, M.D., University of Nebraska Medical Center, Omaha.*)

can be seen throughout the entire GI tract, involving the esophagus, stomach, and intestines. Combination chemoradiotherapy in the conditioning regimen accentuates the severity.[7] The use of methotrexate to prevent acute GVHD also enhances the severity of the mucositis.[23] Clinical symptoms include excessive secretions that vary from being watery to very thick and ropy, difficulty swallowing, anorexia, vomiting, abdominal cramping, and watery diarrhea.[32,46] The varying symptomatology reflects the involvement of different areas of the GI tract. Severe mucositis with excessive secretions, sloughing tissue, and local swelling can require intubation of the patient to facilitate breathing and protect the airway from aspiration.

Reactivation of oral herpes simplex virus (HSV) could further compound the severity of mucositis. Administration of prophylactic oral acyclovir has decreased the risk of oral HSV reactivation.[152] Poor oral hygiene and poor dental health can contribute to oral mucositis. Thrombocytopenia combined with friable, denuded, and ulcerated tissue from mucositis increases the risk for oral bleeding.

Although there is no absolute prevention of mucositis, supportive measures are helpful to decrease toxicity until the body repairs the damaged tissue and healing occurs, which coincides with marrow engraftment.[46] Nursing care focuses on controlling pain, minimizing the risks of infection, cleansing and maintaining the integrity of the oral mucosa and perirectal mucosa, and minimizing the occurrence of significant bleeding.

Pain from mucositis can be extremely severe and often requires the use of a continuous narcotic infusion, usually morphine sulfate. In older children the use of patient-controlled analgesia (PCA) can be effective and provides the patient with some degree of control. Parents and patients may express fears of addiction with the use of a continuous morphine drip. This issue should be approached in an honest and forthright manner, emphasizing that this is the most effective way to manage the child's discomfort associated with severe mucositis and that addiction does not occur in the presence of physical pain. The patient and parents need reassurance that the medication will be discontinued when it is no longer needed. Boluses of narcotic may be administered before mouth care and medication administration to enhance compliance. When a child can cooperate, mouth care is more effective at removing debris and dried secretions, with minimal trauma to the area that could cause bleeding. A regularly scheduled thorough oral assessment and care program decreases the risk of infection.[11,41] Precautions to prevent aspiration must be implemented.

Severe mucositis of the lower GI tract may cause excessive diarrhea, which can compromise skin integrity in the perirectal area. Meticulous skin care using protective creams and emollients, plus daily bathing accompanied by sitz baths, is important to protect this area from breakdown.

Hepatic Complications. Veno-occlusive disease (VOD) of the liver is the most common hepatic complication seen in the immediate post-BMT period.[111] It results from the use of high-dose chemotherapy and radiation in the transplant conditioning regimen.[48,111] Although there are few studies of the incidence of VOD in young children, they have shown the incidence is higher in patients transplanted for malignancies and in patients receiving allogeneic transplants.[111] The incidence of VOD for patients undergoing allo-BMT for malignancy is 20%, whereas that for auto-BMT patients is 9.4%.[40,111] Currently there is no effective therapy to alter the course of VOD.[48,64] Supportive care is the cornerstone of management, and nurses play a key role in the early recognition of VOD symptoms.[48,64]

To understand the clinical manifestations and progression of VOD, a brief description of hepatic anatomy and physiology is useful. The functional unit of the liver is the lobule, which is composed of hepatic cells organized into an elongated cylindrical shape, two cells in diameter.[64,66] Each liver lobule is constructed around a central vein and radiates outward.[66] Individual liver lobules are bordered on either side by hepatic sinusoids. Blood enters the liver from the GI tract by the portal vein and venules and hepatic artery and flows through the central vein, exiting the liver through the hepatic sinusoids into the hepatic veins and then into the inferior vena cava. Because of their close proximity to the hepatic sinusoids, hepatic cells are in constant contact with portal venous blood.[64,66] The endothelial lining of the hepatic sinusoids has large pores, making it extremely permeable. Underneath this lining, between the endothelial cells and the hepatic cells, is a small space called the space of Disse.[129] Large protein molecules and other components of blood plasma diffuse freely in and out of the hepatic sinusoids into the space of Disse where the exchange of nutrients between the blood and hepatic cells takes place.[64,66] Excess fluid diffusing through the sinusoidal endothelium into the space of Disse is removed by the lymphatic system and returned to the bloodstream.

With VOD there is an obstruction to blood flow leaving the liver. It is postulated that the chemotherapy and radiotherapy of the conditioning regimen injure the tissues of the hepatic cells and venous endothelium.[111] Fluid and cellular debris, including exfoliated hepatic cells, collagen, and reticulum fibers, collects and is trapped in the endothelial lining, resulting in fibrosis of the venous walls. Gradual narrowing and occlusion of hepatic venous outflow occur, impairing sinusoidal circulation and causing venous congestion and stasis.[64,111] Because of the extreme permeability, there is a significant outpouring of protein-rich fluid from the sinusoids into the extravascular spaces of the liver. Excessive fluid volume overwhelms the lymphatics and leaks through the outer surface of the liver into the abdominal cavity as ascites. Venous congestion and stasis damage the hepatic cells, impairing their function. Through an undetermined mechanism, the occlusion of portal hepatic blood flow causes a decrease in renal blood flow, which activates aldosterone, causing increased sodium and water retention and intravascular fluid loss.[113]

VOD is a clinical diagnosis based on the patient's clinical status and diagnosis of exclusion. It is characterized by sudden unexplained weight gain, thrombocytopenia refractory to platelet transfusions, jaundice, hepatomegaly, right upper quadrant pain, ascites, and encephalopathy.[112,142] Clinical manifestations of VOD develop early (within 1 to 3 weeks after BMT), and most patients present with some but not all of the symptoms. Subtle weight gain without obvious cause and difficulty in maintaining an adequate platelet count can be present as early as day +6 after transplant.[112,142] Hepatocellular dysfunction with impaired excretion of bilirubin results in jaundice and an increased bilirubin level, which can be evident by day +7. Significant abdominal distension from ascites, with an enlarged painful liver, follows on day +11 or +12. Pleural effusion and respiratory compromise result from ascitic fluid in the peritoneal cavity that leaks into the pleural cavity and from massive abdominal distension.[64] Encephalopathy occurs as hepatocellular damage and/or portal venous shunting leads to inadequate detoxification of portal venous blood ammonia.[88]

The main medical goal is to maintain intravascular volume and renal perfusion while decreasing the accumulation of extravascular fluid.[46] Overall, 53% of the patients recover from VOD with supportive management.[111] Most deaths from progressive VOD occur before day +35.[111] Risk factors that predispose patients to VOD are preexisting liver disease, hepatitis, elevated liver function test results before transplant, older age, and prior intensive chemotherapy.[111]

Nursing interventions center on the collaborative management of fluid volume excess, altered nutritional status, hepatic dysfunction, and impaired gas exchange, provision of comfort measures, and protection of the patient from injury related to refractory thrombocytopenia and encephalopathic changes. Patient teaching and provision of support to patient and family are also important. Supportive measures maintain residual hepatic function while the liver heals.

Renal Complications. Renal insufficiency is a common occurrence after BMT; however, the kidney is rarely the primary site of toxicity after BMT. Renal complications most often occur as a result of various factors that affect renal blood flow and tubular function.[46,91]

In prerenal conditions systemic circulatory disturbances compromise the glomerular filtration rate or blood flow, causing structural failure.[5,91] In a transplant patient there are multiple causes of systemic circulatory disturbances that can adversely affect renal blood flow and kidney function. They include dehydration, third spacing of fluid, VOD, hemorrhage, hypovolemia, septic shock, and hypoproteinemia.[46,91,108]

In intrarenal conditions the functioning structural components of the kidney itself are compromised, impairing renal function and resulting in acute tubular necrosis (ATN). The renal tubules maintain fluid, electrolyte, and acid-base balances by reabsorption and secretion through the epithelial lining.[66,107] Damage to the epithelial lining causes cellular sloughing and tubular obstruction, impairing tubular reabsorption and secretion, altering fluid, electrolyte, and acid-base balances and the elimination of waste products.[66,107] Cytotoxic drugs and radiation therapy used in the conditioning regimen can be nephrotoxic, damaging renal blood vessels, the glomeruli, the nephron, and the tubules.[133] Essential drugs used in transplant pharmacology such as aminoglycoside antibiotics, vancomycin, amphotericin B, cyclosporine, and acyclovir are also nephrotoxic.

Prerenal and intrarenal conditions often coexist during the post-BMT period. Impaired circulatory dynamics and nephrotoxic agents exacerbate renal tissue damage and the occurrence of ATN, resulting in impaired renal function. Loss of renal function can be 75% to 80% before significant laboratory changes or clinical symptoms occur.[96]

Since younger children have a higher basal metabolic rate and larger body surface area in proportion to total body weight, they are more sensitive to body fluid shifts. This has implications for overall management of fluid and electrolyte and acid-base balance.[129,188] Nurses caring for younger children after BMT must be aware of the normal physiologic differences between a child and an adult in the distribution and regulation of water and electrolytes in body fluids and in their ability to maintain acid-base balance. Other important variables are previous treatment with nephrotoxic agents, previous local radiation to or near the kidneys, and a history of nephrectomy. These factors must be integrated into post-transplant nursing assessment and management.[129,188]

Nursing assessment focuses on fluid and electrolyte status as medical interventions are implemented.[47,108,129] Treatment of renal complications involves maintaining adequate intravascular volume and renal perfusion, correcting fluid, electrolyte, and acid-base imbalances, and minimizing the use of nephrotoxic agents while continuing to provide effective treatment and prophylaxis for infections and acute GVHD.[46,91,108]

Acute Graft-Versus-Host Disease in Allo-BMT

GVHD is an immune-mediated response that occurs between the donor's immunocompetent cells and the patient's immunosuppressed cells. It is the major cause of morbidity and mortality in allo-BMT. This immune response is attributed to the genetically determined histocompatibility difference, or disparity, between the tissue type of the donor and recipient. Immunocompetent donor T-lymphocyte cells are capable of mounting an immune reaction against the patient, but the patient is incapable of reacting against the donor cells. The immunocompetent donor T lymphocytes become sensitized to antigens of the patient and generate cytotoxic effector cells targeted at specific host tissues, most notably those of the skin, GI tract, and liver. The clinical findings related to acute GVHD are described in Table 6–7.

Acute GVHD occurs in the first 100 days after transplant and is usually preceded by documented engraftment. Some centers report a 40% to 70% incidence of acute GVHD.[167] Of these patients, 30% to 50% will experience serious to severe GVHD, and 10% to 30% of this group will die from the complications.[37,167] The risks of GVHD increase when there is high MLC reactivity, HLA discordance between the donor and recipient, older age of patient, male sex of recipient, and/or female donor–to–male recipient pairing, which is a significantly higher risk if the female donor was previously alloimmunized through pregnancy or previous blood transfusion.[182]

The hallmark presentation of acute GVHD is a maculopapular rash resembling rubella, which starts on the palmar and plantar sur-

TABLE 6–7. *Clinical Findings of Acute and Chronic GVHD*

CLINICAL	LABORATORY
Acute GVHD	
Maculopapular, pruritic rash	Hyperbilirubinemia
Erythroderma	Elevated transaminase values
Jaundice	Lymphocytosis or lymphocytopenia
Hepatomegaly	Eosinophilia
Diarrhea (guaiac positive)	Thrombocytopenia
Fever	Anemia
Hypertension	Proteinuria
Infection	Pulmonary infiltrates
Chronic GVHD	
Skin desquamation	Hypergammaglobulinemia
Nail ridging	Circulating immune complexes
Scleroderma	Eosinophilia
Musculoskeletal changes	Lymphocytopenia or lymphocytosis
Hepatosplenomegaly	Elevated transaminase values
Malabsorption	
Chronic diarrhea	
Weight loss	
Xerostomia	
Photophobia	
Recurrent infections	
Idiopathic interstitial pneumonitis	

faces of the hands and feet and evolves to a confluent erythematous rash involving most of the body.[59] Lymphocytes and eosinophils infiltrate the skin layers, causing lysis and degeneration of dermal cells and separation of the dermal-epidermal junction. In its most severe form, acute skin GVHD is manifested by desquamation and sloughing of the skin surfaces over part or all of the body.

Acute GVHD is staged by a variety of schema, usually graded I to IV, which allows tailoring the monitoring and treatment to the clinical severity. An example of the classification of progressive GVHD in older children and young adults is illustrated in Table 6–8. The degree of severity is associated with treatment outcome.

Acute liver GVHD involves dysfunction that is cholestatic and related to lymphocyte infiltration into the bile ducts, leading to bile duct and hepatocellular necrosis. Hyperbilirubinemia and elevations in the liver transaminase and alkaline phosphatase levels occur. GI dysfunction is manifested by a char-

TABLE 6–8. *Clinical Staging of Acute GVHD*

STAGE	SKIN	LIVER	GUT
I	Maculopapular rash on <25% body surface	Bilirubin, 2–3 mg/dl	Diarrhea, 500–1000 ml/day (8–15 ml/kg)
II	Maculopapular rash on <25%–50% body surface	Bilirubin, 3–6 mg/dl	Diarrhea, 1000–1500 ml/day (16–25 ml/kg)
III	Generalized erythroderma	Bilirubin, 6–15 mg/dl	Diarrhea, >1500 ml/day (>25 ml/kg)
IV	Desquamation and bullae formation	Bilirubin, >15 mg/dl	Pain or ileus

Data from reference 168.

acteristic diarrhea of green, watery stool that is guaiac positive and has a typical foul odor. The bowel wall becomes thickened, and there is concomitant lymphocyte infiltration with loss of the intestinal mucosal folds, causing mucosal sloughing. It can progress to complete intestinal mucosa denudation. Abdominal cramps, anorexia, nausea, vomiting, malabsorption, ascites, and ileus are related complications that cause much distress to patients.

Acute GVHD is a syndrome that has farreaching and even life-threatening effects. It is critical to differentiate its effects from other BMT-related complications, including those of the preparative regimen, infections, and VOD.

Perhaps the most problematic complication of GVHD is that it increases the risk of infection in the host.[178] This severe risk is amplified by the profound myelosuppression and persistent immunosuppression related to BMT. Acute GVHD can cause compromise of the immune function, suppression of the marrow hematologic recovery, and breakdown of mechanical barriers; and all increase the risk for life-threatening infections, especially coagulase-negative staphylococcal infections from skin contaminants, gram-negative rod infections from enteric pathogens, and cytomegalovirus (CMV).[178]

To prevent GVHD, several chemoprophylaxis regimens are used, depending on the degree of immune suppression desired, the degree of histocompatibility between donor and recipient types, and the preference of the transplant center. Investigation is ongoing to determine the most efficacious protocol. Methotrexate, cyclosporine, and ATG are the most frequently used agents (often used in combination) and have been demonstrated as more effective than single-agent prophylaxis and as improving survival.[177] Physical techniques are also being used to deplete the donor marrow of the T lymphocytes.[177]

Ex vivo techniques have been used to deplete the donor marrow of T lymphocytes before the marrow is infused to the recipient. Newer techniques are being investigated to remove the subset(s) of lymphocytes most responsible for GVHD more selectively while preserving the viability of stem cells. Selective

T-lymphocyte depletion is important because certain T lymphocytes may be responsible for eliminating residual tumor cells and others may be instrumental in promoting engraftment.[169] Currently the ex vivo techniques used include monoclonal anti–T-cell antibodies with attached complement, soybean lectin agglutination, treatment with sheep erythrocytes to stimulate rosette separation, elutriation techniques, and immunotoxic conjugates.[169] Although these techniques may decrease the incidence and severity of acute GVHD, they are associated with graft rejection, stem cell loss, secondary B-cell malignancies, and disease recurrence (particularly leukemia).

Since other complications of allo-BMT can be confused with acute GVHD, histologic confirmation of affected tissue is desired before the initiation of therapy. Treatment of acute GVHD includes topical, oral, and IV corticosteroid administration, depending on the severity of the clinical manifestations. Steroids prevent proliferation of the T lymphocytes. ATG has also been used to destroy the T lymphocytes involved in acute GVHD. This prophylaxis is used cautiously because ATG interferes with platelet function and blood cell production and can cause hypersensitivity reactions in patients. Some transplant centers are using monoclonal antibodies to T cells to treat acute GVHD more selectively, but the toxicities of these regimens are not clearly understood.

Early recognition of the signs and symptoms of acute GVHD are essential for effective therapy and to prevent tissue damage. Aggressive, supportive nursing care makes a significant impact on the comfort of the patient and the progression of the disease. Table 6–6 specifies the nursing diagnoses and related interventions for acute GVHD.

Graft Rejection

Graft rejection, the failure of the donor marrow to sustain engraftment in the recipient is associated with (1) ineffective immunosuppression of the host; (2) damage of the microstromal environment by conditioning treatment; and/or (3) significant discordance between the donor and recipient tissue types.

When immunosuppression is inadequate, functional recipient immune cells are capable of recognizing the foreign T lymphocytes and destroying the graft. Graft rejection is seen in only 5% of HLA phenotypically matched donor and recipient transplants but occurs in approximately 15% to 25% of major mismatched transplants.[8] Graft rejection can also be associated with T-lymphocyte depletion in which those T cells that prevent graft rejection are removed indiscriminately along with those T cells that lead to acute GVHD. It is believed that a subset of T cells in the inoculum may facilitate donor engraftment by destroying residual host cells that mediate rejection.[186] The percentage of graft failures in T-depleted transplants approaches 60%.[160]

Graft Versus Leukemia

It is theorized that there is a relationship between acute GVHD and disease recurrence, most specifically with the leukemias. The phenomenon is called *graft versus leukemia effect*. Allo-BMT patients who experience some degree of acute or chronic GVHD have a lower incidence of leukemic relapse than those patients who do not.[186] This probably is related to the immunocompetent donor T lymphocytes' providing additional tumoricidal activity against residual leukemia cells. For this reason syngeneic (identical twin) BMTs, when the allograft tissue is genetically identical to that of the patient's, have a higher relapse rate than allo-BMTs. Further studies are needed to elucidate this phenomenon.

INTERMEDIATE POST-BMT PERIOD: DAY +30 TO DAY +100

During the intermediate post-transplant phase, patients begin healing and resolving acute toxicities to the GI tract, liver, and kidneys. Engraftment is demonstrated by an increasing white blood cell count (WBC) and absolute neutrophil count (ANC), thus decreasing the risks for bacterial and fungal infections.[126] There is a decreased need for platelet and RBC transfusions as the newly engrafted marrow begins to repopulate and begin cellular production. However, humoral and cellular immune functions remain inad-

equate and can be further suppressed by medications to prevent and treat acute GVHD, leaving patients at risk for opportunistic infections.[126] Nursing care focuses on teaching and preparation for discharge and transfer back to the ambulatory care setting.

The predominant life-threatening complication facing children during this period is the development of interstitial pneumonia. Susceptibility to interstitial pneumonia increases with depressed immune responses. Children with grades II to IV acute GVHD are at the greatest risk to contract interstitial pneumonia.[115,126]

Interstitial Pneumonia

Interstitial pneumonia is a nonbacterial, nonfungal inflammatory process that results in the accumulation of infiltrate in the alveolar walls.[33,78] A chest x-ray film shows a diffuse infiltrative pattern. This can be contrasted to the traditional clinical presentation of pneumonia in which the alveolar air spaces themselves are filled with exudate, which can be seen as consolidation on chest x-ray film.[49] With interstitial pneumonia the walls of the alveoli thicken as a result of cellular infiltrate accumulation, congestion, and edema, resulting in progressively impaired gas exchange, decreased lung volumes, and diminished compliance.[49,78,189] Initially there may be a dry, nonproductive cough with tachypnea, nasal flaring, and fever, which can rapidly progress to dyspnea and hypoxia requiring ventilatory support.[17,32,46,78]

Interstitial pneumonia commonly occurs 30 to 100 days after BMT. Two thirds of the patients have a documented causative infectious agent that is usually viral or protozoal in origin, and the other cases are attributed to the effects of drugs, radiation, or both.[49] Viral infections, most commonly CMV, are the leading causative agents of interstitial pneumonia. Other viral pathogens such as herpes simplex, herpes zoster, and adenovirus account for 5% to 10% of cases.[49,126] *Pneumocystis carinii* pneumonia, a protozoal infection, was once the most common fatal cause of interstitial pneumonia; however, the use of trimethoprim-sulfamethoxazole prophylaxis has significantly minimized this threat.[49]

In severely immunocompromised patients after BMT, CMV interstitial pneumonia remains a major cause of morbidity and mortality.[42] The overall incidence of CMV pneumonia in these patients is approximately 15% to 20%, with a mortality rate approaching 80% or more.[42] The median onset of CMV interstitial pneumonia is roughly 5 to 13 weeks after BMT, with a peak at 8 weeks.[32] Patients who present as CMV seropositive before BMT can progress to active CMV disease with activation of the latent virus. In patients who are CMV seronegative before BMT, acquisition of CMV is from either CMV-infected donor marrow or blood products.[14,49,194]

Until recently there was no effective prevention or treatment of CMV pneumonia after a transplant. The development of the technology to screen blood products for CMV was the first major breakthrough in the prevention of primary CMV infection in patients CMV seronegative before the transplant.[14,15] Bone marrow recipients who had CMV-seronegative donors and received CMV-seronegative blood products had significantly less infection than those who received random donor blood products.[15] For the CMV-seronegative patient, the goal is to prevent exposure to the virus. The use of CMV-negative blood products is a standard practice when the bone marrow donor is also CMV negative.[14] Inline leukopoor blood filters, which remove approximately 99% of the leukocytes in the transfused blood product, provide an alternative way to provide a CMV-"screened" blood product when CMV-negative donors are unavailable. Studies are underway to evaluate the efficacy of these filters in preventing primary CMV infection.[14]

Patients who are CMV seropositive before the transplant have a significantly higher risk of CMV infection.[14,116] The primary concern in these patients is to prevent the progression of latent CMV infection to symptomatic disease.[14] The use of prophylactic high-dose acyclovir (500 mg/m² q8h) significantly decreases the risk of CMV infection and is associated with a significant increase in survival in this patient group.[116]

If patients develop CMV pneumonia, combined treatment with gancyclovir and IV immune globulin (IVIG) has been effective in increasing the survival rate in comparison to historical controls.[43,139] Gancyclovir is a derivative of acyclovir. When it is metabolized to its active form, it prevents viral replication of CMV. The major side effect, unfortunately, is bone marrow suppression. The mechanisms by which IVIG works against CMV is not known. The pathology of CMV pneumonia is thought both viral and host related. IVIG appears effective against the immune response of the host, and gancyclovir is effective against the virus.[194]

Cytomegaloviral interstitial pneumonia remains a major clinical problem for patients undergoing allogeneic transplantation. Patients often experience a rapid deterioration in respiratory status once symptoms appear. The use of bronchoalveolar lavage (BAL) with special culture techniques can provide the diagnosis within 24 hours so that appropriate treatment strategies can be instituted promptly. Astute nursing assessment is important to identify those patients who exhibit subtle signs and symptoms of respiratory compromise. Understanding the risk factors and the pathophysiology of interstitial pneumonia helps the nurse educate the child and family and provide appropriate supportive care. Psychosocial support of the child and family is critical during this potentially perilous and difficult period after BMT. Nursing must keep abreast of the ever-changing advances in prevention, diagnosis, and treatment of CMV pneumonia.

LONG-TERM PERIOD: DAY +100
Discharge Criteria

Discharge criteria vary, depending on the type of transplant performed and the institution. In general, the patient must be afebrile with an ANC of approximately 500 polymorphonuclear (PMN) cells/mm³ for 48 to 72 hours. Some centers use immune reconstitution parameters such as PHA mitogen stimulation assays as discharge criteria. Most centers require patients not to be taking antimicrobials (except for prophylactic agents) at discharge, although other centers are equipped to administer certain antibiotics and antifungal drugs in the outpatient setting. The patient should be blood-product independent or have a replacement schedule that can be accommodated in an outpatient setting. This is theoretically possible if the unsupported platelet count is greater than 15,000 mm³ and the hematocrit is above 25%.[33]

Patients should be ambulatory, able to provide basic, age-appropriate self-care, and maintain an oral nutrient intake that is at least or above 33% of baseline needs.[33] The prescribed discharge diet is a modified regular diet if it can be tolerated. Modifications might include low-lactose, low-fat, sodium restricted, gluten-free, and/or antimicrobial diets. TPN may be necessary in some patients. Nausea, vomiting, and diarrhea are controlled by diet or medication. Fluid intake should equal or be greater than 1500 ml/m²/day or supplemented parenterally to a maintenance level based on the child's height and weight.

The child must be able to take the required oral medications such as prophylactic antimicrobials, immunosuppressant drugs, and antiemetics. The parents and patient, when appropriate, must clearly understand and demonstrate skill in central line care and the administration of medications.

Follow-Up

Follow-up evaluations are based on the type of transplant and clinical course of the patient. Auto-BMT patients are generally discharged sooner and require less follow-up than allogeneic patients who are monitored for complications of GVHD. Both types of patients are evaluated at 3, 6, and 12 months after transplant unless more frequent monitoring is necessary. Studies are done to evaluate hematologic, renal, hepatic, and pulmonary functions. Bone marrow aspiration evaluations are occasionally done to document sustained engraftment and disease status. Lumbar punctures and immune function studies are repeated occasionally. A large portion of the follow-up care can be accomplished at the referring center; therefore communication and coordination between nurses at the referring and transplant centers are necessary.

Autologous transplant patients, who do not receive prolonged immunosuppression, are generally allowed to return to school within 3 to 6 months after the transplant. Allogeneic transplant patients, on the other hand, may be restricted from attending school for 9 to 12 months, at which time their immune function has partially recovered. The decision about when it is safe for a child to return to school is based on immune reconstitution studies, including determination of quantitative immunoglobulin levels and mitogen stimulation assays. Outbreaks of varicella-zoster virus in the school should be reported promptly. Because of the immune reconstitution delay, varicella-zoster immune globulin (VZIG) is administered to all transplant patients exposed to the virus for the first year after BMT. Some centers reimmunize patients who have immune recovery, using attenuated or killed toxin vaccinations. Others elect not to reimmunize if there is a high probability that the majority of the population is vaccinated.

Chronic GVHD in Allo-BMT

Chronic GVHD occurs later in the BMT course and is referred to as the disease that occurs after the first 100 days after infusion. Approximately 25% of allogeneic patients experience chronic GVHD, which resembles an autoimmune or collagen storage disease and is associated with a high rate of morbidity, debilitation, and mortality.[59] There are three patterns of presentation: (1) de novo chronic GVHD has a late onset, may or may not be related to acute GVHD, and is considered the least lethal form; (2) quiescent chronic GVHD follows a benign period or "break" from acute GVHD; and (3) progressive chronic GVHD is a direct extension of acute GVHD and is considered the most serious form.

Skin manifestations progress to dryness, poikiloderma (hyperpigmentation followed by atrophy), and scleroderma. Joint contractures may develop. Liver dysfunction progresses to bile duct destruction, with fibrosis of liver tissue causing severe cholestatic changes. The GI changes are manifested as strictures, malabsorption, xerostomia, and anorexia. Other significant manifestations include dry eyes, pigmentation abnormalities of the skin, vaginal dryness and strictures, sicca syndrome of the lacrimal and salivary glands, and chronic obstructive bronchiolitis. Table 6–7 describes the signs and symptoms related to chronic GVHD.

In chronic GVHD abnormal T-cell and B-cell functions and depressed levels of circulating IgG class II and IV antibodies have been noted.[178] This, combined with denudation of mucosal barriers and functional asplenia, increases the risk for fungal and viral infections. Chronically, infections can be caused by streptococcal bacteria, herpes zoster virus, and *Aspergillus*.

The treatment of chronic GVHD often provides discouraging results. Methotrexate is used to suppress activity of T lymphocytes. Maintenance doses of 1.5 mg/kg/day have been used, given concurrently with prednisone therapy, usually at a dose of 1 mg/kg every other day. Long-term immune suppression and steroid therapy have been associated with deleterious musculoskeletal and metabolic effects. New agents such as thalidomide are being investigated for the treatment of chronic GVHD.

Long-Term Sequelae of BMT

Recognition of survivorship issues after BMT may improve the quality of life for transplant patients and their families. Insurability is an important concern since many children who have undergone BMT reach the lifetime limits of their coverage at the time of the transplant or are terminated from their parents' health care policies when they reach legal age. Health care policies for which they apply may exclude or restrict coverage of preexisting conditions. Life insurance is equally hard to obtain and may be cost prohibitive. Employment barriers such as exclusion from benefits, refusal to hire, and employee fear of transplant patients may lead to job discrimination for young people who have undergone BMT. Political lobbyists and transplant advocate groups such as Candlelighter's Association and the Children's Transplant Association work to empower transplant survivors and eliminate discrimination.

Late Effects

Late effects of BMT have gained increased clinical significance as the number of children achieving long-term disease-free survival after BMT has increased. Many of these late effects are similar to those caused by high-dose chemotherapy and radiation therapy. However, the late effects related to BMT are generally considered impairments that occur after the first 100 days and can be amplified by (1) higher antineoplastic and TBI doses of the ablative therapy, (2) prolonged functional and chemotherapeutic immunosuppression, and (3) complications of chronic GVHD.

Recipients of BMT are at risk for the same constellation of potential late effects as any other pediatric cancer patient. Late effects (see Chapter 17) are persistent adverse organ system dysfunctions, with or without anatomic abnormalities, that are caused by antineoplastic drugs, radiation, and other chemotherapeutic agents (e.g., antimicrobials) used in the treatment of cancer. In addition there are late effects particular to chronic GVHD that may be associated with immunosuppression, corticosteroid therapy, and the autoimmune-like process of the disease (Table 6–9).

Impaired growth is common after TBI, with decreased growth velocity and a lesser increase in height over time for approximately 4 to 5 years after the transplant. This may lead to an average height at least 1 standard deviation below average height for age and sex.[145] Growth may later resume at a normal sex- and age-adjusted rate, but these children never quite "catch up" to their peers. Growth impairment is exacerbated by prolonged corticosteroid therapy and malnutrition. Growth hormone supplementation may improve growth velocity.[145]

Fertility is impaired from damage to the gonads by TBI and ablative chemotherapy, particularly the alkylating agents. Prepubertal girls experience delayed puberty and may fail to achieve menarche.[146] Older girls may resume menarche after the transplant but usually experience early menopause and infertility.[31] Prepubertal boys experience delayed puberty. All boys are generally considered sterilized by the effects of both chemotherapy

TABLE 6—9. *Late Effects of Bone Marrow Transplantation Related to Chronic GVHD*

LATE EFFECT	SIGNS AND SYMPTOMS
Neurologic	
Cyclosporine-related neuro-toxicity	Lethargy, headaches, confusion, parasthesias
Myasthenia gravis	Muscle weakness, ptosis, dysarthria, parasthesias, dyspnea
Pulmonary	
Obliterative bronchiolitis	Decreased activity tolerance, easy fatigue, increased expiratory effort
Integumentary	
Scleroderma	Red discoloration of skin, fibrosis of skin, stiffness of connective tissue
Lichen planus	White, dry patches of skin
Joint contracture	Stiff joints, scar tissue around joints
Mucositis (oral, ocular, esophageal, and vaginal)	Painful, swollen, friable mucous membranes
Dyspigmentation	Changes in normal skin coloration; either decreased or increased coloration
Alopecia	Loss of hair, uneven hair growth, absence of eyebrows, absence or sparsity of pubic hair
Musculoskeletal	
Muscular dystrophy or atrophy	Muscle weakness and wasting
Myositis	Muscle weakness, vague muscular pain
Aseptic osteonecrosis	Painful joints, particularly hips and knees
Hepatic	
Chronic active hepatitis	Jaundice, malaise, icterus, malnutrition
Biliary cirrhosis	Jaundice, icterus, pruritus, spider angiomas
Renal	
Cyclosporine-related renal toxicity	Electrolyte abnormalities, hypertension, decreased urinary output
Oral	
Lichenoid lesions	White, dry, striated patches on buccal mucosa
Stomatitis	Red, swollen, tender oral mucosa
Caries, interrupted dentition	Tooth decay, cavities, absence of deciduous or permanent teeth
Xerostomia	Dry mouth, difficulty swallowing, absence of saliva, oral lesions
Ocular	
Xerophthalmia	Dry, burning, gritty, reddened eyes
Gastrointestinal	
Malabsorption	Weight loss, diarrhea, electrolyte abnormalities
Anorexia	Disinterest in eating, taste disruptions, weight loss
Dysphagia	Difficult mastication, inability to swallow bulk foods, anorexia, narrowing of esophagus
Reproductive	
Vaginal strictures	Inflammation, narrowing of vaginal vault, dyspareunuria, obstruction of menstrual and mucous flow, bleeding with intercourse
Vaginal adhesions	Dry membranes, inflammation, pruritus, vaginal lacerations, dyspareunuria, bleeding
Decreased libido	Disinterest in intercourse or alternate sexual activities, disruptions in relationships with usual sexual partners

Data from references 31 and 167.

and TBI.[31] Reproductive function and sexuality are affected by the patient's energy level, self-esteem, and other complications such as GVHD. Patients with chronic GVHD experience delayed puberty, regardless of whether TBI was used or not.[146]

Pulmonary late effects include restrictive lung disease and infections. Patients with chronic GVHD are at greater risk for pulmonary infections.[92] Infectious agents include CMV, *P. carinii*, varicella-zoster virus, and certain bacteria. Interstitial pneumonitis and obliterative bronchiolitis can occur, with the latter exacerbated by chronic GVHD. Infectious agents, antineoplastics, TBI, and corticosteroid therapy may contribute to chronic interstitial pneumonitis.

Cataract formation is common after TBI, especially if single-dose and/or high-dose TBI is used.[6] Corticosteroid therapy increases the risk. These cataracts can usually be surgically repaired. Xerophthalmia, or dry eyes, can also occur and cause patients to complain of "grittiness" in their eyes. Artificial tears and/or saline solution eye drops can alleviate some of the discomfort.

Skin and mucous membrane changes are usually associated with chronic GVHD. Skin changes are sclerodermatous (thickened and inflamed) in nature and are accompanied by changes in pigmentation. Mucous membranes are affected by sicca syndrome, characterized by dryness and atrophy. Ulcerations can occur. Oral mucosa may be affected by lichenoid (plaquelike) lesions. Alterations in taste result from TBI. Vaginal mucosa may become dry and friable, and vaginal strictures may develop. Steroidal creams and/or skin emollients may be prescribed after careful considering whether they will irritate or destroy tissue further.

Musculoskeletal dysfunction can be manifested by myositis, muscular atrophy, joint contractures, aseptic osteonecrosis, and osteoporosis. These complications are primarily due to the autoimmune-like destruction of chronic GVHD but may also result from treatment with corticosteroids, antineoplastics, or TBI.

Secondary cancers after allogeneic, syngeneic, and autologous transplant have been reported.[190] In a retrospective study of 1926 patients who underwent BMT, 35 patients experienced second malignant neoplasms (SMNs) in a median interval of 1 year after BMT. The common SMNs were non-Hodgkin's lymphomas, solid tumors, and leukemias. They represented an approximately seven times greater increase of SMNs than that of primary cancer in the general population. Risk factors for development of SMNs are ATG therapy, immunosuppression, and TBI. Routine health care maintenance and disease prevention measures should be encouraged with post-BMT patients. Other late effects of BMT include chronic active hepatitis, biliary cirrhosis, nephritis, delayed or persistent hemorrhagic cystitis, polyneuropathy, and prolonged functional immunosuppression.

Emotional late effects involve the entire family. Social isolation, chronic health care needs, the severe financial burden of chronic illness, and disrupted family relationships can contribute to family maladjustment. The stress of BMT strains the function of even the most well-adjusted families and can severely exacerbate problems in dysfunctional family systems. Poor self-esteem, emotional dependence, and an overwhelming sense of uncertainty can occur in the recipients, many of whom display an external focus of control in personal and life decisions.[73] Resentment and fear can develop in the healthy siblings. Studies are being undertaken to determine the emotional impact of allo-BMT on the donor.

PSYCHOSOCIAL IMPLICATIONS

Children and families undergoing BMT encounter numerous psychologic and emotional stresses. These complications are related to the situational stress of evaluation and the transplant process, separation of family members at the time of transplant, financial strain, exorbitant out-of-pocket expenses, role changes within the family, other family burdens associated with catastrophic and life-threatening illness, and societal perceptions of the transplant patient.[68] The child's ability to cope with the hospitalization depends on the child's developmental level.[188] Children react to the increased stress of the parents and staff. In most cases they react negatively, with

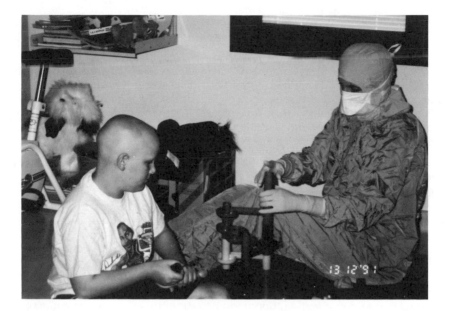

FIGURE 6–7. Patient-nurse interaction. Positive patient interactions can be maintained in spite of strict isolation measures. *(Courtesy Children's Hospital, Los Angeles, California.)*

feelings of anger, isolation, frustration, withdrawal, depression, and fear of the entire BMT process. They can be irritable and uncooperative. Parental stress can escalate, and previous adaptive coping mechanisms of both parent and child may fail (Table 6–10 and Chapter 14).

A multidisciplinary team approach is the best mechanism by which to meet the emotional needs of the child. In addition to the nurses and physicians, social workers, educational (tutorial) therapists, play therapists or child life specialists, and physical therapists are instrumental in developing and reinforcing coping skills that empower the child. Team assessments and follow-up care conferences are usually organized by the nursing team and should include nurses from the BMT unit and outpatient clinic. Play and schoolwork, which normalize the child's experience and imply that the child is expected to recover from the intensive treatment, should be integral components of the transplant process. They also afford the child with an opportunity to exercise control.[61] It is important to advocate for these services in any BMT center that has children as part of their program.

Although the highly intense atmosphere and stressful clinical situations of BMT dramatically affect families, they also affect nursing staff and can influence nursing care. Table 6–11 outlines specific stressors encountered by nurses caring for children and families undergoing BMT. Nurse managers, ethicists, and advocates in inpatient and outpatient BMT settings must be sensitive to these stressors and consider providing institutionally based support mechanisms. Professional nursing organizations and support networks for BMT nurses are emerging and are valuable resources for state-of-the-art information and leadership.

FUTURE TRENDS IN BMT

The knowledge base and clinical practice of pediatric BMT are rapidly expanding. Both an increase in the number of collaborative group transplant clinical trials and in the number of operational transplant centers have contributed to this growth. Advances in basic science technology have also had a major impact on transplantation and will continue to provide direction and support.

Biotherapy and immune technology are being used to expand the application and supportive care of BMT. The relationships be-

TABLE 6–10. *Common Nursing Psychosocial Diagnoses Related to Pediatric BMT*

Activity/Rest

Potential activity intolerance secondary to generalized weakness and/or periodic immobility

Sleep pattern disturbance secondary to interrupted sleep, psychologic stress, chronic illness

Deficit in diversional activity related to prolonged therapeutic isolation and immobility

Potential for disuse syndrome resulting from unavoidable inactivity, pain, altered level of consciousness, physical limitations of therapeutic isolation

Fatigue of child or parent related to altered sleep patterns, psychologic or emotional demands, loss of normal routines

Emotional Reactions

Anxiety of child related to disruption of routine, parental separation, therapeutic isolation practices, invasive procedures, the unknown

Anxiety of parent related to consent, donor identification, disruption of routine, information learning, child's tolerance of BMT, potential toxicities, financial concerns, the unknown

Potential for impaired adjustment of child related to inability to accept transplant process, inability to set pertinent goals, external locus of control, lack of future-oriented thinking

Ineffective individual coping of child or parent

Fear of child related to treatments, hospitalization, pain

Anxiety of donor related to donor testing, donor identification, unsuccessful outcome of BMT, potential graft rejection and/or GVHD, the unknown

Fear of donor related to harvest, hospitalization, pain

Decisional conflict regarding BMT and parental consent process

Disturbance in self-concept (body image, self-esteem, role performance, personal identity) related to lengthy hospitalization, separation from usual support systems, prescribed dependence, steroid effects, loss of body mass

Social isolation secondary to separation from usual support systems and/or therapeutic isolation practices

Powerlessness of child or parent related to prolonged aplasia, life-threatening complications, potential for severe acute GVHD, therapeutic isolation, decreased self-care activities

Hopelessness secondary to prolonged activity restriction, long-term stress, prolonged physical deterioration

Potential for spiritual distress of child or parent related to separation from religious support, life-threatening illness, potential for intense suffering, feelings of distrust and worthlessness

Family Pattern Alterations

Alteration in family processes or role performances related to separation of family, family role changes, inability to communicate in usual patterns, situational traumatic crises and complications of BMT, lack of adaptive skills

Compromised and/or ineffective family coping secondary to miscommunication of information, family separation, family role changes, exhaustion of personal or financial resources

Potential alteration in parenting of ill child and/or healthy siblings related to separation of family support systems, preoccupation with ill child, lack of communication with healthy siblings, parental stress and feelings of helplessness and guilt

Altered growth and development of child related to prescribed dependence, separation from usual support systems, absence from school, lack of play opportunities, therapeutic isolation, and social isolation

Hygiene

Self-care deficit: feeding, bathing, skin care, dressing, venous access care, toileting leading to prescribed dependency on parents or medical personnel

Neurologic

Impaired verbal communication of child secondary to developmental age abilities, lack of environmental stimulation while isolated, severe oral mucositis

---

Data from references 68, 70, and 90.

GVHD = Graft versus host disease; BMT = bone marrow transplant; TBI = total body irradiation; VOD = veno-occlusive disease.

TABLE 6–10. *Common Nursing Psychosocial Diagnoses Related to Pediatric BMT* Continued

Neurologic—cont'd

Alteration in sensory-perception (visual, auditory, kinesthetic, gustatory, tactile, olfactory) related to therapeutic isolation, side-effects of medications (e.g., analgesics), skin breakdown from acute GVHD and/or infection, side-effects of antibiotics (e.g., antibiotic ototoxicity), severe oral mucositis

Alteration in thought processes secondary to prolonged therapeutic isolation, side-effects of medications (e.g., analgesic psychosis), altered sleep patterns

Pain

Alteration in patient's comfort leading to pain related to side-effects of chemotherapy (e.g., vomiting), mucositis, skin breakdown, possible VOD of liver, possible infections

Alteration in donor's comfort leading to pain related to effects of bone marrow harvest on musculo-skeletal tissue

Safety

Impaired physical mobility

Potential for traumatic injury related to developmental age, unsafe or unmonitored isolation environment, generalized weakness, reduced level of consciousness

Teaching/Learning

Knowledge deficit about BMT

Knowledge deficit about bone marrow harvest procedure

Knowledge deficit about mandatory daily care regimens for BMT (e.g., central line care, oral care protocol, physical therapy)

Impaired home maintenance management related to necessary changes in eating, sleep, or isolation patterns, knowledge deficits about home care, anxiety related to separation from BMT center, complex discharge medication regimen

Potential alteration in adherence to treatment secondary to deleterious side-effects (e.g., steroids), complex or inconvenient drug regimens, unrealistic exercise goals, unrealistic or adverse food and fluid requirements

---

tween different components of the immune system and their influence on tumor biology and post-transplant immune reconstitution are being studied. Growth factors such as GM-CSF and G-CSF are being used widely to promote more rapid marrow recovery after transplantation, especially for those patients experiencing delayed or failed engraftment.[79,120]

Biologic response modifiers (e.g., interleukin-2 [IL-2]) have been used to promote antiviral activity of the donor T cells when given concomitantly with an allogeneic marrow infusion. The use of biologic response modifiers incorporated as part of transplant conditioning regimens is expected to increase with the goals of enhancing antitumor response, providing protection against viral reactivation, and eliminating residual malignant disease.[140]

Gene transfer has been an exciting technologic breakthrough at the molecular level. Potentially, normal genes can be transferred by retroviral vectors into autologous cells with defective or absent genetic material to correct a genetically determined disorder such as thalassemia major. Autologous cells could then be harvested, defective genetic material repaired in the laboratory, and the cells replaced by reinfusion. This method theoretically would avoid acute GVHD. It will be necessary to develop efficient processes by which to reintroduce the cells into the patient's cell line while destroying the abnormal cells present in the patient. Major problems with this technology include normal and sustained gene expression.[171]

In spite of successes of BMT in curing patients with hematologic malignancies, a significant number of patients with ALL and AML relapse after BMT. The systematic use of transplantation in patients with selected solid tumors is becoming more widespread, with the most extensive pediatric transplant experience in patients with neuroblastoma.

TABLE 6–11. *Selected Stressors Facing Nursing Staff Who Work in Bone Marrow Transplantation**

STRESSOR	SIGNIFICANCE
Potential for emotional overinvestment in the patient and family by nursing staff	BMT provides a medically intense and complex setting. Patients and families rely heavily on the nurse to explain and deliver complex care regimens. Being a highly specialized procedure, patients and families often travel long distances to undergo a transplant. As a result, patient and families are deprived of their normal support systems and often rely on the nurse for this support. The isolated BMT environment further reinforces and intensifies the bond between patient and families and the nurse. The consequences of emotional overinvestment can lead to decreased objectivity on the part of the nurse and an inability to intervene effectively as a professional.[156] The situation becomes emotionally draining for the staff and can lead to burnout.
Potential for rapid change in patient treatment goals, from attempting cure to providing palliative care	BMT units are ICU-type settings in which there is a tremendous commitment of resources toward aggressive patient management with a curative focus. In this critical care environment nurses are faced with balancing the intense physical care needs with the tremendous psychosocial needs of the patient and family. Characteristic of ICU or critical care settings, the emphasis of patient treatment can change rapidly within days to hours from a curative to a palliative approach. The attitudes and hopes of the nursing staff often cannot change rapidly enough to deal effectively with the situation. Nursing staff who value the goal of cure can feel cheated and defeated. Further, they may feel lacking in the skills needed to feel confident in promoting a dignified death for the patient and his or her family. Nurses who value the goal of caring and a dignified death may feel frustrated at not having adequate time to prepare the patient and family for this outcome.
Potential for patient nonadherence to care	Aggressive care requires patient cooperation and participation. BMT nursing care regimens (hygiene, exercise, and isolation procedures) are designed to minimize the complications of aggressive BMT therapy. Nurses expect patient cooperation and participation with care. Eliciting these is time consuming. Nonadherence because of patient or family factors can be doubly draining for the nursing staff. Staff may question the worth and effectiveness of elaborate protocols (e.g., for mouth care) in minimizing complications that may cause the patient additional distress and discomfort.
Potential for ambivalent feelings resulting from questioning the benefits of treatment as compared to fostering and maintaining quality of life.	Aggressive treatment can result in extreme morbidity for the patient. The BMT nursing staff develops expert nursing skills in attempts to decrease morbidity and prevent mortality. Complications from BMT are usually due to the treatment and not the disease. BMT nurses can feel guilty for being in part responsible for the patient's pain, discomfort, and suffering and as a result question the worth and benefits of this aggressive form of treatment. The

Data from references 16, 22, 24, 100, 156, 166, 192.
*Bone marrow transplantation is a subspecialty characterized by change. In addition to daily responsibilities, BMT nurses must be prepared to deal with issues related to ethical decision making, human rights, prolongation of life, and research-oriented activities. This creates an exciting, challenging but stessful environment within which to work. Some of the stressors encountered by BMT nurses in their job are noted above.

TABLE 6–11. *Selected Stressors Facing Nursing Staff Who Work in Bone Marrow Transplantation* Continued

STRESSOR	SIGNIFICANCE
	BMT environment is infused with high hopes for cure. Intellectually the nursing staff is aware of BMT risks but are often not emotionally prepared for untoward changes that can occur in the patient's status. In these situations nurses may respond paradoxically to the patient and family. Nurses verbally will provide accurate information to the patient framed in a way that continues to promote hope and optimism while their affective interactions convey the sense of pessimism the nurse feels about the patient's condition and potential outcome. A patient's death can lead to unresolved grief on the part of the nursing staff, which is heightened by the close bond that was established with the patient and the family.
Ethical concerns	Informed consent: patients and parents view the option of BMT as choosing between a chance for life versus certain death. The importance of "outcome" takes precedence for patients and families in the informed consent process over information about life-threatening toxicities. BMT nurses strongly believe it is important for the patient and family to take the information about BMT's side-effects and toxicity into account when making the decision to pursue BMT. This can create a frustrating situation for the nurse in which they value different aspects of the BMT process as compared to the patient and family.
Potential for interpersonal conflict among nursing staff and other interdisciplinary team members	The complexity of physical and psychologic care in the BMT setting requires careful nursing planning. Characteristically, BMT nurses are very knowledgeable about their field, and independent nursing judgment in patient care is highly valued. Staff conflict arises when there is lack of collaboration in patient care by nurses and inconsistent follow-through on nursing interventions developed by other colleagues on the unit. The need to manage toxicities and side-effects while maintaining quality care often takes a tremendous amount of cooperation and collaboration from the mulidisciplinary team. The energy spent by the BMT nurses in securing support from other disciplines can detract from patient care.

Consequently, improvement of the efficacy of transplant conditioning regimens is a high priority. Clinical studies are evaluating current regimens, comparing their antitumor efficacy to the side effects leading to morbidity and mortality. The gold standard for the ablation of ALL has been cyclophosphamide and TBI, although other agents such as cytosine arabinoside, busulfan, thiotepa, etoposide, L-phenylalanine mustard, carboplatin, and monoclonal antibodies are being investigated with interest.

Particular focus will be on the treatment of refractory diseases such as advanced rhabdomyosarcoma, brain tumors, recurrent leukemia, and non-Hodgkin's lymphoma. Hyperfractionation of TBI (two to three times daily) and total lymphoid irradiation (TLI) are two modalities of radiation being compared with the standard TBI as methods to deliver effective antitumor immunosuppressive therapy while decreasing side effects such as marked stomatotoxicity. Some centers are using a combination of both TBI and TLI in various doses and schedules. Also, monoclonal antibodies with antileukemic specificities or monoclonal antibodies attached to radioactive isotopes or toxins targeted at certain malignant cells have proved encouraging in early clinical trials of preparative regimens. The increasing intensity of front-line therapy in the treatment of most malignancies increases the challenge in designing preparative regimens to salvage relapsed patients.

The majority of pediatric BMTs performed in the 1980s were allogeneic transplants, although with the advent of new purging and preservation techniques, the application of auto-BMT will increase and perhaps equal that of allo-BMT in the 1990s. Major advances in allo-BMT can be expected in donor identification, less toxic effective preparative regimens, and the management of GVHD, all of which currently are limiting factors of allo-BMT.

More than 70% of all patients lack an HLA-matched sibling donor. This severe limitation in allo-BMT will become more problematic if the decrease in the average size of the family unit continues.[167] Improved methods of identifying HLAs, including DNA analysis, are being tested. Minor histocompatibility antigens are being identified with improved accuracy, and their effect on tolerance and GVHD is being studied. This knowledge will enable transplant centers to match recipients and donors more closely, even within a single family. It is projected that the existing donor pool will expand in several ways:

1. *Unrelated donor pool.* A combined national and international effort is underway among donor registries to recruit more unrelated donors, particularly from ethnic minorities. Currently the time from initiating a formal search to fruition in BMT is several months. Decreasing the time interval from search to transplant, which is especially important for high-risk relapse patients, is the goal. However, the incidence of marrow failure, infection, and acute GVHD will increase the risks for those receiving unrelated donor transplants.[72]

2. *Peripheral stem cell transplantation (PSCT).* In patients receiving autologous transplants, peripheral blood stem cells can be collected by intermittent leukopheresis during the recovery period after chemother-

apy when the cell numbers are sufficient and tumor burden is low. The peripherally collected cells are cryopreserved and infused at a later time.[89] Engraftment and immune reconstitution have been documented with this method.[93] The pluripotent stem cells are capable of engrafting and differentiating in the recipient in the same fashion as if given in an autologous marrow infusion. Possible marrow contamination with circulating tumor cells, time to engraftment, maintenance of sustained engraftment, associated morbidity, long-term outcome, and specific application in the pediatric and allogeneic settings must be explored.

3. *Non-HLA-matched donors.* Early research results show that survival is equivalent between one-antigen mismatched transplants and HLA-identical transplants.[8] Donors who are a one-antigen mismatch should routinely be considered as standard donor sources for candidates requiring bone marrow grafting.[9]

Increased emphasis will be placed on the prevention of acute GVHD, particularly through the application of in vivo and in vitro T-lymphocyte purging. Research is aimed at investigating and describing the immunopathology of acute GVHD and isolating those T cells most responsible. Specific purging techniques will be explored to destroy the implicated T cells selectively while preserving the integrity and function of those responsible for engraftment and other immune functions. However, although T-cell depletion decreases GVHD, it has been associated with unsuccessful engraftment and increased leukemic relapse in a significant number of patients.[122,132] Study of GVHD prophylaxis will continue and is likely to focus on new agents such as IL-2–receptor antibodies and new drug combinations that will lessen the incidence and severity of acute GVHD while maintaining optimal immune function. Likewise, clinical trials will continue to explore and elucidate the best treatment for chronic GVHD.[172] New agents and new applications of old agents such as thalidomide are being studied. The nursing role involves research to identify and implement more applicable and cost-effective assessment tools to facilitate early identification of both acute and chronic GVHD.

For auto-BMT, many controversial issues

surrounding the use of purging must be clarified for future application. In treating malignancies, determining the optimal situations and timing in respective disease states to harvest bone marrow will maximize both the effectiveness of in vivo purging and the efficacy of ex vivo purging methods. The development of more sensitive detection methods for different tumor systems and alternative purging methodologies such as positive stem cell selection are being explored.

Although the future of BMT probably will be exciting and encouraging, the research and treatment developments must take place in a health care milieu of decreasing and/or limited resources. Financial planning and strategies to provide adequate resources (e.g., an appropriate number of BMT beds in qualified BMT centers) will be crucial for the support and development of BMT. Ethical dilemmas regarding allogeneic donor issues, candidate selection, payment structures, and research protocols are complex and must be addressed. Studies are being undertaken to compare the cost effectiveness of BMT and conventional chemotherapy. Early analyses conclude that for select patient groups such as patients with AML, the cost effectiveness of BMT compares favorably with that of chemotherapy, partly owing to increased disease-free survival rates of transplant patients.[58] Future direction will entail reducing the cost of the procedure and reducing the length of stay in specialty care units. Bone marrow transplant nurses will be expected to participate in setting priorities.

Nursing must keep abreast of changes in the field and evaluate the impact on nursing practice and the consequences for patients and families. Emphasis on research to identify and develop more applicable and cost-effective assessment tools and interventions is essential. A focus on developing creative strategies to deliver BMT care in more cost-conscious, efficient methods will involve nurses as an integral part of the multidisciplinary team.

REFERENCES

1. Alexander J. Acral erythema during bone marrow transplantation: A case study. Oncol Nurs Forum 1989; 16:829–831.
2. Armitage JO, Gale RP. Bone marrow autotransplantation—A new direction in cancer therapy? In Gale RP, Champlin RE (eds): Bone Marrow Transplantation: Current Controversies. New York: Alan R Liss, 1989, pp 229–235.
3. Atkins DM, Patenaude AF. Psychosocial preparation and follow-up for pediatric bone marrow transplant patients. Am J Orthopsychiatry 1987; 57:246–252.
4. Bach FH, Albertini RJ, Anderson JL, et al. Bone marrow transplantation in patients with the Wiskott-Aldrich syndrome. Lancet 1968; 2:1364–1366.
5. Badr KF, Ichikawa I. Prerenal failure: A deleterious shift from renal compensation to decompensation. N Engl J Med 1988; 319:623–629.
6. Barrett A, Nicholls J, Gibson B. Late effects of total body irradiation. Radiother Oncol 1987; 9:131–135.
7. Bearman SI, Appelbaum FR, Buckner CD, et al. Regimen-related toxicity in patients undergoing bone marrow transplantation. J Clin Oncol 1988; 6:1562–1568.
8. Beatty PG, Clift RA, Mickelsan EM, et al. Marrow transplantation from related donors other than HLA-identical siblings. N Engl J Med 1985; 313:765.
9. Beatty PG, Anasetti C, Thomas ED, et al. Marrow transplantation from relatives other than HLA-identical siblings. In Gale RP, Champlin RE (eds): Bone Marrow Transplantation: Current Controversies. New York: Alan R Liss, 1989, pp 619–624.
10. Beck D, Maritaz O, Gross N, et al. Immunocytochemical detection of neuroblastoma cells infiltrating clinical bone marrow samples. Eur J Pediatr 1988; 147:609–612.
11. Beck S: Impact of a systematic oral care protocol on stomatitis after chemotherapy. Cancer Nurs 1979; 2:185–199.
12. Benjamin D, Magrath IT, Douglass EC, et al. Derivation of lymphoma cell lines from microscopically normal bone marrow in patients with undifferentiated lymphomas: Evidence of occult bone marrow involvement. Blood 1983; 61:1017–1019.
13. Bleyer WA. The impact of childhood cancer on the United States and the world. CA 1990; 40:355–367.
14. Bowden RA, Meyers JD. Prophylaxis of cytomegalovirus infection. Semin Hematol 1990; 27(suppl 1):17–21.
15. Bowden RA, Sayers M, Flournoy N, et al. Cytomegalovirus immune globulin and seronegative blood products to prevent primary cytomegalovirus infection after marrow transplantation. N Engl J Med 1986; 314:1006–1010.
16. Brack G, LaClave L, Blix S. The psychological aspects of bone marrow transplant; A staff's perspective. Cancer Nurs 1988; 11:221–229.
17. Brochstein JA. Critical care issues in bone marrow transplantation. Crit Care Clin 1988; 4:147–166.
18. Brochstein JA, Kernan NA, Groshen S, et al. Allogeneic bone marrow transplantation after hyperfractionated total-body irradiation and cyclophosphamide in children with acute leukemia. N Engl J Med 1987; 317:1618–1624.
19. Buckner CD, Clift RA, Sanders JE, et al. Protective environment for marrow transplant recipients. Ann Intern Med 1978; 89:893–901.
20. Burgdorf WH, Gilmore WA, Ganick RG. Peculiar acral erythema secondary to high-dose chemotherapy for acute myelogenous leukemia. Ann Intern Med 1982; 97:61–62.
21. Carl W, Higby DJ. Oral manifestations of bone marrow transplantation. Am J Clin Oncol 1985; 8:81–87.
22. Carney B. Bone marrow transplantation: Nurses'

and physicians' perceptions of informed consent. Cancer Nurs 1987; 10:252–259.

23. Champlin RE, Gale RP. The early complications of bone marrow transplantation. Semin Hematol 1984; 21:101–108.

24. Chauvenet AR, Smith NM. Referral of pediatric oncology patients for marrow transplantation and the process of informed consent. Med Pediatr Oncol 1988; 16:40–44.

25. Cheson BD, Lacerna L, Leyland-Jones B, et al. Autologous bone marrow transplantation: Current status and future directions. Ann Intern Med 1989; 110:51–65.

26. Children's Hospital of Los Angeles: BMTU Patient and Family Teaching Guidelines, 1983.

27. Clifford P, Clift RA, Duff JK. Nitrogen mustard therapy combined with autologous marrow infusion. Lancet 1961; 1:687–690.

28. Coccia PF, Krivit W, Cervenka J, et al. Successful bone marrow transplantation for infantile malignant osteoporosis. N Engl J Med 1980; 302:701–708.

29. Coccia PF, Strandjord SE, Warkentin PI, et al. High-dose cytosine arabinoside and fractionated total-body irradiation: An improved preparative regimen for bone marrow transplantation of children with acute lymphoblastic leukemia in remission. Blood 1988; 71:88–93.

30. Collins L. Veno-Occlusive Disease. Childrens Hospital of Los Angeles, 1989.

31. Corcoran-Buchsel P. Long-term complications of allogeneic bone marrow transplantation: Nursing implications. Oncol Nurs Forum 1986; 13:61–70.

32. Corcoran-Buchsel P. Bone marrow transplantation. In Groenwald SL, Frogge MH, Goodman M, et al. (eds): Cancer Nursing—Principles and Practice, 2nd ed. Boston: Jones & Bartlett, 1990, pp 307–337.

33. Corcoran-Buchsel P, Parchem C. Ambulatory care of the bone marrow transplant patient. Semin Oncol Nurs 1988; 4:41–46.

34. Crider MK, Jansen J, Norins AL, et al. Chemotherapy-induced acral erythema in patients receiving bone marrow transplantation. Arch Dermatol 1986; 122:1023–1027.

35. Damon LE, Mass R, Linker CA. The association between high-dose cytarabine neurotoxicity and renal insufficiency. J Clin Oncol 1989; 7:1563–1568.

36. Deeg HJ. How should marrow transplantation be approached? In Deeg HJ, Klingemann HG, Phillips GL (eds): A Guide to Bone Marrow Transplantation. Berlin-Heidelberg: Springer-Verlag, 1988, pp 7–17.

37. Devergie A, Esperou H, Traineau R, et al. Role of immunosuppressive drugs for prevention of graft-v-host disease after bone marrow transplantation. Nouv Rev Fr Hematol 1989; 31:73–75.

38. Doney KC, Buckner CD. Bone marrow transplantation: Overview. Plasma Ther Transfusion Technol 1985; 6:149–161.

39. Dujak LA. HLA typing implications for nurses. Oncol Nurs Forum 1984; 11:20–36.

40. Dulley FL, Kanfer EJ, Appelbaum FR, et al. Veno-occlusive disease of the liver after chemoradiotherapy and autologous bone marrow transplantation. Transplantation 1987; 43:870–873.

41. Eilers J, Berger A, Petersen M. Development, testing and application of the oral assessment guide. Oncol Nurs Forum 1988; 15:325–330.

42. Emanuel D. Treatment of cytomegalovirus disease. Semin Hematol 1990; 27(suppl 1):22–27.

43. Emanuel D, Cunningham I, Jules-Elysee K, et al. Cytomegalovirus pneumonia after bone marrow transplantation successfully treated with the combination of ganciclovir and high-dose intravenous immune globulin. Ann Intern Med 1988; 109: 777–782.

44. Fefer A, Clift RA, Thomas ED, et al. Allogeneic marrow transplantation for chronic granulocytic leukemia. J Natl Cancer Inst 1986; 76:1295–1299.

45. Foley MK. Children with cancer: Ethical dilemmas. Semin Oncol Nurs 1989: 5:109–113.

46. Ford R, Ballard B. Acute complications after bone marrow transplantation. Semin Oncol Nurs 1988; 4:15–24.

47. Ford R, Eisenberg S. Bone marrow transplant: Recent advances and nursing implications. Nurs Clin North Am 1990; 25:405–422.

48. Ford R, McClain K, Cunningham BA. Veno-occlusive disease following marrow transplantation. Nurs Clin North Am 1983; 18:563–568.

49. Fort JA, Graham-Pole J. Pulmonary complications of bone marrow transplantation. In Johnson FL, Pochedly C (eds): Bone Marrow Transplantation in Children. New York: Raven Press, 1990, pp 397–411.

50. Freedman SE. An overview of bone marrow transplantation. Semin Oncol Nurs 1988; 4:3–8.

51. Frei E. Curative cancer chemotherapy. Cancer Res 1985; 45:6523–6537.

52. Frei E, Antman K, Teicher B, et al. Bone marrow autotransplantation for solid tumors—Prospects. J Clin Oncol 1989; 7:515–526.

53. Furman WL, Feldman S. Infectious complications. In Johnson FL, Pochedly C (eds): Bone Marrow Transplantation in Children. New York: Raven Press, 1990, pp 427–450.

54. Gallagher MT. Experimental basis. In Blume KG, Petz LD (eds): Clinical Bone Marrow Transplantation. New York: Churchill-Livingstone, 1983, pp 33–64.

55. Gardner GG, August CS, Githens J. Psychological issues in bone marrow transplantation. Pediatrics 1977; 60:625–631.

56. Gatti RA, Meuwissen HJ, Allen HD, et al. Immunological reconstitution of sex-linked lymphopenic immunological deficiency. Lancet 1968; 2:1366–1369.

57. Gee AP. Bone marrow purging and processing—A review of ancillary effects. In Gross S, Gee AP, Worthington-White DA (eds): Bone Marrow Purging and Processing. New York: Alan R Liss, 1990, pp 507–521.

58. Gilbert HG, Larson EB. Cost effectiveness of bone marrow transplantation in acute nonlymphocytic leukemia. N Engl J Med 1989; 321:807–812.

59. Glucksberg H, Storb R, Fefer A, et al. Clinical manifestations of graft-versus-host-disease in human recipients of marrow from HLA-matched sibling donors. Transplantation 1974; 18:295–304.

60. Gorin NC, Aegerter P, Auvert B. Autologous bone marrow transplantation for acute leukemia in remission: An analysis of 1322 cases. Haematol/Bluttransfus 1990; 33:660–666.

61. Gottlieb SE, Portnoy S. The role of play in a pediatric bone marrow transplantation unit. Child Health Care 1988; 16:177–181.

62. Graeve JLA, De Alarcon PA, Sato Y, et al. Miliary pulmonary neuroblastoma. A risk of autologous bone marrow transplantation? Cancer 1988; 62:2125–2127.

63. Graham-Pole J, Casper J, Elfenbein G, et al. High-dose chemoradiotherapy supported by marrow infusions for advanced neuroblastoma: A pediatric oncology group study. J Clin Oncol 1991; 9:152–158.

64. Grant NC. Hepatic veno-occlusive disease following bone marrow transplantation. Oncol Nurs Forum 1989; 16:813–817.

65. Gress RE. Purged autologous bone marrow transplantation in the treatment of acute leukemia. Oncology 1990; 4:35–47.

66. Guyton AC. Textbook of Medical Physiology, 6th ed. Philadelphia: WB Saunders, 1981.

67. Haberman MR. Psychosocial aspects of bone marrow transplantation. Semin Oncol Nurs 1988; 4:55–59.

68. Hanigan MJ. Complex problems of children following allogeneic bone marrow transplantation. J Pediatr Oncol Nurs 1990; 7:73–75.

69. Hanigan MJ. Unrelated bone marrow transplantation: Past, present, and future. J Pediatr Oncol Nurs 1991; 8:80–81.

70. Hanigan MJ. Unrelated bone marrow transplantation and the national marrow donor program: An update. J Pediatr Oncol Nurs 1992; 9:71–75.

71. Hansen JA. Donor selection for marrow transplantation. HLA polymorphism and matching. In Gale RP, Champlin RE (eds): Bone Marrow Transplantation: Current Controversies. New York: Alan R Liss, 1989, pp 607–618.

72. Hansen JA, Anasetti C, Beatty PG, et al. Marrow transplantation from unrelated HLA-matched volunteer donors. Transplantation Proc 1989; 21:2993–2994.

73. Hare J, Skinner D. Family systems approach to pediatric bone marrow transplantation. Children's Health Care 1989; 18:30–36.

74. Hartmann O, Benhamou E, Beaujean F, et al. Repeated high-dose chemotherapy followed by purged autologous bone marrow transplantation as consolidation therapy in metastatic neuroblastoma. J Clin Oncol 1987; 5:1205–1211.

75. Herzig RH, Lazarus GP, Herzig PF, et al. Central nervous system toxicity with high-dose cytosine arabinoside. Semin Oncol 1985; 12(suppl 3):233–236.

76. Herzig RH, Wolff SN, Lazarus HM, et al. High-dose cytosine arabinoside therapy for refractory leukemia. Blood 1983; 62:361–369.

77. Hill HF, Chapman CR, Jackson TL, et al. Assessment and management of donor pain following marrow harvest for allogeneic bone marrow transplantation. Bone Marrow Transplantation 1989; 4:157–161.

78. Ho M. Cytomegalovirus. In Mandell GL, Douglas RG, Bennett JE (eds): Principles and Practice of Infectious Disease, 3rd ed. New York: Churchill Livingstone, 1990, pp 1159–1171.

79. Hoang I, Nara N, Wong G, et al. Effects of recombinant GM-CSF on the blast cells of acute myeloblastic leukemia. Blood 1986; 68:313–316.

80. Hobbs JR, Barrett AJ, Chambers D, et al. Reversal of clinical features of Hurler's disease and biochemical improvement after treatment by bone marrow transplantation. Lancet 1981; 2:709–712.

81. Hutchinson MM, King AH. A nursing perspective on bone marrow transplantation. Nurs Clin North Am 1983; 18:511–522.

82. International Autologous Bone Marrow Transplant Registry. Bone marrow autotransplantation in man. Lancet 1986; 2:960–962.

83. Jacobson LO. Evidence for a humoral factor (or factors) concerned in recovery from radiation injury: A review. Cancer Res 1952; 12:315–325.

84. Jacobson LO, Marks EK, Robson MJ, et al. The effect of spleen protection on mortality following x-irradiation. J Lab Clin Med 1949; 34:1538–1543.

85. Johnson FL, Look AT, Gockerman J, et al. Bone marrow transplantation in a patient with sickle cell anemia. N Engl J Med 1984; 31:780–783.

86. Joshi SS, Kessinger A, Mann SI, et al. Detection of malignant cells in histologically normal bone marrow using culture techniques. Bone Marrow Transplant 1987; 1:303–310.

87. Kampmann KK, Graves T, Rogers SD. Acral erythema secondary to high-dose cytosine arabinoside with pain worsened by cyclosporine infusions. Cancer 1989; 63:2482–2485.

88. Keith JS. Hepatic failure: Etiologies, manifestations and management. Crit Care Nurse 1985; 5:60–86.

89. Kessinger A, Armitage JO, Landmanrk GD, et al. Autologous peripheral hematopoietic stem cell transplantation restores hematopoietic function following marrow ablative therapy. Blood 1988; 71:723–727.

90. Kim MJ, McFarland GK, McLane AM (eds). Pocket Guide to Nursing Diagnoses, 4th ed. St. Louis: CV Mosby, 1991.

91. Klingemann HG. Acute transplant related problems: Urinary tract. In Deeg HJ, Klingemann HG, Phillips GI (eds). A Guide to Bone Marrow Transplantation. Berlin-Heidelberg: Springer-Verlag, 1988, pp 135–139.

92. Kolb HJ, Bender-Gotze CH. Late complications after allogeneic bone marrow transplantation for leukemia. Bone Marrow Transplant 1990; 6:61–72.

93. Korbling M, Dorken B, Ho AD, et al. Autologous transplantation of blood derived hemopoietic stem cells after myeloablative therapy in a patient with Burkitt's lymphoma. Blood 1986; 67:529–562.

94. Krzysko A, Erdel S, Greiner M, et al. Impaired gas exchange. In McNally JC, Stair JC, Somerville ET (eds): Guidelines for Cancer Nursing Practice. Orlando, Fla: Grune & Stratton, 1985, pp 291–295.

95. Kurnick NC, Montano A, Gerdes JC, et al. Preliminary observations and the treatment of post irradiation haematopoietic depression in man by the infusion of stored autologous marrow. Ann Intern Med 1958; 49:969.

96. Lancaster LE. Renal failure: Pathophysiology, assessment and intervention. Nephrol Nurs 1983; 5:38–51.

97. Lass JH, Lazarus HM, Reed MD, et al. Topical corticosteroid therapy for corneal toxicity from systemically administered cytarabine. Am J Ophthalmol 1982; 94:617–621.

98. Leitman SF. Posttransfusion graft-versus-host disease. In Smith DM, Silvergleid AJ (eds): Special Considerations in Transfusing the Immunocompromised Patient. Arlington, Va.: American Association of Blood Banks, 1985, pp 15–37.

99. Lenarsky C, Parkman R. Bone marrow transplantation for the treatment for immune deficiency states. Bone Marrow Transplant 1990; 6:361–369.

100. Lesko LM. Patients', parents', and oncologists' perceptions of informed consent for bone marrow transplantation. Med Pediatr Oncol 1989; 17:181–187.

101. Levine AS, Siegel SE, Schreiber AD, et al. Protected environments and prophylactic antibiotics. N Engl J Med 1973; 288:477–483.

102. Lindsley DL, Odell TT, Tausche FG. Implantation of functional erythropoietic elements following total-body irradiation. Proc Soc Exp Biol Med 1955; 90:512–515.

103. Lingren PS. The laminar air flow room: Nursing practices and procedures. Nurs Clin North Am 1983; 18:553–561.

104. Lipton JM, Nathan DG. The anatomy and physiology of hematopoiesis. In Nathan DG, Oski FA (eds): Hematology of Infancy and Childhood, 3rd ed. Philadelphia: WB Saunders, 1987, pp 128–158.

105. Lorenz E, Congdon C, Uphoff D. Modification of acute irradiation injury in mice and guinea pigs by bone marrow injections. Radiology 1952; 58:863–877.

106. Lucarelli G. Bone marrow transplantation in patients with thalassemia. N Engl J Med 1990; 312:417–421.

107. Luttrell JS. Genitourinary tract: Implications of inflammation, obstruction and structural abnormalities. In Mott SR, James SR, Sperhac AM (eds): Nursing Care of Children and Families, 2nd ed. Redwood City: Addison-Wesley, 1990, pp 1446–1498.

108. Lydon J. Assessment of renal function in the patient receiving chemotherapy. Cancer Nurs 1989; 12:133–143.

109. Marshall D. Care of the pediatric oncology patient in a laminar air flow setting; A conceptual framework for nursing practice. Nurs Clin North Am 1985; 20:67–82.

110. McCullough J, Hansen J, Perkins H, et al. The national marrow donor program. Oncology 1989; 3:63–68.

111. McDonald GB, Sharma P, Matthews DE, et al. Venoocclusive disease of the liver after bone marrow transplantation: Diagnosis, incidence, and predisposing factors. Hepatology 1984; 4:116–122.

112. McDonald GB, Sharma P, Matthews DE, et al. The clinical course of 53 patients with venoocclusive disease of the liver after marrow transplantation. Transplantation 1985; 39:603–608.

113. McDonald GB, Shulman HM, Sullivan KM, et al. Intestinal and hepatic complications of human bone marrow transplantation, parts 1 and 2. Gastroenterology 1986; 90:460–477, 770–784.

114. McGlave PB, Beatty P, Ash R, et al. Therapy for chronic myelogenous leukemia with unrelated donor bone marrow transplantation: Results in 102 cases. Blood 1990; 75:1728–1732.

115. Meyers JD, Flournoy N, Thomas ED. Risk factors for cytomegalovirus infection after human marrow transplantation. J Infect Dis 1986; 153:478–488.

116. Meyers JD, Reed EC, Shepp DH, et al. Acyclovir for prevention of cytomegalovirus infection and disease after allogeneic marrow transplantation. N Engl J Med 1988; 318:70–75.

117. Moore I, Kramer R, Ablin A. Late effects of central nervous system prophylactic leukemia therapy on cognitive functioning. Oncol Nurs Forum 1986; 13:45–51.

118. Morrison M, Samwick AA. Intramedullary (sternal) transfusion of human bone marrow. JAMA 1940; 115:1708–1711.

119. Moss TJ, Seeger RC, Kindler-Rohrborn A, et al. Immunohistologic detection and phenotyping of neuroblastoma cells in bone marrow using cytoplasmic neuron specific enolase and cell surface antigens. Prog Clin Biol Res 1985; 175:367–378.

120. Motoji T, Takanashi M, Fuchinoue M, et al. Effect of recombinant GM-CSF and recombinant G-CSF on colony formation of blast progenitors in acute myeloblastic leukemia. Exp Hematol 1989; 17:56–60.

121. Nand S, Messmore HL, Patel R Jr, et al. Neurotoxicity associated with systemic high-dose cytosine arabinoside. J Clin Oncol 1986; 4:571–575.

122. O'Reilly RJ, Kernan NA, Cunningham I, et al. T cell depleted transplants for the treatment of leukemia. In Gale RP, Champlin RE (eds): Bone Marrow Transplantation: Current Controversies. New York: Alan R Liss, 1989, pp 477–493.

123. Osgood EE, Riddle MC, Mathews TJ. Aplastic anemia treated with daily transfusions and intravenous marrow: Case report. Ann Intern Med 1939; 13:357–367.

124. Peters WP. The effect of recombinant human colony-stimulating factors on hematopoietic reconstitution following autologous bone marrow transplantation. Semin Hematol 1989; 26:18–23.

125. Philip T, Armitage JO, Spitzer G, et al. High-dose therapy and autologous bone marrow transplantation after failure of conventional chemotherapy in adults with intermediate grade or high grade non-Hodgkin's lymphoma. N Engl J Med 1987; 316:1493–1498.

126. Phillips GL. Acute transplant related problems: Management of infection. In Deeg HJ, Klingemann HG, Phillips GI (eds): A Guide to Bone Marrow Transplantation. Berlin-Heidelberg: Springer-Verlag, 1988, pp 107–113.

127. Phillips GL. Preparation for marrow transplantation. In Deeg HJ, Klingemann HG, Phillips GL: A Guide to Bone Marrow Transplantation. Berlin-Heidelberg: Springer-Verlag, 1988, pp 26–42.

128. Pick TE. Autologous bone marrow transplantation in children. Crit Rev Oncol Hematol 1988; 8:311–337.

129. Piggott KS. Fluid and electrolytes: Implications of imbalance. In Mott SR, James SR, Sperhac AM (eds): Nursing Care of Children and Families, 2nd ed. Redwood City: Addison-Wesley, 1990, pp 907–954.

130. Pizzo PA. Infectious complications in the child with cancer. I. Pathophysiology of the compromised host and the initial evaluation and management of the febrile cancer patient. J Pediatr 1981; 98:341–354.

131. Pizzo PA. The value of protective isolation in preventing nosocomial infections in high risk patients. Am J Med 1981; 70:631–637.

132. Poynton CH. T cell depletion in bone marrow transplantation. Bone Marrow Transplant 1988; 3:265–279.

133. Prescott LF. Assessment of nephrotoxicity. Br J Clin Pharmacol 1982; 13:303–311.

134. Quine WE. The remedial application of bone marrow. JAMA 1896; 26:1012–1013.

135. Quinn JJ. Bone marrow transplant in the management of childhood cancer. Pediatr Clin North Am 1985; 32:811–833.

136. Ramsay NKC. Bone marrow transplantation in pediatric oncology. In Pizzo PA, Poplack DG (eds): Principles and Practice of Pediatric Oncology, 2nd ed. Philadelphia: JB Lippincott, 1993, pp 315–334.

137. Ramsay NKC. Use of bone marrow transplantation in bone marrow failure. In Johnson FL, Pochedly C (eds): Bone Marrow Transplantation in Children. New York: Raven Press, 1990, pp 181–202.

138. Rappeport JM, Ginns EI. Bone marrow transplantation in severe Gaucher's disease. N Engl J Med 1984; 311:880–888.

139. Reed EC, Bowden RA, Dandliker PS, et al. Treatment of cytomegalovirus pneumonia with ganciclo-

vir and intravenous cytomegalovirus immunoglobulin in patients with bone marrow transplants. Ann Intern Med 1988; 109:783–788.

140. Reittie JE, Gottlieb D, Heslop HE, et al. Endogenously generated activated killer cells circulate after autologous and allogeneic marrow transplantation but not after chemotherapy. Blood 1989; 7:1351–1358.

141. Reynolds CP, Moss TJ, Feig SA, et al. Treatment of poor prognosis neuroblastoma with intensive therapy and autologous bone marrow transplantation. In Dicke K, Spitzer G, Jagannath S (eds): Autologous Marrow Transplantation: Proceedings of Fourth International Symposium. Houston: University of Texas MD Anderson Hospital & Tumor Institute, 1989, pp 575–582.

142. Rio B, Andreu G, Nicod JP, et al. Thrombocytopenia in venoocclusive disease after bone marrow transplantation or chemotherapy. Blood 1986; 67:1773–1776.

143. Rohaly J. The use of busulfan therapy in bone marrow transplantation: A nursing overview. Cancer Nurs 1989; 12:144–152.

144. Sanders J, Buckner CD, Bensinger WI, et al. Experience with marrow harvesting from donors less than two years of age. Bone Marrow Transplant 1987; 2:45–50.

145. Sanders J, Sullivan K, Witherspoon R, et al. Long-term effects and quality of life in children and adults after bone marrow transplantation for leukemia. Bone Marrow Transplant 1989; 4(suppl 4):27–29.

146. Sanders JE. Effects of bone marrow transplantation on reproductive function. Buffalo, N.Y.: International Conference on Complications of Treatment of Children and Adolescents for Cancer, June 22–24, 1990.

147. Sanders JE, Flournoy N, Thomas ED, et al. Marrow transplant experience in children with acute lymphoblastic leukemia: An analysis of factors associated with survival, relapse and graft-v-host disease. Med Pediatr Oncol 1985; 13:165–172.

148. Sanders JE, Buckner CD, Sullivan K, et al. Growth and development after bone marrow transplantation. In Buckner CD, Gale RP, Lucarelli G (eds): Advances and Controversies in Thalassemia Therapy: Bone Marrow Transplantation and Other Approaches. New York: Alan R Liss, 1989, pp 375–382.

149. Santos GW. Immunosuppression for clinical marrow transplantation. Semin Hematol 1974; 11:341–351.

150. Santos GW. History of bone marrow transplantation. Clin Haematol 1983; 12:611–639.

151. Santos GW, Tutschka PJ, Brookmeyer R, et al. Marrow transplantation for acute nonlymphocytic leukemia after treatment with busulfan and cyclophosphamide. N Engl J Med 1983; 309:1347–1353.

152. Saral R, Burns WH, Laskin OL, et al. Acyclovir prophylaxis of herpes-simplex virus infections. N Engl J Med 1981; 305:63–67.

153. Seeger RC, Reynolds CP. Treatment of high risk solid tumors of childhood with intensive therapy and autologous bone marrow transplantation. Pediatr Clin North Am 1991; 38:393–424.

154. Seeger RC, Reynolds CP, Moss TJ, et al. Autologous bone marrow transplantation for poor prognosis neuroblastoma. In Dicke KA, Spitzer G, Jagannath S (eds): Autologous Bone Marrow Transplantation: Proceedings Third International Symposium. Houston: University of Texas MD Anderson Hospital & Tumor Institute, 1987, pp 375–382.

155. Seeger RC, Villablanca JG, Matthay KK, et al. Intensive chemoradiotherapy and autologous marrow transplantation for poor prognosis neuroblastoma. In Evans AE, D'Angio GJ, Knudson AG, et al. (eds): Advances in Neuroblastoma Research 3. New York: Wiley-Liss, 1991, pp 351–357.

156. Shedd P. Nursing staff stresses and ethical dilemmas in caring for bone marrow transplant patients. In Whedon MB (ed): Bone Marrow Transplantation: Principles, Practice, and Nursing Insights. Boston: Jones & Bartlett, 1991, pp 349–361.

157. Spruce WE. Bone marrow transplantation: Use for aplastic anemia, hereditary diseases, and hemoglobinopathies. Am J Pediatr Hematol Oncol 1983; 5:295–300.

158. Spruce WE. Bone marrow transplantation: Use in neoplastic diseases. Am J Pediatr Hematol Oncol 1983; 5:287–294.

159. Spruce WE. Supportive care in bone marrow transplantation. In Johnson FL, Pochedly C (ed): Bone Marrow Transplantation in Children. New York: Raven Press, 1990, pp 69–85.

160. Storb R. Graft rejection and graft-versus-host disease in marrow transplantation. Transplant Proc 1989; 21:2915–2918.

161. Storb R, Buckner CD. Human bone marrow transplantation. Eur J Clin Invest 1990; 20:119–132.

162. Storb R, Deeg H, Pepe M, et al. Methotrexate and cyclosporine versus cyclosporine alone for prophylaxis of graft-versus-host disease in patients given HLA-identical marrow grafts for leukemia: Long-term follow-up of a controlled trial. Blood 1989; 73:729–734.

163. Storb R, Prentice RL, Buckner CD, et al. Graft-versus-host disease and survival in patients with aplastic anemia treated by marrow grafts from HLA-identical siblings; Beneficial effect of a protective environment. N Engl J Med 1983; 308:302–307.

164. Storb R, Thomas ED. Allogeneic bone marrow transplantation. Immunol Rev 1983; 71:77–102.

165. Storb R, Thomas ED, Buckner CD, et al. Allogeneic marrow transplantation for the treatment of aplastic anemia. Blood 1974; 43:157–180.

166. Stutzer C. Work-related stresses of pediatric bone marrow transplant nurses. J Pediatr Oncol Nurs 1989; 6:70–78.

167. Sullivan KM. Graft versus host disease. In Blume KG, Petz LD (eds): Clinical Bone Marrow Transplantation. New York: Churchill Livingstone, 1983, pp 91–129.

168. Sullivan KM. Acute and chronic graft-versus-host disease in man. Int J Cell Cloning 1986; 4(suppl 1):42–93.

169. Sullivan KM. Congress review: Progress and prospects in bone marrow transplantation. Transplant Proc 1989; 21:2919–2922.

170. Tavassoli M, Hardy C. Molecular basis of homing of intravenously transplanted stem cells to the marrow. Blood 1990; 76:1059–1070.

171. Thomas ED. Marrow transplantation and gene transfer as therapy for hematopoietic diseases. In Molecular biology of homosapiens. Cold Springs Harb Symp Quant Biol 1986; 51:1009–1011.

172. Thomas ED. The future of bone marrow transplantation. Semin Oncol Nurs 1988; 4:74–78.

173. Thomas ED, Buckner CD, Banji M, et al. One-hundred patients with acute leukemia treated by chemotherapy, total body irradiation and allogeneic bone marrow transplantation. Blood 1977; 49:511–533.

174. Thomas ED, Buckner CD, Sanders JE, et al. Marrow transplantation for thalassemia. Lancet 1982; 2:227–229.
175. Thomas ED, Clift RA, Fefer A, et al. Marrow transplantation for the treatment of chronic myelogenous leukemia. Ann Intern Med 1986; 104:155–163.
176. Thomas ED, Storb R, Clift R, et al. Bone marrow transplantation, part 1. New Engl J Med 1975; 292:832–843.
177. Tollemar J, Ringdin O, Backman L, et al. Results of four different protocols for prophylaxis against graft-versus-host disease. Transplant Proc 1989; 21:3008–3010.
178. Tutschka PJ. Chronic infections and immunodeficiency in bone marrow transplantation. Pediatr Infect Dis J 1988; 7:s22–s29.
179. van der Meer JWM, Guiot HF, van den Broek PJ, et al. Infections in bone marrow transplant recipients. Semin Hematol 1984; 21:123–140.
180. van der Wal R, Nims J, Davies B. Bone marrow transplantation in children: Nursing management of late effects. Cancer Nurs 1988; 11:132–143.
181. Vassal G, Hartmann O, Benhamou E. Busulfan and veno-occlusive disease of the liver. Ann Intern Med 1990; 112:881.
182. Vega RA, Franco CM, Abdel-Mageed AMS, et al. Bone marrow transplantation in the treatment of children with cancer: Current status. Hematol Oncol Clin North Am 1987; 1:777–800.
183. Von Fliender V, Higby DJ, Kim U. Graft versus host reaction following blood product transfusion. Am J Med 1982; 72:951–961.
184. Wagner JE, Yeager AM, Beschorner WE. Pathology of bone marrow transplantation. In Johnson FL, Pochedly C (eds): Bone Marrow Transplantation in Children. New York: Raven Press, 1990, pp 141–164.
185. Waskerwitz MJ, Wiley FM, Perin GA. Nursing communication between local and referral cancer centers for pediatric bone marrow transplant patients. J Assoc Pediatr Oncol Nurses 1984; 1:26–34.
186. Weiden PL, Flournoy N, Thomas ED, et al. Antileukemic effect of graft-versus-host disease in human recipients of allogeneic-marrow grafts. N Engl J Med 1979; 300:1068–1073.
187. Weinberg KI, Parkman R. Bone marrow transplantation for genetic diseases. In Johnson FL, Pochedly C (eds): Bone Marrow Transplantation in Children. New York: Raven Press, 1990, pp 243–260.
188. Wiley FM, House KU. Bone marrow transplant in children. Semin Oncol Nurs 1988; 4:31–40.
189. Wilson LA, Price SA. Restrictive patterns of respiratory disease. In Price SA, Wilson LA (ed): Pathophysiology: Clinical Concepts of Disease Processes. New York: McGraw-Hill, 1978, pp 430–446.
190. Witherspoon RP, Fisher LD, Schoch G, et al. Secondary cancers after bone marrow transplantation for leukemia or aplastic anemia. N Engl J Med 1989; 321:784–789.
191. Yeager A. Autologous bone marrow transplantation in patients with acute nonlymphocytic leukemia, using ex vivo marrow treatment with 4-hydroperoxycyclophosphamide. N Engl J Med 1986; 315:141–147.
192. Younger SJ, Allen M, Montenegro H, et al. Resolving problems at the intensive care unit/oncology unit interface. Perspect Biol Med 1988; 31:299–308.
193. Zaia JA. Infections. In Blume KG, Petz LD (eds): Clinical Bone Marrow Transplantation. New York: Churchill-Livingstone, 1983, pp 131–176.
194. Zaia JA. Epidemiology and pathogenesis of cytomegalovirus disease. Semin Hematol 1990; 27(suppl 1):5–10.

BIOLOGIC RESPONSE MODIFIERS

Myra Woolery-Antill
Constance Colter

For more than a century scientists and researchers have been intrigued by the intricate and complex functions of the body's immune system, especially the role(s) it plays in disease development and disease prevention. Early scientific manipulation of the immune system was referred to as *immunotherapy*. The earliest clinical reports concerning the use of immunotherapy date back to the late 1800s; however, research and extensive exploration were hindered by scientific technology, limited quantities and crude preparations of immune substances, and inconsistent, often disappointing clinical results.[81,99,109] Researchers' interest with immunotherapy has been like a roller coaster, directly influenced by technologic advances.[99]

Many cancer researchers have postulated that advances in the understanding of the immune system will assist in the identification of risk factors and the prevention and/or treatment of many cancers. Researchers have known for decades about the existence of substances occurring in minute quantities in the body that influence immune system functioning. Many of these substances, now referred to as *biologic response modifiers (BRMs)*, encompass a variety of agents (e.g., colony-stimulating factors [CSFs], interleukins, monoclonal antibodies, tumor necrosis factor, interferons).[1,60,85,109] They are named according to cellular origin and function. Several BRMs are interdependent and belong to the cytokine network (Fig. 7–1).[73,74] Cytokines are naturally occurring glycoproteins produced by a variety of cells. They are responsible for the regulation and function of other cells in the body.[75]

The term *biologic response modifiers* includes not only agents but also therapeutic approaches capable of modifying physiologic and/or immune responses. Although the terms *biologic, BRM, immunotherapy*, and *biotherapy* are often used interchangeably, they are not necessarily synonymous. As a direct result of clinical trials, the biologic activities of specific BRMs have been identified, and new BRMs have been discovered. Since the activities and clinical responses elicited in patients receiving BRMs are not necessarily confined to the immune system, as once speculated, many researchers no longer consider the term *immunotherapy* reflective of the diverse activities and responses elicited. Therefore many refer to this expanding field of knowledge and technology as *BRMs* or *biotherapy*.[81]

Scientific advances of the late 1970s and early 1980s (e.g., molecular biology, genetic engineering, and immunology) have led to a reemergence of the concept of immunotherapy and a renewed enthusiasm in conducting

179

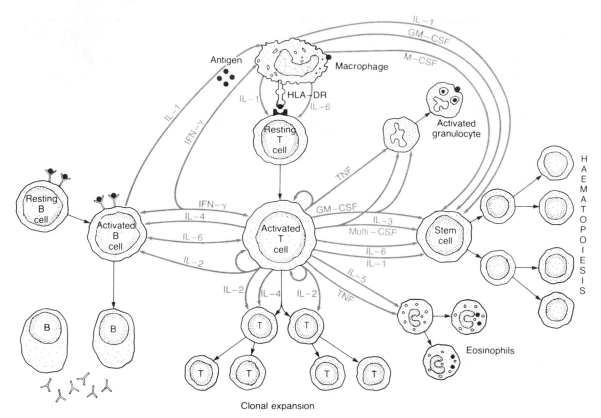

FIGURE 7–1. Positive interactions in the cytokine network when antigen is encountered. *(From Balkwill FR. Cytokines in Cancer Therapy. Oxford: Oxford University Press, 1989, p 215, by permission of Oxford University Press.)*

research using BRMs to modulate or alter the individual's immune system for the treatment of various diseases and their side effects.[6,10,18,60,99] As a direct result of scientific advances, the use of BRMs in laboratory and clinical research has increased rapidly. One example of an important scientific advance in the field of biotherapy is hybridization technology (Fig. 7–2), which spawned the development of monoclonal antibodies (MoAbs).[114] This technology is based on the immune system's response to a foreign antigen. When stimulated, B cells can differentiate to plasma cells and secrete a specific antibody. The spleen is a reservoir for these antibody-secreting lymphocytes. Using a mouse that has been injected with tumor cells (acting as the antigen), researchers can induce antibody production. The foreign tumor cells incite an immune response in the mouse, initiating antibody production. Antibody-secreting B cells, removed from the spleen of

the mouse, are fused with a cell from a malignant myeloma cell line to combine the immortal properties of the cancer cell with the antibody-producing properties of the spleen cell. The result of this fusion is the hybridoma, which can indefinitely produce a specific antibody. The antibodies produced from this single clone are MoAbs.[141] Once the technology was refined in vitro, hybridization technology and MoAb production were used in many clinical trials in the diagnosis and treatment of cancer. In fact, MoAbs can be produced to screen proteins made by recombinant DNA molecules, demonstrating the interrelatedness of the many advances in techniques of biotechnology.[116]

Further examples of scientific advances are the techniques developed through genetic engineering. They have opened an exciting new field involving recombinant DNA technology (Fig. 7–3).[37,114] Basically, this technology involves identifying the genes on a par-

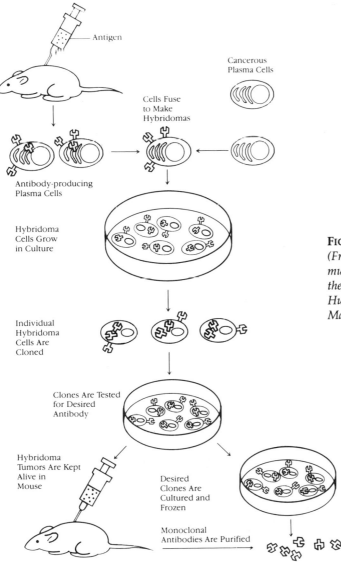

Antigen

Cancerous
Plasma Cells

Cells Fuse
to Make
Hybridomas

Antibody-producing
Plasma Cells

Hybridoma
Cells Grow
in Culture

Individual
Hybridoma
Cells Are
Cloned

Clones Are Tested
for Desired
Antibody

Hybridoma
Tumors Are Kept
Alive in
Mouse

Desired
Clones Are
Cultured and
Frozen

Monoclonal
Antibodies Are Purified

FIGURE 7–2. Hybridization technology. *(From Schindler LW. Understanding the immune system. NIH publication 90-529. Bethesda, Md.: U.S. Department of Health and Human Services, National Institutes of Health, March 1990, p 29.)*

ticular area of a DNA strand that code for a specific cell function such as protein synthesis. Using an enzyme preparation, the DNA can be broken at the ends of the area of interest and removed from the strand. This portion of DNA is inserted into a plasmid, a spliced ring of DNA, and introduced into a chosen host organism such as *Escherichia coli.* After subsequent cloning procedures, multiple copies of the DNA fragment are produced within the vector, unaffected by the host cell's chromosomes. The molecules constructed by this method are called *recombinant DNA.* Researchers can further manipulate these molecules for use in laboratory and clinical set-

tings, including drug production (e.g., colony-stimulating factors), study of genetic diseases, and cancer research.

The increased availability of recombinant preparations has sparked rapid progress in this field of study. The use of BRMs in phase I, II, and III clinical trials has increased dramatically and will continue to do so. Most of what is currently known about BRMs results from clinical trials conducted in the adult population. Although this information provides a valuable foundation to guide possible applications in children, it cannot be assumed the same applications will elicit comparable responses. What exact role this treatment mo-

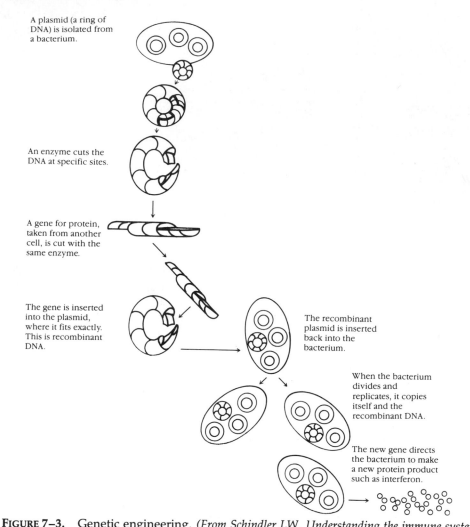

A plasmid (a ring of DNA) is isolated from a bacterium.

An enzyme cuts the DNA at specific sites.

A gene for protein, taken from another cell, is cut with the same enzyme.

The gene is inserted into the plasmid, where it fits exactly. This is recombinant DNA.

The recombinant plasmid is inserted back into the bacterium.

When the bacterium divides and replicates, it copies itself and the recombinant DNA.

The new gene directs the bacterium to make a new protein product such as interferon.

FIGURE 7–3.   Genetic engineering. *(From Schindler LW. Understanding the immune system. NIH Publication 90-529. Bethesda, Md.: U.S. Department of Health and Human Services, National Institutes of Health, March 1990, p 32.)*

dality will have in children will become more evident as research continues. Nevertheless, it is clear from early studies that children do not necessarily experience the same therapeutic effects and/or side effects with BRMs as adults.

The pediatric oncology nurse caring for patients receiving BRMs must have a basic understanding of the concepts of immunology, hematopoiesis, and biotherapy. Unlike other cancer treatment modalities (i.e., chemotherapy, radiation, bone marrow transplantation regimens), which have direct cytotoxicity, BRMs possess a variety of biologic actions and may or may not be directly cy-

totoxic. Even in its infancy, BRMs, or biotherapy, is being recognized as the fourth modality for cancer treatment.[10,77]

COLONY-STIMULATING FACTORS
Hematopoietic Cascade

Hematopoiesis is a dynamic process involving the proliferation, differentiation, and maturation of stem cells (found in the bone marrow) into circulating blood cells (red blood cells [RBCs], white blood cells [WBCs], and platelets).[17] The complex set of hierarchical events responsible for this process is known as the *hematopoietic cascade*. All hematopoietic lineages are derived from a small pool of pluripotent stem cells that are uncommitted to any blood cell lineage. These cells have the ability to self-replicate (reproduce stem cells), proliferate, and differentiate (develop into any blood cell lineage). As differentiation proceeds, cells take on the specific cell lineage characteristics and no longer have the capacity for self-renewal.[35] Pluripotent stem cells (the most primitive cells of the bone marrow) can become multipotent progenitors of myeloid or lymphoid lineage. The myeloid progenitor gives rise to the colony-forming unit of granulocytes, erythrocytes, monocytes, and megakaryocytes (CFU-GEMM). The CFU-GEMM leads to the development of colony-forming units (CFUs) of various cell lineages and eventually to precursors. Precursors are the earliest recognizable cells of various blood cell lineages. For example, the proerythroblast is the earliest recognizable cell in erythrocyte, or RBC, lineage. Through the process of differentiation, precursors develop into the functional components of circulating blood, which have a limited life span and must be continually replaced.[19] Alterations in production of blood cells can occur as a result of a crisis (e.g., infection, bleeding), certain disease processes, and certain medical treatments.

Overview

CSFs are naturally occurring cytokines responsible for stimulating and regulating the complex process of hematopoiesis.[29] Each cytokine exerts its influence at a different point in the hematopoietic cascade[31,35,57,76,83,84] (Fig. 7–4). CSFs can exhibit either multilineage (affecting uncommitted precursors) or single lineage (affecting committed precursors) effects. Examples of CSFs having multilineage effects are interleukin-3 (IL-3) and granulocyte-macrophage colony-stimulating factor (GM-CSF). Examples of single-lineage CSFs are granulocyte colony-stimulating factor (G-CSF), macrophage colony-stimulating factor (M-CSF), and erythropoietin (EPO). In addition, many CSFs augment the various functions of mature blood cells. Examples of the vital uses CSFs have in pediatrics include (1) acceleration of hematopoietic reconstitution;

(2) amelioration of the side effect of myelosuppression; (3) reduction in length of hospitalization secondary to fever and neutropenia; and (4) facilitation of aggressive dose-intensive regimens without the need for bone marrow reinfusion.

CSFs play a primary therapeutic role in alleviating the severity of myelosuppression associated with the disease process and/or treatment. This is important since the longer patients are neutropenic with absolute neutrophil counts below 500, the greater is the risk for the development of infection and/or septicemia. CSFs alleviate the severity of neutropenia by shortening the period of myelosuppression and decreasing the depth of the nadir (the point of the lowest neutrophil count). As a result, patients are less susceptible to opportunistic infections. Clinical trials have been aimed at evaluating the effects of CSFs on a variety of disease processes and in conjunction with a variety of treatment modalities.[4,5,7,44,47,52,53,55,132] The CSF dose is titrated (increased, decreased, or discontinued) to maintain the white blood cell count (WBC) and differential or hemoglobin level within a specified range. Therefore children receiving CSFs require frequent monitoring of their blood counts to evaluate the response to CSF therapy. The optimal timing and duration of therapy for the various CSFs to produce the desired effects and the interactions between CSFs have not been clarified. Patients receiving CSFs that affect the production of WBCs usually experience a rapid increase in their WBCs over the first few days after beginning CSF therapy. After a few days, they experience a decrease or stabilization of their blood counts. After cessation of CSF therapy, the WBCs return to baseline in 4 to 7 days.[106]

With the change in how new BRMs are named, many of the newer CSFs are also known as interleukins. Those interleukins that act as hematopoietic CSFs are discussed in this section.

Interleukin-3. Naturally occurring IL-3 is produced primarily by T lymphocytes.[64] The gene for this complex glycoprotein is located on chromosome 5q23-31. IL-3 has multilineage effects. It is capable of supporting the formation of various types of single and mul-

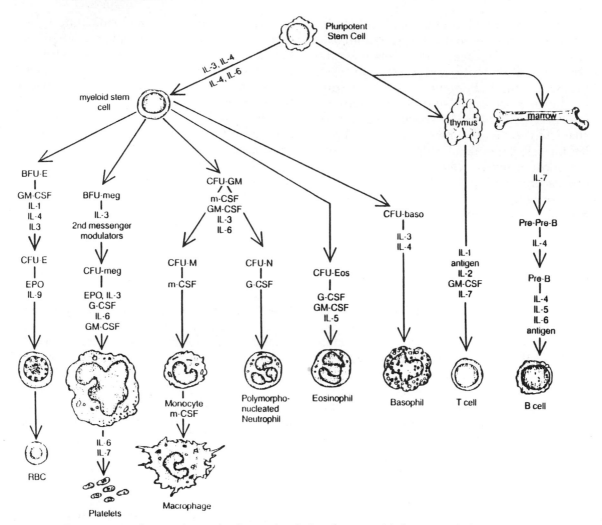

FIGURE 7–4.   Interactions of colony-stimulating factors with hematopoietic precursors. *(From Delmonte L. Demystifying blood growth factors. Oncology Times 1990; 12:11.)*

tilineage colonies (Table 7–1). Since it is capable of stimulating multipotential hematopoietic stem cells to differentiate, it has often been called multi-CSF. IL-3 can counteract the myelosuppressive effects of radiation and chemotherapy, thereby reducing the incidence of infection, perhaps to a greater extent than GM-CSF or G-CSF.[124,134] Early clinical results suggest IL-3 may also enhance the acceleration of platelet reconstitution.

Thus far, clinical trials using IL-3 have focused on adult patients with bone marrow failure (e.g., with aplastic anemia) and malignancies. There have been attempts to stimulate hematopoiesis in children with aplastic anemia and myelodysplastic syndrome. Ad-

ditionally, in the pediatric setting increasing numbers of dose-intensive protocols incorporate myeloablative chemotherapy or radiation therapy or both for the treatment of high-risk or resistant childhood cancers. Children treated with these regimens may benefit from the administration of IL-3 during the recovery period to reduce the degree and duration of neutropenia.

Potential side effects of IL-3 include fever, flulike symptoms, including malaise and myalgias, swelling of the face and extremities, mild splenomegaly, a pruritic papular rash, and injection site inflammation. Headaches have been a dose-limiting toxicity associated with IL-3 administration. Eosinophilia and

TABLE 7–1. *Human Hematopoietic Colony-Stimulating Factors (CSFs)*

FACTOR	CHROMOSOME	CELLULAR SOURCE	TARGET CELL	ACTION
IL-3 (multi-lineage)	5q23–31	T cells	CFU-GEMM CFU-GM BFU-E CFU-MEG CFU-EO Monocytes	Stimulates early growth of granulocyte, monocyte, erythroid, and megakaryo-cyte precursors Supports mast cell growth
GM-CSF (multi-lineage)	5q23–32	T cells Endothelial cells Fibroblasts	CFU-GEMM CFU-GM BFU-E Granulocytes Monocytes	Stimulates granulocyte, macrophage, eo-sinophil, and early erythroid precur-sors Activates mature granulocytes and monocytes Enhances antibody-dependent, cell-mediated cytotoxicity
G-CSF (single lineage)	17q11.2–21	Monocytes Fibroblasts	CFU-G Granulocytes	Stimulates mature granulocyte precursors Activates mature granulocytes Increases antibody-dependent, neutro-phil-mediated cytotoxicity
M-CSF (single lineage)	5q33.1	Monocytes Fibroblasts	CFU-M Monocytes Endothelial cells	Stimulates macrophage precursors and macrophage colonies Activates mature monocyte Enhances antibody-dependent, mono-cyte-mediated cytotoxicity
EPO (single lineage)	7q11–22	Renal cells	BFU-E CFU-E	Stimulates proliferation and maturation of erythroid precursors Increases red blood cell production

Data from references 6, 7, 17, 29, 47, 52, 57, 83, and 84.
CFU = colony-forming unit; BFU = burst-forming unit; GEMM = granulocyte, erythroid, macrophage, megakaryocyte; GM = granulocyte, macrophage; G = granulocyte; M = macrophage; E = erythroid; EO = eosinophil; EPO = erythro-poietin; Meg = megakaryocyte.

basophilia can also occur and may lead to a rise in plasma histamine.[46,74] Nursing obser-vation and documentation during clinical trials will result in a more comprehensive de-scription of side effects and nursing interven-tions appropriate for pediatric patients re-ceiving IL-3.

Granulocyte-Macrophage Colony-Stimulat-ing Factor. GM-CSF is the cytokine re-sponsible for regulating the production of granulocytes, monocytes, and eosinophils. This glycoprotein is produced by T cells, endothelial cells, and fibroblasts. The gene for this cytokine is located on chromosome 5q23-32[8,13,17,33] (see Table 7–1). GM-CSF has multilineage effects because it stimulates the proliferation, differentiation, and maturation

of granulocytes, monocytes, and eosinophils. Its other biologic activities include inducing mature neutrophils and monocytes to in-crease phagocytosis, augmenting antibody-dependent cellular cytotoxicity (ADCC), in-creasing tumorcidal killing, stimulating other cytokine production, and enhancing mono-cyte tumor necrosis factor (TNF).

Since 1987 when recombinant GM-CSF first became available, multiple studies have been conducted in a variety of disease pro-cesses.[4,5] Initial human trials validated obser-vations from animal trials that GM-CSF in-creased neutrophils, monocytes, and eosin-ophils, which return to baseline with discontinuation of therapy. GM-CSF de-creases the duration of myelosuppression af-ter chemotherapy and accelerates hematopoietic reconstitution after bone marrow transplantation.

GM-CSF has been administered by a variety of routes (subcutaneously and intravenously by continuous infusion or bolus) and in various dosages. The maximal tolerated dose (MTD) varies slightly according to the recombinant preparation used. Subcutaneous doses as low as 5 μg/kg/day stimulate bone marrow reconstitution. The side effects observed clinically with low-dose administration include a flulike syndrome (or constitutional symptoms), low-grade fever, chills, fatigue, myalgia, bone pain, nausea, anorexia, rash, and occasional thrombocytopenia.[12,33,78,106] Erythema at the injection site has been noted in patients receiving subcutaneous administration. Serious side effects observed with high doses of GM-CSF include fluid retention, pleural effusions, and capillary leak syndrome (i.e., a fluid shift caused by increased vascular permeability).[33] Eosinophilia has been observed. The potential long-term effects need further exploration. An event associated with GM-CSF, known as the *first-dose phenomenon,* has been identified. It is characterized by facial flushing, the urge to defecate, changes in blood pressure, dyspnea, and transient oxygen desaturation.[80] This reaction generally occurs on the first day of administration and can occur on subsequent cycles, even if the patient has not had a previous reaction. Patients should be monitored for approximately 2 hours after administration. Vital signs are generally taken at baseline, 15 minutes, 1 hour, and 2 hours after subcutaneous administration. This phenomenon has been observed in adults and to a lesser extent in the pediatric population. It demonstrates the importance of nursing assessment and careful, thorough documentation of side effects (observed and patient reported) and interventions. With Food and Drug Administration (FDA) approval in 1991, GM-CSF has become more widely available in the clinical setting.

Granulocyte Colony-Stimulating Factor.
This cytokine is responsible for regulating the production of granulocytes. The G-CSF gene is located on chromosome 17q11.2-21 (see Table 7–1). G-CSF is considered lineage specific because it stimulates the late proliferation and differentiation of progenitor cells committed to granulocyte lineage. In addition, it increases neutrophil phagocytosis and enhances the activity of erythropoietin. Recombinant forms are available for clinical trials. The first clinical trials were designed to evaluate the ability of G-CSF to accelerate neutrophil recovery after chemotherapy.[76] Children who received subcutaneous administration of G-CSF experienced fewer episodes of fever and neutropenia, a shortened nadir period, and fewer treatment delays caused by myelosuppression. Results of clinical trials indicate G-CSF is better tolerated than GM-CSF, with medullary bone pain (a dull transient ache) the only consistent side effect. Unlike GM-CSF, a dose-limiting toxicity was not reached with G-CSF.[45] Subcutaneous doses range from 3 to 20 μg/kg/day. G-CSF received FDA approval for the treatment of myelosuppression in 1991.[74,139]

Macrophage Colony-Stimulating Factor.
The cytokine that regulates the production of macrophages is M-CSF. The gene for this glycoprotein is located on chromosome 5q33.1. M-CSF is lineage specific because it stimulates the proliferation and differentiation of progenitor cells committed to the macrophage lineage (see Table 7–1). In addition, M-CSF activates mature macrophages and augments host defenses by enhancing the antimicrobial-tumoricidal properties of macrophages. This factor has been the most difficult of all the CSFs to synthesize to date, but recombinant preparations are now available. In one animal trial the administration of M-CSF after pretreatment with chemotherapy induced hematopoietic progenitor cells to enter the cell cycle, resulting in an increased number of progenitor cells in the marrow and the spleen. In another animal study a continuous infusion of M-CSF for 14 days resulted in an increase in monocytes.[61]

The potential use in human trials is less clear with M-CSF than with the other CSFs. Enhanced tumor infiltration by macrophages stimulated with M-CSF is one of many interesting areas being researched. Clinical trials using recombinant M-CSF in adults and children have only recently been initiated and therefore are limited.

Erythropoietin. EPO was first identified more than 30 years ago as an important regulatory factor in erythropoiesis (the development of erythrocytes). The gene for EPO is located on chromosome 7q11-22 (see Table 7–1). This factor is produced primarily by the kidneys in response to the amount of oxygen available to the tissues and renal cells. Therefore increased EPO levels are produced in the presence of anemia or tissue hypoxia. EPO induces RBC production by stimulating proliferation, differentiation, and maturation of erythroid progenitors. However, the proliferation of immature progenitors into mature erythrocytes requires the presence of EPO plus IL-3 and GM-CSF. EPO is the most lineage restricted of all the hematopoietic CSFs identified to date.[38,83,84]

Successful cloning and expression have resulted in adequate supplies for clinical trials. EPO was the first hematopoietic growth factor used clinically. Initial trials with recombinant EPO were conducted in a group of patients with anemia and in another group with end-stage renal disease who required hemodialysis and frequent transfusions. Results of these studies demonstrated that erythropoiesis was stimulated by EPO and patients' transfusion requirements were minimized or eliminated after as little as 1 week of EPO therapy.[39]

Clinical trials have been conducted that studied children with human immunodeficiency virus (HIV) who were anemic secondary to treatment with zidovudine (AZT). Clinical use of EPO for this indication alleviated the distressing side effects related to anemia, thus increasing tolerance to therapy with zidovudine.

Others. Several other hematopoietic CSFs have been identified. They include interleukin-1 (IL-1), or hematopoietin, which is involved in the early differentiation of hematopoietic pluripotent stem cells, interleukin-5 (IL-5), which plays a role in eosinophil differentiation, and interleukin-6 (IL-6), or thrombopoietin, which is involved in the production of platelets. It is too early to ascertain what role, if any, these factors will play in cancer therapy.

Clinical Applications

CSFs are being used increasingly as an adjunct to cancer and HIV treatments. It is anticipated that the use of CSFs alone and in combination is likely to increase over the next few years. The optimal timing of administration to produce the desired outcome will be identified and refined as a result of ongoing clinical investigations.

Adjunct to Intensive Chemotherapy. Most of the CSFs currently under investigation in children are used in conjunction with chemotherapy. For example, one of the most challenging problems of treating aggressive cancers such as Burkitt's lymphoma is the ability to give chemotherapy in rapid pulses. The intensive chemotherapeutic regimens often result in prolonged neutropenia, leading to delays between cycles of therapy. With the addition of CSFs such as GM-CSF, the time planned between cycles can be maintained as designed by decreasing the period of aplasia. This may lead to more effective therapy and increase the long-term survival time of children diagnosed with aggressive lymphomas and other cancers.

Adjunct to Bone Marrow Transplantation
PERIPHERAL STEM CELL HARVEST. One of the difficulties encountered in autologous bone marrow transplantation (BMT) is obtaining adequate stem cells. Until recently the only way to obtain stem cells was from multiple bone marrow aspirations with the patient under general anesthesia (harvesting). Children with aggressive hematologic malignancies were often at risk of relapsing before harvesting or during the time between the harvesting procedure and the start of the preconditioning regimen. With the advent of peripheral stem cell harvesting, these children often remain in remission during the collection procedure. This procedure involves the administration of chemotherapy followed by

the administration of a CSF such as G-CSF. Once the peripheral WBC count is greater than 1000/mm³, the stem cells can be harvested (see Chapter 6 for details on peripheral stem cell harvesting).[9,79]

POST BONE MARROW REINFUSION. For the last several years BMT centers have used CSFs to accelerate hematopoietic reconstitution and decrease the period of aplasia. In many cases this has led to reduced hospital stays for recipients of bone marrow transplants. Clinical trials have evaluated GM-CSF, G-CSF, and M-CSF after high-dose cytotoxic therapy with autologous BMT. Reports of reduced incidence of bacteremia have encouraged investigators to explore the use of these CSFs in a variety of marrow transplant settings.[9,79]

Adjunct to HIV Management. Many children with HIV infection experience myelosuppression at some point during their disease trajectory. The administration of antiviral therapies such as zidovudine to treat HIV infections often results in neutropenia and anemia, requiring a decrease in dosage or discontinuation of therapy. Clinical trials incorporating a combination of EPO and either GM-CSF or G-CSF have begun in an effort to treat myelosuppression associated with therapy and/or secondary to the disease process itself.[48,87,89]

INTERLEUKINS

The class of cytokines called *interleukins* includes protein molecules that send messages between leukocytes. The many types of interleukins are grouped according to their biologic activities. The nomenclature system that assigns a number to each interleukin was devised by participants at the Sixth International Congress of Immunology in 1986.[10,19] The group decided to name newly discovered substances according to their biologic actions. After establishing the human amino acid sequence, the molecule is given an interleukin number corresponding to the order in which it was identified. Often researchers in different laboratories "discover" the same substance performing different functions in separate experiments at the same time. When the amino acid sequence is unveiled, the researchers can then determine if the substance truly is a newly identified cytokine. If the unique properties of a substance are confirmed, another numbered interleukin is added to the list.

Although all of the substances assigned to the growing list of interleukins may not directly affect cancer cells, their activities as cytokines may indirectly assist in cancer therapy. The interleukins are produced by and regulate many cell types. Each has a specific function within the immune system. Ongoing clinical trials and in vitro research have yet to determine the way these immunoregulators can best be used as adjuvants in pediatric cancer therapy. The administration of interleukins has as its goal the enhancement of the body's natural immune system.

Interleukin-1

Researchers originally discovered the cytokine known as *interleukin-1 (IL-1)* in the 1940s when it was named *endogenous pyrogen*. Since that time numerous sources and functions of the IL-1 molecule have been identified. It is also known as *lymphocyte-activating factor (LAF)*, *hemopoietin-1*, and *mononuclear cell factor (MCF)*. Although nearly all cell types can produce it, monocytes and macrophages are generally considered the most important sources of IL-1.[121]

IL-1 is involved in almost all regulatory aspects of the immune response. The ability of IL-1 to activate T cells directly implicates this substance in stimulating the events of the cytokine cascade, a chain reaction beginning with the stimulation of the immune system by a foreign antigen and concluding with the intricate network of activities known as the *humoral* and *cellular immune responses* (see Fig. 7–1).

Laboratory studies in animals have revealed therapeutic uses for IL-1. IL-1 can protect normal cells against the effects of radiation.[92] It can stimulate recovery of bone marrow after myelosuppression caused by chemotherapy and radiation.[41,90] Its ability to stimulate platelet production and differentiation in thrombocytopenic patients has been demonstrated in the clinical setting, but further research is needed to determine its benefit in treatment schemas. Side effects reported in preliminary trials include fever with chills or rigors, tachycardia, hypertension, headache, and mild myalgias. These symptoms resolve shortly after completion of the infusion.[125]

Interleukin-2

The cytokine now known as *interleukin-2* *(IL-2)* was originally known as T-cell growth factor when it was identified in 1976.[118] Researchers have validated its potential as a potent immunotherapeutic agent. Since 1983 when the DNA sequence of the gene coding for IL-2 was established, researchers have had access to a large supply of IL-2 produced by recombinant gene technology.[21] Studies have shown that the presence of IL-2 stimulates cells known as lymphokine-activated killer (LAK) cells to lyse fresh tumor cells while sparing normal cells.[110] LAK cells may proliferate in the lungs, liver, spleen, kidneys, and mesenteric lymph nodes.[21] Controlling this proliferation is the goal of incorporating IL-2 into cancer therapy.

The regression of certain experimental tumors in animals in the presence of IL-2 has paved the way for use of this substance in clinical trials. The first human studies involved metastatic malignant melanoma and renal cell carcinoma. Treatment with IL-2 depends on its potential to promote direct cell-mediated destruction of tumor cells and to mobilize cells capable of destroying neoplasms.[15] These cells include LAK cells, activated natural killer (NK) cells, tumor-infiltrating lymphocytes (TILs), and certain T and B cells. TILs and LAK cells are used in the technique of adoptive cellular therapy, which relies on IL-2 to stimulate certain immune system cells in the laboratory; then the cells are readministered to cause tumor regression in the host organism.[127] IL-2 enhances the cytotoxic activity of NK cells against solid tumors such as neuroblastoma and rhabdomyosarcoma in children.[3] Researchers have begun to use information about dosage and scheduling to combine IL-2 with other recombinant cytokines to optimize antitumor immunotherapy.

IL-2 has been incorporated into therapeutic regimens with chemotherapeutic agents such as cyclophosphamide, dimethyl triazenol imidazole carboxamide (DTIC) and 5-fluorouracil (5-FU). Studies have used IL-2 with other biologic agents, including interferon, MoAbs, TNF, and adoptive cells such as LAK cells and TILs.[21,82,93,110] Further research with these combinations is necessary to identify their clinical use in anticancer therapy.

IL-2 has been implicated in augmenting the graft-versus-leukemia (GVL) effect (activity of infused T cells against leukemia) in autologous BMT. Clinical investigators suggest that the administration of IL-2–activated bone marrow followed by therapy with IL-2 in the immediate post-transplant period will optimize the GVL response by stimulating the T cells administered with the infused marrow against residual leukemia cells.[22]

The clinical use of IL-2 in pediatrics is emerging. Treatment designs designate administration of IL-2 by intravenous bolus or continuous infusion, subcutaneous injection, intrahepatic infusion, or intraperitoneal infusion.[66] The child receiving IL-2 must have a thorough pretreatment examination since IL-2 affects many body organs. Documented toxicities in children receiving low-dose IL-2 therapy (1×10^6 U/m^2 three times weekly for 3 weeks) included fever, nausea, vomiting, and mild hypotension. Toxicity with higher dose therapy (3×10^6 U/m^2 three times weekly for 3 weeks) was more severe, including fluid retention, significant hypotension, increased creatinine, oliguria, and elevated liver enzymes.[96] Most toxicities of IL-2 are dose related and reversible. Peripheral edema is treated by administering diuretics. Although the classic flulike syndrome usually resolves after the IL-2 is discontinued, associated myalgias, malaise, and anorexia can last for several weeks.

The results of pediatric clinical trials have shown that IL-2 has the lowest response rate in children who have been heavily pretreated with intensive high-dose chemotherapy such as those who have had unsuccessful treatment with multidrug regimens. However, children who have not been affected by the toxicities of multiple antineoplastic agents may be able to tolerate a more aggressive dose schedule of IL-2 and receive the full benefit of this biologic response modifier without eliciting early multisystem toxicities. In addition, when administered to children with a small tumor burden, IL-2 elicits the best response because of the desirable effector-to-target ratio (i.e., a large amount of IL-2–activated cells [effectors] compared to a small number of tumor cells [targets]).[96]

Interleukin-3

Interleukin-3 (IL-3) is a hematopoietic CSF widely known as *multi-CSF*. Refer to the section on CSFs for further detail.

Interleukin-4

Interleukin-4 (IL-4) was first named *B cell growth factor-1 (BCF-1)*. It later emerged as T-cell growth factor-2 *(TCGF-2)*. The function of IL-4 is to enhance the cytotoxic activity of activated B and T cells. This capability enables it to play a role in the body's fight against mutated cells. IL-4 has the potential to initiate activity in any TIL, which can infiltrate tumor cells and cause cell lysis under the appropriate immunologic conditions.[10,100]

Interleukin-5

IL-5 primarily regulates the differentiation of eosinophils. As a cytokine, its importance as an adjuvant to chemotherapy has not been described. However, levels of IL-5 may be increased by certain tumors in which eosinophilia is a clinical finding. In addition, IL-5 is associated with the presence of IL-2 receptors on activated B cells, but the significance of this association is still not clear.[19,121,123,129]

Interleukin-6

The discovery of IL-6 was made by several separate research teams investigating various immunologic functions. It has been named *B-cell differentiating factor (BCDF), beta-2 interferon (INFb2), plasmacytoma growth factor, hybridoma growth factor (HGF), hepatocyte-stimulating factor (HSF),* and *T-activating factor (TAF).*[10] IL-6 is similar to IL-1 in its ability to

regulate the immune response of nonimmune cells. Its role in cancer therapy is in stimulating the pluripotent hematopoietic stem cell. It can also promote killer T-cell production.[121,129] Studies suggest that IL-6 plays an important, yet unclear, role in megakaryocytopoiesis, the production of platelets.[68]

Interleukin-7

Extensive investigation into the regulation and differentiation of events governing hematopoiesis in bone marrow led to the identification of the factor supporting the proliferation of precursor B cells.[98] The substance, now known as *interleukin-7 (IL-7)* and also called *lymphopoietin-1*, is secreted by cells in the spleen, thymus, and kidney.[94,95] Subsequent studies indicate that IL-7 also regulates cytotoxic T lymphocytes (CTL) and LAK cells.[2,50,91,122] Much has yet to be learned about IL-7, its interactions with other cytokines, and its potential therapeutic applications.

The significance of IL-1, IL-4, IL-5, IL-6, IL-7, and other emerging interleukins and their place in pediatric cancer therapy will become more evident as research results become available.

TUMOR NECROSIS FACTOR

In the late nineteenth century William Coley,[30] a New York surgeon, began researching the necrosis and regression of tumors in patients with concurrent bacterial infections. His treatment with a conglomeration of bacterial cultures, known as *Coley's mixed toxin*, was widely used as the sole mode of systemic cancer therapy through the early 1900s.[10] Interest in pursuing this research treatment abated as radiotherapy and chemotherapeutic agents emerged.

In the 1970s interest in the antitumor activity of endotoxin preparations was once again sparked. Researchers found that a protein serum factor was produced in response to the presence of lipopolysaccharide present in the cell walls of gram-negative bacteria.[117] Hemorrhagic necrosis of tumors was induced by this protein, hence the name *tumor necrosis factor (TNF).*

Purification and cloning techniques have isolated two specific proteins: TNF, which is derived mainly from macrophages, and lymphotoxin (LT), also called *TNF-β*, which is derived from activated lymphocytes.[135] Although the production of each arises from a response to a different stimulus, they share the same receptor site on the surface of tumor cell membranes and can cause tumor necrosis when they can bind to this site.[101]

The antitumor activity of TNF occurs in several ways. TNF exerts direct cytotoxicity by disrupting the vascular endothelium of the cancer cell, resulting in hemorrhagic necrosis. Indirectly, TNF blocks tumor blood vessels, promotes inflammatory response in the host, and stimulates cytotoxicity of macrophages and tumor-specific antibodies.[10]

Researchers have determined that not all human tumor cells are receptive to TNF. However, since TNF acts selectively, its toxicity to most normal cells is less than to those recognized as foreign.[120] Pharmacokinetically, TNF is cell cycle specific, effectively arresting cells in the G_2 phase of the cell cycle. TNF acts synergistically with other cytokines and chemotherapy. For these reasons, TNF has a potential role in multimodal treatment regimens.[103]

In adult and pediatric clinical trials patients have received TNF in various dosage and administration schedules. TNF is administered intravenously, intramuscularly, or subcutaneously.[120] Patients commonly experience fever and chills and occasionally fatigue, anorexia, nausea, and vomiting. Dose-limiting toxicities include pronounced thrombocytopenia, leukopenia, hypotension, and hepatotoxicity.[32]

Clinical responses in studies using TNF alone have been minimal. There have been significant toxicities at high dosages, with limited tumor regression.[121] The antitumor activity of this agent remains under investigation in adult and pediatric clinical trials. Synergistic cytotoxicity has been reported when TNF has been administered in combination with interferon-γ. This may be related to the ability of interferon to increase the number of TNF receptors on the cell membrane, making the tumor cell more susceptible to the cytotoxic effects of TNF.[32] Chemotherapeutic agents such as doxorubicin, actinomycin D, or cyclophosphamide can be administered sequentially with TNF to augment the activity of this protein by advantageously using the known effects of such antineoplastic agents on the cell cycle.[135,136] IL-2 and interferon are two biologic agents that have been administered with TNF to augment its cytotoxic activity against cancer cells.[117,120,135]

MONOCLONAL ANTIBODIES

The Nobel Prize–winning introduction of hybridoma technology by Kohler and Milstein[72] in 1975 resulted in the development of highly specific agents called *monoclonal antibodies (MoAbs)* (see Fig. 7–2). This technique involves injecting a target antigen into a mouse, which then makes an antibody to the injected antigen. Antibody-secreting B lymphocytes from the mouse's spleen are removed and placed in a culture with a single strain of immortal cancer cells. The B lymphocytes and cancer cells, including their nuclei, fuse to form a hybridoma, which shares the genetic information of both the B lymphocytes and the cancer cell. The immortal hybridoma can produce a perpetual supply of cancer-specific antibody, the MoAb.[43] The MoAb produced is specific for a target antigen, usually a glycoprotein, expressed on the surface of a particular type of cancer cell.[89] Thus researchers have mimicked the immune system's response to foreign substances, resulting in antigen-antibody complex formation, by applying this lock-and-key concept to cancer-targeted interventions with anticancer MoAbs.

Target-specific MoAbs are used to detect the presence of tumors. Using a sample of a patient's blood, an oncologist can more specifically test for the presence of tumors that have specific antigen markers or secrete identifiable antigens. Small amounts of tumor-associated antigen such as carcinoembryonic antigen (CEA) can be identified using MoAbs in laboratory immunoassays.[107]

The first cancer-specific MoAbs were developed to detect certain lymphocytic leukemia cells, melanoma cells, and lymphoma cells. Of special interest in pediatrics is the MoAb 3F8, which recognizes ganglioside GD2 expressed on neuroblastoma cells.[25,138]

The GD2 antigen is selectively expressed on some brain tumors, melanoma, and some osteogenic sarcoma cells, making them targets for 3F8 as well.[59] Ideally, MoAbs can be developed for many more cancer types.

Researchers have been able to couple MoAbs with radioisotopes such as iodine 131 and indium 111 and the lower-energy radionuclides iodine 123 and technetium 99.[16] These radioimmunoconjugates, which combine a MoAb with a radioisotope, have greatly enhanced the diagnostic capabilities of MoAbs. Radioimaging techniques, using total body gamma scan or single photon emission computed tomography (SPECT), can detect tumors in primary and metastatic sites marked by an injected radioimmunoconjugate, which may not be detected by other currently available means. The diagnostic workup is thus more thorough and allows monitoring of disease sites more accurately during and after therapy. Researchers in Japan and the United States have reported using this technique with iodine 131–labeled antibody during the diagnosis, treatment, and follow-up in children with neuroblastoma.[27,40,86]

The effectiveness of MoAbs as single agents in treatment plans has not generally been impressive.[103] Through the process of opsinization (making bacteria and tumor cells susceptible to phagocytosis), MoAbs are capable of activating complement and stimulating ADCC.[20,93] Although some tumor regression may occur, larger tumor burdens are not significantly affected by this process.[103]

To overcome this limitation in treatment, researchers have linked MoAbs to chemotherapy (chemoimmunoconjugates); radioactive particles, including iodine preparations (radioimmunoconjugates); cytotoxic agents such as Ricin A (immunotoxins), or other biologic agents. Treatment with immunoconjugates potentially allows the accurate administration of toxins, radiation, or antineoplastic agents to the sites of disease while limiting the destruction of surrounding tissue.[20,27,51,115] This seek-and-destroy concept, whereby the target-specific antibody delivers a lethal agent to the cancer cell, brings to life Paul Ehrlich's image of MoAbs as "magic bullets."[62] Clinical trials using radiolabeled MoAb 3F8 in children

with chemotherapy-resistant or disseminated neuroblastoma are setting the stage for using radioactive, or "hot," target-specific antibodies for other malignancies.[26]

MoAbs are usually administered intravenously through the bloodstream or subcutaneously through the lymphatic system.[137] They have been given intra-arterially through the hepatic artery when used to treat neoplastic liver disease.[107] Research is being conducted using intrathecally administered radiolabeled MoAbs for neural tumors with leptomeningeal disease.[67] In addition, radiolabeled MoAb is used to purge a patient's harvested marrow in some bone marrow transplant protocols, thus diminishing the likelihood of reseeding by affected marrow.[105] The peritoneal route is another area that probably will be studied for these highly specific targeting techniques of therapy. Toxicities of intravenously administered unconjugated MoAb 3F8 observed in clinical trials include pain, hypertension, urticaria, and depletion of serum complement. Adverse side effects can be managed with treatment using analgesics, diuretics, antihypertensives, and antihistamines to alleviate the symptoms as they occur.[24]

Early clinical trials with radiolabeled MoAb 3F8 demonstrated that more than 10 mg/m² of 3F8 antibody can be administered with more than 12 mCi/kg of iodine 131. Although there were minimal acute radiation side effects, prolonged myelosuppression with marked thrombocytopenia was observed.[23] This marrow toxicity has necessitated the incorporation of bone marrow rescue with previously harvested marrow into the design of protocols using treatment with multiple infusions of radiolabeled MoAbs.

Safety issues must be considered when children receive radiolabeled MoAb preparations. The institution's radiation safety department must work with the medical and nursing teams to develop appropriate guidelines to maintain a safe environment. Depending on the type and amount of radioisotope administered, patients may need isolation in a manner similar to those implanted with radioactive sources. The implications when the patient is very young are especially important since parents may need to minimize close contact with their developing child. Using an absorbing shield at the bedside and establishing organized sequences for interactions while the child's level of radio activity is high will decrease the risks of radiation exposure to the family and health care team while providing essential contact and support to the isolated child. The restricted contact is determined by monitoring the radioactivity levels daily. This is done by a member of the radiation safety department. The expected amount of time necessitating isolation varies by treatment protocol and may range from several days to weeks, based on the amount and administration sequence of the isotope. In some cases there may be a period just before administration of a scheduled dose of radioimmunoconjugate when a child's radioactivity is at a safe level; this time may be used to allow the child to "escape" isolation briefly. The nurse and family can determine if this would benefit the child and plan an appropriate activity outside of the isolation room.

The production of human antimouse antibodies (HAMA) in patients treated with murine (mouse) MoAbs appears responsible for most of the reported side effects of MoAb administration. These side effects include hypotension, dyspnea, fever, chills, diarrhea, bronchospasm, tachycardia, and pruritus. Serologically detectable HAMAs in children receiving MoAb therapy signal an increased risk for anaphylaxis in subsequent administrations. Some studies use skin testing or the monitoring of complement levels to predict allergic reactions, but these techniques have not been universally recommended because of their unreliable predictor value.[36]

To bypass the interspecies reactions and reduce the side effects caused by infusing mouse MoAbs, researchers have produced human MoAbs and human-mouse chimeric, or combination, MoAbs. The advantages of using these hybridomas include a diminished risk of sensitization and an increased capability of activating a more appropriate and effective human immune response. New technologies have had varying success in producing new hybrids, and in vivo studies have yet to determine their diagnostic and therapeutic feasibility.[11,116] As these techniques are refined, increased quantities and types of human MoAbs can be developed and tested. The elimination of the hypersensitivity reaction will enable clinicians to use MoAbs for longer periods in therapies without the risk of anaphylactic shock.

INTERFERONS

Interferon was first described in 1957 by Isaacs and Linderman as a single soluble protein with antiviral activity. Since its initial discovery, several types of interferons (alpha, beta, and gamma) and a broad spectrum of properties have been identified (Table 7–2).[42,69,71,112] Interferons (INFs), members of the cytokine network, are part of a complex family of proteins and glycoproteins capable of inhibiting viral replication, modulating immune responses, and altering cellular proliferation; however, the precise mechanism of action is still not clearly understood.

In addition to their antiviral properties, which may play a role in HIV therapy, INFs' antiproliferative and immunomodulatory properties may play a role in cancer therapy.[70] For instance, INFs prolong the cell cycle by delaying the entry of cells into the S phase, thereby increasing the number of cells in the G_0 phase. This is an important phenomenon when considering using the combination of INFs with other treatment modalities to achieve the maximal therapeutic effect. The majority of cells contain two different types of INF cell receptors; however, the number varies from approximately 100 to 1000 receptors per cell. What role, if any, this variation in the number of INF cell receptors plays has not been determined.

Since only minute amounts of INFs are synthesized in the body, extensive clinical trials could not be conducted until 1981 when recombinant forms of interferon (rINF) became available.[102] The goal of phase I, II, and III trials was to define the maximal tolerated dose, optimal schedule, route of administration, and maximal biologic response. The side effects and their intensity were found to vary with each type of INF, the dose, route of administration, and patient factors (e.g., age, clinical condition).[104] However, the majority

TABLE 7–2. *Interferons*

CYTOKINE	CHROMOSOME	CELLULAR SOURCE	ACTION
Interferon alpha (INF-α)	9	T cells B cells Null cells Macrophages Natural killer (NK) cells	Antiviral activity Antiproliferative properties Augments NK cell activity Augments monocyte tumor activity Enhances HLA classes I and II antigen expression Induces MHC class I antigen expression
Interferon beta (INF-β) β1 β2	 9 7	Fibroblasts Macrophages Epithelial cells	Antiproliferative properties Antiviral activity Induces MHC class I antigen expression
Interferon gamma (INF-γ)	12	T cells NK cells	Immunomodulatory properties Antiviral activity Augments NK cell activity Augments expression of Fc receptors Augments ADCC Stimulates monocyte-macrophage function Antibody synthesis Enhances MHC class II expression Stimulates lymphocytes, IL-2, and tumor necrosis factor

Data from references 10, 42, 69, 71, 74, and 99.
MHC = major histocompatibility complex; ADCC = antibody-dependent cellular cytotoxicity; HLA = human leukocyte antigen.

of the side effects (Table 7–3) were manageable and reversible. Chronic side effects associated with INF administration include fatigue and anorexia.

Interferon Alpha

Naturally occuring interferon alpha (INF-α) is derived primarily from leukocytes and is often referred to as a type I interferon. Thus far 20 different subtypes of INF-α have been identified.[49,88,111,119] The genes encoding INF-α are located on the short arm of chromosome 9. INF-α was the first recombinant INF available and is the most widely studied of all the INFs.[28] It has been used to treat a variety of cancers; however, the hematologic malignancies (e.g., hairy cell leukemia) appear the most responsive. Results of clinical trials indicate that INF-α may be more effective in patients with minimal tumor burden than in patients with extensive tumor burden; therefore it may play an active role as adjuvant therapy after the tumor burden is reduced by another treatment modality (e.g., chemotherapy, radiation, surgery). In 1986 INF-α became the first cytokine to receive FDA approval for the treatment of hairy cell leukemia, Kaposi's sarcoma, and condyloma acuminatum.[34] Although the role INF-α will play in pediatric oncology is not yet known, it is currently being studied in a variety of other settings. Clinical trials examining the potential role of INF-α in the treatment of juvenile laryngeal papillomatosis (a benign tumor of the larynx) have been ongoing in the pediatric population, and results are encouraging. INF-α is also being studied as a treatment option for non-A, non-B (type C) hepatitis.[28]

INF-α has been administered by a variety of routes (subcutaneous, intramuscular, intraperitoneal) and in different dosages. The MTD is 5 to 100 × 10⁶ U/m² or 25 to 500 m². The side effects include flulike syndrome (also referred to as constitutional symptoms): fever, chills, fatigue, headache, malaise, nausea, diarrhea, and leukopenia. Fevers associated with INF-α usually peak within 6 hours of administration and resolve within 4 to 8 hours. Although the symptoms may be severe initially, the patient's body adjusts to the INF-α over time. Premedicating the patient with acetaminophen and then remedicating every 4 hours for the first 24 hours benefits many patients. Fatigue, often a dose-limiting side effect, can be minimized by administering INF-α at bedtime.[104]

Interferon Beta

Interferon beta (INF-β; also referred to as a type I interferon) is derived primarily from fibroblasts and epithelial cells.[130] It is similar to INF-α genetically, structurally, and in activity; they also compete for the same cell surface receptor.[20,63,130,140] Two subtypes of INF-β have been identified. The gene encoding INF-β1 is located on chromosome 9, whereas the gene encoding INF-β2 is located on chromosome 7.[54] INF-β2 has also been called B-cell differentiation factor and IL-6. The multiple names for this substance further illustrate the complexities of identifying biologics and BRMs based on their cellular activities and properties. Clinical trials to date are limited and thus far have not demonstrated any superiority of INF-β over INF-α in efficacy. Currently there are no ongoing trials in pediatrics; therefore the unique functions of INF-β and its role(s) in pediatric oncology and HIV treatment have not yet been determined.

Interferon Gamma

Interferon gamma (INF-γ) is produced primarily by T cells and NK cells and is often referred to as a type II interferon.[130] The genes responsible for encoding INF-γ production are located on chromosome 12, and the genes responsible for encoding INF-γ receptors are located on chromosome 21. Although this cytokine has functions similar to those of the other INFs, its immunomodulatory functions apparently are more prominent (see Table 7–2).[14] In vitro and in vivo studies have revealed synergy between INF-γ and several other cytokines (e.g., INF-α, INF-β, TNF,

IL-2) and with chemotherapy and/or radiation.[6,19,28,34,49,113]

The side effects associated with INF-γ are similar to those observed with INF-α. However, more frequent headaches, prolonged fevers, and an increase in liver enzymes and serum triglycerides have also been observed.[104] The role of INF-γ in cancer therapy will probably not be as a cytotoxic agent but as an adjuvant to therapy by modulating host responses, altering cellular structure, and/or inhibiting cellular growth. Results of phase I and II studies exploring the use of INF-γ in the treatment of chronic granulomatous disease have revealed significantly fewer bacterial and fungal infections.[6] This result may indicate a potential role for INF-γ in the management of fever and neutropenia associated with cancer therapy.

SIDE EFFECTS

BRM therapy often results in significant toxicities that can occur acutely or chronically and are generally noncumulative. The side effects associated with each BRM often are influenced by the dose, route of administration, and schedule.[65,106] Additionally, many of the side effects reported from the adult clinical trials have not been found to occur in children to the same degree. As always, it is best to keep in mind that there are differences in the immune systems of adult and pediatric patients, and a thorough assessment of each individual will ensure the identification of unexpected findings. In general, the side effects related to BRM therapy in children do not overlap those associated with chemotherapy and/or radiation and are generally reversible once administration of the agent is stopped.[18] Prolonged, severe fatigue, widely observed as a significant side effect in adult patients treated with BRMs, has not been universally reported or documented in the pediatric population. Recovery from the effect(s) may occur instantaneously or take several weeks. The most unique side effect associated with BRMs, occurring to some degree with almost all BRM therapy, is known as the flulike syndrome. It is characterized by fever, chills, rigors, myalgias, headache, and fatigue.[56,58] The immunologic, hematologic, and endo-

TABLE 7–3. *Side Effects Associated with BRMs*

SIDE EFFECTS	INTERFERONS			INTERLEUKINS	
	ALPHA	BETA	GAMMA	IL-2	IL-3
Flulike Syndrome					
Fever	Common	Common	Common	Common	Common
Chills and rigors	Common	Common	Common	Common	
Myalgias	Common	Common	Common	Common	Rare
Headache	Common	Common	Common	Common	Common
Bone pain					
Cardiopulmonary					
Capillary leak				Common Dose related	
Hypotension		Dose related		Common	
Hypertension					
Dyspnea				Occasional	
Fluid retention				Common	
Facial edema				Occasional to common	Common
Gastrointestinal					
Nausea and vomiting	Occasional			Common	
Diarrhea	Occasional			Common	
Mouth sores				Occasional	
Renal					
Oliguria				Common	
Increase in creatinine				Common	
Neurologic					
Lethargy	Common			Occasional	
Confusion	Occasional			Occasional	
Integumentary					
Erythema			Injection site	Common	
Urticaria				Rare	
Pruritus				Common	
Rash				Common	Common
Anaphylaxis					

Note: Many side effects are dose related and reversible.

crine effects of systemic treatment with BRMs contribute to the appearance of these symptoms. The severity of this syndrome is variable.[140] Edema, resulting from vascular leakage, combined with lymphocytic mobilization and infiltration, compounds the symptoms ascribed to this phenomenon (see Table 7–3).

Nursing Management

The management of the side effects associated with BRMs presents a unique challenge for nursing. Much can be extrapolated from the knowledge about the management of side effects associated with chemotherapy and radiation. These interventions can serve as a

| COLONY-STIMULATING FACTORS | | | | | |
GM-CSF	G-CSF	M-CSF	EPO	MoAb	TNF
Low grade	Low grade		None	Common Various patterns	Common Biphasic pattern
Rare or mild	Rare		None	Common	Common
Common	Rare		Nonc	Arthralgias	Severe
Transient or mild	Rare		None	Rare	Common
Common	Common				
Rare				Common	
Occasional		Occasional		Occasional Occasional	Dose limiting
		Occasional		Occasional Common Common	
Occasional				Occasional	Rare
Occasional				Rare	Rare
At injection site					
				Occasional	
Rare				Common	
					Irritation at in- jection site
				Occasional	

starting point in the management of side effects associated with BRMs; however, they may prove ineffective in dealing with the unique manifestations exhibited by the interactions BRMs have on the patient's immune system. Emphasis should be placed on comprehensive ongoing assessment, including establishment of the child's baseline physiologic and psychologic functioning, daily physical assessment, observation for subtle changes in physical status or behavior, and documentation of observed and patient-reported side effects. Following these criteria will enable nurses to establish trends and devise plans of action for expected clinical situations.

Many of the interventions fall into one of three categories.[81,106] The first includes the implementation of preventive measures such as patient teaching or administration of premedications to prevent allergic reactions or pain. The second incorporates the measures to reduce side effects as they are manifested. This includes correction of fluid or electrolyte imbalances, administering analgesics, antipyretics, or antihistamines, and adjusting therapy administration if allowable. Third, individual strategies must be devised to provide for patient comfort. Although reducing side effects will improve patient comfort in most cases, there are many nonprescriptive ways of manipulating the environment to relax the patient and improve tolerance to therapy. They can range from providing quiet surroundings or an age-appropriate roommate to identifying distracting activities. Two of the most important measures are the ongoing explanation of nursing and medical activities related to the therapy and the emotional support from the primary health care team before, during, and after treatment. For more details about potential nursing diagnoses and nursing interventions for the child receiving BRM therapy, see Table 7–4. Despite becoming more knowledgeable about the acute side effects and their management, further research is needed to identify and refine effective symptom management interventions. In addition, research is needed to determine long-term side effects associated with this therapy and their impact on quality of life.

TABLE 7–4. *Potential Nursing Diagnoses For Patient Receiving Biologic Response Modifiers (BRMS)*

NURSING DIAGNOSIS	EXPECTED OUTCOME	NURSING INTERVENTIONS
General		
Knowledge deficit related to treatment with BRMs	Child and family will verbalize: Purpose of BRM treatment Side effects and complications of treatment Interventions to alleviate side effects.	1. Provide opportunities for and encourage questions. 2. Assess readiness for learning. 3. Assess understanding of illness and plan of treatment. 4. Assess understanding of information frequently; reinforce and repeat instructions as needed. 5. Provide instruction on purpose, side effects, and interventions of BRM therapy. Reinforce with written materials.
Altered family processes related to an ill family member	Child and family will verbalize their feelings, fears and concerns about diagnosis and BRM therapy. Child and family will identify appropriate resources to seek and how to mobilize them.	1. Encourage expression of feelings, fears, and concerns about treatment with BRMs. 2. Assess: a. Prior experience with hospitalization b. Disease trajectory c. Coping abilities and strategies that have been effective in the past d. Available resources. 3. Promote family strengths. 4. Refer for counseling as indicated.
Altered thought processes related to BRM therapy	Child will demonstrate minimal disorientation to person, place, and time.	1. Assess baseline neurologic and mental status. 2. Monitor mental status frequently. Note any changes (e.g., confusion, agitation, anxiety, lethargy). 3. Instruct family about potential mental status changes. Reassure them that changes are

TABLE 7—4. *Potential Nursing Diagnoses For Patient Receiving Biologic Response Modifiers (BRMS)* Continued

NURSING DIAGNOSIS	EXPECTED OUTCOME	NURSING INTERVENTIONS
General *(cont)*		related to treatment and will subside after treatment. 4. Instruct family to report any changes in mental or neurologic status. 5. Orient child to person, place, and time as indicated. 6. Assess potential for harm and initiate appropriate interventions to protect patient from harm.

Integumentary
Impaired skin integrity related to administration of BRMs
	Child will maintain intact skin.
	Child and family will demonstrate proper skin care measures to protect skin integrity.
		1. Inspect skin for color and areas of irritation, redness, breakdown, scaling, moisture.
		2. Skin care measures:
		  a. Provide daily bath or shower using gentle soaps (e.g. Basis) or bath oils (e.g., Alpha Keri, Domol). Aveeno oatmeal bath may be used for pruritus.
		  b. Apply lotions or creams to skin as needed.
		  c. Minimize sun exposure.
		3. Monitor need for medications to relieve itching (e.g., diphenhydramine, hydroxyzine).

Cardiopulmonary Potential for injury related to immune-mediated anaphylaxis secondary to: Murine monoclonal antibody (MoAb) therapy or toxin therapy Adverse or allergic response to biotherapy	Child will tolerate therapy without adverse response. Signs of adverse reaction will be recognized and controlled.	1. Obtain baseline physical assessment, including vital signs. 2. Place oxygen, airway, and emergency medications in appropriate calculated dosages at bedside 3. Premedicate when ordered by physician. 4. Monitor vital signs every 15–30 min during treatment and every 2–4 hr for 24 hr after treatment. 5. Assess peripheral pulses, color of skin and mucous membranes, and mental status. 6. Notify physician if adverse symptoms occur: increase or decrease in blood pressure, heart rate, or respiratory rate, rash, edema, hives, wheezing, chest pain. Interrupt treatment if medication is infusing. 7. Remain with patient until condition has stabilized. 8. Report adverse drug reaction according to institutional or protocol guidelines.
Alteration in fluid volume related to capillary leak syndrome secondary to interleukin-2 administration	Child will maintain normal body fluid and electrolyte balance.	1. Assess respiratory and cardiovascular status before, during, and after therapy. 2. Assess intake and output; monitor IV fluids. 3. Monitor serum electrolytes and blood gas values.

Table continued on following page.

TABLE 7—4. *Potential Nursing Diagnoses For Patient Receiving Biologic Response Modifiers (BRMS)* Continued

NURSING DIAGNOSIS	EXPECTED OUTCOME	NURSING INTERVENTIONS
Cardiopulmonary *(cont)*		
		4. Monitor vital signs for evidence of tachycardia and/or hypotension. 5. Assess for edema; elevate edematous extremities. 6. Weigh patient BID. 7. Measure abdominal girth, head circumference. 8. Administer albumin 5% as ordered for oliguria and/or hypotension if indicated. 9. Ensure safe environment; instruct patient and family to report any dizziness or change in level of consciousness.
Activity intolerance related to orthostatic hypotension secondary to decreased peripheral vascular resistance	Child will tolerate treatment in a safe environment. Child and family will state safety measures to observe during treatment.	1. Monitor orthostatic blood pressure with vital signs every 3–4 hr. 2. Monitor intake and output. 3. Monitor serum electrolyte values. 4. Inform patient and family that dizziness may occur. 5. Provide instructions for minimizing discomfort related to dizziness such as slowly changing from horizontal to vertical position. 6. Ensure safe environment by keeping siderails up when patient is unattended in bed; keep call bell nearby; check patient frequently.
Impaired gas exchange related to pulmonary complications of treatment	Child will maintain normal tissue oxygenation and perfusion.	1. Monitor baseline pulmonary functions. 2. Perform daily assessment of cardiorespiratory status. 3. Monitor for symptoms associated with impaired pulmonary function: dusky color, cyanosis, stridor, dyspnea, cough, adventitious respiratory sounds, use of accessory muscles, nasal flaring. 4. Keep head of bed elevated 30 degrees. 5. Monitor serum oxygenation via blood gas values or pulse oximetry. 6. Monitor hemoglobin and hematocrit values.
Comfort/Pain Alteration in comfort related to flulike syndrome (fever, chills, aches) associated with BRM therapy	Child will tolerate therapy with minimal discomfort.	1. Assess physical parameters; monitor vital signs. 2. Monitor for adequate hydration and nutrition. 3. Observe for fever, chills, aches. 4. Assess ability to perform routine activities of daily living. 5. Assess for causes of fever or discomfort. 6. Administer premedication such as acetaminophen or diphenhydramine if indicated.

TABLE 7–4. *Potential Nursing Diagnoses For Patient Receiving Biologic Response Modifiers (BRMS) Continued*

NURSING DIAGNOSIS	EXPECTED OUTCOME	NURSING INTERVENTIONS
Comfort/Pain *(cont)*		7. Assess for rigors and need for meperidine. 8. Administer antipyretics or prostaglandin inhibitors as ordered for pyrexia. 9. Facilitate comfortable environment. 10. Provide audio or visual distraction; use relaxation techniques. 11. Encourage frequent rest periods. 12. Refer to physical therapy; follow up on recommendations.
Alteration in comfort related to bone pain and headaches secondary to colony-stimulating factor (CSF) therapy	Child will tolerate therapy with minimal discomfort.	1. Assess patient's history of pain; note onset, location, sensation, duration. 2. Obtain baseline vital signs and monitor every 4 hr. 3. Inform patient and family that headaches and/or bone pain are frequent side effects of CSF therapy. 4. Monitor for signs and symptoms of pain. 5. Facilitate comfortable environment. 6. Use distraction, relaxation techniques. 7. Medicate as needed.
Alteration in comfort related to abdominal cramping and pain at tumor sites secondary to MoAb therapy	Child will tolerate therapy with minimal discomfort.	1. Perform pretreatment assessment of pain status and vital signs. 2. Inform patient and family that abdominal cramping and pain around tumor sites may occur with MoAb therapy. 3. Monitor signs and symptoms of pain during and after administration of MoAb. 4. Assess pain when it occurs; note onset, location, duration, sensation. 5. Administer analgesics to alleviate pain. 6. Use relaxation and diversional techniques. 7. Provide comfortable environment. 8. Support patient and family through painful episodes.

RESEARCH ACTIVITIES AND FUTURE DIRECTIONS

True science always stands upon a frontier. It probes at the edges of our knowledge and our ignorance, and we accept its contributions as valuable, its continuation as a necessity. Perceived as a gradual extension of the sphere of knowledge, science is accepted and praised as both our benefactor and our servant.[126]

The emergence of BRMs on the therapeutic horizon has led to the exciting promise of biotherapy as the fourth modality in cancer therapy; as a result, a challenging new frontier awaits the pediatric oncology nurse.

Many BRMs (e.g., IL-2) have demonstrated antitumor activity for a variety of cancers when administered alone. Differences in mechanism of action provide a rationale for combining biotherapies with each other or as adjuvants with cytotoxic regimens. Another rationale for using BRMs in combination therapy is that activity of any one cytokine may induce the emergence of target cell membrane receptor sites or stimulate activity in other cytokines.[19,103] Researchers are now investigating the optimal use and exact role of each BRM in multimodal therapeutic regimens. It is becoming increasingly apparent that biotherapeutic agents exert their greatest effect when used in concert with other cytotoxic modalities. Complimentary activity and synergistic effects are being observed and documented for a growing list of combinations, which are expected to become more complex as the data base expands.

The complex nature of BRM interactions make the determination of the most effective routes of administration, dose levels, and dose scheduling essential.[65] Clinical trials of this decade will be designed to determine whether BRMs alone, in combination with each other, or as adjuvants with other treatment modalities are efficacious in the treatment of pediatric oncologic diseases and their associated side effects. Many combination clinical trials to address these issues are currently being conducted in the pediatric population. Some of the more widely used combinations involve BRMs with other BRMs, BRMs with chemotherapy, and BRM with radiotherapy.[11,97,128,133] The physician data query (PDQ), a computerized data base of clinical trials funded by the National Cancer Institute, is an excellent resource for ascertaining information about active clinical trials using biologics and/or BRMs in cancer treatment. It can be accessed through the toll-free number 1-800-4-CANCER. Current and future research will help to clarify the many interrelated functions and activities of BRMs.

As the excitement of new cancer therapies builds and research in the clinical setting becomes more aggressive, the pediatric oncology nurse's role takes on new dimensions and more responsibilities. The nurse must always consider child and family safety, education, and support; data collection and documentation; and peer education.[108,131] The pediatric oncology nurse must develop an understanding of the components of the immune system and the process of hematopoiesis and an understanding of the intimate interactions of BRMs with each other and with other elements of the immune system. In addition, excellent assessment skills are necessary to recognize the subtle changes that can occur in the patient receiving BRM therapy. The nurse must be aware of the particular side effects most commonly associated with each biologic agent, although many side effects are similar and are experienced in varying degrees for any patient receiving BRM therapy. As new combination therapies are developed, many unexpected side effects can occur.

In addition to the challenges of physical care, the nurse also must recognize the child and family's need for psychosocial support. Often children receiving biologic agents are participating in experimental therapy or clinical trials, which adds another component to the child and family's physical and psychosocial care. Families may have experienced multiple unsuccessful treatment attempts before the use of a BRM. The nurse will be relied on to provide information and reassurance to the child and family, who look to the nurse for answers, guidance, and hope.

Clinical application of protocols using biotherapy beckons nurses to become involved in nursing research. Much has been published to guide nurses who care for adult patients who are enrolled in investigational protocols and/or are receiving BRM therapies. Pediatric oncology nurses are in a unique position to contribute to this body of knowledge from a different perspective. Thorough assessment and documentation before, during, and after the treatment period will enable the collection of important data necessary to develop policies, procedures, and standards of care for the child receiving therapy with BRMs. Patient information (e.g., teaching booklets) for the child and family must be developed for patients receiving BRMs. It is the responsibility of the pediatric oncology nurse to collect, analyze, and disseminate information about experiences with biotherapy to colleagues. The professional nurse who accepts this challenge welcomes the opportunity to contribute to the body of science on this new frontier.

GLOSSARY

adoptive cellular therapy technique of passive immunity whereby immune system cells possessing antitumor capabilities are manipulated in the laboratory and then transferred to the tumor-bearing organism to stimulate tumor regression; LAK cells and TILs are used in adoptive cellular therapy.

antibody-dependent cell-mediated cytotoxicity (ADCC) process by which neutrophils, monocytes, macrophages, and lymphocytes recognize bound antibody on a target cell and kill that cell.

biologic response modifiers (BRMs) naturally occurring or synthesized substances that can enhance, regulate, or restore functions of the immune system.

biotechnology science that uses living specimens to create or modify a substance.

capillary leak syndrome phenomenon of increased vascular permeability; vascular fluid leakage occurs most often in the lungs, liver, spleen, kidney, and thymus.

cell surface receptor site unique structure on the membrane of the cell body where binding can occur.

colony-forming unit (CFU) hematopoietic progenitor cell that has the ability for self-renewal.

colony-stimulating factors (CSFs) family of glycoproteins responsible for stimulating and regulating hematopoiesis.

commitment process by which a hematopoietic stem cell loses the ability for self-renewal and develops the characteristics of a specific blood cell lineage.

cytokines glycoproteins that are produced by a variety of cells; they are responsible for regulation and function of other cells.

cytotoxic T lymphocytes cells that directly attack malignant or infected cells.

erythropoiesis production of red blood cells (erythrocytes).

erythropoietin (EPO) lineage-specific glycoprotein responsible for stimulating the proliferation, differentiation, and maturation of red blood cells (erythrocytes) from committed erythroid precursors.

flulike syndrome (FLS) collection of symptoms, including fever, myalgia, malaise, and anorexia, frequently observed in patients receiving biotherapy; also known as *constitutional symptoms.*

genetic engineering technology that enables scientists to combine gene segments from two separate organisms.

granulocyte colony-stimulating factor (G-CSF) lineage-specific glycoprotein responsible for the production and maturation of white blood cells known as granulocytes or neutrophils from committed precursor cells.

granulocyte-macrophage colony-stimulating factor (GM-CSF) multilineage specific glycoprotein responsible for the proliferation, differentiation, and maturation of granulocytes, monocytes, macrophages, and eosinophils.

hematopoiesis dynamic process involving the proliferation, differentiation, and maturation of blood cells; steps involved in hematopoiesis are referred to as the *hematopoietic cascade.*

hybridoma cell created by fusing a secretory cell with an immortal cancer cell that can indefinitely produce a desired immune system product.

interleukin-3 (IL-3) multilineage-specific glycoprotein, also known as multicolony-stimulating factor (multi-CSF); it stimulates the early proliferation and differentiation of granulocyte, monocyte, erythrocyte, and megakaryocyte precursors.

interleukins cytokines that relay information between leukocytes to modulate their activities.

lymphokine-activated killer (LAK) cells lymphocytes that have been cultured with IL-2 to produce cells with cytolytic capabilities.

lymphokine glycoproteins produced by lymphocytes.

macrophage colony-stimulating factor (M-CSF) lineage-specific glycoprotein responsible for the proliferation, differentiation, and maturation of monocytes and macrophages from committed precursor cells.

myeloablative term that describes agents and treatment modalities that affect bone marrow production; patients receiving myeloablative therapy are profoundly neutropenic for several weeks, often requiring marrow reinfusion for blood cell counts to recover.

myelosuppressive term to describe agents or treatment modalities that have a transient effect on the production of blood cells; a decrease in any or all of the blood cell lines can occur.

natural killer (NK) cells large granular lymphocytes that are not antigen specific and attack cells that appear foreign such as tumor cells and infected cells.

opsinization process whereby foreign substances are coated by antibodies to enhance their recognition and destruction by phagocytic cells.

pluripotent stem cell most primitive cell in the bone marrow that has the potential to self-replicate or differentiate into myeloid or lymphoid cell lineages.

precursor cell most primitive and recognizable cell of a specific blood cell lineage; precursors are cells that are intermediate between pluripotent stem cells and mature blood cells; they are unable to self-replicate but produce mature blood cells through differentiation and maturation.

stem cell gives rise to various precursors of the different blood cell lineages and has the ability to self-replicate and differentiate.

tumor-infiltrating lymphocytes (TILs) lymphoid cells produced in response to stimulation with IL-2 that are capable of infiltrating solid tumors and exerting lytic activity.

REFERENCES

1. Abernathy E. Biological response modifiers: An introductory overview. Oncol Nurs Forum 1987; 14(suppl):13–15.
2. Alderson MR, Sassenfeld HM, Widmer MB. Interleukin-7 enhances cytolytic T lymphocyte generation and induces lymphokine activated killer cells from human peripheral blood. J Exp Med 1990; 172:577–587.
3. Alverado CS, Findley HW, Chan WC. Natural killer cells in children with malignant solid tumors. Effect of recombinant interferon-alpha and interleukin-2 on natural killer cell function against tumor cell lines. Cancer 1989; 63:83–89.
4. Amgen. Colony-stimulating factors: Literature service, vol 1, 1989–1990. Langhorne, Penn.: Adis International, 1990.
5. Amgen. Colony-stimulating factors: Literature service, vol 2, 1991. Langhorne, Penn.: Adis International, 1991.
6. Ammann AJ. Biologic and immunomodulating factors in the treatment of pediatric AIDS. In Pizzo P, Wilfert C (eds): Pediatric AIDS: The Challenge of HIV Infection in Infants, Children and Adolescents. Baltimore: Wilkes, 1990, pp 495–515.
7. Andreeff M, Welte K. Hematopoietic colony-stimulating factors. Semin Oncol 1989; 16:211–229.
8. Antman KS, Griffin JD, Elias A, et al. Effect of recombinant human granulocyte-macrophage colony-stimulating factor on chemotherapy-induced myelosuppression. N Engl J Med 1988; 319:593–598.
9. Aurer I, Ribas A, Gale RP. What is the role of recombinant colony stimulating factors in bone marrow transplantation? Bone Marrow Transplantation 1990; 6:79–87.
10. Balkwill FR. Cytokines in Cancer Therapy. Oxford: Oxford University Press, 1989.
11. Barker E, Mueller BM, Handgretinger R. Effect of a chimeric anti-ganglioside GD2 antibody on cell-mediated lysis of human neuroblastoma cells. Cancer Res 1991; 51:144–149.
12. Betcher DL, Burnham N. Granulocyte-macrophage colony-stimulating factor. J Pediatr Oncol Nurs 1991; 8:134–135.
13. Bonnem EM, Morstyn G. Granulocyte macrophage colony stimulating factor (GM-CSF) current status and future development. Semin Oncol 1988; 15:46–51.
14. Bonnem EM, Oldham RK. Gamma-interferon: Physiology and speculation on its role in medicine. J Biol Response Mod 1987; 6:275–301.
15. Borden EC, Sondel PM. Lymphokines and cytokines as cancer treatment: Immunotherapy realized. Cancer 1990; 65:800–814.
16. Brady LW, Markoe AM, Woo DV. The present and future role of monoclonal antibodies in the management of cancer. Front Radiat Ther Oncol 1990; 24:247–259.
17. Cannistra SA, Griffin JD. Regulation of the production and function of granulocytes and monocytes. Semin Hematol 1988; 25:173–188.
18. Cetus. Immunotherapeutics—A new direction in cancer treatment. In Herberman RB (ed): Cetus Immunoprimer Series, part 2. Emeryville, Calif.: Cetus, 1989.
19. Cetus. Cytokines. In Herberman RB (ed): Cetus Immunoprimer Series, part 3. Emeryville, Calif.: Cetus, 1989.
20. Cetus. Tumor immunology. In Herberman RB (ed): Cetus Immunoprimer Series, part 4. Emeryville, Calif.: Cetus, 1989.
21. Chang AE, Rosenberg SA. Overview of interleukin-2 as an immunotherapeutic agent. Semin Surg Oncol 1989; 5:385–390.
22. Charak BS et al. Induction of graft versus leukemia effect in bone marrow transplantation: Dosage and time schedule dependency of interleukin-2 therapy. Cancer Res 1991; 51:2015–2020.
23. Cheung N-KV. Immunotherapy: Neuroblastoma as a model. Pediatr Clin North Am 1991; 38:425–441.
24. Cheung N-KV, Lazarus H, Miraldi FD. Ganglioside GD2 specific monoclonal antibody 3F8: A phase 1 study in patients with neuroblastoma and malignant melanoma. J Clin Oncol 1987; 5:1430–1440.
25. Cheung N-KV, Saarinen UM, Neeley JE. Monoclonal antibodies to a glycolipid antigen on human neuroblastoma cells. Cancer Res 1985; 45:2642–2649.
26. Cheung N-KV, Landmeier B, Neeley JE. Complete tumor ablation with iodine 131–radiolabeled disialoganglioside GD-2-specific monoclonal antibody against human neuroblastoma xenografted in nude mice. J Natl Cancer Inst 1986; 77:739–745.
27. Cheung N-KV, Neeley JE, Landmeier B. Targeting of ganglioside GD2 monoclonal antibody to neuroblastoma. J Nucl Med 1987; 28:1577–1583.
28. Clark JW, Longo DL. Interferons in cancer therapy. In DeVita VT, Hellman S, Rosenberg SA (eds): Cancer Principles and Practice of Oncology Updates 1987; 1:1–16.

29. Clark SC, Kamen R. The human hematopoietic colony-stimulating factors. Science 1987; 236:1229–1237.

30. Coley WB. The treatment of malignant tumors by repeated inoculations of erysipelas: With report of ten original cases. Am J Med Sci 1893; 105:487.

31. Delmonte L. Demystifying blood growth factors. Oncol Times 1990; 12:11–13.

32. Demetri GD, Spriggs DR, Sherman ML. A phase I trial of recombinant human tumor necrosis factor and interferon-gamma: Effects of combination cytokine administration in vivo. J Clin Oncol 1989; 7:1545–1553.

33. Devereux S, Linch DC. Granulocyte-macrophage colony stimulating factor. Biotherapy 1990; 2:305–313.

34. Deyton L, Walker R, Kovacs J, et al. Reversible cardiac dysfunction associated with interferon alpha therapy in AIDS patients with Kaposi's sarcoma. N Engl J Med 1989; 321:1246–1249.

35. DiJulio J. Hematopoiesis: An overview. Oncol Nurs Forum 1991; 18(suppl):3–6.

36. Dillman RO, Beauregard JC, Halpern SE. Toxicities and side effects associated with intravenous infusions of murine monoclonal antibodies. J Biol Response Mod 1986; 5:73–84.

37. Emery AELH. Recombinant DNA technology. Lancet 1981; 19:1406–1409.

38. Eridani S. Erythropoietin. Biotherapy 1990; 2:291–298.

39. Eschbach JW, Egrie JC, Downing MR, et al. Correction of the anemia of end-stage renal disease with recombinant human erythropoietin. N Engl J Med 1987; 316:73.

40. Etoh T, Takahashi H, Maie M. Tumor imaging by antineuroblastoma monoclonal antibody and its application to treatment. Cancer 1988; 62:1282–1286.

41. Fibbe WE, Schaafsma MR, Falkenburg JH. The biological activities of interleukin-1. Blut 1989; 59:147–156.

42. Figlin R. Biotherapy with interferon in solid tumors. Oncol Nurs Forum 1987;14(suppl):23–26.

43. Foon KA. Monoclonal Antibodies in the Diagnosis and Treatment of Cancer. Seattle: NeoRx, 1989.

44. Gabrilove JL. Colony stimulating factors: Clinical status. In DeVita VT, Hellman S, Rosenberg SA (eds): Biologic Therapy of Cancer. Philadelphia: JB Lippincott, 1991, pp 445–463.

45. Gabrilove JL, Jakubowski F, Scher H, et al. Effect of granulocyte colony stimulating factor on neutropenia and associated morbidity due to chemotherapy for transitional-cell carcinoma of the urothelium. N Engl J Med 1988; 318:1414–1422.

46. Gillio AP, Gasparetto C, Laver J. Effects of interleukin-3 on hematopoietic recovery after 5-fluorouracil or cyclophosphamide treatment of cynomolgus primates. J Clin Invest 1990; 85:1560–1565.

47. Glaspy JA, Amerbsley JM. The promise of colony-stimulating factors in clinical practice. Oncol Nurs Forum 1990; 17(suppl):20–26.

48. Glapsy JA, Golde DW. Clinical trials of myeloid growth factors. Exp Hematol 1990; 18:1137–1141.

49. Goldstein D, Laszio J. The role of interferon in cancer therapy: A current perspective. CA 1988; 38:258–277.

50. Grabstein KH, Namen AE, Shanebeck K. Regulation of T cell proliferation by IL-7. J Immunol 1990; 144:3015–3020.

51. Griener JW, Guadagni F, Naguchi P. Recombinant interferon enhances monoclonal antibody-targeting of carcinoma lesions in vivo. Science 1987; 235:895–898.

52. Griffin D. Clinical applications of colony-stimulating factors. Oncology 1988; 2:15–23.

53. Groopman JE. Colony-stimulating factors: Present status and future applications. Semin Hematol 1988; 25:30–37.

54. Gutterman J. Clinical and biological activity of the interferons in hematologic malignancies. Immunity Cancer 1989; 2:337–348.

55. Haeuber D. Future strategies in the control of myelosuppression: The use of colony-stimulating factors. Oncol Nurs Forum 1991; 18(suppl):16–21.

56. Haeuber D. Recent advances in the management of biotherapy-related side effects: Flu-like syndrome. Oncol Nurs Forum 1989; 16(suppl):35–41.

57. Haeuber D, DiJulio JE. Hematopoietic colony stimulating factors: An overview. Oncol Nurs Forum 1989; 16:247–255.

58. Hahn MB, Jassak P. Nursing management of patients receiving interferon. Semin Oncol Nurs 1988; 4:95–101.

59. Heiner JP, Miraldi F, Kallick S. Localization of GD2-specific monoclonal antibody 3F8 in human osteosarcoma. Cancer Res 1987; 47:5377–5381.

60. Herberman RB. Cancer therapy by biological response modifiers. Clin Physiol Biochem 1987; 5:238–248.

61. Herrmann F, Lindermann A, Mertelsmann R. G-CSF and M-CSF: From molecular biology to clinical application. Biotherapy 1990; 2:315–324.

62. Himmelweit B (ed). The Collected Papers of Paul Ehrlich. Oxford: Pergamon Press, 1975.

63. Hu E, Horning S. Phase I study of recombinant human interferon beta in patients with advanced cancer. J Biol Response Mod 1986; 6:121–129.

64. Ihle JN, Keller J, Henderson L, et al. Procedures for the purification of interleukin-3 to homogeneity. J Immunol 1982; 129:231–235.

65. Irwin MM. Patients receiving biological response modifiers: Overview of nursing care. Oncol Nurs Forum 1987; 14(suppl):32–37.

66. Jassek PF, Stickin LA. Interleukin-2: An overview. Oncol Nurs Forum 1986; 13:17–22.

67. Kemshead JT, Coakham HB, Lashford LS. Clinical experience of iodine-131 monoclonal antibodies in treating neural tumors. In Vaeth JM, Meyer JL (eds): The present and future role of monoclonal antibodies in the management of cancer. Front Radiat Ther Oncol 1990; 24:166–181.

68. Kioke K, Nakahata T, Kubo T. Interleukin-6 enhances murine megakaryocytopoiesis in serum-free culture. Blood 1990; 75:2286–2291.

69. Kirkwood JM, Ernstoff M. Interferons in the treatment of human cancer. J Clin Oncol 1984; 2:336–352.

70. Kirkwood JM, Ernstoff M. Potential applications of the interferons in oncology: Lessons drawn from studies of human melanoma. Semin Oncol 1986; 13:48–56.

71. Known SE. Interferons and interferon inducers in cancer treatment. Semin Oncol 1986; 13:207–217.

72. Kohler G, Milstein C. Continuous cultures of fused cells secreting antibody of predefined specificity. Nature 1975; 256:495–497.

73. Krakoff IH. Cancer chemotherapeutic and biologic agents. CA 1991; 41:264–278.

74. Kurtzberg J, Miller L, Enama M, et al. Treatment

approaches with recombinant cytokines. In Pizzo P, Poplack D (eds): Principles and Practice of Pediatric Oncology, 2nd ed. Philadelphia: JB Lippincott, 1993, pp 371–408.

75. Lange W, Brugger W, Rosenthal R, et al. The role of cytokines in oncology. Int J Cell Cloning 1991; 9:252–273.

76. Laver J, Moore MAS. Clinical use of recombinant human hematopoietic growth factors. J Natl Cancer Inst 1989; 81:1370–1382.

77. Leventhal BG, Wittes RE. Biologic response modifiers. In Research Methods in Clinical Oncology. New York: Raven Press, 1988, pp 171–190.

78. Lieschke GJ, Burgess AW. Granulocyte colony stimulating factor and granulocyte-macrophage colony-stimulating factor (part 1). N Engl J Med 1992; 327:28–35.

79. Lieschke GJ, Burgess AW. Granulocyte colony stimulating factor and granulocyte-macrophage colony-stimulating factor (part 2). N Engl J Med 1992; 327:99–106.

80. Lieschke GH, Ceban J, Morstyn G. Characterization of the clinical effects after the first dose of bacterially synthesized recombinant human granulocyte-macrophage colony-stimulating factors. Blood 1989; 74:2634–2643.

81. Mayer D. Biotherapy: Recent advances and nursing implications. Nurs Clin North Am 1990; 25:291–308.

82. McIntosh JK, Mule JJ, Merino MJ. Synergistic antitumor effects of immunotherapy with recombinant interleukin-2 and recombinant tumor necrosis factor-alpha. Cancer Res 1988; 48:4011–4102.

83. Metcalf D. Hematopoietic growth factors. Lancet 1989; 825–827.

84. Metcalf D, Morstyn G. Colony-stimulating factors: General biology. In DeVita VT, Hellman S, Rosenberg SA (eds): Biologic Therapy of Cancer. Philadelphia: JB Lippincott, 1991, pp 417–444.

85. Mihich E. Future perspectives for biological response modifiers: A viewpoint. Semin Oncol 1986; 13:234–254.

86. Miraldi FD, Nelson AD, Kraly C. Diagnostic imaging of human neuroblastoma with radiolabeled antibody. Radiology 1986; 161:413–418.

87. Mitsuyasu RT. Hematopoietic growth factors in the treatment of patients with HIV infection. Biotherapy 1990; 2:173–181.

88. Mitsuyasu RT. The role of alpha interferon in the biotherapy of hematologic malignancies and AIDS-related Kaposi's sarcoma. Oncol Nurs Forum 1988; 15(suppl):7–12.

89. Moldawer NP, Murray JL. The clinical uses of monoclonal antibodies in cancer research. Cancer Nurs 1985; 8:207–213.

90. Moore MA et al. Cytokine networks involved in the regulation of hematopoietic stem cell proliferation. Ciba Found Symp 1990; 148:43–58.

91. Morrissey P, Goodwin RG, Nordan RP. Recombinant interleukin-7, pre-B cell growth factor, has costimulatory activity on purified mature T cells. J Exp Med 1989; 169:707–716.

92. Morrissey P, Charrier K, Bressler L. The influence of IL-1 treatment on the reconstitution of the hematopoietic and immune systems after sublethal radiation. J Immunol 1988; 140:4204–4210.

93. Munn DH, Cheung N-KV. Interleukin-2 enhancement of monoclonal antibody-mediated cellular cytotoxicity against human melanoma. Cancer Res 1987; 47:6600–6605.

94. Namen AE, Schmierer AE, March CJ, et al. B cell precursor growth promoting activity: Purification and characterization of growth factor on lymphocyte precursors. J Exp Med 1988; 167:988–1002.

95. Namen AE, Lupton S, Hjerrild K, et al. Stimulation of B cell progenitors by cloned murine interleukin-7. Nature 1988; 333:571–573.

96. Nasr S, McKolanis J, Pais R, et al. A phase I study of interleukin-2 in children with cancer and evaluation of clinical and immunologic status during therapy. Cancer 1989; 64:783–788.

97. Nelson BE, Borden EC. Interferons: Biological and clinical effects. Semin Surg Oncol 1989; 5:391–401.

98. O'Garra A. Interleukins and the immune system. Lancet 1989; 1:1003–1005.

99. Oettgen HF, Old LJ. The history of cancer immunotherapy. In DeVita VT, Hellman S, Rosenberg SA (eds): Biologic therapy of cancer. Philadelphia: JB Lippincott, 1991, pp 87–119.

100. Paul WE, Ohara J. B-cell stimulatory factor-1/interleukin-4. Annu Rev Immunol 1987; 5:429–459.

101. Pennica D, Nedwin GE, Hayslick JS, et al. Tumor necrosis factor: Precursor structure, expression, and homology to lymphotoxin. Nature 1984; 312:724–729.

102. Pestka S. The purification and manufacture of human interferons. Sci Am 1983; 249:36–43.

103. Quesada JR. Biological response modifiers in cancer therapy: A review. Tex Med 1989; 85:42–47.

104. Quesada JR, Talpa M, Rios A, et al. Clinical toxicity of interferons in cancer patients: A review. J Clin Oncol 1986; 4:234–243.

105. Reynolds CP, Seeger RG, Vod D, et al. Model system for removing neuroblastoma cells from bone marrow using monoclonal antibodies and magnetic immunobeads. Cancer Res 1986; 46:5882–5886.

106. Rieger PT. Biotherapy. In Otto SE (ed): Oncology Nursing. St. Louis: Mosby–Year Book, 1991, pp 318–348.

107. Rieger PT. Monoclonal antibodies. Am J Nurs 1987; 87:469–471.

108. Rieger PT, Rumsey K. Responding to the educational needs of patients receiving biotherapy. In Carroll-Johnson RM (ed): The Biotherapy of Cancer. Pittsburgh: Oncology Nursing Press, 1992, pp 10–15.

109. Roper M. Biologics and biological response modifers. In Pizzo P, Poplack D (eds): Principles and Practice of Pediatric Oncology. Philadelphia: JB Lippincott, 1989, pp 295–308.

110. Rosenberg SA. The development of new immunotherapies for the treatment of cancer using interleukin-2. Ann Surg 1988; 208:121–135.

111. Roth MS, Foon KA. Alpha interferon treatment of hematologic malignancies. Am J Med 1986; 81:871–882.

112. Roth MS, Foon KA. Biotherapy with interferon in hematologic malignancies. Oncol Nurs Forum 1987; 14(suppl):16–22.

113. Schiller J, Bittner G, Storer B, et al. Synergistic antitumor effects of tumor necrosis factor and γ-interferon on human colon carcinoma cell lines. Cancer Res 1987; 47:2809–2813.

114. Schindler LW. Understanding the immune system. NIH publication 90–529. Bethesda, Md.: U.S. Department of Health and Human Services, National Institutes of Health, March 1990.

115. Schlom J. Basic principles and applications of monoclonal antibodies in the management of carcinomas:

The Richard and Hilda Rosenthal Foundation Award Lecture. Cancer Res 1986; 46:3225–3238.

116. Schook LB (ed). Monoclonal Antibody Production: Techniques and Applications. New York: Marcel Dekker, 1987.

117. Semenzato G. Tumor necrosis factor: A cytokine with multiple biological activities. Br J Cancer 1990; 61:354–361.

118. Smith KA. Interleukin-2: Inception, impact, and implications. Science 1988; 240:1169–1176.

119. Spiegel RJ. The alpha interferons: Clinical overview. Semin Oncol 1987; 14(suppl):1–12.

120. Spriggs DR, Sherman ML, Frei E, et al. Clinical studies with tumor necrosis factor. Ciba Found Symp 1987:206–227.

121. Staren ED, Essner R, Economou JS. Overview of biological response modifiers. Semin Surg Oncol 1989; 5:379–384.

122. Stotter H, Custer MC, Bolton ES, et al. IL-7 induces human lymphokine activated killer cell activity and is regulated by IL-4. J Immunol 1991; 146:150–155.

123. Takatsu K, Kikuchi Y, Takahashi T, et al. Interleukin-5, a T-cell derived B-cell differentiation factor also induces cytotoxic T lymphocytes. Proc Natl Acad Sci U S A 1987; 84:4234–4238.

124. Takaue Y, Kawano Y, Reading CL, et al. The effects of recombinant human G-CSF, GM-CSF, IL-3, and IL-1 alpha on the growth of purified human peripheral blood progenitors. Blood 1990; 76:330–335.

125. Tewari A, Buhles WC, Starnes HF. Preliminary report: Effects of interleukin-1 on platelet counts. Lancet 1990; 336:712–714.

126. Thorton R. Science policy implications of DNA recombinant molecule research. Washington, D.C.: U.S. Government Printing Office, 1977.

127. Topalian SL, Rosenberg SA. Adoptive cellular therapy: Basic principles. In DeVita VT, Hellman S, Rosenberg SA (eds): Biologic Therapy of Cancer. Philadelphia: JB Lippincott, 1991, pp 178–196.

128. Torrisi J, Berg C, Bonnem E, et al. The combined use of interferon and radiotherapy in cancer management. Semin Oncol 1986; 13:78–83.

129. Tosato G, Seamon KB, Goldman ND, et al. Monocyte-derived human B-cell growth factor identified as interferon-2 (BSF-2), IL-6. Science 1987; 239:502–504.

130. Trotta P. Preclinical biology of alpha interferons. Semin Oncol 1986; 13(suppl):3–12.

131. Tsevat JG, Lacasse CL. Understanding the special needs of patients receiving biotherapy: A conceptual model. In Carroll-Johnson RM (ed): The Biotherapy of Cancer. Pittsburgh: Oncology Nursing Press, 1992, pp 5–9.

132. Vadhan-Raj S. Clinical applications of colony-stimulating factors. Oncol Nurs Forum 1989; 16(suppl): 21–26.

133. Wadler S, Schwartz EL. Interferons as modulators of cytotoxic drugs. Mediguide Oncol 1990; 10:1–6.

134. Wagemaker G, Burger H, Van Gils FCJM, et al. Interleukin-3. Biotherapy 1990; 2:337–345.

135. Wanebo HJ. Tumor necrosis factors. Semin Surg Oncol 1989; 5:402–413.

136. Watanabe N, Niitsu Y, Yamauchi N, et al. Synergistic cytotoxicity of recombinant human TNF and various anti-cancer drugs. Immunopharmacol Immunotoxicol 1988; 10:117–127.

137. Woolfenden JM, Larson SM. Radiolabeled monoclonal antibodies for imaging and therapy. In Foon KA, Morgan AC (eds): Monoclonal Antibody Therapy of Human Cancer. Boston: Martinus Nijhoff, 1985.

138. Wu Z-L, Schwartz E, Seeger R, et al. Expression of GD2 ganglioside by primary human neuroblastomas. Cancer Res 1986; 46:440–443.

139. Wujcik D. Overview of colony-stimulating factors: Focus on the neutrophil. In Carroll-Johnson RM (ed): A Case Management Approach to Patients Receiving G-CSF. Pittsburgh: Oncology Nursing Press, 1992, pp 8–13.

140. Yasko JM, Dudjak LA (eds). Biological response modifier therapy: Symptom management. Emeryville, Calif.: Cetus Corporation & Park Row, 1990.

141. Zola H. Monoclonal Antibodies: A Manual of Techniques. Boca Raton, Fla.: CRC Press, 1987.

8

LEUKEMIA IN CHILDREN AND ADOLESCENTS

▪ ACUTE LYMPHOCYTIC LEUKEMIA

Debra Gaddy Cohen

Leukemia is the most common malignancy of children less than 15 years of age. It accounts for approximately 500 deaths annually in these children.[20] Each year there are 40 newly diagnosed cases per million white children and 20 cases per million African-American children.[115] The peak incidence occurs at 4 years of age, with the incidence in males greater than in females (1.3:1). Approximately 2500 new cases occur in the United States each year, and the approximate risk of any white child younger than 15 years of age developing leukemia is one in 2880.[115] Although leukemia is an uncommon disease in childhood, its seriousness and the age of the affected population draw much attention. The survival rates for the major types of childhood leukemia—acute lymphocytic and acute nonlymphocytic—were 4% and 3%, respectively, in the early 1960s. By the 1980s survival rates for acute lymphocytic leukemia (ALL) had risen to 72% and to 25% to 40% for acute myelocytic leukemia (AML).[16,100] Children diagnosed with ALL in 1990 are projected to have a long-term survival rate of 80%.[13] A small subset of children with certain cytogenetic characteristics in their leukemic cells have an expected survival rate as high as 90%.[40,103]

ETIOLOGY

Despite the expenditure of much effort by many investigators, the cause of leukemia remains elusive. The origin of leukemic transformation of cells most likely results from a fundamental alteration in the genetic makeup of a progenitor (stem) cell. All cells that come from the progenitor cell will have the same defect, resulting in a malignant "clone" (cells with common ancestry) of immature (blast) cells. The blasts lack the capacity to differentiate in response to normal hormonal signals and cellular interactions. The blasts divide at a rate similar to or even slower than normal lymphocytes.[110] Agents that can induce leukemia in animal models include viruses, radiation, chemical and drug exposure, familial predisposition, and a variety of chromosomal aberrations. It is possible that any or some combination of these agents could also produce leukemia in children. However, there is no way to determine if and how any of them cause leukemia in a particular child. Certainly a single universal cause of all cases of leukemia is not known.

Infection as a cause for childhood leukemia has drawn much attention since the discovery that viruses were the cause of some animal (feline and bovine) leukemias. More recently some adult malignancies have been closely linked with viruses: adult T-cell leukemia with the retrovirus human T-cell lymphotropic virus type I (HTLV-I), Kaposi's sarcoma with HTLV-III (now called human immunodeficiency virus [HIV]), and hairy cell leukemia with HTLV-II. None of these diseases affect children less than 15 years old except in very rare cases.

Although clusters or outbreaks in children have been interpreted by some as evidence of viral transmission, sophisticated epidemiologic studies have not supported this theory.[73] What appears as case clustering probably reflects either (1) chance occurrence of an unlikely event; (2) exhaustive case finding in suspected areas; (3) post hoc defining of time and space boundaries that accentuate supposed grouping; (4) or environmental exposures. Other data mitigate against an infectious cause for leukemia. Neither children of women with leukemia, their breastfed infants, nor their marital partners have an increased incidence of leukemia.[54]

One notable example of case clustering occurred in Woburn, Massachusetts, where 18 cases of leukemia occurred in a small geographic area between 1979 and 1985. Statisticians from Harvard University in Cambridge, Massachusetts, implicated a water supply contaminated by chemicals from factory water.[52] Investigations continue in an effort to explain this apparent cluster of leukemias.

The evidence for ionizing radiation as a causative agent in leukemia has seemed compelling since March[62] reported in 1944 that leukemia was the cause of death in radiologists 10 times more often than in other physicians. In the 1950s radiation was used for relatively benign childhood disorders such as enlarged thymus, tonsillar hypertrophy, and tinea capitis. It was also used in department stores to determine foot size when shoes were purchased.

Prenatal maternal irradiation has been suggested as a cause of childhood leukemia since 1958, but the data are conflicting.[58,68] A more recent study of in utero exposure to diagnostic x-rays and the development of leukemia in twin sets seems to confirm this association.[41,59] Receiving small doses of irradiation (<300 cGy) over long periods of time, as occurs with diagnostic radiology, has not been shown to increase the risk of developing leukemia.[6]

The question remains whether or not other forms of low-dose irradiation are leukemogenic to children. There is much speculation about the possible relationships between natural background radiation, radon levels in the home, living distance from nuclear installations, and an increased risk of leukemia. It is widely accepted that hematologic cancers result from a single cell that has undergone multiple mutations that are sequential and specific. Constant exposure to low-level radiation could produce some of the mutations that lead to leukemia.[43,45] Research studies continue to explore the relationship between radiation and leukemia.

Electromagnetic field exposure has been studied as a cause of ALL. Two successive case-controlled studies in Denver, Colorado, showed an increased risk for ALL and other cancers among children living near electromagnetic fields.[95,111] However, other studies have not been able to confirm these data.[77] There is evidence supporting an association between leukemia and occupational exposure (e.g., among telegraph, radio, and radar operators, power and telephone linemen) to electromagnetic fields.[93] One study demonstrated a small but significant relationship between prenatal and postnatal electric blanket use and later development of childhood leukemia.[94] This observation warrants further study.

The possible carcinogenic nature of the chemical benzene was identified when several workers who used it occupationally developed leukemia.[107] Other bone-marrow–depressive agents used industrially may also have leukemogenic potential, but they have not yet been clearly identified. In children contact with leukemia-producing chemicals most often occurs during drug therapy. For example, the immunosuppressive drugs associated with organ transplantation (e.g., azathioprine and cyclophosphamide) have been correlated with an increased incidence of leukemia.[47] There is also an increased incidence of leukemia as a second malignancy in patients with Hodgkin's disease.[19,104] Although diethylstilbestrol (DES) has been associated with some cancers, it has not been associated with an increased risk of leukemia.

A genetic basis for leukemia has also been suggested, but it is probably erroneous to think of leukemia as *either* environmental *or* genetic. At the level of the transformation of the single first cancer cell, cancer is always a genetic disease. However, the genetic transformation takes place from a complex interaction of environmental factors and genetic variations.[8,55,108] A new term coined to describe this interaction is *ecogenetics*, which is the study of the genetic variations that occur in response to environmental agents.[70]

Two genetically transmitted diseases, Fanconi's anemia and Bloom syndrome, carry a high risk of leukemia, usually of the myelocytic type.[65,73] Both of these conditions are characterized by chromosomal fragility. The incidence of leukemia in children with Down syndrome (trisomy 21) is 1 in 95, or 10 to 20 times greater than the incidence in normal children.[32,66] The age of onset is bimodal, with peaks occurring in the newborn period and at 3 to 6 years. When fibroblasts (cells that will develop into connective tissue) from children with Down syndrome are exposed to oncogenic viruses in vitro (in a test tube), they undergo leukemic transformation much more readily than fibroblasts from normal children.[32]

Advanced maternal age, even when cases of Down syndrome are excluded, has also been associated with ALL.[37] Numerous studies have attempted to relate other prenatal and perinatal events to an increased risk of leukemia. However, none has been confirmed.

At greatest risk for developing leukemia is an infant whose identical twin has leukemia. Most of these children become ill within weeks or months of the sibling's diagnosis.[67] If one twin develops leukemia before age 5 years, the likelihood of the second twin acquiring the disease is 10% to 20%. The risk then decreases with increasing age. At 6 to 7 years and older, the risk is similar to that for other siblings. Several theories attempt to explain this high concordance rate. They include genetic predisposition, simultaneous exposure to a leukemogenic event either prenatally or postnatally, or migration of malignant cells from one twin to another via placental circulation while in utero.

Nontwin siblings of leukemic children are also more likely (1:720) than other children (1:2880) to develop leukemia. However, many of these cases of siblings come from high-risk families (e.g., those with Fanconi's anemia).

In summary, why any one child has leukemia is rarely known. But an interesting study was recently undertaken with parents of 175 Australian children with leukemia.[60] The question, "What do you feel caused your child's illness?" was asked of each parent. Parents believed that 80% of the cancers were due to environmental agents such as insecticides, chemical exposures, or radiation.

CLINICAL PRESENTATION

Children with leukemia usually have been symptomatic for less than 1 or 2 weeks before diagnosis,[82] although some report symptoms for several weeks or months. The typical clinical presentation of leukemia in children results from bone marrow failure and infiltration of other organs and tissues by leukemic cells. In general, the most common symptoms are pallor, bleeding, fever, and pain.[106]

Anemia resulting from inadequate erythrocyte production is present at diagnosis in most children with leukemia. Often the symptoms of anemia (weakness, lassitude, pallor, and dyspnea) lead parents to seek medical attention.

Symptoms caused by decreased platelet production and the resultant thrombocytopenia are present in approximately 75% of these children.[80] They include petechiae, purpura, and bruising after even minimal trauma. These symptoms are well recognized by the lay public, and many parents fear leukemia whenever they see signs of increased bruising. If the platelet count is below 20,000/mm^3, nasal, oral, and scleral bleeding may be prominent. Hematuria and gastrointestinal (GI) hemorrhage may also occur but are very rare. Central nervous system (CNS) bleeding may occur during thrombocytopenic periods, and the risk is increased if the peripheral white blood count (WBC) is extremely high (>300,000/mm³)[30] This bleeding results from rupture of intracerebral vessels damaged or occluded by leukocyte sludging or by nodules of leukemic cells.

Fever is present at diagnosis in approximately 60% of children with leukemia.[80] Therefore leukemia must be considered in any child with fever of unknown cause. Children with leukemia commonly have fever associated with infection since bone marrow failure results in decreased neutrophil production and increased susceptibility to infection. Rapid growth and destruction of leukemic cells can cause a hypermetabolic state and "tumor fever."

Pain, usually in bones or joints, is another common presenting symptom. It usually results from bone destruction by leukemic infiltration and from pressure exerted by masses of leukemic cells within the medullary space.[80] Other common presenting complaints include anorexia, abdominal pain, and weight loss. These GI symptoms may be due to the proliferation of leukemic cells in the abdominal viscera, liver, and/or spleen. Another relatively common abnormality is lymphadenopathy. The involved organs and other reticuloendothelial tissues (e.g., liver and spleen) become infiltrated by leukemic cells; massive enlargement is associated with a large tumor burden.

Although the peripheral blood count in a child with leukemia may be normal, it usually is not. The leukocyte count can range from less than 1000/mm³ to more than 1 million/mm³. The hemoglobin level can be as low as 2 g/dl and the platelet count as low as 1000/mm³, or either or both may be normal. The lactic dehydrogenase (LDH) level may be increased, and there may be a mild elevation in the serum glutamic oxaloacetic transaminase (SGOT [AST]) and serum glutamic pyruvic transaminase (SGPT [ALT]) levels related to leukemia in the liver. The blood urea nitrogen (BUN) and creatinine levels may also be increased, and results of the coagulation studies (especially in AML) may be abnormal. An elevated uric acid level may occur, indicating increased turnover of the malignant cells.

Death of cells results in release of nucleic acid purines, potassium, and other intracellular elements into the bloodstream. Depending on the level of elevation, emergency treatment may be required to prevent or treat uric acid nephropathy.[25] Results of radiologic studies are usually normal. Some patients may have a mediastinal mass, increased kidney size caused by leukemic infiltration, lytic bone lesions resulting from destruction by lymphoblasts, or leukemic lines at the ends of long bones.[79]

Leukostasis (WBC clumping) as a result of hyperleukocytosis is a medical emergency. Many of these patients have headaches, blurred vision, and respiratory problems resulting from the plugging of capillaries and small vessels and leukemic infiltration in the CNS and lungs; and cerebrovascular accidents associated with hyperleukocytosis have substantial mortality. The metabolic abnormalities hyperkalemia, hypocalcemia, hyperuricemia, and hyperphosphatemia are common when the WBC is greater than 100,000/mm³ and/or there is massive organ infiltration by leukemia cells.

The diagnosis of leukemia can be confirmed only by examination of the bone marrow. The specimen usually reveals hypercellularity with 60% to 100% blast cells, which results in a reduction of healthy cells. Using a three-point grading system, an M_3 marrow indicates more than 25% blasts in the bone marrow and denotes uncontrolled disease (at diagnosis or relapse).[33] An M_2 marrow shows 5% to 25% blasts and indicates partial remission or a preleukemic syndrome. A normal or remission (no active leukemia) marrow specimen has less than 5% blasts and is designated an M_1 marrow. An M_1 marrow must also have representation of all cell series, even though the cellularity may be decreased.

Although the diagnosis of leukemia is relatively easy to make, the differentiation within this diagnostic category is sometimes more difficult. With a variety of cytomorphologic, cytochemical, and immunologic studies, the abnormal cells can be categorized into clinically significant subgroups, including acute lymphocytic or lymphoblastic leukemia (ALL), acute myelocytic leukemia (AML), or chronic myelogenous leukemia

(CML). Since the specific cell type is an important prognostic factor and a determinant of therapy, the identification must be unequivocal. Figure 8–1 shows the cell lineages of the hematopoietic system. Hematopoietic malignancies are identified by the nomenclature of this system.

Mixed lineage, or biphenotypic, leukemia, in which the cells have characteristics of both myeloid and lymphoid lineage, may occur in as many as 20% of children with leukemia.[48] In mixed lineage leukemia the blast cells can each express surface antigens of different lineages, or two different populations of blast cells with distinct morphology or surface antigens can coexist. They result from malignant transformation of a pluripotent stem cell (a stem cell that is not yet committed to a specific cell line) or from abnormal gene expression.[8]

A classification system for ALL is based on the cellular characteristics relating to the thymic (T-cell) and bursal equivalent (B-cell) origin of normal lymphocytes. At most large centers immunologic studies are performed on each patient's bone marrow and peripheral blood to classify the malignant cells on the basis of cell origin and differentiation.[49] This classification has been facilitated by the discovery of a variety of cell membrane surface markers.[17,28] These markers have made it pos-

sible to identify several major phenotypic subgroups of ALL: T cell, B cell, early pre-B cell, and pre-B cell.[3,15,109]

Age at onset is another way to classify leukemia. *Neonatal* or *congenital* usually refers to diagnosis before 1 month of age. *Infant leukemia* is variously identified as onset below either 12 or 24 months of age. The upper age for *childhood leukemia* is between 15 and 20 years.

A discussion of ALL is presented below and is followed by discussions of the other types of childhood leukemia (i.e., AML and CML).

ACUTE LYMPHOBLASTIC LEUKEMIA

ALL accounts for approximately 80% of childhood leukemias. In this form of the disease the lymphocyte cell line is affected. It can now be cured in more than 70% of cases.[13,103]

Originally the terms *acute* and *chronic* leukemia referred to the natural course of the diseases. Acute leukemia was rapidly fatal (within a few weeks or months). Chronic leukemia was also fatal but not as quickly (months to a few years). Effective treatments have changed these definitions. Now *acute leukemia* refers to those diseases with a predominance of immature blast cells and *chronic*

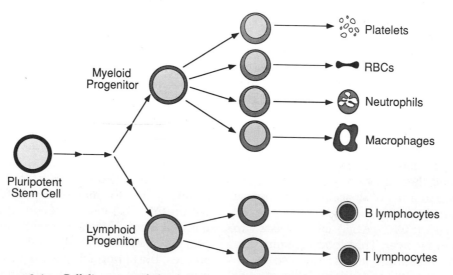

FIGURE 8-1. Cell lineages of the hematopoietic system showing common pluripotent stem cell and lineage-committed intermediates. Hematopoietic malignancies are identified by the nomenclature of this system. (*Modified from Sawyers CL, Denny CT, Witte ON. Leukemia and the disruption of normal hematopoiesis. Cell 1991, 64:337–350. © Cell Press.*)

leukemia refers to an expansion of more mature marrow elements.[89,91]

The French-American-British (FAB) cooperative group has established a classification system of acute leukemias based primarily on the morphology (form, structure, and cytochemistry) of the blast cells. Malignant cells vary from patient to patient according to cell size and shape, amount of cytoplasm, appearance of chromatin, intensity of cytoplasmic staining (basophilia), and the number, size, and prominence of vacuoles.[110] The FAB classification identifies three types, termed L_1, L_2, and L_3.[7] The cell type commonly found in childhood ALL (80%) is L_1. The cytoplasm is scanty and pale blue and usually has no granules. The lymphoblasts are small and uniform and have no or only one indistinct nucleolus. The nucleus is regular with homogeneous chromatin. L_2 cells are more commonly found in adult leukemias and are large and heterogeneous with moderately abundant cytoplasm and more distinct nucleoli. The nucleus is irregular with clumped chromatin. L_3 cells are associated with B-cell lineage (Burkitt-type) leukemia and are large and homogeneous with numerous prominent nucleoli, moderately large amounts of deep blue cytoplasm, and striking vacuolation. The nucleus is regular with homogeneous chromatin.

The role of cytochemical stains in differentiating ALL from other types of leukemia has diminished in favor of cytogenetic and immunologic studies.[74] Monoclonal antibodies (MoAbs) are now used to detect the presence of the common ALL antigen (CALLA) on leukemic cells. Positivity for CALLA has been associated with a favorable prognosis and is present in 75% to 80% of the B-lineage ALL patients.[17] It is positive in early pre-B cell ALL (see below).

Cytogenetic studies of leukemic cells are routinely performed at most major institutions. Structural and numerical (ploidy) abnormalities of chromosomes have been identified.[56,102] Cells are *hypodiploid* if the chromosome complex is low (<46) and *hyperdiploid* if it is high (>46). *Pseudodiploid* describes cases in which the correct number (46) of chromosomes is present but there are structural abnormalities or chromosome substitutions. All of these abnormalities occur only in the malignant cells. They are not found in normal cells.

A small number (5%) of children with ALL have a chromosomal abnormality similar to that seen with CML. This cytogenetic marker, the Philadelphia (Ph) chromosome, is the result of a translocation t(9;22), although the actual break point is different from that of CML. The Ph chromosome–positive cells are found in patients with B-cell or T-cell lineage ALL. These patients have a poor prognosis compared to other ALL patients and are treated with more aggressive therapy.

Molecular studies of these and other cytogenetic abnormalities have begun to identify specific chromosomal break points and specific genes (oncogenes) important to the development of malignancy.[42,114] The specific biologic mechanisms producing these abnormalities are not known. There is also no explanation why the individual chromosomal abnormalities detected in children with ALL are associated with different clinical outcomes. Hyperdiploidy (excessive amounts of DNA) has been associated with a good prognosis in childhood ALL, whereas chromosomal translocations such as t(1;19), t(4;11), and t(8;14) are associated with a worse prognosis.[42]

Approximately 10% to 15% of children with ALL have blast cells with T-cell surface markers.[28] At 37° C, T cells form heat-stable rosettes with sheep erythrocytes (E-rosette positive) and react with antisera against human T lymphocytes. T-cell leukemia is seen predominantly in older children, particularly males.[69] T-cell ALL is often associated with a mediastinal mass, a high WBC, and hepatosplenomegaly.

It is now clear that leukemia cells in T-cell ALL undergo malignant transformation at various stages along the T-lymphocytic pathway (Fig. 8–2). Widespread disease or large clusters of cells in one area are usually found outside the marrow in sites where T lymphocytes are found. Lymphoma-like disease is common to this subgroup of ALL. T-cell leukemia is a more aggressive form of leukemia and has a poorer prognosis unless aggressively treated. Patients with T-cell leukemia also appear to develop CNS involvement

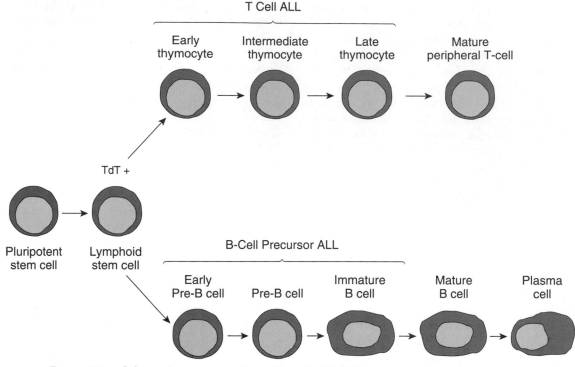

FIGURE 8-2. Schematic representation of lymphoid differentiation seen with childhood acute lymphocytic leukemia.

more frequently and sooner in their disease. A number of specific chromosomal translocations are associated with T-cell ALL.[2]

A very small percentage (1% to 2%) of children with ALL have B-cell leukemia. The blasts have surface immunoglobulin (Ig) detectable by direct immunofluorescent staining and bind immune complexes.[17] They also lack T-cell markers. In children B-cell-derived leukemia usually represents bone marrow infiltration by Burkitt's or other B-cell lymphomas, and the prognosis is poor.[49]

Sophisticated immunologic techniques have been developed to examine closely the group of leukemias previously termed *null cell* or *not classified*. It is accepted that the majority of non-T, non-B leukemias are of early B-cell lineage (also called *B-progenitor ALL*) (see Fig. 8–2). Pre-B-cell leukemia was first described as a subcategory of childhood ALL in the late 1970s.[109] It is apparent that 80% to 85% of childhood ALL cases develop from malignant monoclonal transformation of B-cell precursors.[27,28] With pre-B-cell ALL 10% of marrow lymphoblasts have cytoplasmic immunoglobulin. Those that do not yet show evidence of immunoglobulin are called *early pre-B-cells*. They both react with MoAbs specific to cells of B-cell lineage.

Even though pre-B cell leukemia and early pre-B cell leukemia arise from precursors of B cells, they are very different clinically. In general, the more mature the cell of origin, the less favorable is the prognosis. Of the B-lineage leukemias, the outcome for children with early pre-B-cell ALL is most favorable; that for pre-B cell ALL is slightly worse, and mature B-cell ALL carries an extremely poor prognosis.[27]

Recent studies have shown that chromosomal translocations are not uncommon in pre-B and mature B-cell ALL, and this fact, rather than the B-cell lineage, may account for the worse outcome seen in these patients. The most common abnormality seen in pre-B ALL is the translocation of one arm of chromosome 1 to chromosome 19 (t[1;19]).[85] Investigators have postulated that the break point of chromosome 19 alters a particular genetic transcriptional unit, resulting in a leukemia-producing gene.[21,102] Although this explanation applies to a very small subset of children with acute leukemia, it is a striking example how new data is being used to define the genetic basis of cancer. Very aggressive therapy for children with pre-B-cell ALL and t(1;19) can improve the prognosis to a level comparable to that of other pre-B-cell patients.[102]

CENTRAL NERVOUS SYSTEM DISEASE

CNS leukemia is an infiltration of the meninges by leukemic cells (although at times the brain may be involved). It can be present at the time of diagnosis or can occur later in the disease. Hemorrhagic petechiae, or infiltration in and around small vessels, or both provide entry of leukemic cells into the subarachnoid space at times when blasts are circulating in the peripheral blood.[112] It is a major cause of morbidity associated with leukemia and is an obstacle to cure.

In one series of patients CNS leukemia was documented at diagnosis in 9 of 123 (8%) children.[99] The incidence of leukemia in the CNS is more common at diagnosis in infants, children with a high WBC, thrombocytopenia, very large lymph nodes, or a mediastinal mass.[76] Each of these characteristics suggests a large tumor burden.

Often the child with CNS leukemia is asymptomatic. The blasts are discovered during routine lumbar punctures performed at the beginning or during the course of treatment. If signs and symptoms of CNS disease are present, they usually reflect increased intracranial pressure and may include headaches, vomiting, papilledema, and blurred or double vision. Symptoms of cranial nerve involvement, focal neurologic signs, or seizures may be present. A rapid weight gain, presumably caused by hypothalamic involvement, may be the only symptom.[38]

Since blasts are not normally in the CSF, the presence of any blasts in association with an elevated CSF WBC confirms the diagnosis of CNS leukemia. The precise determination of the number of blasts and the level of pleocytosis (total CSF WBC) required to make the diagnosis of CNS leukemia remains under discussion. The finding of five or more cells with blasts presents sufficient evidence to make the diagnosis. The CSF protein level and the CSF pressure may be elevated or normal. The CSF glucose level may be normal or slightly decreased.

As systemic chemotherapy during the 1960s and 1970s improved and prolonged the length of bone marrow remission, CNS leukemia became more common. Blood-borne blasts probably invade the CNS early in the disease and lie dormant with potential viability, protected from the action of systemic chemotherapeutic agents.[51,112] Malignant cells from the CNS can reseed the marrow and lead to hematologic relapse.[11]

GONADAL LEUKEMIA

The increase in survival rates of children with leukemia is also associated with an increase in testicular leukemia. Eight percent to 16% of boys treated for ALL during the 1970s developed testicular disease as their first site of relapse, but this number has decreased with modern therapy.[80] Testicular ALL usually presents as a painless gonadal enlargement. It is usually not noticed until the testicle becomes larger than normal. The enlargement may be unilateral or bilateral, and there can be firmness or scrotal discoloration. These changes are frequently discovered during a physical examination, so clinicians must be compulsive about including testicular inspection and palpation in each assessment.

Testicular involvement has been found at the time of the initial diagnosis of leukemia, during the course of therapy, and several months or even years after therapy is completed. Occult (no pain or swelling) testicular disease was found in up to 10% of asymptomatic males who underwent wedge biopsies of the testicles before stopping maintenance therapy.[72] The practice of "off-therapy" biopsies was once routine but recently has been called into question.[64,72] The practice was discontinued because of the high false negative rate (10%) and because a negative result does not mean relapse will not occur later.[64,84]

These late relapses without concurrent bone marrow disease suggest the existence of a blood-gonad barrier. The testes may be a pharmacologic sanctuary comparable to the CNS.[90] It is also possible that blasts are present in the testes early in the disease course but remain dormant for long periods of time. This makes them less susceptible to cytotoxic agents that destroy dividing cells.[113] Several studies have demonstrated that the testicles can act as sanctuaries because of other local factors (e.g., hypothermia) and a lower concentration of immunoglobulins.[105] It is also possible that the testicles only seem to be the first site of failure in some patients because disease is easy to detect in this site.

The term *isolated testicular relapse* may be a misnomer.[5] Exploratory laparotomies done in conjunction with positive testicular biopsies have found leukemia in the spleen, liver, and abdominal lymph nodes in some patients.[105] Factors associated with an increased risk of testicular disease are a high initial WBC (>20,000/mm³), massive splenomegaly and lymphadenopathy, and thrombocytopenia (<30,000/mm³).[113] Just as CNS leukemia is more common with T-cell disease, the frequency of testicular involvement in patients with this cell marker also is increased.

The frequency of ovarian leukemia is difficult to quantitate, although occasional cases have been reported.[22] The inability to examine the ovaries easily makes enlargement more difficult to recognize than testicular disease. Clinical ovarian relapse is very rare.

TREATMENT

The first encouraging treatment reports for childhood ALL were made in 1948 by Farber et al.,[31] who treated 16 children with a folic acid antagonist. Ten children showed "clinical, hematologic, and pathologic" evidence of improvement. With this early clinical trial, effective treatment for leukemia began. Most current treatment strategies are based on several principles: rapid remission induction, early intensification (several weeks or months of very aggressive therapy), continued maintenance with combination (multiple-drug) chemotherapy, early CNS prophylaxis, aggressive supportive care, and more intensive

therapy for high-risk groups (i.e., patients with clinical and/or laboratory features associated with a poorer prognosis) (see Table 8–1).

Treatment begins by quickly addressing presenting symptoms such as profound anemia, infection, hemorrhage, or metabolic abnormalities. The release of nucleic acid purines from lysed neoplastic cells can lead to an elevated uric acid level and acute renal failure.[25] Prevention of hyperuricemia is achieved by intravenous (IV) hydration, urinary alkalinization to a pH of 7 or 8, and administration of allopurinol. The importance of diligent nursing attention to this early phase of therapy cannot be overemphasized. When destruction of large numbers of malignant cells is expected (e.g., with a high WBC or nodal and organ enlargement), this care is even more critical.

Remission Induction

Reduction of the leukemic cell burden to an undetectable level (remission) is the first objective of therapy. Several combinations of drugs and treatment schedules can achieve this, but the most frequently used combination includes vincristine, prednisone, and L-asparaginase. Anthracyclines and cyclophosphamide are also used in some protocols. These regimens induce complete remission in 98% of children with ALL, usually within 4 weeks.[44,46,88] Remission-induction therapy is usually well tolerated, and the mortality rate is less than 5%.[88] The most common causes of death during induction are hemorrhage, infection, and tumor lysis syndrome.

A speedy response to therapy is important. Children who are in remission between day 7 and day 14 have a superior rate of disease-free survival compared to those who achieve it later.[34] A recent Childrens Cancer Group (CCG) study showed that the number of blasts present on day 7 is a very strong predictor of eventual outcome.[36]

Tailored Therapy

Remission induction is relatively standard for most ALL patients. However, recognition of the heterogenous nature of childhood ALL has profoundly affected other phases of therapy. T-cell ALL is an excellent example. During the late 1970s the dismal prognosis for children with T-cell leukemia caused oncologists to give them more aggressive therapy such as the 10-drug regimen, LSA_2-L_2, originally designed at Memorial Sloan-Kettering Cancer Center, New York. Other regimens have followed, most including alkylating agents, anthracyclines, epipodophyllins, and/or cytosine arabinoside. Now children with T-cell disease who are aggressively treated have a 60% chance of survival.[2,57]

A number of cooperative groups around the world study ALL, and each has a unique system for determining risk groups. Table 8–1 shows how certain clinical and laboratory features are used to place children in prognostic categories. The intermediate (or standard) risk group is the largest group. Children in this group have a 70% to 75% chance of cure.[13] Low (or good) risk suggests a better prognosis than that of the intermediate-risk group, and the high (or poor)-risk group has a worse prognosis than the standard-risk group. Grouping patients in categories according to their chance of cure facilitates the provision of "tailored" therapy. Tailored therapies allow aggressive treatment for children who need it. Conversely, children who will do well with less therapy are spared the ill effects of treatment they do not need.

As therapies have been designed to meet the needs of each group, prognoses have improved. But at times it has been difficult to determine if this improvement is therapy related or is due to a statistical phenomenon that occurs from shifting patients from one prognostic group to another.[12]

Intensification

Even when clinical remission is attained, blasts are still present, although they are undetectable.[29] The amount of residual disease at this point is variable. In some children the leukemic burden can be as great as 10^8 or 10^9 cells per kilogram.[53] If therapy is discontinued at this time, most children will relapse within 3 to 4 months. Therefore a consolidation, or intensification, phase is begun immediately after remission is attained. The goals at this point are to decrease or eliminate the minimal residual disease further while simultaneously ridding sanctuary sites of any remaining leukemia. This phase may overlap the CNS prophylactic phase or be given at the same time. High-dose L-asparaginase is an example of a successful consolidation agent.[24]

The German cooperative group (Berlin-Frankfurt-Muenster [BFM]) used a very intensive consolidation phase for several months after induction.[46] They had an overall event-free survival (EFS) rate of 67% to 74%. These data are impressive because all subgroups—good-, intermediate-, and poor-risk patients—are included. A recent study by the CCG used modified BFM therapy for children with unfavorable prognoses.[35] The 4-year EFS rate was 62%, with a median follow-up of 3½ years. These studies show that aggressive therapy, primarily during the consolidation phase, can cure a high percentage of even poor-risk patients. This is one of the most remarkable improvements in ALL treatment in the last 20 years.

CNS Therapy

As mentioned, prophylactic therapy to the CNS is a necessary part of ALL therapy. The "gold standard" of CNS prophylactic therapy was pioneered by St. Jude Children's Research Hospital, Memphis, Tenn., in the early 1970s. It included 2400 cGy of cranial irradiation and several doses of intrathecal (into the spinal canal) methotrexate (IT MTX).[4] This route of therapy is necessary because leukemia cells easily cross the blood-brain barrier but most chemotherapeutic agents do not. This regimen decreased the rate of CNS leukemia from greater than 50% to less than 10%.[4] Further studies have modified this regimen somewhat, decreasing the amount of cranial irradiation to 1800 cGy (or eliminating it in some low-risk patients) and varying the amount of IT MTX given.[75] A change in this regimen that raised the dose of IT MTX for younger children further reduced the CNS relapse rate to 2% to 5% overall and to only 6% in high-risk patients.[10]

A study between the National Cancer Institute (NCI) and the CCG investigated differences between high-dose intravenous methotrexate (IV MTX) and a regimen that combined 2400 cGy cranial irradiation with five doses of IT MTX.[78] There was no difference in CNS relapse rate between the two groups at a median follow-up time of 64 months. The high-dose IV MTX arm was associated with significantly less long-term toxicity than regimens including cranial irradiation. High-dose MTX alone has not yet been tested against other regimens that also lack radiation therapy.

After almost 20 years of experience in the prophylactic treatment of the CNS of children with leukemia, certain principles of CNS prophylaxis have been defined.[12,99] All children need CNS prophylaxis, even if they meet all the low-risk criteria. IT MTX alone is as good as multidrug IT therapy; and CNS radiotherapy is valuable in children with high-risk factors. In children with a low risk of CNS leukemia, CNS radiotherapy can be deleted if IT MTX or a combination of IT MTX and IV MTX is continued during the maintenance phase of therapy. Children with intermediate-risk ALL do well with IT MTX and intermediate-dose IV MTX in some studies. However, the Pediatric Oncology Group (POG) has used triple intrathecal therapy (methotrexate, cytosine arabinoside, and hydrocortisone without radiation) for more than 10 years, with CNS remission rates equal to those cited above. Induction and maintenance with high-dose IV MTX (because it crosses the blood-brain barrier in high doses) can be used instead of IT medications and radiotherapy for low- and intermediate-risk children.

Adverse reactions to CNS therapy can be immediate, delayed, or very late. Children undergoing CNS radiation can experience vomiting, anorexia, drowsiness, fatigue, and headache. Five to 7 weeks later many also develop a somnolence syndrome characterized by a recurrence of the initial symptoms, particularly drowsiness. Some children have fever and mild ataxia and are irritable.

IT MTX is sometimes associated with a chemical meningitis that develops within the first 12 hours after treatment. Children may experience nausea and vomiting, headache, fever, back pain, stiff neck, and dizziness. Some youngsters never experience any of these symptoms, and others do so consistently.

Delayed reactions to IT MTX usually occur only after multiple doses. Seizures have been reported in rare patients, and a few have developed paraplegia.[18] The most serious sequela to CNS treatment—progressive leukoencephalopathy—is very rare now that changes have been made in drug and radiotherapy doses and schedules. Other problems include diminished intelligence quotient scores, learning disabilities, and attention problems.

The adverse effects of CNS therapy are of grave concern. Both prophylactic CNS therapy and treatment for overt CNS disease are associated with serious long-term sequelae. These problems are addressed in detail in Chapter 17. However, when the consequences of uncontrolled leukemia are considered, effective CNS therapy seems worth the risk. The best CNS regimens are those that prevent or cure disease and result in the fewest acute and delayed toxicities.

Maintenance

The goals of this phase of therapy are to maintain disease control, both medullary (bone marrow) and extramedullary, and to prevent the development of drug-resistant clones (groups of cells descended from a single parent cell) of cells. Although a variety of agents and schedules are used, most regimens for non-T, non-B ALL include weekly oral or intramuscular (IM) MTX and daily oral 6-mercaptopurine to the maximal tolerated doses. Vincristine and prednisone administered at intervals add to remission duration. The addition of other agents such as cyclophosphamide, cytosine arabinoside, and daunorubicin or the use of intermittent reinductions may be useful in some patients. Their benefit must be balanced against the increased risk of serious infections and other toxicities.

The choice of which agents and what level of intensity depends on prognostic subgrouping. Drug dosing and metabolism also play key roles in response to therapy. Several studies have concluded that problems with compliance, absorption, and metabolism account for some of the relapses seen in low- and intermediate-risk children.[1,81] The POG was concerned enough by these studies to change from using oral weekly MTX to using parenteral MTX in all front-line leukemia studies. However, no scientific evidence exists proving that IM MTX is superior to oral MTX.

Most treatment plans continue therapy for 30 to 36 months in patients who maintain a continuous complete remission.[63] The CCG stops therapy at 24 months for girls with low-risk ALL because they are less likely to relapse. However, the intensity of therapy influences the optimal length of therapy. The German regimen (BFM), which featured intensive early therapy, used a maintenance regimen of only 24 months.[46]

RELAPSE

Despite the successes of modern therapy, 30% of children with ALL will relapse.[13] Relapse is defined as the presence of leukemic cells in any site or having more than 25% blast cells in the bone marrow. As discussed previously, the gonads and CNS are the most common sites of extramedullary relapse. Other rare sites include the vitreous of the eye, lungs, bone cortex, skin, and abdomen.

Children who experience repeated relapses have an increasingly difficult time being reinduced into clinical remission, and each remission is shorter than the one that preceded it, probably because of the development of drug resistance.[1] A number of new regimens and new agents are being tested for use in relapsed children. But even with aggressive therapy, relapse while receiving therapy portends a very poor prognosis. Seventy percent of children will achieve a second remission,[87] but children who relapse during therapy or within 6 months of stopping therapy have less than a 10% to 25% chance of being cured.[29] This chance drops to 5% if the relapse occurs in the first 18 months of therapy.[18] Children who relapse early into therapy have a median duration of second remission of only 7 months, and only 10% of those who achieve a second remission are free of disease 2 years later.[18]

If a child has CNS leukemia at diagnosis or relapses in the CNS during therapy, successful CNS remission can still be achieved.[75] The POG study from 1983 to 1988 showed that virtually 100% of patients achieve a second CNS remission.[97] However, the duration of remission is short, approximately 12 to 24

months. The treatment of CNS overt disease always requires radiation therapy and maintenance IT MTX. The occurrence of CNS leukemia at diagnosis or early in the disease is a poor prognostic sign.

Children whose CNS disease develops at least 1 year after their original diagnosis and whose initial CNS preventive therapy did not include CNS radiation have a 30% long-term survival rate.[75] This compares to only 11% for those who relapsed before 1 year. The majority of children will have another CNS relapse or a recurrence in the bone marrow, testicles, or multiple sites.

The use of intraventricular reservoirs as a delivery system for MTX in this clinical setting seems to have some advantages over intrathecal administration. It minimizes patient discomfort and allows more equal distribution of drug within the CNS. The primary disadvantages are that placement requires general anesthesia and the subcutaneous port is aesthetically displeasing to some patients and parents.

Patients who relapse first in the testes may rapidly relapse in the bone marrow, CNS, or both. Radiation in a dose of 1200 cGy to 2400 cGy is delivered to each testicle since both are usually involved, even if only one is enlarged. Although this dose renders the patient sterile, it does effectively destroy local testicular disease. Systemic reinduction with chemotherapy, along with retreatment of the CNS, is also necessary to prevent hematologic relapse.[98]

One study demonstrated a 70% 3-year EFS rate with isolated occult (only microscopic) testicular disease, compared to 90% among those who had overt (enlarged testicles) relapse.[98] The ability to provide extended second remissions to two thirds of the boys with testicular disease is very encouraging. There is no explanation for the unexpected differences in EFS rate between boys who had overt disease and boys who had occult disease. Prognosis for boys who have simultaneous or subsequent bone marrow relapse is very poor.

Approximately 10% of children treated for ALL in the 1980s relapsed after therapy was discontinued.[63] The highest rates of relapse occurred during the first year off therapy.[18] The relapse rate was higher among males, partially because of the risk of testicular leukemia. The rate of relapse for all children declined exponentially over the next 2 to 3 years and leveled off. Relapse was rare after the fourth year (7 years from diagnosis). Prolonged second remissions (>2 years) could be obtained in only one third of children who relapsed after their initial 3-year course of treatment.[18]

A disturbing observation was reported in 1989 at St. Jude Children's Research Hospital. An exceptionally high risk of developing AML after treatment for T-cell ALL was recognized.[83] A subsequent POG study has suggested that the increased risk may be associated with treatment regimens containing VM26, an epipodophyllotoxin.[50] The role of epipodophyllotoxins in the development of secondary AML requires further study.

Further study also is necessary to explain the significantly higher failure rates during second remission for children who receive anthracyclines during their first remission.[97,98]

PROGNOSIS

Before the era of chemotherapy, 84% of patients with ALL died within 8 weeks of the onset of their symptoms.[69] This compared to the 50% five-year survival rate in 1975.[96] Currently the overall survival rate is 70% to 73%,[13,34,86] and the survival rate for certain low-risk patients may be as high as 90%.[40,103]

Important prognostic criteria have been elucidated to allow prediction of the EFS rate for various risk categories (Table 8–1). These criteria include physical and basic laboratory data and sophisticated immunologic and molecular genetic data.[26] However, although there has been incredible progress in the refinement of prognostic criteria, there is little agreement about a common "staging" classification. The major leukemia study groups around the world are working to develop a way to compare treatment regimens used for similar groups of patients.[14,39,61]

The WBC at diagnosis has consistently been considered the single most important predictor of treatment response and survival. The best survival rate occurs in the 30% of patients who have an initial WBC of less than 5000/mm³.[39] Children with a WBC exceeding 100,000/mm³ have the worst prognosis, showing that WBC is a continuous variable and is inversely proportional to remission duration. The remission duration of patients with very high WBCs (>300,000/mm³) is short (median, 6 months), even though the leukemia is very sensitive to initial therapy. Early responsiveness to treatment may be due to very active metabolic pathways associated with a rapidly dividing leukemic population. This rapid genetic division allows them to overcome quickly metabolic blocks induced by the chemotherapy.[101]

Age at diagnosis is the second most important prognostic variable. The chances for survival decrease as the child's age increases except for the very poor prognosis for children less than 12 months of age. In one study only 16% of children less than 12 months of age lived for 1 year after diagnosis.[29] The interrelationship between other prognostic factors is also important. In the infant group 64% have a WBC greater than 50,000/mm³ at diagnosis compared to only 13% of the 1- to 9-year-old age group.[92] CNS disease at diagnosis, chromosomal abnormalities, and marked organomegaly are overrepresented in this group as well. The immature immune system of infants may also play a role. Infants have three times the remission induction failure rate of the 1- to 9-year-old group.

Children greater than 10 years of age also do poorer than the midchildhood age group.[39] The long-term disease-free survival rate for children 10 and over is 41%. The older group is more likely to have an elevated WBC, mediastinal mass, CNS disease at diagnosis, T-cell disease, L_2 morphology, and hepatosplenomegaly.

Hepatomegaly, splenomegaly, mediastinal enlargement, and lymphadenopathy are evidence of a large tumor burden and are associated with a poor prognosis. However, since these conditions correlate positively with WBC, their importance as independent variables is limited.

The number of chromosomes (ploidy) in the lymphoblasts of children with ALL has important prognostic significance.[42,56] The 30% of children with ALL who have hyperdiploidy (cells that contain more than 46 chromosomes) have a better prognosis than chil-

TABLE 8–1. *Relative Importance and Relative Comparison of Prognostic Variables in ALL*

	LEVEL OF IMPORTANCE		
	MOST FAVORABLE (LOW RISK)	INTERMEDIATE (STANDARD RISK)	LEAST FAVORABLE (HIGH RISK)
Major			
WBC/mm³	<10,000	10,000–50,000	>100,000
DNA index	>1.16		
<1			
Blast morphology	L1		L3
Immunologic markers	CALLA positive, early pre-B	Early pre-B, pre-B	T or B
Age (yr)	3–5	1–9	<12 mo >10 yr
Chromosonal abnormalities			t(1;19) t(4;11) t(8;14) Philadelphia
Moderate			
Sex	Female		
Time to remission (days)	≤14	≤28	≥28
CNS disease	Absent		
Minor			
Adenopathy	Absent		
Splenomegaly	Absent		
Race	White		

dren with fewer than 46 chromosomes (hypodiploidy) or an abnormal structure to their chromosomes (pseudodiploidy). Hyperdiploidy is often associated with other good prognostic features. Some studies describe ploidy by DNA index, which compares the DNA content of the normal cells to that of the blast cells. Hyperdiploid cells have a DNA index of more than 1, meaning they have more DNA than normal cells. Hypodiploid cells have a DNA index of less than 1. A DNA index of more than 1.16 has been strongly associated with a better prognosis.[40,42,56]

Cytogenetic abnormalities also have prognostic significance. Patients with translocation of portions of one chromosome onto another have more frequent relapses.

As previously mentioned, children with T-cell surface markers on their leukemic lymphoblasts have a poor prognosis. Several of the initial clinical features suggesting adverse outcomes are often also present in patients with T-cell disease. These features include CNS involvement, older age, mediastinal mass, male sex, and high WBC. Children with B-cell surface markers have a poor prognosis and often fail to achieve even an initial remission.[26] Children with a low initial WBC who are between the ages of 2 and 10 years with early pre-B cell, CALLA-positive ALL and a DNA index greater than 1.16 have a long-term EFS rate approaching 90%.[103] Patients within this group likely will achieve a cure with therapy that produces few significant late effects.

The route by which these and other prognostic factors exert an influence on survival is still unclear. It is possible that some play no direct role but are simply related to the basic biology of the involved leukemia cell line. The truest indicator of prognosis is response to therapy. As treatment regimens improve, various biologic and clinical indicators may decrease in importance.

Future Progress

The central challenge facing leukemia researchers is to design rational preventive programs. For example, if household radon is actually a cause of ALL, efforts to limit exposure can be aggressively instituted. If retroviruses are implicated, the search for effective vaccines will quickly follow.

However, since prevention is not in the foreseeable future, other problems must be addressed.

Prognostic subgrouping should be standardized to facilitate comparisons among treatment trials. There must be prospective recognition of the subgroup of patients who will do poorly even with aggressive "high-risk" therapy. Treatment plans for this "super-high-risk" group can then be instituted.

More studies about the impact of pharmacokinetics and drug metabolism on treatment response are needed.[23] This information must then be integrated into study designs in an effort to prevent treatment failure. Intensive efforts must be made to design "safe" treatment protocols that limit the adverse effects of drug treatment and radiotherapy.

These efforts will improve therapy, but they will be in vain if children fail to take their medications. Studies to determine ways to improve adherence to treatment, especially among teenagers, are needed.

All practitioners must diligently attempt to eliminate unnecessary, painful procedures performed in the course of care. The pain and stress of bone marrow aspirations and spinal taps are almost always viewed as the most difficult part of therapy for children and their parents.

Studies aimed at improving the detection of minimal residual disease must be made a priority.[22] This will allow treatment of children who have active disease but normal bone marrow examination results.

Progress must be made in the ability to determine which patients need marrow transplantation and when they need it. Some centers transplant certain high-risk children as soon as their disease is under control. Other centers treat with aggressive chemotherapy until there is evidence of marrow relapse.

The appropriate role of biologic response modifiers as a treatment modality for ALL must be determined.

A transfer of knowledge and information from cancer centers and university hospitals to community facilities and local physicians and nurses must be actively pursued. As treatment of children with low-risk ALL becomes more "routine" and less intensive, much of their care will be done locally. Although their care may seem ordinary to oncologists and oncology nurses, it will not be ordinary to health care workers in the community, and it will never be ordinary to the affected child and family.

REFERENCES

1. Adamson PD, Poplack DG, Balis FM. Pharmacology and drug resistance in childhood lymphoblastic leukemia. Hematol Oncol 1990; 4:871–894.
2. Amylon MD. Treatment of T-lineage acute lymphoblastic leukemic. Hematol Oncol 1990; 4:937–949.
3. Anderson JK, Bates MP, Slaughenhoupt BL, et al. Expression of human B cell associated antigens on leukemia and lymphomas: A model of human B cell differentiation. Blood 1984; 63:1424–1433.
4. Aur RJA, Simone JV, Hustu HO. Comparison of two methods of preventing central nervous system leukemia. N Engl J Med 1974; 291:1230–1233.
5. Baum E, Heyn R, Nesbit M, et al. Occult abdominal involvement with apparently isolated testicular relapse in children with ALL. Am J Pediatr Hematol Oncol 1984; 6:343–346.
6. Baverstam U, Holmberg M. Are low doses of radiation leukemogenic in children. Leuk Res 1989; 13:515–517.
7. Bennett JM. Proposals for the classification of the acute leukemias. French-America-British Cooperative Group. Br J Haematol 1976; 33:451.
8. Bishop JM. The molecular genetics of cancer. Science 1987; 235:304–311.
9. Bizzozero OJ, Johnson KG, Ciocco A. Radiation-related leukemia in Hiroshima and Nagasaki 1946–64. I. Distribution, incidence, and appearance time. N Engl J Med 1966; 274:1095.
10. Bleyer WA. Intrathecal methotrexate versus central nervous system leukemia. Cancer Drug Deliv 1984; 1:157–167.
11. Bleyer WA. Central nervous system leukemia. Pediatr Clin North Am 1988; 35:789–814.
12. Bleyer WA. Remaining problems in the staging and treatment of childhood acute lymphoblastic leukemia. Am J Pediatr Hematol Oncol 1989; 11:371–379.
13. Bleyer WA. The impact of childhood cancer in the United States and the world. CA 1990; 40:355–367.
14. Bleyer WA, Satler H, Coccia P, et al. The staging of childhood ALL: Strategies of CCSG and a 3 dimensional technique of multivariate analysis. Med Pediatr Oncol 1984; 14:271–280.
15. Borella L, Sen L. T cell surface markers on lymphoblasts from acute lymphoblastic leukemia. J Immunol 1973; 111:1257–1260.

16. Boring CC, Squires TS, Tong T. Cancer Statistics, 1991. CA 1991; 41:19–36.

17. Borowitz MJ. Immunologic markers in childhood acute leukemia. Hematol Oncol 1990; 4:743–766.

18. Buchanan G. Diagnosis and management of relapse in acute lymphoblastic leukemia. Hematol Oncol 1990; 4:937–949.

19. Byrd R. Late effects of treatment of cancer in children. Pediatr Clin North Am 1985; 32:835–857.

20. Cancer Facts and Figures—1992. American Cancer Society publication 92-425 M—No. 5008.92-LE, 1992.

21. Carroll AJ, Crist WM, Parmley RT. Pre-B cell leukemia associated with chromosome translocation 1;19. Blood 1984; 63:721.

22. Cepalupo AJ, Frankel LS, Sullivan MP. Pelvic and ovarian extramedullary leukemia relapse in young girls. A report of four cases and a review of the literature. Cancer 1982; 50:587–593.

23. Civin C. Directions for future research in childhood lymphoblastic leukemia. Hematol Oncol 1990; 4:1009–1018.

24. Clarell LA, Gelber RD, Cohen HJ, et al. Four agent induction and intensive asparaginase treatment of childhood acute lymphoblastic leukemia. N Engl J Med 1986; 315:657–663.

25. Cohen DG. Metabolic complications of induction therapy for leukemia and lymphoma. Cancer Nurs 1983; 6:307–310.

26. Crist W, Boyett J, Pullen J, et al. Clinical and biological features predict poor prognosis. Med Pediatr Oncol 1986; 13:135–139.

27. Crist W, Boyett J, Jackson J, et al. Prognostic importance of the pre-B cell immunophenotype and other presenting factors in B-cell lineage childhood acute lymphoblastic leukemia: A POG Study. Blood 1989; 74:1252–1259.

28. Crist WM, Grossi CE, Pullen DJ, et al. Immunologic markers in childhood acute lymphocytic leukemia. Semin Oncol 1985; 12:105–121.

29. Crist WM, Pullen J, Rivera GK. Acute lymphoblastic leukemia. In Fernbach DJ, Vietta TJ (eds): Clinical Pediatric Oncology, 4th ed. St. Louis: Mosby–Year Book, 1991.

30. Dearth J, Salter M, Wilson E, et al. Early deaths in acute leukemia in children. Med Pediatr Oncol 1983; 11:225–228.

31. Farber S, Diamond L, Merser R. Temporary remissions in acute leukemia in children produced by folic acid antagonists, 4-aminopteroyl-glutoamic acid (Aminopterin). N Engl J Med 1948; 238:787–793.

32. Fong CT, Brodeur GM. Down's syndrome and leukemia: Epidemiology, genetics, cytogenetics and mechanism of luekemogenesis. Cancer Genetics 1987; 28:55–76.

33. Foucar K. Bone marrow examination in the diagnosis of acute and chronic leukemias. Hematol Oncol Clin North Am 1990; 2:567–584.

34. Gaynon PS. Primary treatment of childhood ALL of non-T cell lineage (including infants). Hematol Oncol 1990; 4:915–936.

35. Gaynon PS, Bleyer WA, Steinherz PG, et al. Modified BFM 76/79 for children with previously untreated ALL and unfavorable prognostic features: Report of CCSG. Am J Pediatr Hematol Oncol 1988; 10:42–50.

36. Gaynon PS, Bleyer WA, Steinherz PG, et al. Day 7 marrow response and outcome for children with ALL and unfavorable presenting factors. J Med Pediatr Oncol 1990; 18:273–279.

37. Greenberg RS, Shuster JL. Epidemiology of cancer in children. Epidemiol Rev 1985; 7:22–48.

38. Greydanus DE, Burgert ED, Gilchrist GS. Hypothalamic syndrome with acute lymphocytic leukemia. Mayo Clin Proc 1978; 63:217.

39. Hammond D, Satler H, Nesbit M, et al. Analysis of prognostic factors in acute lymphoblastic leukemia. Med Pediatr Oncol 1986; 14:124–134.

40. Harris MB, Shuster JJ, Carroll A, et al. Trisomy of leukemic cell chromosomes 4 and 10 identifies children with B-progenitor cell acute lymphoblastic leukemia with a very low risk of treatment failure: A Pediatric Oncology Group study. Blood 1992; 79:3316–3324.

41. Harvey EB, Boice JD, Honeyman M, et al. Prenatal x-ray exposure and childhood cancer in twins. N Engl J Med 1985; 312:531–545.

42. Heerema NA. Cytogenetic abnormalities and molecular markers of acute lymphoblastic leukemia. Hematol Oncol Clin North Am 1990; 4:795–820.

43. Henderson ES. Etiology of leukemia: A persisting puzzle. In Henderson ES, Lister TA (eds): Leukemia, 5th ed. Philadelphia: WB Saunders, 1990.

44. Henderson ES, Hoelzer D, Freeman AI. The treatment of ALL. In Henderson ES, Lister TA (eds): Leukemia, 5th ed. Philadelphia: WB Saunders, 1990, pp 443–484.

45. Henshaw DL, Eatough JP, Richardson RB. Radon as a causative factor in induction of myeloid leukemia and other cancers. Lancet 1990; 355:100–112.

46. Henze G, Langermann J, Ritter J, et al. Treatment strategy for different risk groups in childhood ALL: A report from the BFM group. In Neth R, Gallo RC, Graf R, et al. (eds): Modern Trends in Human Leukemia. IV. Berlin: Springer-Verlag, 1991, p 87.

47. Hoover R, Fraumeni JF. Risk of cancer in renal-transplant recipients. Lancet 1973; 2:55.

48. Hurwitz CA, Mirro J. Mixed lineage leukemia and asynchronous antigen expression. Hematol Oncol Clin North Am 1990; 4:767–794.

49. Kalwinsky DK, Roberson P, Dahl G, et al. Clinical relevance of lymphoblast biologic features in children with ALL. J Clin Oncol 1985; 3:477–484.

50. Kreissman SG, Gelber RD, Sallan SE, et al. Secondary AML in children treated for ALL. Proc Am Soc Clin Oncol 1990; 9:219. (Abstract.)

51. Kuo AH, Yataganas X, Galacich JH. Proliferative kinetics of central nervous system leukemia. Cancer 1975; 36:232.

52. Lagakos SW, Wessen BJ, Zelen M. An analysis of contaminated well water and health effects in Woburn, Massachusettes. J Am Stat Assoc 1986; 81:583–596.

53. Lance B, Rivera G. Detection of minimal residual disease in acute lymphoblastic leukemia. Hematol Oncol Clin North Am 1990; 4:895–914.

54. Li FP, Bader J. Epidemiology of cancer in childhood. In Oski F, Nathan DG (eds): Hematology of Infancy and Childhood, 3rd ed. Philadelphia: WB Saunders, 1987, pp 918–941.

55. Li FP, Jamieson DS, Meadows AT. Questionnaire study of cancer etiology in 503 children. J Natl Cancer Inst 1986; 76:31–36.

56. Look AT, Robertson PK, Williams DL, et al. Prognostic importance of blast cell DNA content in childhood ALL. Blood 1985; 65:1079–1086.

57. Ludwig WD, Seibt H, Hiddermann W, et al. Clinical significance of immunophenotyping in childhood ALL: Experience of BFM. ALL-83 study. Proc Am Assoc Cancer 1988; 29:A850. (Abstract.)

58. MacMahon B. Susceptibility to radiation-induced leukemia? N Engl J Med 1975; 287:144.

59. MacMahon B. Prenatal x-ray exposure and twins. N Engl J Med 1985; 312:576–577.

60. McWhirter WR, Kirk D. What causes childhood leukemia? Some beliefs of parents of affected children. Med J Aust 1986; 145:121–123.

61. Mantrangelo R. The problem of "staging" in childhood ALL: A review. Med Pediatr Oncol 1986; 14:121–123.

62. March HG. Leukemia in radiologists. Radiology 1944; 43:275.

63. Miller DR, Leikin SL, Albo VC, et al. Three versus five years of maintenance therapy are equivalent in childhood ALL: A report from CCSG. J Clin Oncol 1989; 7:316–325.

64. Miller DR, Leikin SL, Albo VC, et al. The prognostic value of testicular biopsy in childhood acute lymphoblastic leukemia. A Report from CCSG. Clin Oncol 1990; 8:57–66.

65. Miller RW. Persons with exceptionally high risk of leukemia. Cancer Res 1967; 27:2420.

66. Miller RW. Neoplasia and Down's syndrome. Ann N Y Acad Sci 1970; 171:637.

67. Miller RW. Deaths from childhood leukemia and solid tumors among twins and other sibs in the United States. 1960-67. J Natl Cancer Inst 1971; 46:203–209.

68. Miller RW, Boice JD. Radiogenic cancer after prenatal or childhood exposure. In Upton AC, Albert RE, Burns FJ, et al. (eds): Radiation Carcinogenesis. New York: Elsevier, 1986, pp 379–386.

69. Mitchell CD, Gordon I, Chessells JM. Clinical, hematological, and radiological features in T cell lymphoblastic malignancy in childhood. Clin Radiol 1986; 37:257–261.

70. Mulvihill JJ. Childhood cancer, the environment and heredity. In Pizzo P, Poplack DG (eds): Principles and Practices of Pediatric Oncology, 2nd ed. Philadelphia: JB Lippincott, 1993, pp 11–28.

71. Myers MH, Heize HW, Li FP, et al. Trends in cancer survival among US white children. J Pediatr 1975; 87:815.

72. Nachman J, Palmer NF, Sather HN, et al. Open-wedge testicular biopsy in childhood ALL after 2 years of maintenance therapy: Diagnostic accuracy and influence on outcome. A report from CCSG. Blood 1990; 175:1051–1055.

73. Neglia J, Robinson J. Epidemiology of childhood acute leukemia. Pediatr Clin North Am 1988; 35:657–692.

74. Nelson D. Leukocytic disorders. In Henry JB, Davidson I, Bernard HJ, et al. (eds): Todd-Sanford-Davidson Clinical Diagnosis and Management by Laboratory Methods, 16th ed. Philadelphia: WB Saunders, 1979.

75. Ortega JA, Nesbit ME, Sather HN, et al. Long-term evaluations of a CNS prophylaxis trial—Treatment comparisons and outcome after CNS relapse in childhood ALL. A report from CCSG. J Clin Oncol 1987; 5:1646–1654.

76. Pochedly C. Prevention of meningeal leukemia: Review of 20 years of research and current recommendations. Hematol Oncol Clin North Am 1990; 4:951–970.

77. Pool R. Is there an EMF-cancer connection? Science 1990; 249:1096–1098.

78. Poplack D, Reaman G, Bleyer A, et al. Central nervous system preventive therapy with high dose methotrexate in ALL: A preliminary report. Proc Am Soc Clin Oncol 1984; 3:204.

79. Poplack DG. Acute lymphoblastic leukemia in childhood. Pediatr Clin North Am 1985; 32:669–697.

80. Poplack DG. Acute lymphoblastic leukemia. In Pizzo PA, Poplack DG (eds): Principles and Practices of Pediatric Oncology, 2nd ed. Philadelphia: JB Lippincott, 1993, pp 431–482.

81. Poplack DG, Balis FM, Zimm S. The pharmacology of orally administered chemotherapy: A reappraisal. Hematol Oncol 1990; 4:895–914.

82. Poplack DG, Reaman G. Acute lymphoblastic leukemia in childhood. Pediatr Clin North Am 1988; 35:903–932.

83. Pui C-H, Behm FG, Raimondi SC, et al. Secondary acute myeloid leukemia in children treated for ALL. N Engl J Med 1989; 321:136–142.

84. Pui CH, Dahl J, Bowman WP. Elective testicular biopsy during chemotherapy for childhood leukemia is of no clinical value. Lancet 1985; 2:410.

85. Ramondi S, Bohn F, Roberson PK, et al. Cytogenetics of pre-B cell acute lymphoblastic leukemia with emphasis on prognostic implications of the t(1;19). J Clin Oncol 1990; 8:1380–1388.

86. Ries LAG, Hankey BF, Miller BA, et al. Cancer Statistics Review. 1973-1988. NIH publication 91-2789. Bethesda, Md.: National Cancer Institute, 1991.

87. Rivera GK, George SL, Williams D, et al. Early results of intensified induction chemotherapy for childhood acute lymphocytic leukemia. Med Pediatr Oncol 1986; 14:177–181.

88. Rivera GK, Pui CH, Mirro J, et al. Rotational combination chemotherapy for childhood ALL: St. Jude Study X1. Proc ASCO 1990; 9:218.

89. Ruccione K. Acute leukemia in children: Current perspectives. Issues Compr Pediatr Nurs 1983; 6:329–362.

90. Russo A, Schiliro G. The enigma of testicular leukemia. A critical review. Med Pediatr Oncol 1986; 14:300–306.

91. Sallan SE, Weinstein HJ. Childhood acute leukemia. In Nathan DG, Oski FA (eds): Hematology of Infancy and Childhood, 3rd ed, vol 2. Philadelphia: WB Saunders, 1987, pp 1028–1063.

92. Sather HN. Age at diagnosis in childhood acute lymphoblastic leukemia. Med Pediatr Oncol 1986; 13:172–178.

93. Savitz DA, Calle EE. Leukemia and occupational exposure to electromagnetic fields: A review of epidemiological surveys. J Occup Med 1987; 29:47–51.

94. Savitz DA, John EM, Kleckner RC. Magnetic field exposure from electric appliances and childhood cancer. Am J Epidemiol 1990; 131:763–772.

95. Savitz DA, Wachtel H, Barnes F. Case-control study of childhood cancer and electromagnetic field exposure. Am J Epidemiol 1987; 126:780.

96. Simone JV, Aur RJA, Hustu HO. Combined modality therapy of acute lymphocytic leukemia. Cancer 1975; 35:25.

97. Smith SD, Winick N, Shuster J, et al. Treatment of isolated central nervous system relapse in children with ALL. A POG study. Proc Am Soc Clin Oncol 1990.

98. Smith SD, Woffard M, Shuster J, et al. Treatment of testicular leukemia in children with ALL. A POG study. Proc Am Soc Clin Oncol 1990; 9:218. (Abstract.)

99. Steinherz PG. Acute lymphoblastic leukemia of childhood. Hematol Oncol 1987; 1:549–566.

100. Steuber CP, Krischer J, Colbert S, et al. Prognostic factors and treatment outcome in childhood acute myeloid leukemia (AML): The POG experience. In Gale RD (ed): Acute Myelogenous Leukemia: Prog-

ress and Controversies. New York: Wiley Liss, 1989, pp 193–203.

101. Sullivan MP, Hrgovic M. Extramedullary leukemia. In Sutow WW, Vietti TJ, Fernbach DJ (eds): Clinical and Pediatric Oncology, 2nd ed. St. Louis: CV Mosby, 1977.

102. Swansbury GJ, Secker-Walker LM, Lawler SD, et al. Chromosomal findings in acute lymphoblastic leukemia of childhood. An independent prognostic factor. Lancet 1981; 2:249.

103. Trueworthy R, Shuster J, Look AT, et al. Ploidy of lymphoblasts is the strongest predictor of treatment outcome in B-progenitor cell acute lymphoblastic leukemia in childhood: A Pediatric Oncology Group Study. J Clin Oncol 1992; 10:606.

104. Tucker MA, Meadows AT, Boice JD, et al. Leukemia after therapy with alkylating agents from childhood cancer. J Natl Cancer Inst 1987; 78:459–464.

105. Vderzo C, Zurol MG, Adamoloi L, et al. Treatment of isolated testicular relapse in childhood acute lymphoblastic leukemia: An Italian Multicenter Study. J Clin Oncol 1990; 8:672–677.

106. Vietti TJ, Land VJ, Ragab AH. Management of acute leukemia. In Sutow WW, Vietti TJ, Fernbach DJ (eds): Clinical Pediatric Oncology, 2nd ed. St. Louis: CV Mosby, 1977.

107. Vigliani E, Saita G. Benzene and leukemia. N Engl J Med 1964; 271:872.

108. Vincent P. Pathophysiology. In Henderson ES, Lister TA (eds): Leukemia, 5th ed. Philadelphia: WB Saunders, 1990, pp 19–34.

109. Vogler LB, Crist WM, Bockman DE. Pre-B cell leukemia. A new phenotype of childhood lymphoblastic leukemia. N Engl J Med 1978; 298:872–878.

110. Weinstein HJ. The childhood leukemias. In Moossa AR, Schimpff SC, Robson MC (eds): Comprehensive Textbook on Oncology, vol 2. Baltimore: Williams & Wilkins, 1991, pp 1486–1498.

111. Wertheimer D, Leeper E. Electrical wiring configuration and childhood cancer. Am J Epidemiol 1979; 109:270–284.

112. West RJ, Graham-Pole J, Hardisty RM, et al. Factors in pathogenesis of central nervous system leukemia. Br Med J 1972; 3:311.

113. Wong K, Ballard ET, Strayer FH. Clinical and occult testicular leukemia in long-term survivors of ALL. J Pediatr 1980; 96:569–574.

114. Wright JJ, Poplack DC, Bakhski A, et al. Gene rearrangements as markers of clonol variation and minimal residual disease in ALL. J Clin Oncol 1987; 5:535–541.

115. Young JL, Ries LG, Silverberg E. Cancer incidence, survival and mortality for children younger than 15 years. Cancer 1986; 58:598–602.

ACUTE MYELOGENOUS LEUKEMIA

Frances McKinney Wiley

The term *acute myelogenous leukemia (AML)* includes a heterogeneous group of hematologic malignancies characterized by the accumulation of leukemic blasts in marrow and extramedullary sites.[17] As in the lymphoblastic form, AML develops in the bone marrow and is characterized by the presence of immature, relatively undifferentiated cells that proliferate and replace healthy marrow elements.[28,29] The term *acute nonlymphoblastic leukemia (ANLL)* was previously used, particularly in the pediatric literature, to designate any leukemia that was not clearly lymphoid, but *acute myelogenous leukemia* has recently become the accepted nomenclature for this group of leukemias.

The reported incidence of AML is 15% to 25% of leukemia in childhood.[11,14,23] There is a relatively constant incidence from birth through adolescence. Approximately 10% of childhood AML occurs in infants under 2 years of age. In neonates less than 1 month of age true monoclonal leukemia, as distinguished from a polyclonal leukemoid reaction (marked elevation of WBC), is most often AML.[17] There are no consistently reported differences between sexes nor ethnic groups. Even though a great deal of progress has been made in the last decade, AML still accounts for 30% to 50% of deaths from childhood leukemia.[13,20]

ETIOLOGY

The etiology of AML is unknown. Most children with AML have no obvious predisposing conditions, although certain children are at greater-than-average risk. These risk groups include the identical twins of children with acute leukemia (particularly before the age of 6 years), children with certain genetically determined disorders, and children exposed to certain environmental factors.[7,11,20,27,28]

Ionizing radiation produced myeloid leukemia in survivors of the Hiroshima and Nagasaki atomic bombs.[20,24] Treatment with alkylating agents, particularly in combination with radiation, has been associated with an increased incidence of AML.[2] One study from the Children's Cancer Group reported a tenfold risk of AML in infants born to mothers who used marijuana while pregnant.[17,22,26] Research is ongoing to study environmental exposure to chemicals, especially benzene, pesticides, and drugs, as they may relate to the development of AML in children.[6,17,20,26]

Children with certain congenital or inherited disorders are at higher risk for developing leukemia. Trisomy 21 (Down syndrome), Fanconi's anemia, Bloom syndrome, Kostmann's syndrome, and Diamond-Blackfan syndrome all are associated with an increased risk.[11,20] Neurofibromatosis and Klinefelter's syndrome have also been associated with AML.[17] The interaction between genetic abnormalities and environmental risk factors as a cause for leukemia is unknown.[20]

No specific oncogene has been identified in AML. Fifty percent to 100% of patients with AML have chromosomal abnormalities in the malignant (blast) cells.[11,13–15,25,36] Appreciation of the frequency of chromosomal abnormalities has increased over time as cytogenetic techniques have improved. Certain abnormal bone marrow karyotypes are associated with specific histologic subtypes of AML.[17,25,35,36] It is not known whether the chromosomal changes result from factors causing AML or whether these changes are the cause of the leukemic process.[25,31] The bone marrow karyotype returns to normal during remission, and usually the same abnormality returns if relapse occurs.

TYPES OF AML

Classification of this heterogenous group of diseases is important in the design and evaluation of therapies and allows more precise study of the epidemiology and etiology. Theoretically, any cell along the pathway from a pluripotent stem cell can become transformed.[11,31] Figure 8–3 illustrates cell lines from which the malignant clone in various types of AML originates. Along with mor-

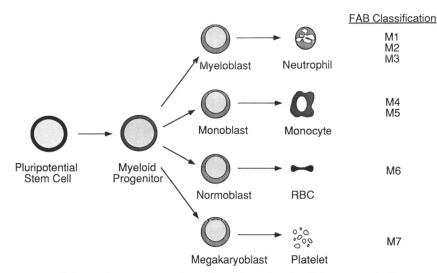

FIGURE 8-3. Schematic representation of nonlymphoid cell lines in which a malignant clone arises showing FAB subtypes of AML. *(Modified from Sawyers CL, Denny CT, Witte ON. Leukemia and the disruption of normal hematopoiesis. Cell 1991, 64:337–350. © Cell Press.)*

phologic and cytogenetic characterizations, a variety of cell surface markers and biochemical markers are used to define subtypes.

The French-American-British (FAB) system classifies the subtypes of AML according to the morphologic and cytochemical characteristics of the malignant cells and has been used extensively to report and standardize data[3,11] (Table 8–2). This system is not related to the M_1, M_2, and M_3 marrow ratings discussed in the ALL section.

In M1 leukemia (myeloblastic without differentiation) the blasts are poorly differentiated, lack maturation, and may have occasional Auer rods (abnormal lysosomes). Auer rods are frequently seen in M2 (myeloblastic with differentiation) blasts, which also show differentiation beyond the promyelocyte stage. M3 (acute promyelocytic) blasts have bundles of Auer rods and are packed with azurophilic granules. M4 (myelomonocytic) blasts have both myeloblastic and monoblastic differentiation. M5 (monocytic) blast cells are large monoblasts with folded nuclei, basophilic vacuolated cytoplasm, and pseudopods. In the M5 type of AML subgroups are categorized by the degree of differentiation; the more poorly differentiated variant is more commonly seen in children.[22] The M6 type (erythroleukemia) is characterized by bizarre dyserythropoiesis with an excess of erythro-

TABLE 8—2. *French-American-British (FAB) Classification of ANLL*

FAB CLASSIFICATION	COMMON NAME
M1	Acute myeloblastic leukemia without differentiation
M2	Acute myeloblastic leukemia with differentiation
M3	Acute promyelocytic leukemia
M4	Acute myelomonocytic leukemia
M5	Acute monocytic leukemia
M6	Erythroleukemia
M7	Acute megakaryoblastic leukemia

blasts, which are also often present in the peripheral blood. Auer rods may be present. The M7 type (megakaryoblastic) is characterized by megakaryoblasts that are undifferentiated and lymphoid in appearance. Standard staining techniques of bone marrow samples are not adequate to characterize M7 clearly. Electron microscopy and ultracytochemistry are used to make the diagnosis.[12,29]

Approximately one half of pediatric AML

is M1 or M2. Another one third is M4 or M5. The remaining cases are the far more rare M3, M6, or M7.

PROGNOSTIC FACTORS

Prognostic factors in AML are less clearly defined than in ALL because of the historically poor overall survival rate and because AML is a heterogeneous group of leukemias.[10,17] Since AML is a rare disease without a large population of survivors, it is difficult to define prognostic variables consistently.

As an example, most investigators associate a high WBC at presentation with a poor outcome.[10,17] A recent analysis of more than 1000 children with AML demonstrates that there is a *progressive* increase in risk, proportional to the WBC at diagnosis, without a threshold effect. That is, patients do not fall naturally into *groups* at high risk and low risk based on WBC, but that risk increases with increasing counts.[4]

Reports conflict about the effect of age on outcome. Neonates (<1 month of age) uniformly have a poor prognosis. Some studies, but not all, show a poorer prognosis for infants (<2 years of age) than for older children. This prognosis may be related to the increased incidence of FAB M4 and M5 types in this age group.[4,11,17,23,24,29]

An increasing ability to assess cell lineage and differentiation may lead to the definition of subtypes that are biologically and prognostically meaningful. As yet, morphologic types have not been consistently associated with outcome, with the possible exception of M5 in infants, which has a poorer prognosis.[4,10,17,22]

The presence or absence of abnormal chromosomes has not consistently been shown to affect outcome in children. Of those with abnormalities (approximately 80%), certain karyotypes have been associated with poorer outcomes, whereas others seem to have a more favorable prognosis.[15,17,25,36] A rapid response to therapy, as measured by a day 7 bone marrow examination showing hypocellularity and no residual leukemia, may be an important favorable prognostic variable.[18,20]

The lack of well-defined prognostic factors in AML reflects the fact that most analyses

are done on relatively small numbers of patients. Different treatment regimens may demonstrate equally valid but different prognostic variables.[10,17] Outcome may be related to the intensity of therapy and specific modalities and may or may not always relate to prognostic factors. The ability to improve outcome by choosing therapy based on stratification according to clinical or biologic prognostic variables awaits an improved understanding of these factors.

CLINICAL PRESENTATION

Children with AML may present with a wide spectrum of findings, from being virtually asymptomatic to a sudden onset of life-threatening hemorrhage or sepsis.[11,13,19] As in ALL, presentation usually reflects diminished bone marrow function with signs of infection, bleeding, and/or anemia.

Children often present with fever (42%), sore throat (18%), or other respiratory symptoms (23%). Recurrent or persistent bacterial infections may be the presenting symptom (3%) because of the frequently depressed absolute neutrophil count.[13] Sepsis may occur at presentation or soon after treatment is begun. Anemia with the resultant pallor, weakness, and fatigue is also common (44%). Congestive heart failure, dyspnea, headache, and tinnitus can also be present as a result of the anemia.

Bleeding is a presenting symptom in 33%.[13] Petechiae, bruising, epistaxis, and gingival oozing are the most common sites of bleeding at presentation. Bleeding, including cutaneous, mucosal, and menorrhagic, is usually associated with thrombocytopenia but may also result from disseminated intravascular coagulation (DIC). DIC may occur in any subtype of AML. It nearly always occurs in M3, acute promelocytic leukemia, because of alterations in the coagulation process caused by release of abnormal intracellular granules in the promyelocytic leukemic cells.[13] The DIC can become worse with the start of therapy as the cells lyse and release additional granules.[6,9,21]

The WBC and percentage of circulating blasts at diagnosis are quite variable. The WBC may range from relatively normal to hyperleukocytosis (WBC >100,000), which is seen in approximately 22% of children with AML.[5,6,12]

Extramedullary AML can occur in any organ or tissue.[21] The overall incidence of CNS disease at diagnosis has been reported from 10% to 25%.[13,34] Children with a high leukocyte count, those under 2 years of age, and those with acute myelomonocytic (M4) or acute monocytic (M5) types have a higher incidence of CNS involvement. CNS disease in AML is usually meningeal infiltration and may be asymptomatic or have either diffuse or focal neurologic findings.

Hepatomegaly or splenomegaly is present in over one half of the children at diagnosis. Less than 25% of children present with significant lymphadenopathy. Most of these patients have M4 or M5 type AML.[11,34] Gingival infiltration leading to gum hypertrophy is characteristically seen in M4 and M5 AML. Testicular involvement may be seen at diagnosis or relapse.[13,17]

Chloromas are localized tumors of malignant cells also called *granulocytic sarcomas* or *myeloblastomas*. Chloromas may appear before signs of bone marrow involvement, either at diagnosis or relapse. Multiple skin nodules (leukemia cutis) and subcutaneous chloromas are more common in infants, particularly those with the M5 phenotype, but the exact incidence is unknown. Rarely, chloromas can occur in the brain or as epidural tumors. Children may present with ptosis secondary to a periorbital chloroma or with cord compression from an epidural lesion.[11,13,17]

Infants (<2 years of age), when compared to older children, are more apt to have monoblastic M5 or myelomonoblastic M4 leukemia; they often present with chloromas, hepatomegaly, and high WBC.[24] Neonates (<1 month of age) often present with an initial WBC greater than 100,000, and nodular infiltration of the skin, lungs, liver, and spleen is common.[23,24]

A myelodysplastic syndrome (MDS) may precede the development of AML, although it is less common in children than adults. MDS involves disorders of stem cell maturation and encompasses a variety of clinical conditions.[32,34] MDS (sometimes referred to as *preleukemia*) is defined as less than in the bone marrow, circulating blasts with Auer rods, chromosomal abnormalities, and dysfunction in at least two of the three cell lines.[17] MDS may be present for several months or years before progressing to AML.

TREATMENT

Immediate therapy must be directed toward management of any life-threatening complications that may be present. Bleeding, hyperleukocytosis, and sepsis all require immediate intervention.[11,13,19] DIC can occur with any type of AML but is a common problem in M3. Tumor lysis syndrome is less frequent in AML than in ALL, but careful medical management is still required to prevent or treat it.

Leukostasis, intravascular clumping of blasts, causes hypoxia, hemorrhage, and infarction of the affected tissues. It is rare except in the presence of hyperleukocytosis (<200,000/mm³).[11] When it does occur, it is a medical emergency. Many of these patients will have headaches, blurred vision, and respiratory problems due to the leukostasis and leukemic infiltration in the CNS and lungs. Cerebrovascular accidents (CVA) associated with hyperleukocytosis have a substantial mortality rate. The metabolic abnormalities hyperkalemia, hypocalcemia, hyperuricemia, and hyperphosphatemia may be present because of renal compromise secondary to leukostasis.[13]

The treatment of choice for hyperleukocytosis remains controversial. Leukopheresis is one approach to reduce viscosity and numbers of circulating blasts but is technically difficult in infants and very small children, and its effects are not long lasting. Double-volume exchange transfusion may be used. Emergency low-dose cranial irradiation has also been used in an attempt to prevent CVAs, but its efficacy remains unproved.[11] Hydroxyurea may be given to decrease the circulating blasts, often in conjunction with irradiation.[11,17] Definitive treatment for the leukemia must be started as soon as possible in patients with hyperleukocytosis, with exceptionally careful monitoring and supportive care.

Antileukemic therapy is designed to use

combinations of drugs that attack leukemic cells by different mechanisms.

Cytosine arabinoside (ara-C) and one of the anthracyclines, daunorubicin (Daunomycin) or doxorubicin (Adriamycin), are included in most induction regimens.[5,10,17,28,34,37]

Daunorubicin is used more often than doxorubicin because there is a lower incidence of severe GI toxicity.[5,11,13] In addition to an anthracycline and cytosine arabinoside, specific regimens may include an etoposide, vincristine, prednisone or another steroid, 6-thioguanine, cyclophosphamide, 5-azacytidine, and other drugs.[11,13,19,21,33]

Successful remission induction can be achieved in 70% to 80% of patients with AML.[5,17,19,21] Less intense regimens have a higher rate of failure of remission induction or of early relapse, and more intense early treatment is associated with increased toxicity.[13] Of those children who do not achieve remission, approximately one half die from infection, leukostasis, or bleeding, and the other half die of resistant leukemia.[29]

Tretinion (all-*trans*-retinoic acid), a differentiation agent that induces blast cells to differentiate and mature, has been successful in obtaining remission in patients with M3, acute promyelocytic leukemia. Marrow aplasia does not occur with this approach. Transient hyperleukocytosis may occur. The role of tretinion in maintaining remission has not been determined.[7,35]

CNS prophylaxis using intrathecal cytosine arabinoside and/or methotrexate with or without cranial irradiation is an element of most pediatric AML protocols. CNS prophylaxis is included to avoid the morbidity of CNS relapse, even though it has not been convincingly shown to improve overall disease-free survival.[11,17,37] The exact schedule and timing of CNS prophylaxis are variable.

Once remission is achieved, further treatment, often referred to as *continuation therapy*, is necessary. Investigation of several strategies is ongoing. The duration, intensity, and timing of continuation therapy remain controversial. Most protocols call for intensification and/or consolidation phases with high doses of chemotherapy or maintenance therapy that is less myelosuppressive. Some protocols call for bone marrow transplantation (BMT) as consolidation.[11,13,19,21,34,37]

BMT is an important modality in childhood AML (see Chapter 6). Many treatment centers recommend BMT in first remission when a fully matched human leukocyte antigen (HLA)-compatible sibling donor is available.[12,14] Others reserve BMT for patients who relapse.[11,13,29]

Randomized trials have shown allogeneic BMT is slightly more effective in maintaining remission than continuation chemotherapy.[11,19] As both induction and continuation chemotherapy become more effective, the advantage of BMT over chemotherapy is less apparent.[19]

Approaches to patients without a compatible sibling donor are under investigation. The use of less than perfectly matched family members and matched unrelated donors for BMT have increased problems with nonengraftment or severe graft-versus-host disease (GVHD).

Autologous BMT (using the patient's own bone marrow) is being studied as an approach to patients without an appropriate donor.[11] Autologous BMT has the potential disadvantages of transplanting residual leukemia cells in the marrow and losing an antileukemic graft-versus-leukemia effect (see Chapter 6). Advantages include a high rate of engraftment and diminished risk of GVHD.

Studies are ongoing to compare intensive chemotherapy and allogeneic and autologous BMTs. When remission is achieved, HLA testing of patient and family is appropriate to determine if a potential donor exists. Harvesting, cryopreserving, and storing of remission marrow also increase the options for an individual patient should relapse occur.

With intensive treatment, approximately 50% of relapsed patients can achieve a second remission.[11,13,17] As with ALL, patients who relapse off therapy have a better prognosis than those who relapse while on treatment. Second remissions usually are of shorter duration, and there are few long-term survivors with chemotherapy alone. The poor prognosis for relapsed patients underscores the importance of frontline therapy and the need to eradicate the disease with effective initial treatment.[4]

BMT, allogeneic or autologous, offers the best chance for survival in relapsed patients. It is unclear whether it is preferable to attempt a second induction or do a bone marrow transplant in early relapse if a matched sibling donor or previously cryopreserved autologous marrow is available.[11,13,29]

For children with a MDS, the optimal strategy for treatment is unknown. If a donor is available, BMT offers the best chance for survival.[30] Other approaches include using both low-dose and aggressive chemotherapy, agents to induce maturation and differentiation of blast cells, and biologic response modifiers.[32,34]

PROGNOSIS

Although AML continues to have a poorer outlook than ALL, there has been significant progress in the last 10 years. Approximately 75% of children newly diagnosed with AML achieve a complete remission. Despite these advances, only 25% to 40% of pediatric patients are long-term survivors, whether treated with intensive chemotherapy or BMT.[4,11,16,17,37] Prognosis for children who do not respond well to initial therapy and those who relapse remains very poor.[4,5,10,16,17]

FUTURE DIRECTIONS

An understanding of the pathogenesis and cause of AML may improve through multidisciplinary epidemiologic studies that examine environmental, genetic, and immunologic factors. As causative factors are precisely identified, certain risks may be reduced or eliminated.[20]

Several different strategies are being evaluated to improve the outlook for children with AML. Evaluation of response to initial treatment to allow earlier introduction of alternative therapy is important.[11,16,17] Development of new drugs and of new uses for established drugs continues. Targeting plasma concentrations of drugs and adjusting doses to achieve these concentrations in individual patients are being explored.[21]

The use of colony-stimulating factors (CSF) to stimulate normal marrow elements to proliferate (to shorten hematopoietic toxicity) or to recruit quiescent cells into the cell cycle and thus increase their responsiveness to chemotherapy is an approach under investigation.[9] A differentiation agent (tretinion) is safe and highly effective in inducing remission in acute promyelocytic leukemia (M3) by causing leukemic cell differentiation. The exact mechanism is unclear, and it is unknown whether receptor sites for this or other differentiation agents are on other types of malignant cells.[7,35]

The ability to support patients through the prolonged periods of marrow aplasia necessary for successful therapy will be enhanced by improvements in blood products, antibiotics, antiviral and antifungal therapies, and nutritional support. Technical advances in pediatric intensive care, including respiratory support, dialysis, and venous access, continue to improve management of both disease-related and therapy-related toxicities—leukostasis, renal failure, infection, and bleeding. Nursing will continue to play a pivotal role in meeting the challenges of supportive care.

CHRONIC MYELOCYTIC LEUKEMIA

Chronic myelocytic leukemia (CML) is a disorder characterized by the proliferation of relatively mature cells. It is a rare disease in children, representing only 1% to 5% of all childhood leukemia.[1,8,34] It is characterized by marrow hyperplasia, extramedullary hematopoiesis, high WBC, granulocyte precursors in the peripheral blood, and a specific cytogenetic marker, the Philadelphia (Ph) chromosome.[1,34]

ETIOLOGY

Little is known about the etiology of most leukemias. Even less is known about CML, especially in children.[20] The only known risk factor clearly associated with CML is ionizing radiation, and this is rarely implicated in pediatric cases.[1,20] The Ph chromosome is the result of a reciprocal translocation t(9;22)(q34;q11). Due to the association of the Ph translocation in most cases of CML, it is suggested that environmental agents that cause chromosomal breaks may be important.

TYPES

There are two distinct types of CML. The adult type usually occurs in older children and adolescents. In 90% of cases the Ph chromosome is present in all myeloid cells but not in somatic cells. There is usually a high WBC, eosinophilia, and basophilia.

Juvenile CML (JCML) is very rare. It is almost always seen in infants (<2 years of age). It is distinguished from the adult form by age at onset, cutaneous manifestations, lymphadenopathy, thrombocytopenia, elevated fetal hemoglobin and immunoglobulin levels, prominent involvement of the monocyte series, and a relatively rapid course.[1] There are an absence of the Ph chromosome and no consistent karyotypic abnormality.[34]

CLINICAL PRESENTATION

In adult type CML chronic, accelerated, and blast phases represent the natural history of the disease as it progresses from hyperproliferation of mostly mature cells to a differentiation arrest with proliferation of immature cells.[1,34] Most children are diagnosed in the chronic phase. They usually have splenomegaly and may have fever, night sweats, pallor, weight loss, and bone pain. The spectrum of symptoms can range from asymptomatic mild splenomegaly to massive hepatosplenomegaly, lymphadenopathy, and extreme elevations of WBC. In those children with hyperleukocytosis, focal or diffuse neurologic findings, respiratory distress, metabolic disturbances, or priapism may be present. Response to therapy to lower the WBC is rapid, but there is no loss of the Ph chromosome in the myeloid cells. The chronic phase lasts, on the average, 3 to 4 years.[1,8,34]

Eventually an accelerated phase occurs. This phase may happen gradually or abruptly and is characterized by an increasing WBC with more immature forms and increasing resistance to therapy. The early symptoms of fever, night sweats, and weight loss can recur. CNS leukemia or chloromas may develop. An abrupt evolution to the accelerated phase, with a rapidly increasing population of peripheral blasts and concurrent neutropenia and thrombocytopenia, is referred to as *blast crisis.*

New chromosomal abnormalities develop during the accelerated phase and usually involve the duplication of the Ph chromosome. Other abnormalities, including isochromosome 17 and trisomy 8, can occur.[1,20]

The blast phase is characterized by having more than 30% blasts in the bone marrow.[1] The leukemic clone loses the ability to differentiate. Since CML affects the stem cells, the blast transformation may involve any lineage. Most often, in 60% to 70% of cases, the cells are myeloblastic, but lymphoblastic and mixed lineage transformation can also occur. Clinically, this phase resembles acute leukemia, with anemia, thrombocytopenia, and increased blasts in the marrow and peripheral blood.

JCML usually presents before age 2 years, with cutaneous lesions (eczema, xanthomata, and cafe-au-lait spots), generalized lymphadenopathy, marked splenomegaly, hepatomegaly, and hemorrhagic problems. Respiratory symptoms, including cough, expiratory wheezing, and tachypnea, may be present.[1,8] A facial rash (erythematous, maculopapular, or desquamative) is common and may be present for several months before the appearance of the leukemic manifestations. Increased fetal hemoglobin values and mild anemia often occur.[34]

PROGNOSTIC FACTORS

For adult type CML, the duration of the chronic phase is the major determinant of length of survival since most patients die within months of transformation to the accelerated or blast phase. In adults certain prognostic factors present at diagnosis predict early transformation. They include splenomegaly, hepatomegaly, thrombocytopenia (<150,000/mm³), thrombocytosis (>500,000/mm³), marked leukocytosis (>100,000/mm³), greater than 1% circulating blasts, or greater than 20% circulating immature granulocytes. In children the prognostic factors are less clear.[1]

TREATMENT

BMT is the only curative treatment available for either adult or juvenile CML.[8,23,30,34] BMT is available to only a minority of patients because of the lack of a suitable donor. The results of BMT are best if the transplant is done in the first chronic phase (50% to 70% long-term survival)

In adult type CML the goal of therapy in the chronic phase is to provide symptomatic relief by lowering the WBC and reducing liver and spleen size. Hydroxyurea or busulfan, given as single agents, is used to regulate leukocytosis. Splenic irradiation and, rarely, splenectomy may be used for symptomatic relief of painful, massive splenomegaly, but they are usually reserved for palliation in patients resistant to chemotherapy.

The goal of treatment in the accelerated, or blast, phase is to obtain reversion to the chronic phase. Intensive, multiagent chemotherapy may return some patients to chronic phase. Those with lymphoblastic transformation are more likely to enter a second chronic phase.

JCML is generally resistant to therapy, although occasional short remissions have been reported with intensive multiagent chemotherapy, and a few children are surviving after BMT.[1,30,34]

PROGNOSIS

Nearly all children with CML will eventually die from the disease. In the adult type, once an initial cytoreduction has been accomplished, the quality of life may be quite good during a chronic phase that may last several years (average, 3 to 4 years). Eventually a blast phase resistant to all therapy will occur and lead to death from leukostasis, bleeding, or infection.[1]

The prognosis in JCML is very poor, with median survival length less than 9 months from diagnosis. Most patients die from infection.[1,34]

FUTURE DIRECTIONS

Autologous BMT using marrow harvested during the chronic phase and subjected to long-term culture techniques to deplete the marrow of Ph cells is a possible approach to patients without a BMT donor.[1]

Both interferons alpha and gamma have shown some ability to induce remission in the chronic phase of CML.[1]

Differentiation of leukemic cells in vitro by tretinion and low-dose cytosine arabinoside has led to clinical trials to determine whether these drugs can delay or prevent transformation to the blast phase.[1]

CML was the first form of leukemia recognized as a distinct clinical entity (in 1844). The Ph chromosome was the first specific chromosomal abnormality associated with a human malignancy (in 1960), and its discovery ushered in the era of cancer cytogenetics.[1] Hopefully, continued research into the biology and pathogenesis of these and other rare leukemias will lead to improved treatment strategies.

REFERENCES

1. Altman AJ. Chronic leukemias of childhood. In Pizzo PA, Poplack DG (eds): Principles and Practice of Pediatric Oncology, 2nd ed. Philadelphia: JB Lippincott, 1993, pp 501–518.
2. Andrieu JM, Ifrah N, Payen C, et al. Increased risk of secondary acute nonlymphocytic leukemia after extended-field radiation therapy combined with MOPP chemotherapy for Hodgkin's disease. J Clin Oncol 1990; 8:1148–1154.
3. Bennett JM, Catovsky D, Daniel MT, et al. Proposals for the classification of the acute leukemias. Br J Haematol 1976; 33:451–458.
4. Buckley JD, Chard RL, Baehner RL, et al. Improvement in outcome for children with acute nonlymphocytic leukemia: A report from the Children's Cancer Study Group. Cancer 1989; 63:1457–1465.
5. Buckley JD, Lampkin BC, Nesbit ME, et al. Remission induction in children with acute non-lymphocytic leukemia using cytosine arabinoside and doxorubicin or daunorubicin: A report from the Children's Cancer Study Group. Med Pediatr Oncol 1989; 17:382–390.
6. Buckley JD, Robison LL, Swotinsky R, et al. Occupational exposures of parents of children with acute nonlymphocytic leukemia: A report from the Children's Cancer Study Group. Cancer Res 1989; 49:4030–4037.
7. Castaigne S, Chomienne C, Daniel MT, et al. All-trans retinoic acid as a differentiation therapy for acute promyelocytic leukemia. I. Clinical Results. Blood 1990; 76:1704–1709.
8. Castoria HA, Harris M. Childhood leukemias. In Hockenberry MJ, Coody DK (eds): Pediatric Oncology and Hematology—Perspectives on Care. St. Louis: CV Mosby, 1986, pp 14–42.
9. Estey E, Kurzrock R, Talpaz M, et al. Use of CSFs in AML. In Gale RP (ed): Acute Myelogenous Leukemia: Progress and Controversies. New York: Wiley-Liss, 1989, pp 441–446.
10. Grier HE, Gelber RD, Camitta BM, et al. Prognostic factors in childhood acute myelogenous leukemia. J Clin Oncol 1987; 5:1026–1032.
11. Greier HE, Weinstein HJ. Acute myelogenous leukemia. In Pizzo PA, Poplack DG (eds): Principles and Practice of Pediatric Oncology, 2nd ed. Philadelphia: JB Lippincott, 1993, pp 483–500.
12. Hirt A, Luethy AR, Mueller B, et al. Acute megakaryoblastic leukemia in children identified by im-

munological marker studies. Am J Pediatr Hematol Oncol 1990; 12:27–33.

13. Kalwinsky DK, Mirro J Jr, Dahl GV. Biology and therapy of childhood acute nonlymphocytic leukemia. Pediatr Ann 1988; 17:172–190.

14. Kalwinsky DK, Raimondi SC, Schell MJ, et al. Cytogenetic abnormalities in childhood AML. In Gale RP (ed): Acute Myelogenous Leukemia: Progress and Controversies. New York: Wiley-Liss, 1989, pp 133–139.

15. Kalwinsky DK, Raimondi SC, Schell MJ, et al. Prognostic importance of cytogenetic subgroups in de novo pediatric acute nonlymphocytic leukemia. J Clin Oncol 1990; 8:75–83.

16. Krischer JP, Steuber CP, Vietti TJ, et al. Long-term results in the treatment of acute nonlymphocytic leukemia: A Pediatric Oncology Group study. Med Pediatr Oncol 1989; 17:401–408.

17. Lampkin BC, Lange B, Bernstein I, et al. Biologic characteristics and treatment of acute nonlymphocytic leukemia in children. Pediatr Clin North Am 1988; 35:743–764.

18. Lampkin BC, Woods W, Strauss R, et al. Current status of the biology and treatment of acute nonlymphocytic leukemia in children (report from the ANLL strategy group of the Children's Cancer Study Group). Blood 1983; 61:215–228.

19. Lange B, Lampkin B, Woods W, et al. Children's Cancer Study Group trials for acute non-lymphoblastic leukemia (ANLL) in children. In Gale RP (ed): Acute Myelogenous Leukemia: Progress and Controversies. New York: Wiley-Liss, 1989, pp 205–217.

20. Linet MS. The Leukemias: Epidemiologic Aspects. New York: Oxford University Press, 1985.

21. Mirro J, Crom W, Santana VM, et al. AML trials at St. Jude Children's Research Hospital. In Gale RP (ed): Acute Myelogenous Leukemia: Progress and Controversies. New York: Wiley-Liss, 1989, pp 219–227.

22. Odom L, Lampkin BC, Tannous R, et al. Acute monoblastic leukemia: A unique subtype—A review from the Children's Cancer Study Group. Leuk Res 1990; 10:1–10.

23. Poplack DG, Kun LE, Cassady JR, et al. Leukemias and lymphomas of childhood. In De Vita VT Jr, Hellman S, Rosenberg SA (eds): Cancer Principles and Practice of Oncology, 3rd ed, vol 2. Philadelphia: JB Lippincott, 1989, pp 1671–1695.

24. Pui C-H, Kalwinsky DK, Schell MJ, et al. Acute nonlymphoblastic leukemia in infants: Clinical presentation and outcome. J Clin Oncol 1988; 6:1008–1013.

25. Raimondi SC, Kalwinsky DK, Hayashi Y, et al. Cytogenetics of childhood acute nonlymphocytic leukemia. Cancer Genet Cytogenet 1989; 40:13-27.

26. Robison LL, Buckley JD, Daigle AE, et al. Maternal drug use and risk of childhood nonlymphoblastic leukemia among offspring—An epidemiologic investigation implicating marijuana. Cancer 1989; 63:1904–1911.

27. Ruccione K. Acute leukemia in children: Current prospectives. Issues Compr Pediatr Nurs 1983; 6:329–363.

28. Ruccione K. Impaired cellular function and alterations. In Servonsky J, Opas SR (eds): Nursing Management of Children. Boston: Jones & Bartlett, 1987, pp 1068–1154.

29. Sallan SE, Weinstein HJ. Childhood acute leukemia. In Nathan DG, Oski FA (eds): Hematology of Infancy and Childhood, 3rd ed, vol 2. Philadelphia: WB Saunders, 1987, pp 1028–1063.

30. Sanders JE, Buckner CD, Thomas ED, et al. Allogeneic marrow transplantation for children with juvenile chronic myelogenous leukemia. Blood 1988; 71:1144–1146.

31. Sawyers CL, Denny CT, Witte ON. Leukemia and the disruption of normal hematopoiesis. Cell 1991; 64:337–350.

32. Schwartz CL, Cohen HJ. Myeloproliferative and myelodysplastic syndromes. In Pizzo PA, Poplack DG (eds): Principles and Practice of Pediatric Oncology, 2nd ed. Philadelphia: JB Lippincott, 1993, pp 519–536.

33. Steuber CP, Krischer J, Culbert S, et al. Prognostic factors and treatment outcome in childhood acute myeloid leukemia (AML): The POG experience. In Gale RP (ed): Acute Myelogenous Leukemia: Progress and Controversies. New York: Wiley-Liss, 1989, pp 193–203.

34. Steuber CP, Mahoney DH Jr, Ogden AK. Acute myeloid leukemias and myeloproliferative disorders. In Fernbach DJ, Vietti TJ (eds): Clinical Pediatric Oncology, 4th ed. St. Louis: CV Mosby, 1991, pp 377–396.

35. Warrell RP Jr, Frankel SR, Miller WH Jr, et al. Differentiation therapy of acute promyelocytic leukemia with tretinoin (all-*trans*-retinoic acid). N Engl J Med 1991; 342:1385–1393.

36. Woods WG, Nesbit ME, Buckley J, et al. Correlation of chromosome abnormalities with patient characteristics, histologic subtype, and induction success in children with acute nonlymphocytic leukemia. J Clin Oncol 1985; 3:3–11.

37. Woods WG, Ruymann FB, Lampkin BC, et al. The role of timing of high-dose cytosine arabinoside intensification and of maintenance therapy in the treatment of children with acute nonlymphocytic leukemia. Cancer 1990; 66:1106–1113.

MALIGNANT TUMORS OF CHILDHOOD AND ADOLESCENCE

■ INTRODUCTION

Linda Wofford

Pediatric solid tumors encompass all the malignancies of childhood except the leukemias. Age-adjusted incidence rates of selected pediatric malignancies are detailed in Tables 9–1, 9–2, and 9–3.[2] Table 9–1 reveals a statistically significant overall increase in incidence. Leukemias and brain tumors are the main diseases causing this increase.[1] Table 9–2 and 9–3 note differences based on race, age, and sex. Leukemia, the most common childhood malignancy, is discussed in Chapter 8. Central nervous system (CNS) tumors are the most commonly diagnosed solid tumors.

Childhood solid tumors are typically sarcomas in which tumor cells divide rapidly. This rapid division contributes to the positive treatment response of pediatric solid tumors since many therapies work best on a dividing cell population. Adult solid tumors are usually carcinomas or adenomas, which contain slowly dividing tumor cells. The long latency period of most adult solid tumors contrasts with the more rapid onset of solid tumors in children. Environmental factors have been linked to the onset of adult malignancies but are not strongly associated with cancer in children. Many times the pediatric cancers do not have indentifiable causes, whereas adult cancers often do (e.g., adult lung cancer after years of exposure to cigarette smoke).

As a group the solid tumors have responded well to advances in treatment. The success stories of children diagnosed with Wilms' tumor and retinoblastoma are particularly encouraging. Treatment of CNS tumors and neuroblastomas continues to present formidable challenges.[1]

Multidisciplinary team management has been critical to improved patient outcomes. Because of the complexity of childhood solid tumors, initial treatment planning must be coordinated by a pediatric solid tumor specialist, usually a pediatric oncologist, working in conjunction with other specialists. Information from diagnostic and staging procedures must be assimilated and integrated into a comprehensive plan. The sequence of therapies is more than the sum of the parts. The placement and timing of chemotherapy, radiation, and surgery can be synergistic. Cooperation between the teams is essential for the maximal therapeutic benefit and the well-being of the child.

This chapter is a series of tumor-specific reviews written by an expert(s) in the field of each particular pediatric tumor. Latest available information about each solid tumor's di-

TABLE 9–1. *Age Specific Cancer Incidence Rates and 16-Year Trends, 1973–88, by Race, Sex, and Age Group (All Primary Cancer Sites Combined)**

| | ALL RACES | | | |
| | AVERAGE RATE | | % CHANGE | EAPC |
SEX/AGE (YR)	1973–1974	1987–1988	1973–1988	1973–1988
Males and females				
0–14	12.8	13.4	4.5	0.7†
Males				
0–14	14.2	14.3	0.5	0.6
Females				
0–14	11.3	12.4	9.7	0.8†

Data from reference 2.
*Rates are per 100,000 and are age adjusted to the 1970 U.S. standard population. Each rate has been age adjusted by
†EAPC is significantly different from zero (*p* <.05).
SEER = Surveillance Epidemiology and End Results; average rate = average annual rate over the specified 2-year period;

TABLE 9–2. *Age-Adjusted Cancer Incidence Rates by Primary Site and 5-Year Age Group, White and African-American Males and Females, SEER Program, 1984–1988**

| | WHITE | | | | | | | |
| | MALES | | | | FEMALES | | | |
DISEASE	0–4	5–9	10–14	15–19	0–4	5–9	10–14	15–19
Brain and nervous system	4.2	3.8	2.3	2.4	3.6	3.2	2.3	2.1
Hodgkin's disease	0.1	0.8	1.5	3.9	—	0.3	1.5	4.7
Non-Hodgkin's lymphoma	0.7	1.4	1.9	1.9	0.4	0.7	0.7	1.2
Bone and joint	0.1	0.5	1.6	1.8	0.1	0.6	1.4	1.2
Kidney and renal pelvis	1.8	0.6	0.2	0.1	1.9	0.6	0.1	0.2
Soft tissue	1.4	0.5	0.5	0.8	1.2	0.4	0.7	0.8
Eye and orbit	1.1	0.3	—	0.1	1.3	0.1	—	—
Liver	0.5	0.1	—	0.1	0.5	—	0.2	0.2
Melanoma of skin	0.1	0.1	0.2	1.0	0.2	0.1	0.3	1.9
All sites, including leukemias	21.5	13.0	12.0	20.7	18.8	9.8	11.9	21.0

Data from reference 2.
*Rates are per 100,000 and are age adjusted to the 1970 U.S. standard population. Each rate has been age adjusted

WHITES				AFRICAN-AMERICANS			
AVERAGE RATE		% CHANGE	EAPC	AVERAGE RATE		% CHANGE	EAPC
1973–1974	1987–1988	1973–1988	1973–1988	1973–1974	1987–1988	1973–1988	1973–1988
13.2	13.7	4.1	0.7†	10.3	11.5	11.7	0.9
14.6	14.4	−1.4	0.6	10.3	12.5	21.3	0.9
11.7	13.0	11.3	0.9†	10.3	10.6	2.2	0.9

5-yr age groups.

EAPC = estimated annual percent change over the 16-yr interval.

AFRICAN-AMERICAN							
MALES				FEMALES			
0–4	5–9	10–14	15–19	0–4	5–9	10–14	15–19
3.5	3.1	1.3	3.1	3.7	3.1	2.1	0.2
—	0.6	1.1	1.8	—	—	0.4	1.7
0.2	0.6	1.3	1.5	0.6	0.4	0.4	0.4
—	0.4	0.4	2.0	—	0.2	1.4	0.6
1.5	0.6	0.2	—	2.3	1.2	—	0.7
2.2	0.4	0.4	0.7	1.6	0.4	0.8	1.5
1.3	0.2	—	—	1.4	—	—	—
0.2	—	0.2	0.2	—	—	0.2	0.2
—	—	—	—	—	—	—	—
13.2	10.8	8.2	15.3	15.0	8.3	9.7	13.0

by 5-yr age groups.

TABLE 9–3. *Age-Adjusted Cancer Incidence Rates by Primary Site and 5-Year Age Group, Both Sexes, SEER Program, 1984–1988**

DISEASE	WHITE				AFRICAN-AMERICAN			
	0–4	5–9	10–14	15–19	0–4	5–9	10–14	15–19
Brain and nervous system	3.9	3.5	2.3	2.2	3.6	3.1	1.7	1.7
Hodgkin's disease	—	0.6	1.5	4.3	—	0.3	0.8	1.8
Non-Hodgkin's lymphoma	0.6	1.0	1.3	1.5	0.4	0.5	0.9	0.9
Bone and joint	0.1	0.5	1.5	1.5	—	0.3	0.9	1.3
Kidney and renal pelvis	1.9	0.6	0.2	0.1	1.9	0.9	0.1	0.4
Soft tissue	1.3	0.4	0.6	0.8	1.9	0.4	0.6	1.1
Eye and orbit	1.2	0.2	—	—	1.3	0.1	—	—
Liver	0.5	—	0.1	0.2	0.1	—	0.2	0.2
Melanoma of skin	0.1	0.1	0.2	1.4	—	—	—	—
All sites, including leukemias	20.1	11.4	12.0	20.8	14.1	9.5	9.0	14.2

Data from reference 2.

*Rates are per 100,000 and are age adjusted to the 1970 U.S. standard population. Each rate has been age adjusted by 5-year age groups.

agnosis, prognosis, treatment options, team management and specific long-term effects is summarized. (Chapter 17 deals exclusively with long-term sequelae.) Specific nursing care issues are raised. Chapters 11 through 14 may be consulted for general nursing care.

REFERENCES

1. Bleyer AW. The impact of childhood cancer on the United States and the world. CA 1990; 40:355–367.
2. Ries LAG, Hankey BF, Miller BA, et al. Cancer Statistics Review 1973–88. NIH publication 91-2789. Bethesda, Md.: National Cancer Institute, 1991.

CENTRAL NERVOUS SYSTEM TUMORS

Mary McElwain Petriccione

Primary brain tumors are the most common solid tumors occurring in children, second only to leukemia among all the childhood neoplasms. The annual age-adjusted incidence in children under 15 years of age has increased slightly to 3.3 per 100,000.[53] There are approximately 1000 to 1500 newly diagnosed cases in the United States each year.[71] In the pediatric population several histologic types of tumor occur with varying incidence. The number of each particular type of brain tumor is small. Approximately half of all pediatric brain tumor patients are treated in cancer specialty centers or university hospitals,[17] yet even these centers and cooperative study groups have difficulty accruing large sample sizes.[19] The incidence of brain tumors for Af-

rican-American and white children and for both sexes (except for medulloblastomas and intracranial germ cell neoplasms, for which the male-female ratio is approximately 3:2) is statistically similar. There are, however, different peak ages at which certain histologic types of tumors are most commonly seen.

The classification of brain tumors is difficult because of the lack of a universally accepted grading system. In 1979 the World Health Organization[72] formulated an international histologic classification that helps define the various subgroups of brain tumors. A modification of this system, made by a group of neuropathologists specifically for pediatrics, is in Table 9–4.[54] The diagnosis of "brain tumor" includes many histologic cat-

TABLE 9–4. *WHO Classification of Brain Tumors (Modified for Pediatrics)*

I. Tumors of neuroepithelial tissue
   A. Glial tumors
      1. Astrocytic tumors
         a. Astrocytoma (fibrillary, protoplasmic, gemistocytic, pilocytic, xanthomatous)
         b. Anaplastic astrocytoma
         c. Subependymal giant cell tumors (tuberous sclerosis)
         d. Gigantocellular glioma
      2. Oligodendroglial tumors
         a. Oligodendroglioma
         b. Anaplastic oligodendroglioma
      3. Ependymal tumors
         a. Ependymoma
         b. Anaplastic ependymoma
         c. Myxopapillary ependymoma
      4. Choroid plexus tumors
         a. Choroid plexus papilloma
         b. Anaplastic choroid plexus tumor (carcinoma)
      5. Mixed gliomas
         a. Oligoastrocytoma: anaplastic oligoastrocytoma
         b. Astroependymoma: anaplastic ependymoastrocytoma
         c. Oligoastroependymoma: anaplastic oligoastroependymoma
         d. Oligoependymoma: anaplastic oligoependymoma
         e. Subependymoma-subependymal glomerate astrocytoma
         f. Gliofibroma
      6. Glioblastomatous tumors
         a. Glioblastoma multiforme
         b. Giant cell glioblastoma
         c. Gliosarcoma
      7. Gliomatosis cerebri

From Rorke LB, Giles FH, Davis RL, et al. Revision of the World Health Organization classification of brain tumors for childhood brain tumors. Cancer 1985; 56:1869–1886.

Table continued on following page.

TABLE 9–4. *WHO Classification of Brain Tumors (Modified for Pediatrics)* Continued

B. Neuronal tumors
    1. Gangliocytoma
    2. Anaplastic gangliocytoma
    3. Ganglioglioma
    4. Anaplastic ganglioglioma
C. "Primitive" neuroepithelial tumors
    1. "Primitive" neuroectodermal tumor, not otherwise specified (NOS)
    2. "Primitive" neuroectodermal tumor with
        a. Astrocytes
        b. Oligodendrocytes
        c. Ependymal cells
        d. Neuronal cells
        e. Other (melanocytic, mesenchymal)
        f. Mixed cellular elements
    3. Medulloepithelioma
        a. Medulloepithelioma, NOS
        b. Medulloepithelioma, with
            (1) Astrocytes
            (2) Oligodendrocytes
            (3) Ependymal cells
            (4) Neuronal cells
            (5) Other (melanocytic, mesenchymal)
            (6) Mixed cellular elements
D. Pineal cell tumors
    1. Primitive neuroectodermal tumor (see C above) (pineoblastoma)
    2. Pineocytoma
II. Tumors of meningeal and related tissues
  A. Meningiomas
    1. Meningiomas, NOS
    2. "Papillary" meningioma
    3. Anaplastic meningioma
  B. Meningeal sarcomatous tumors
    1. Meningeal sarcoma, NOS
    2. Rhabdomyosarcoma or leiomyosarcoma
    3. Mesenchymal chondrosarcoma
    4. Fibrosarcoma
    5. Others
  C. Primary melanocytic tumors
    1. Malignant melanoma
    2. Melanomatosis
    3. Melanocytic tumors, miscellaneous
III. Tumors of nerve sheath cells
  A. Neurilemmoma (schwannoma, neurinoma)
  B. Anaplastic neurilemmoma (schwannoma, neurinoma)
  C. Neurofibroma
  D. Anaplastic neurofibroma (neurofibrosarcoma, neurogenic sarcoma)
IV. Primary malignant lymphomas (classify according to local current standards)
V. Tumors of blood vessel origin
  A. Hemangioblastoma
  B. Hemangiopericytoma
  C. Neoplastic angioendotheliosis-angiosarcoma
VI. Germ cell tumors
  A. Germinoma
  B. Embryonal carcinoma
  C. Choriocarcinoma

TABLE 9–4. *WHO Classification of Brain Tumors (Modified for Pediatrics)* Continued

      D. Endodermal sinus tumor
      E. Teratomatous tumors
          1. Immature teratoma
          2. Mature teratoma
          3. Teratocarcinoma
      F. Mixed
  VII. Malformative tumors
      A. Craniopharyngioma
      B. Rathke's cleft cyst
      C. Epidermal cyst
      D. Dermoid cyst
      E. Colloid cyst of third ventricle
      F. Enterogenous or bronchial cyst
      G. Cyst, NOS
      H. Lipoma
      I. Granular cell tumor
      J. Hamartoma
          1. Neuronal
          2. Glial
          3. Neuronoglial
          4. Meningioangioneurinomatosis
 VIII. Tumors of neuroendocrine origin
      A. Tumors of anterior pituitary
          1. Adenoma
          2. Pituitary carcinoma
      B. Paraganglioma
  IX. Local extensions from regional tumors (specify according to primary diagnosis)
   X. Metastatic tumors
  XI. Unclassified tumors

egories. Each is distinct in regard to the clinical presentation, specific treatment, and overall prognosis. Pediatric brain tumors differ from those seen in the adult population. Histologically, approximately 60% of pediatric tumors are of glial origin (e.g., astrocytoma or oligodendroglioma), but the percentage of tumors of glial origin is much smaller in the adult population.[67] Of all pediatric tumors, astrocytomas represent approximately 50%, followed by medulloblastomas (25%), brainstem gliomas (11%), and ependymomas (9%) (Table 9–5).[26] More than half of these tumors are highly malignant and have traditionally responded poorly to treatment. Pediatric brain tumors also differ by location from adult brain tumors (Fig. 9–1).[1] The majority of childhood brain tumors (approximately 60%) arise in the posterior fossa, whereas approximately 75% of adult brain tumors are supratentorial (Table 9–6).[67]

TABLE 9–5. *Distribution of Childhood Brain Tumors*

TUMOR	PERCENT
Astrocytoma	
High grade	11
Cerebellar astrocytoma	13
Cerebral astrocytoma (low grade)	23
Medulloblastoma	25
Brainstem glioma	10
Ependymoma	9
Others	9

From Finlay JL, Goins SC, Uteg R, et al. Progress in the management of childhood brain tumors. Hematol Oncol Clin North Am 1987; 1:753–776.

The cause of childhood brain tumors is unknown, although hereditary and environmental factors have been implicated. Direct correlations exist between certain hereditary

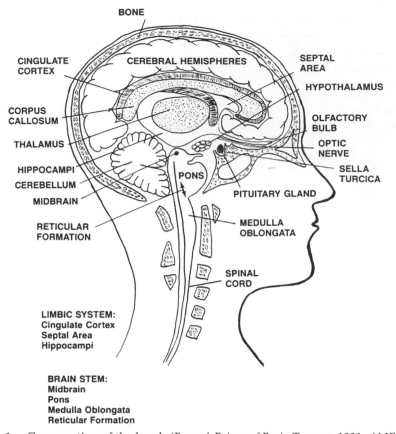

FIGURE 9–1. Cross section of the head. *(From A Primer of Brain Tumors, 1991. AMERICAN BRAIN TUMOR ASSOCIATION, Chicago. Reproduced with permission.)*

TABLE 9–6. *Location of Pediatric Brain Tumors*

LOCATION	PERCENT
Posterior fossa	60
Supratentorial	40
Midline region	15
Cerebral hemisphere	25

From Walker RW, Allen JC. Pediatric brain tumors. Pediatr Ann 1983; 12:385.

and familial syndromes and the occurrence of brain tumors. Neurofibromatosis, tuberous sclerosis, von Hippel-Lindau disease, and retinoblastoma are all autosomal-dominant illnesses associated in varying degrees with tumors of the CNS.[8] Children with neurofibromatosis have a significantly increased risk of developing CNS tumors such as optic gliomas (particularly in children <10 years of age), other types of astrocytomas, acoustic neuromas, and meningiomas.[3] There have been several reports of families with more than one child developing a CNS neoplasm. When examining the oncogenesis of these tumors, the role of heredity needs further study.[35,57]

Environmental agents such as industrial and chemical toxins have been postulated as risk factors in the development of brain tumors. Studies have investigated prenatal and perinatal episodes that may correlate with the increased incidence of brain tumors. Associations have been made between certain parental occupations, particularly those of the father, and a higher incidence of CNS neoplasms.[30] Ionizing radiation is associated with the development of a brain tumor, and there are several documented cases of children who develop a second primary intracranial neoplasm after receiving cranial irradiation.[58] Further investigation of the epidemiology of primary brain tumors is needed, for if specific risk factors are understood, preventive strategies can be developed.

DIAGNOSTIC EVALUATION

Any child suspected of having a CNS neoplasm must receive both a thorough physical and a neurologic examination. Obtaining an accurate history from the parent and child (age appropriate) is crucial. A typical scenario is that of a previously healthy child with a relatively short history of a rapidly progressing local neurologic symptom or increased intracranial pressure (ICP).[46]

The development of computerized tomography (CT) has revolutionized the diagnosis and management of brain tumors. Suspicion of a CNS mass warrants a CT scan with and without iodinated contrast (1 ml/kg given intravenously). Cuts on the scan should be small enough (i.e., not more than 5 mm) to enhance the detection of small lesions. A noncontrast CT scan may reveal relative hypodensity in the area of a brain tumor as compared to normal adjacent tissue, compression of adjacent structures, peritumoral edema due to a disrupted blood-brain barrier, and hydrocephalus. Presence of calcification, cysts, or hemorrhage may suggest certain types of tumors.[26] The enhancement of the mass after the contrast infusion improves detection by localizing and describing the nature and extent of the mass and by distinguishing between edema and hypodense tumor. It may also "light up" tumors that are isodense with surrounding tissue on the unenhanced scan.

Magnetic resonance imaging (MRI) enhanced by the administration of gadolinium diethylenetriaminepentaacetic acid (DTPA), a paramagnetic contrast material, optimally defines neuroanatomy and tumor margins. This technique is superior to that of unenhanced MRI or enhanced CT.[7] Because of its ability to image in three planes, the MRI is particularly helpful in diagnosing infiltrative tumors of the brainstem, and there are no ionizing radiation and no imaging artifacts that obscure CT images in the posterior fossa.

There are disadvantages, however, with the MRI. It does not image calcification unless it is quite extensive. The actual imaging time is longer than with a CT scan and requires the child to stay motionless inside a darkened tube. While the scan is in progress, there is a loud clanging noise, which can frighten a child. It is difficult to monitor a seriously ill child during the scan because of the child's placement in the tube. Currently data from both the CT and MRI give the most comprehensive information about a CNS neoplasm.[4]

Myelography is an important tool used in the detection of tumor dissemination. The myelogram can distinguish tumor nodules along the spinal column and the thickness and abnormality of nerve roots. A follow-up CT scan through areas in question further clarifies the extent of disease. Samples of cerebrospinal fluid (CSF) taken during the procedure are evaluated for the presence of tumor cells or in the case of germ cell tumors, for the presence of specific tumor markers. Tumors that require myelography as part of the initial evaluation are those known to disseminate throughout the neuraxis such as medulloblastomas, high-grade ependymomas, and germ cell tumors.[23] Recently a gadolinium-enhanced MRI of the spine has been demonstrated as an effective means of evaluating neuraxis dissemination of tumor.

Angiography is performed occasionally in situations in which an arteriovenous malformation or aneurysm is suspected. It can also contribute to preoperative evaluation of the neoplasm's vascularity.

Studies currently in the investigational stage are being used in limited clinical situations. The positron-emission tomography (PET) and thallium single photon emission computed tomography (SPECT) scanning techniques provide some insight into whether residual abnormalities seen with CT or MRI after treatment represent live or necrotic tumor cells, a distinction not possible with CT or MRI.

CLINICAL PRESENTATION

The clinical presentation of each child with a CNS neoplasm varies, depending on the tumor's location and the child's age and stage of development.[18] Because the majority of childhood brain tumors arise in the posterior fossa (see Table 9–6),[67] the initial symptoms indicate increased ICP and hydrocephalus caused by compression of the fourth ventricle. The child who presents with increased ICP at the time of diagnosis usually complains of headache. These headaches may be generalized or focal and are usually worse in the morning, although they may also be nocturnal.[56] Vomiting is commonly present, usually without nausea, and may help to relieve the headaches temporarily. Activities such as coughing, straining with a bowel movement, or in severe situations, changing the position of the head aggravate the headache. There is frequently a history of changes in personality, marked by irritability, apathy, depression, fatigue, or lethargy. If the ICP increases, drowsiness may occur, leading to actual somnolence, depression of cardiac and respiratory systems, and ultimately coma. A child less than 3 years of age will present in a similar fashion, with marked irritability, disrupted sleep patterns, resistance to being held or comforted, and anorexia. The child may exhibit developmental delays or begin to lose acquired milestones. Increased head circumference is a sign of increased pressure. Although normal closure of the anterior fontanelle occurs usually between age 8 and 18 months, this may be delayed. When ICP is increased, the fontanelle may lose its normal

pulsation and become elevated tensely above the skull. Double vision may or may not be detected by the child, but dysconjugate eye movements are often found on examination, most commonly due to sixth cranial nerve palsies. Papilledema (usually bilateral) may exist, as may optic atrophy and varying degrees of visual loss. Transient blurring or "greying out" can occur.[33,48,55]

A variety of symptoms specific to certain tumor locations (Table 9–7) assist in localizing the particular tumor area in the brain (see Fig. 9–1). Cerebellar tumors can cause symptoms of gait ataxia and truncal ataxia. Nystagmus, which is a rhythmic movement of the eyes directed toward the side of the lesion, may occur. Head tilt is a common presenting symptom of cerebellar tumors, although the exact mechanism is unknown. Decreased muscle tone, abnormal reflexes, and abnormal speech (specifically scanning speech, characterized by pauses between syllables) may also be present. Symptoms of increased ICP may present early, with rapid onset. Brainstem tumors generally infiltrate the fragile brainstem and rarely cause increased ICP until late in the course of the disease. These tumors more commonly cause multiple cranial nerve abnormalities, a spastic gait, hemi-

TABLE 9–7. *Signs and Symptoms of Brain Tumors According to Location*

BRAINSTEM TUMORS	TUMORS OF CEREBRAL HEMISPHERE	MIDLINE TUMORS	CEREBELLAR TUMORS
Cranial neuropathies	Hemiparesis	Visual loss	Truncal ataxia
Long tract signs	Hemisensory loss	Endocrinopathies Increased appetite Decreased appetite Precocious puberty	Appendicular ataxia
Ataxia	Hemivisual loss	Personality changes	Scanning speech
Late development of increased intracranial pressure	Cognitive changes	Nonlocalizing signs of increased intracranial pressure	Hypotonia
	Seizures		Pendular reflexes Nystagmus toward the involved hemisphere Early development of increased intracranial pressure

From Duffner PK, Cohen MF, Freeman A. Pediatric brain tumors: An Overview. CA. 1985; 35:287–301.

paresis, and upgoing toes (positive Babinski sign).

Supratentorial tumors have multiple symptoms, depending on the involved hemisphere and whether or not hydrocephalus is present as a result of blocked CSF pathways. A focal loss such as a hemiparesis, a partial sensory loss, or visual disturbance may occur. Lesions in the temporal lobe can cause focal seizures, and temporoparietal lesions in the dominant hemisphere can cause aphasia. Frontal lobe lesions can produce personality changes, and occipital lesions affect vision. Midline tumors such as germ cell tumors, optic gliomas, and craniopharyngiomas can cause visual loss or multiple endocrine abnormalities such as thyroid dysfunction, diabetes insipidus, and precocious puberty.[18,23,33]

TREATMENT MODALITIES

The treatment of brain tumors, in general, involves the use of surgery, radiotherapy, and chemotherapy. The actual plan of treatment is specific for each child and depends on the age of the child, the pathology, the location of the tumor, and the degree of tumor dissemination.

Surgery

Once a brain tumor has been evaluated, a neurosurgical procedure is commonly the next step in the plan of care. The goal of the neurosurgeon is to remove as much of the tumor as possible, tempered by the need to preserve neurologic function. At the very least, however, a biopsy should be performed, even in those tumors that are deep-seated and considered inoperable. The only exceptions are the brainstem lesions, where biopsy has proved of little value to the overall prognosis and often has damaged the child, and certain germ cell tumors that can be diagnosed by the presence of specific tumor markers in the CSF. The greater the amount of tumor removed, the better are the child's chances to tolerate further therapy with fewer complications. Significant neurosurgical advances have been made; thus gross total resection of large tumor masses or tumors located in a delicate area of the brain often can be accomplished. The value of aggressive surgical debulking of both low-grade and high-grade primary brain tumors of childhood is well recognized.[26] Certain tumors, including cerebellar juvenile pilocytic astrocytoma and some low-grade astrocytomas, are surgically curable if completely removed.

Advances in presurgical evaluations with the use of enhanced CT and MRI allow the surgeon to plan the operative approach better. Microsurgical techniques such as using the operating microscope provide greater accessibility to deeper neural lesions. Bipolar coagulation allows the maintenance of sufficient hemostasis in delicate areas such as the brainstem, the ventricles, and those in close proximity to the cranial nerves. With the use of brainstem auditory-evoked potentials, the surgeon can monitor the functioning of the auditory nerve intraoperatively. The use of intraoperative ultrasound tumor localization minimizes the need for exploration through normal brain tissue. Intraoperative laser therapy, which destroys tumor cells by vaporizing them, decreases the chances of microscopic tumor cells remaining at the primary tumor site. Photoradiation therapy may be cytotoxic to the exposed tumor cells during the operative procedure. The ultrasonic surgical aspirator enhances the possibility of removing tumors adjacent to fragile structures without inducing permanent damage. The stereotactic placement of a needle directly into the lesion makes it possible to obtain tumor tissue in delicate regions such as the pineal area.[26,27,70]

Once a pathologic diagnosis is made, a specific, complete treatment plan including rehabilitation needs is decided by the neuro-oncology team and is presented to the family. Treatment may consist of either radiation alone, chemotherapy alone, or a combination of radiation and chemotherapy. A child less than 4 years of age usually receives chemotherapy alone.

Radiation Therapy

As early as 1930 improved survival rates were achieved in children who received adjuvant radiotherapy after resection of high-grade tumors.[26] This form of therapy has been the mainstay in the treatment of all brain tumors not surgically curable. The ability to give increasingly more accurate irradiation to the tumor site has greatly improved with the advancements of both CT and MRI.

The planning of an individual radiation treatment course is very intricate and is determined, in part, by tumor pathology and potential to disseminate to other areas of the CNS. Precision is required to maximize the dose of irradiation to the tumor and to minimize the dose of irradiation to surrounding normal tissue.[38] The child's position and complete immobility during treatment are crucial. Maintaining immobility usually requires the use of sedation in the young child. Individually designed casts or molds are used to ensure correct positioning. The length of irradiation is usually 6 to 7 weeks, with daily or twice-daily treatments given consecutively 5 days each week.

Standard treatment for tumors such as medulloblastomas is craniospinal irradiation with doses of 3500 to 4500 cGy to the neuraxis, with a boost to the posterior fossa for a total of 5500 cGy. This is given in daily fractions of 180 cGy. Recent studies have suggested that a lower dose of 2500 cGy to the spinal cord may be sufficient treatment for these children.[27,34] This lower dose may lessen some of the long-term sequelae produced by the higher doses.

Children with high-grade astrocytomas receive high doses of irradiation, 5500 to 6000 cGy, to the focal tumor area. Anaplastic ependymomas have generally received high doses of focal brain irradiation. Debate continues about whether the entire neuraxis should be irradiated.[68] Recent studies with ependymomas, however, have indicated that the site of recurrence usually is the primary site; therefore only involved field irradiation may be necessary.[32] The course of radiotherapy is followed by intensive chemotherapy.

Among the newer techniques for delivering radiotherapy is hyperfractionated irradiation. This method currently is used primarily in the treatment of brainstem gliomas. Children are treated twice a day at 100 cGy per fraction to a total dose of 7200 to 7800 cGy to the tumor bed. Hyperfractionation permits a greater total dose delivery without concurrent increased adverse sequelae.[20] Another newer technique under study is interstitial radiation (brachytherapy) for the treatment of high-grade supratentorial astrocytomas. It involves the surgical implantation of small radioactive seeds within the tumor bed, either temporarily or permanently.

Although a vital part of brain tumor treatment, radiation is not without sequelae that are categorized as *acute, subacute,* and *chronic*. An increase in cerebral edema can occur acutely after one treatment, causing an increase in a present neurologic deficit or, if severe enough, a cerebral herniation. The use of corticosteroids such as dexamethasone (Decadron) usually minimizes the amount of edema. The somnolence syndrome is a subacute reaction that usually occurs 4 to 10 weeks after completion of therapy and lasts 4 days to 3 weeks. Symptoms include increased lethargy (children may sleep up to 20 hours a day), anorexia, vomiting, and the presence of a low-grade fever. The syndrome eventually resolves completely, usually without sequelae, but symptomatic relief can be accomplished by a few days of corticosteroid therapy.[60,67] Chronic sequelae are usually permanent and can occur several months after completion of therapy. They range from learning disabilities to tissue necrosis, which can cause death if it is progressive. An overview of chronic sequelae is presented later in this chapter.

Chemotherapy

Major cooperative study groups such as Children's Cancer Group (CCG), Pediatric Oncology Group (POG), and International Society for Pediatric Oncology (SIOP) have conducted studies that demonstrated the beneficial role of chemotherapy, either alone or in combination with radiation therapy.

Several studies have demonstrated the value of chemotherapy in the treatment of medulloblastoma both initially and at the time of recurrence.[22,43,64] Chemotherapy in conjunction with radiotherapy has prolonged survival time in children with high-grade astrocytoma, although the 5-year survival rate is not as good as with medulloblastoma.[24] The use of chemotherapy with brainstem glioma has not proved effective.

A new method of chemotherapy administration is to give one or two courses after surgery and before radiation (neoadjuvant chemotherapy) to permit evaluation of response to a drug alone and provide the theoretic advantage of better penetration into tumor tissue. In the young child chemotherapy is given for a longer time period to delay the initiation of radiotherapy and therefore lessen the adverse sequelae.[37] The use of neoadjuvant chemotherapy can in some cases permit a decrease in the amount of radiation given. In patients with germ cell tumors, which are extremely chemosensitive, new chemotherapeutic protocols may eliminate the need for radiation therapy. Autologous bone marrow "rescue" after marrow-ablative doses of chemotherapy is currently under investigation for the treatment of high-grade malignant tumors at the time of presentation and at recurrence. Although it is too early to assess the overall efficacy of this approach, early data are promising, and studies continue.[25]

Prognosis

The prognosis of a child with a brain tumor depends on a variety of factors, including tumor histology, amount resected, degree of dissemination, age, general physical status, and neurologic condition. Survival rates vary greatly, from 90% in the child with cerebellar astrocytoma to less than 20% in the child with a brainstem tumor.

Since the management of a child with a brain tumor depends on the specific diagnosis, the four most commonly seen tumors are discussed individually.

MEDULLOBLASTOMA

Medulloblastoma accounts for approximately 25% of all pediatric brain tumors and is the most common malignant primary CNS tumor of childhood. It is a highly cellular, soft, friable tumor composed of small round or oval cells with hyperchromatic nuclei. It is usually located in the midline of the cerebellum but may occur in the cerebellar hemispheres as well.[49]

Medulloblastoma is a rapidly growing tumor in which the duration of symptoms is usually short. As a result of its location in the posterior fossa, obstruction of the fourth ventricle and consequent hydrocephalus result in symptoms of increased ICP. Headache and vomiting (usually worse in the morning), lethargy, ataxia, and diplopia are common. In the infant there may be an increase in head circumference.

The lesion is demonstrated by a CT or MRI scan and is enhanced with contrast administration. Usually disease is confined to the primary site, but it may be disseminated at diagnosis. The first line of treatment is surgery, with a gross total resection as the goal. A postoperative CT or MRI scan (within 72 hours), myelogram, examination of the spinal fluid (cytology), and bone marrow aspiration help establish extent of disease.[45,49]

The Chang staging system is generally used to quantitate tumor size at diagnosis using T stage and to delineate the degree of metastasis using M stage (Table 9–8).[42] Controversy surrounds the T stage because this is a preoperative-operative observation. The question remains whether the relationship between the tumor size and prognosis changes when a complete resection is achieved. Using the Chang classification and other factors, a child's disease can be categorized as either average (standard) or poor (high) risk. In prior studies poor-risk patients have had large invasive tumors (T_3 or T_4) and disseminated disease at diagnosis. Children less than 4 years of age tend to do worse than their older counterparts.[29,49] After staging evaluation, the next treatment step is irradiation to the entire craniospinal axis. The amount varies, depending on the child's age and the risk category. However, the posterior fossa dose must be 5000 to 5500 cGy. In those patients who are poor risk, chemotherapy also is given. In the very young child chemotherapy is given initially to avoid early irradiation of the craniospinal axis.

The greatest strides in the treatment of medulloblastoma have occurred over the last decade. The 5-year overall disease-free survival rate is 55%,[22] and even higher survival rates are being reported for average-risk patients.

TABLE 9–8. *Chang Operative Staging System for Cerebellar Medulloblastoma (PNET)*

T_1	Tumor less than 3 cm diameter and limited to the classic midline position in the vermis, the roof of the fourth ventricle, and less frequently to the cerebellar hemispheres
T_2	Tumor 3 cm or greater in diameter further invading one adjacent structure or partially filling the fourth ventricle
T_3	Stage divided into T_{3A} and T_{3B}
	T_{3A}—tumor further invading two adjacent structures or completely filling the fourth ventricle with extension into the aqueduct of Sylvius, foramen of Magendie or foramen of Luschka, thus producing marked internal hydrocephalus
	T_{3B}—tumor arising from the floor of the fourth ventricle or brainstem and filling the fourth ventricle
T_4	Tumor further spreading through the aqueduct of Sylvius to involve the third ventricle or midbrain or tumor extending to the upper cervical cord
M_0	No evidence of gross subarachnoid or hematogenous metastasis
M_1	Microscopic tumor cells formed in cerebrospinal fluid
M_2	Gross nodular seeding demonstrated in cerebellar, cerebral subarachnoid space or in the third or lateral ventricles
M_3	Gross nodular seeding in spinal subarachnoid space
M_4	Metastasis outside the cerebrospinal axis

From Laurent JP, Chang CH, Cohen ME. A classification system for primitive neuroectodermal tumors (medulloblastoma) of the posterior fossa. Cancer 1985; 56:1807–1809.
PNET = primitive neuroectodermal tumor.

ASTROCYTOMA

Astrocytomas comprise the largest category of pediatric brain tumors (see Table 9–5). They occur at any age in the cerebellum (35%), cerebral hemispheres (23%), brainstem (15%), optic nerve (11%), and hypothalamus (7%).[6] Astrocytomas are classified into three categories based on an increasing degree of anaplasia: astrocytoma, anaplastic astrocytoma, and glioblastoma multiforme. The greater the degree of anaplasia, the more difficult the disease is to control.[2] Therefore there are wide variations between the different grading classifications.

Cerebellar Astrocytomas

Cerebellar astrocytomas represent 13% of all pediatric brain tumors (see Table 9–5). They are the second most common tumor occurring in the cerebellum and can involve the vermis, the hemispheres, or both regions.

Children with this midline tumor present with signs of increased ICP such as headache and vomiting (usually worse in the morning), ataxia, and irritability. The history of symptoms is usually short. If the lesion is located in a particular hemisphere, the child may develop extremity weakness marked by a clumsy arm and leg. The ataxia may involve falling to one side.

CT demonstrates which type of cerebellar astrocytoma is present: a large cystic lesion with a single enhancing mural nodule; a lesion with an irregular, diffusely enhanced, thick wall; or a solid lesion with smaller cystic areas.[41] The microscopic appearance greatly affects prognosis. The juvenile pilocytic cerebellar astrocytoma is more common, and children with it have a projected survival rate of 94% (>25 years); whereas children with diffuse astrocytoma, which is similar to low-grade astrocytomas in other locations, have a projected survival rate of 38%.[31]

A total surgical resection is crucial and greatly enhances the disease-free survival rate. If a complete resection is achieved, no further treatment is needed. Follow-up CT scans are done routinely. If the resection is incomplete, there is controversy about the ideal plan of treatment. The lesion is observed and another resection performed should growth occur. Local radiotherapy is used in some institutions for residual tumors, those that infiltrate the brainstem, or recurrent tumors.[41,65] Should a tumor recur after an initial complete resection, surgery should again be performed. Chemotherapy has not proved useful in the treatment of these tumors.

Low-Grade Astrocytoma

Low-grade astrocytomas account for approximately 23% of childhood brain tumors (see Table 9–5).[26] The initial symptoms depend on the location of the tumor. Generally there is a history of progressive symptoms increasing over months or, in some instances, years. The most common symptoms are headache, vomiting, and seizures. Papilledema is often present at diagnosis.

The diagnosis is easily made with a CT or MRI scan. Most children with these tumors present with hypodense lesions on precontrast CT that do not always enhance after contrast is given. A complete surgical resection is the ideal treatment and may provide long-term cure.[14] Radiotherapy may prolong survival in patients with an incomplete resection. The field of radiation depends on the extent of disease. A chemotherapy protocol for recurrent or progressive low-grade tumors using carboplatinum and vincristine, now in clinical practice, may delay the immediate need for radiotherapy.

Several factors that indicate a favorable prognosis include seizures on presentation, young age, minimal neurologic deficits after surgery, low-grade pathology, slow onset of symptoms before diagnosis, and the presence of giant cells during pathologic examination.[10] Five-year survival rates range from 58% to 88%. Total resection is the best predictor of long-term survival.

Anaplastic Astrocytoma and Glioblastoma Multiforme

The high-grade astrocytoma commonly occurs supratentorially, occasionally in the brain stem, and less often in the cerebellum. Approximately 11% of all pediatric brain tumors are high-grade astrocytomas (see Table 9–5).[26]

The presenting symptoms depend on the tumor's location and size. Generally there is a shorter history of symptom onset than with the lower grade astrocytomas because these lesions grow rapidly. They become quite large and infiltrate vital adjacent structures. Initial symptoms range from signs of increased ICP to focal seizures. Rarely patients present acutely with a rapid neurologic deterioration caused by intratumoral hemorrhage.[15]

A CT or MRI scan will demonstrate an infiltrating, contrast-enhanced lesion, usually with significant edema. Surgery is the initial form of treatment, with a complete resection the goal; however, a complete resection often is not possible because of the infiltrative nature of these tumors. Histologically, anaplastic astrocytomas are characterized by increased cellularity with pleomorphism, vascular hyperplasia, and increased mitoses. In addition to these findings, glioblastomas have tumor necrosis, which is diagnostic.[15,69]

Radiotherapy is the mainstay of treatment of high-grade astrocytomas. The recommended area of treatment is a broad focal port with large margins rather than whole brain. A radiation dose of 5500 cGy to 6000 cGy should be given over a 5- to 6-week period.[15] Intensive chemotherapy follows radiotherapy. Historically, although chemotherapy has lengthened the time before tumor progression, it has not significantly improved overall survival rates.[15,52] Several multiagent chemotherapy protocols are now under study.[62] Autologous bone marrow rescue after intensive chemotherapy is also being studied in the treatment of high-grade astrocytoma and glioblastoma multiforme.[25]

Historically, the survival rates for children with high-grade astrocytomas have been dismal. Only 20% to 30% of patients with an anaplastic astrocytoma will survive for 5 years without disease progression, whereas most children with glioblastoma multiforme will die from disease progression within 2 years.[25] Investigators hope that the addition of intensive chemotherapy protocols will improve these survival statistics while maintaining good quality of life for these children.

BRAINSTEM GLIOMA

Brainstem gliomas represent approximately 10% of all childhood brain tumors and occur most frequently in the younger child (infancy to 10 years). The pons is the most common location, although the tumors can arise in the medulla and midbrain. Children usually present with multiple cranial nerve palsies and experience weakness of the face and extremities, diplopia, and ataxia. There may be personality changes such as irritability or depression. Headaches and vomiting may occur but are unusual. Parents usually report the onset of clumsiness anywhere from weeks to several months before diagnosis. Typically the onset of crossed eyes due to a sixth cranial nerve palsy results in medical attention and diagnosis.

The optimal diagnostic tool is MRI, which is able to distinguish between glioma and the vascular malformations that may mimic a tumor on CT scan. An enlarged brainstem is seen best on sagittal views and may or may not enhance with the administration of contrast (gadolinium). Some brainstem gliomas are intensely contrast enhancing and have an exophytic component that extends out of the brainstem into the fourth ventricle. These children may benefit from a debulking surgical procedure, and in many of these cases the pathology is low grade. This particular group of children has a slightly better prognosis.[21] The vast majority of these tumors are not surgically resectable because of their location in this vital area of the brain. The risks of surgery are unacceptably high.[63]

Conventional treatment consists of focal irradiation. Newer radiation therapy is given in twice-daily fractionated dosages to a total as high as 7800 cGy. Initial results demonstrate prolonged survival time with this hyperfractionated method.[20] Although there have been documented cases of spine metastases associated with brainstem gliomas,[59] the incidence is small, and neuraxis radiotherapy is not recommended. Chemotherapy has not been effective.[66] There are, however, ongoing institutional studies using multidrug protocols and the autologous bone marrow rescue protocol.[25,36] The overall survival rate remains at 20%, with a median survival time of 15 months.[12]

EPENDYMOMA

Ependymomas account for approximately 10% of all pediatric brain tumors; 25% to 40% occur above the tentorium, and 60% to 75% occur below the tentorium. Spinal cord ependymomas occur very rarely in childhood.[61] These tumors occur predominantly in the young child (≤10 years of age), with a marked

increase in the less than 3 years of age group.[47,61] A slight male predominance has been noted with spinal cord lesions.

Ependymomas are derived from ependymal cells and are histologically separated into two main groups. Low-grade ependymomas are very cellular tumors with a diagnostic pattern of ependymal rosettes around blood vessels. Anaplastic, or high-grade, ependymomas have, in addition to the characteristic formation, pleomorphism, necrosis, mitoses, and increased cellularity. The high-grade lesions are more commonly found supratentorially.[9,61] No universal grading system is used for ependymomas.

The presenting signs and symptoms vary according to the tumor's location, although papilledema is the most common finding in these children, regardless of the tumor's location. If the tumor is in the posterior fossa, the child will present with symptoms of increased ICP such as nausea, vomiting, headache, and ataxia. Supratentorial lesions usually cause focal motor weakness, visual disturbances, and seizures (present in approximately 25% of children). The duration of symptoms varies with the pathology and location of the tumor, with a shorter symptomatic history in patients with anaplastic lesions because of the increased growth rate. Diagnostic evaluation begins with a CT or MRI scan, which shows a contrast-enhanced lesion with, possibly, a cystic component. Myelography or spinal MRI to detect seeding of the spinal cord and CSF cytology are recommended for use in children with infratentorial high-grade lesions or in any child who has symptoms of spinal cord disease.

A complete surgical resection, when possible, is the first line of treatment, followed by radiation. A wide range of radiation doses is given, depending on pathology and location. Children with high-grade posterior fossa lesions receive neuraxis irradiation, and those with a supratentorial lesion receive focal therapy. There is controversy about the optimal treatment for supratentorial high-grade lesions or infratentorial low-grade lesions, which may or may not require neuraxis irradiation, respectively.[47] Historically, chemotherapy has not been advantageous in the treatment of ependymomas. Recently, however, extended survival time has been documented with certain chemotherapeutic regimens. Cisplatinum and etoposide (VP-16)-containing regimens have induced responses in children with recurrent disease.[32] Although disease dissemination is always a possibility, local recurrence is usually the area of failure.[32,47,51,61] At relapse, children with low-grade ependymomas should have a second surgery, radiation if it has not already been given, and chemotherapy. Relapse in a child with an anaplastic ependymoma indicates a dismal prognosis. These children are currently treated with a variety of intensive chemotherapeutic protocols.

The overall survival rate of a child with an ependymoma depends on histology, degree of dissemination, and age of the child. A child with a low-grade ependymoma who receives a complete resection followed by irradiation has a 50% chance of a long disease-free survival time.[61] A child with a low-grade ependymoma who experiences a first relapse may again do well for an extended period if aggressively treated. On the contrary, few children with malignant ependymomas survive for a significant time period after recurrence.[32]

LONG-TERM SEQUELAE OF TREATMENT

Children with brain tumors are surviving for longer periods of time. With the advances in multimodal therapy (surgical techniques, radiation, and chemotherapy), more children will survive. Improved survival rates are accompanied by concern for the long-term sequelae of treatment.

The long-term effects of cranial irradiation have been well studied in children with leukemia. The amount of radiation received by brain tumor patients is considerably larger than that given to children with leukemia. The post-treatment sequelae are therefore more detrimental. Several studies have shown that all children who receive radiation therapy to the cranium have some degree of intellectual impairment.[16,39,50] Children who receive whole-brain treatment as opposed to treatment to a focal area have increased dif-

ficulties as do children less than 2 years of age. Significant deficiencies are noted both in verbal intelligence quotient (IQ) and memory function.[16,50] The addition of certain chemotherapeutic agents (e.g., methotrexate) may have a synergistic effect on declining intellectual development.[39] Learning disabilities can be progressive over time.[16] One study found that children irradiated in adolescence maintained an average IQ but had more subtle cognitive dysfunction.[40]

Other important long-term sequelae result from neuraxial radiation, which directly affects the growing spinal column causing short sitting height, and from radiation to the pituitary, which affects growth hormone production leading to short stature and hypothyroidism with reduced thyroxine (T_4) and/or elevated thyroid-stimulating hormone.[44] Second malignancies can occur as sequelae of both radiotherapy and chemotherapy.[13,29]

Disfiguring physical sequelae (e.g., a facial palsy) can directly affect the development of self-esteem. Social withdrawal in these individuals is not uncommon. Research has found that psychologic-emotional dysfunction more than the physical disabilities was responsible for a lower self-reported quality of life.[40]

A thorough follow-up plan of care is essential for each child receiving therapy for a brain tumor. It should include a baseline neuropsychologic evaluation, ideally at the time of diagnosis, which is then repeated at regular intervals. Baseline endocrine studies, including thyroid function and growth hormone studies, should be performed and monitored systematically. Gonadotropin evaluation is necessary if puberty is delayed. Films to determine bone age should be obtained, prior growth curves evaluated, and linear growth closely monitored, especially during the first 2 years after diagnosis.

The value of comprehensive psychosocial care of both the children and their families cannot be overly stressed. Both parents and teachers need education to help them recognize the early warning signs of difficulties these children may experience and to identify the supports needed to enhance optimal functioning.[5]

REFERENCES

1. A Primer of Brain Tumors: A Patient's Reference Manual, 5th ed. Chicago: American Brain Tumor Association, 1991.

2. Allen JC. Childhood brain tumors: Current status of clinical trials in newly diagnosed and recurrent disease. Pediatr Clin North Am 1985; 32:641–643.

3. Baptiste M, Nasca P, Metzger MS, et al. Neurofibromatosis and other disorders among children with CNS tumors and their families. Neurology 1989; 39:487–492.

4. Barnes PD. Magnetic resonance in pediatric and adolescent neuroimaging. Neurol Clin 1990; 8:741–757.

5. Baron MC. Advances in the care of children with brain tumors. J Neurosci Nurs 1991; 23:39–43.

6. Becker LE, Jay V. Tumors of the central nervous system in children. In Deutsch M (ed): Management of Childhood Brain Tumors. Boston: Kluwer Academic Publishers, 1990, pp 17–23.

7. Cohen BH, Bury E, Packer RJ, et al. Gadolinium-DTPA enhanced magnetic resonance imaging in childhood brain tumors. Neurology 1989; 39:1178–1183.

8. Cohen ME, Duffner PK. Introduction. In Brain Tumors in Children: Principles of Diagnosis and Treatment. International Review of Child Neurology Series. New York: Raven Press, 1984, p 3.

9. Cohen ME, Duffner PK. Ependymomas. In Brain Tumors in Children: Principles of Diagnosis and Treatment. International Review of Child Neurology Series. New York: Raven Press, 1984, pp 136–155.

10. Cohen ME, Duffner PK. Supratentorial hemispheric astrocytomas. In Brain Tumors in Children: Principles of Diagnosis and Treatment. International Review of Child Neurology Series. New York: Raven Press, 1984, pp 173–192.

11. Cohen ME, Duffner PK. Current therapy in childhood brain tumors. Neurol Clin 1985; 3:147–164.

12. Cohen ME, Duffner PK, Heffner RR, et al. Prognostic factors in brain stem gliomas. Neurology 1986; 36:602–605.

13. D'Angio GJ, Rorke LB, Packer R, et al. Key problems in the management of children with brain tumors. Int J Radiat Oncol Biol Phys 1990; 18:805–809.

14. Deutsch M. Cerebral hemisphere glioma. In Management of Childhood Brain Tumors. Boston: Kluwer Academic Publishers, 1990, pp 325–342.

15. Dropcho EJ, Wisoff JH, Walker RW, et al. Supratentorial malignant gliomas in childhood: A review of fifty cases. Ann Neurol 1987; 22:355–364.

16. Duffner PK, Cohen ME. The long-term effects of central nervous system therapy on children with brain tumors. Neurol Clin 1991; 9:479–495.

17. Duffner PK, Cohen ME, Flannery JR. Referral patterns of childhood brain tumors in the state of Connecticut. Cancer 1982; 50:1636–1640.

18. Duffner PK, Cohen ME, Freeman A. Pediatric brain tumors: An overview. CA 1985; 35:287–301.

19. Duffner PK, Cohen ME, Myers MH, et al. Survival of children with brain tumors: SEER program, 1973-1980. Neurology 1986; 36:597–601.

20. Edwards MS, Wara WM, Urtasuri RC, et al. Hyperfractionated radiation therapy for brain stem glioma: A phase I-II trial. J Neurosurg 1989; 70:691–700.

21. Epstein F. A staging system for brain stem gliomas. Cancer 1985; 56(suppl):1804–1806.

22. Evans AE, Jenkin RD, Sposto R, et al. The treatment of medulloblastoma: Results of a prospective randomized trial of radiation therapy with and without CCNU, vincristine and prednisone. J Neurosurg 1990; 72:572–582.

23. Finlay J, Goins SC. Brain tumors in children. I. Advances in diagnosis. Am J Pediatr Hematol Oncol 1987; 9:246–255.

24. Finlay J, Goins SC. Brain tumors in children. III. Advances in chemotherapy. Am J Pediatr Hematol Oncol 1987; 9:264–267.

25. Finlay JL, August C, Packer R, et al. High-dose multiagent chemotherapy followed by bone marrow "rescue" for malignant astrocytomas of childhood and adolescence. J Neurooncol 1990; 9:239–248.

26. Finlay JL, Goins SC, Uteg R, et al. Progress in the management of childhood brain tumors. Hematol Oncol Clin North Am 1987; 1:753–776.

27. Finlay JL, Uteg R. Geise WL. Brain tumors in children. II. Advances in neurosurgery and radiation oncology. Am J Pediatr Hematol Oncol 1987; 9:256–263.

28. Fraser MC, Tucker MA. Late effects of cancer therapy: Chemotherapy-related malignancies. Oncol Nurs Forum 1988;15:67–75.

29. Friedman HS, Oakes WJ, Bigner SH, et al. Medulloblastoma: Tumor biological and clinical perspectives. J Neurooncol 1991; 11:1–15.

30. Giuffré R, Liccardo G, Pastroe FS, et al. Potential risk factors for brain tumors in children: An analysis of 200 cases. Child's Nerv Syst 1990; 6:8–12.

31. Gjerris F, Klinken L. Long-term prognosis in children with benign cerebellar astrocytoma. J Neurosurg 1978; 49:179–184.

32. Goldwein JW, Glauser TA, Packer RJ, et al. Recurrent intracranial ependymomas in children: Survival, patterns of failure and prognostic factors. Cancer 1990; 66:557–563.

33. Gomez MR, Groover RV, Mellinger JF. Tumors of the brain and spinal cord. In Swainman KF, Wright FS (eds): The Practice of Pediatric Neurology, vol 2, 2nd ed. St. Louis: CV Mosby, 1982, pp 823–871.

34. Hughes EN, Shillito J, Sallan SE, et al. Medulloblastoma at the Joint Center for Radiation Therapy between 1968 and 1984. The influence of radiation dose on the patterns of failure and survival. Cancer 1988; 61:1992–1998.

35. Hung KL, Wu CM, Huang JS, et al. Familial medulloblastomas in siblings: Report in one family and review of the literature. Surg Neurol 1990; 35:341–346.

36. Jenkin RD, Bosel C, Ertel I, et al. Brain-stem tumors in childhood: A prospective randomized trial of irradiation with and without adjuvant CCNU, vincristine and prednisone. A report of the Children's Cancer Study Group. J Neurosurg 1987;66:227–233.

37. Kretschmar CS, Tarbell NJ, Kupsky W, et al. Pre-irradiation chemotherapy for infants and children with medulloblastoma: A preliminary report. J Neurosurg 1989; 71:820–825.

38. Kun LE, Principles of radiation therapy. In Cohen ME, Duffner PK (eds): Brain Tumors in Children: Principles of Diagnosis and Treatment. New York: Raven Press, 1984, pp 47–70.

39. Kun LE, Mulhern RK, Crisco JS. Quality of life in children treated for brain tumors: Intellectual, emotional and academic function. J Neurosurg 1983; 58:1–5.

40. Lannering B, Marky I, Lundberg A, et al. Long-term sequelae after pediatric brain tumors: Their effect on disability and quality of life. Med Pediatr Oncol 1989; 18:304–310.

41. Lapras C, Patet JD, Lapras CK Jr, et al. Cerebellar astrocytomas in childhood. Child's Nerv Syst 1986; 2:55–59.

42. Laurent IP, Chang CH, Cohen ME. A classification system for primitive neuroectodermal tumors (medulloblastoma) of the posterior fossa. Cancer 1985; 56:1807–1809.

43. Lefkowitz IB, Packer RJ, Siegel KR, et al. Results of treatment of children with recurrent medulloblastoma/primitive neuroectodermal tumors with lomustine, cisplatin and vincristine. Cancer 1990; 65:412–417.

44. Meadows AT, Silber J. Delayed consequences of therapy for childhood cancer. In Vouse PA, Bloom HJG, Lemerle J (eds): Cancer in Childhood: Clinical Management. Berlin: Springer-Verlag, 1986, pp 70–81.

45. Milstein J. Medulloblastoma. Historical, diagnostic and prognostic factors. In Zeltzer PM, Pochedly C (eds): Medulloblastoma in Children: New Concepts in Tumor Biology, Diagnosis and Treatment. New York: Praeger Publishers, 1986, pp 76–86.

46. Milstein JM. Neurological assessment. In Deutsch M (ed): Management of Childhood Brain Tumors. Boston: Kluwer Academic Publishers, 1990, pp 121–135.

47. Nazar GB, Hoffman HJ, Becker LE, et al. Infratentorial ependymomas in childhood: Prognostic factors and treatment. J Neurosurg 1990; 72:408–417.

48. Pack B, Maria BL. Neurological emergencies in pediatric oncology. J Assoc Pediatr Oncol Nurses 1987; 4:12–14.

49. Packer RJ, Finlay JL. Medulloblastoma: Presentation, diagnosis and management. Oncology 1988; 2:35–49.

50. Packer RJ, Sutton LN, Atkins TE, et al. A prospective study of cognitive function in children receiving whole-brain radiotherapy and chemotherapy: 2-year results. J Neurosurg 1989; 70:707–713.

51. Papadopoulos DP, Shankar G, Evans RG. Prognostic factors and management of intracranial ependymomas. Anticancer Res 1990; 10:689–692.

52. Phupanich S, Edwards MS, Levin VA, et al. Supratentorial malignant gliomas of childhood: Results of treatment with radiation therapy and chemotherapy. J Neurosurg 1984; 60:495–499.

53. Ries LAG, Hankey BF, Miller BA, et al. Cancer Statistics Review 1973-1988. NIH publication 91-2789. Bethesda, Md.: National Cancer Institute, 1991.

54. Rorke LB, Giles FH, Davis RL, et al. Revision of the World Health Organization classification of brain tumors for childhood brain tumors. Cancer 1985; 56:1869–1886.

55. Rosman PN. Increased intracranial pressure. In Swainnan KF, Wright FS (eds): The Practice of Pediatric Neurology, vol 1, 2nd ed. St. Louis: CV Mosby, 1982, pp 188–205.

56. Rossi LN, Vassella N. Headache in children with brain tumors. Child's Nerv Syst 1989; 5:307–309.

57. Savard ML, Gilchrist DM. Ependymomas in two sisters and a maternal male cousin with mosaicism with monosome 22 in tumor. (Review.) Pediatr Neurosci 1989; 15:80–84.

58. Shapiro S, Mealey J Jr, Sartorius C. Radiation-induced intracranial malignant gliomas. J Neurosurg 1989; 71:77–82.

59. Silbergeld D, Berger M, Griffin B, et al. Brain stem glioma with multiple intraspinal metastases during life: Case report and review of the literature. Pediatr Neurosci 1988; 14:103–107.

60. Silverman CL, Palkas H, Talent B, et al. Late effects of radiotherapy on patients with cerebellar medulloblastoma. Cancer 1984; 4:825–829.

61. Silverman CL, Thomas PR, Cox W. Ependymomas. In Deutsch M (ed): Management of Childhood Brain Tumors. Boston: Kluwer Academic Publishers, 1990, pp 369–382.

62. Sposto R, Ertel IJ, Jenkin RD, et al. The effectiveness of chemotherapy for treatment of high grade astrocytoma in children: Results of a randomized trial (a report from the Children's Cancer Study Group). J Neurooncol 1989; 7:165–177.

63. Stroink AR, Hoffman HJ, Hendrick EB, et al. Diagnosis and management of pediatric brain-stem gliomas. J Neurosurg 1986; 65:745–750.

64. Tait DM, Thorton-Jones J, Bloom HJG, et al. Adjuvant chemotherapy for medulloblastoma: The first multi-centre control trial of the International Society of Paediatric Oncology (SIOP I). Eur J Cancer 1990; 24:464–469.

65. Undjian S, Marinov M, Georgiev K. Long-term follow-up after surgical treatment of cerebellar astrocytomas in 100 children. Child's Nerv Syst 1989; 5:99–101.

66. Van Eys J, Baram TZ, Cangir A, et al. Salvage chemotherapy for recurrent brain tumors in children. J Pediatr 1988; 113:601–606.

67. Walker RW, Allen JC. Pediatric brain tumors. Pediatr Ann 1983; 12:383–394.

68. Wallner KE, Wara WM, Sheline GE, et al. Intracranial ependymomas: Results of treatment with partial or whole brain irradiation without spinal irradiation. Int J Radiat Oncol Biol Phys 1986; 12:1937–1941.

69. Woo SY, Donaldson SS, Cox RS. Astrocytoma in children: 14 years' experience at Stanford University Medical Center. J Clin Oncol 1988; 6:1001–1007.

70. Yasargi MG, Cravens GF, Roth P. Surgical approaches to "inaccessible" brain tumors. Clin Neurosurg 1986; 34:42–110.

71. Young JL, Ries LG, Silverberg E, et al. Cancer incidence, survival and mortality for children younger than age 15 years. Cancer 1986; 58:598–602.

72. Zulch KJ. Histological Typing of Tumors of the Central Nervous System. Geneva: World Health Organization, 1979.

■ HODGKIN'S DISEASE

Patricia Liebhauser

Hodgkin's disease is a malignancy of the lymphoid system first described as an entity by Thomas Hodgkin in 1832. It differs from the other lymphomatous diseases in its histology, behavior, and response to treatment.

Hodgkin's disease accounts for 5% of malignancies diagnosed in children in the United States. The incidence is approximately 7.3 per million in white children and 5.2 per million in African-American children or approximately 290 white children and 30 African-American children under 15 years of age diagnosed each year in the United States.[52] It has been reported in infants and very young children but is considered rare before the age of 5 years.[22,37,43] The number of cases increases significantly in the second decade of life in the United States.[37,43] Hodgkin's disease occurs more frequently in boys than in girls. In studies of children under 15 years of age, the ratio of boys to girls has ranged from 1.1 to 3.9:1.[7,10,43,46] This preponderance in boys diminishes in the preteen years. In adults a sex ratio of approximately 1.3:1 is seen.[3]

The highest incidence rates of Hodgkin's disease in children have been observed in some countries in Central and South America, Africa, and the Middle East. The incidence of Hodgkin's disease is lowest in East Asia and particularly rare in Japan and the Philippines.[37]

ETIOLOGY

The cause of Hodgkin's disease is unknown; however, epidemiologic studies suggest possible influential factors. In most developed countries there is a bimodal age-incidence curve, with a primary peak occurring in the late twenties and a secondary peak after age 50 years. This bimodal curve suggests a dual cause, with Hodgkin's disease in the young caused by an infectious agent and that in the elderly with a cause similar to that of other lymphomas.[31] The bimodal curve could reflect a variation in response over age to a single causative process.[35] Whether Hodgkin's disease has one or more different etiologic processes remains unresolved.

In children and young adults, age distribution patterns vary with geographic location and socioeconomic condition. In developed countries or higher socioeconomic groups, the overall incidence of Hodgkin's disease is higher, but it is rare in early childhood, increases in adolescence, and peaks in young adulthood. The most frequent histologic type in these populations is nodular sclerosis.[35,43] In underdeveloped countries or lower socioeconomic groups, the overall incidence of Hodgkin's disease is lower but peaks before 15 years of age. Mixed cellularity and lymphocytic depletion are the most frequent histologic types in these populations.[35,40,43] The pattern of early childhood disease is also found in the low incidence areas of East Asia.[37] These patterns suggest an infectious cause with social class factors affecting when exposure occurs.[16,35,37]

Numerous studies have reported an increased risk of disease in close relatives of patients with Hodgkin's disease, especially same sex siblings.[15,35] This higher risk may be related to environmental or genetic factors associated with immunocompetence. Hodgkin's disease is one of the few malignancies in which multicase occurrences involving siblings and cousins revealed concordant human leukocyte antigen (HLA) types more frequently than expected.[20,36,38] Hodgkin's disease apparently is more common in persons with immunodeficiency diseases such as ataxia-telangiectasia and Wiskott-Aldrich syndrome. Lymphomas, including Hodgkin's disease, may develop in patients with immunodeficiency syndromes such as acquired immunodeficiency syndrome (AIDS).[27,42]

Viruses and bacteria have been investigated for their role as causative agents. Indirect associations between Epstein-Barr virus (EBV) and Hodgkin's disease have been reported: case reports of Hodgkin's disease developing in association with primary EBV infection; increased incidence of Hodgkin's disease in persons with a history of infectious mononucleosis; and elevated EBV titers found in patients with Hodgkin's disease.[35] However, EBV DNA has not been isolated in tumor tissue. Results of antibody studies for cytomegalovirus (CMV) in patients with Hodgkin's disease have been inconsistent, and research is continuing.[35]

A history of tonsillectomy, occupational exposure to wood or sawdust, or exposure to chemicals (e.g., phenoxy acids and chlorophenols) has been associated with an increased risk of Hodgkin's disease in some studies, but these findings have not been confirmed in others.[18,35]

CLINICAL PRESENTATION

In 60% to 90% of cases the presenting sign is cervical or supraclavicular adenopathy.[8,27,45,46,48] The lymph nodes are characteristically painless, firm, and movable in the surrounding tissue. More than half of the patients with cervical adenopathy will also have mediastinal involvement, which can cause pressure on the trachea or bronchi and subsequent symptoms of airway obstruction. Axillary or inguinal adenopathy is an unusual presenting sign. The presence of splenomegaly or hepatomegaly may indicate generalized disease. Infiltration of nonlymphoid organs is rare. When unexplained lymphadenopathy persists after a trial of antibiotic therapy, further evaluation and biopsy are indicated.

Anorexia, weight loss, malaise, and lethargy are commonly seen in children. Approximately 30% of children have fever, with intermittent elevations of 1° to 2° C.[2,48] As opposed to the adult presentation, children infrequently complain of night sweats and pruritus.

Certain systemic symptoms are considered of prognostic significance. Patients with unexplained weight loss of more than 10% of body weight in the previous 6 months, unexplained fever with temperatures above 38° C, or night sweats are classified *B* in the staging procedure.[4,28] The absence of these symptoms is the *A* classification. Approximately one third of children staged for Hodgkin's disease has been reported to have B classification.[27,46]

The percentage of children with the B classification increases in advanced disease.[46,48] Pruritis does not have prognostic significance and is not included as a B symptom.

Evaluation begins with a thorough history and physical examination. Particular attention is directed to the peripheral lymph nodes and abdomen. The presence of small, soft lymph nodes may be misleading in children. Only lymph nodes that have been increasing in size or are significantly enlarged are considered important in estimating involvement. Retroperitoneal disease usually cannot be palpated.

Laboratory studies in the diagnostic workup include a complete blood count (CBC), erythrocyte sedimentation rate (ESR), serum copper and iron levels, serum ferritin and transferrin determinations, renal and liver function tests, and baseline thyroid function tests. Anemia may indicate advanced disease. Hemolysis and impaired mobilization of iron stores are known causes of anemia in patients with Hodgkin's disease.[27,48] The white blood count (WBC) is markedly decreased only in advanced disease. It is usually normal in children. Abnormal liver function test results suggest liver involvement. Although nonspecific for Hodgkin's disease, tests that reflect activation of the reticuloendothelial system such as ESR and serum copper may be increased at diagnosis and when disease recurs.[27,49,50]

Patients with Hodgkin's disease frequently have an immunodeficiency characterized by altered functioning of T and B lymphocytes. Altered T-cell function is shown in impaired cell-mediated immunity. Patients demonstrate decreased, delayed hypersensitivity reactions to skin test antigens such as tuberculin (purified protein derivative [PPD]), diphtheria toxoid, streptokinase-streptodornase, mumps, *Trichophyton,* and *Candida albicans.*[41,48] Total anergy, a complete lack of reactivity, may occur in advanced stages of disease. T-lymphocyte counts are normal in most patients. T lymphopenia may be found in patients with marked lymphocytopenia, systemic symptoms, or advanced disease.[41] A reduced number of circulating T-helper or inducer cells has been found in patients with initial or advanced disease. Patients with advanced disease and lymphocytopenia may have a decreased number of T-cytotoxic or suppressor cells.[41] Lymphocytes show impaired proliferation when stimulated by phytohemagglutinin and other T-cell mitogens. This defect can be detected in patients with limited disease and is more pronounced with advanced disease.

Antibody responses may remain intact until disease is advanced. B-lymphocyte counts are normal in most patients.[41] Antibody production may be normal or decreased. Impaired antibody production results in decreased resistance to infections. Increased serum immunoglobulin (IgG, IgA, IgD, and IgE) levels and elevated serum titers of antiviral antibodies (EBV and CMV) have been reported.[41]

A chest x-ray film may show mediastinal or hilar node involvement. CT is especially useful for evaluating mediastinal, pulmonary, and upper abdominal disease.[2,6] CT scan of the chest, abdomen, and pelvis should be done with images at 1 cm intervals.[28] A CT scan can detect enlarged nodes but cannot visualize lymph node architecture or filling defects or differentiate reactive hyperplasia from lymphoma. Lymph nodes greater than 1.5 cm in diameter are considered abnormal on CT scan. Ultrasound imaging of the neck and abdomen can determine bulky tumor margins, spleen size, and liver masses. The location of the kidneys can be determined by CT or ultrasonography before radiotherapy is given. Isotope scanning (e.g., gallium for nodes or technetium for bone) can confirm the extent of involvement at a site.[28] MRI may provide information on soft tissue disease, but its role is not yet defined in staging.

A lymphangiogram (LAG) may be done to evaluate retroperitoneal involvement. Lymph node size, architecture, and filling defects can be visualized, and specific nodes can be identified for biopsy. LAG has demonstrated unsuspected involvement in patients and has an overall accuracy of 70% in pediatric patients.[11] It may be helpful for designing radiotherapy treatment fields. Since the radiopaque dye is retained in the lymph nodes for several months, follow-up radiographs can monitor the residual nodes for response to treatment. LAG is technically difficult to perform in small children; some centers elect to omit it, especially when advanced disease has been documented or when treatment will be unaffected by results. LAG is contraindicated when there is massive mediastinal or pulmonary involvement because of the risk of pulmonary oil embolism.[2]

The diagnosis is determined by biopsy of a lymph node and histologic classification by the pathologist. Needle biopsies and frozen section diagnoses, which distort or do not reveal the normal architecture of the lymph node, are contraindicated.

TYPES

The description of a characteristic cell by Sternberg in 1898 and Reed in 1902 differentiated Hodgkin's disease from the other lymphomatous diseases. The histologic diagnosis of Hodgkin's disease is determined by the presence of Reed-Sternberg cells in an appropriate background; however, the presence of Reed-Sternberg cells alone is not diagnostic because similar cells have been described in infectious mononucleosis, other reactive lymphoid hyperplasias, and other neoplastic diseases. The Reed-Sternberg cell has a lobulated nucleus or is multinucleated; each lobe or nucleus contains a large prominent nucleolus. These cells have been described as "owl's eyes."

Hodgkin's disease is classified by the predominating cells. A modification of the Lukes and Butler classification was adopted at the 1965 symposium on Hodgkin's disease held in Rye, New York, and is currently used.[30] The histologic classification of Hodgkin's disease is described in Table 9–9.

Strum and Rappaport[44] examined sequential biopsy specimens and demonstrated a histologic progression in Hodgkin's disease. Disease may remain unchanged or evolve from lymphocytic predominance (LP) to mixed cellularity (MC) to lymphocytic depletion (LD). A reversal of this progression was not found. The nodular sclerosis (NS) type does not follow this evolution; untreated patients with

TABLE 9–9. *Histologic Classification of Hodgkin's Disease*

HISTOLOGIC TYPE	DESCRIPTION
Lymphocytic predominance	Numerous small lymphocytes and/or reactive histiocytes Nodular or diffuse No necrosis Usually no fibrosis Reed-Sternberg cells rare and difficult to find
Nodular sclerosis	Collagen bands dividing lymphoid tissue into nodules Nodules containing atypical histiocytic cells lying in clear spaces (lacunar cells) Eosinophils usually present Necrosis frequently present Reed-Sternberg cells difficult to find
Mixed cellularity	Intermediate between lymphocytic predominance and lymphocytic depletion Variety of histologic components (eosinophils, plasma cells, mature neutrophils, lymphocytes, histiocytes, and Reed-Sternberg cells) Possible necrosis Possible fibrosis
Lymphocytic depletion	Decreased number of lymphocytes with Diffuse fibrosis with decreased number of all other cells against a background of disorderly connective tissue *or* Reticular type with atypical histiocytes and increased number of Reed-Sternberg cells

Data from references 27, 29, and 30.

NS show a progressive depletion of lymphocytes.[48]

In pooled series from U.S. treatment centers, the frequency of the histologic types of Hodgkin's disease in 800 children was as follows: NS, 63%; LP, 10%; MC, 25%; LD, 1%; and unclassified or unknown, 1%.[27,33,45,46]

STAGING

Staging is the determination of the extent of disease at the time of diagnosis. A standardized staging system was developed for Hodgkin's disease at the Rye symposium in 1965, modified at the Ann Arbor conference in 1971, and further defined at a meeting held in the Cotswolds, England, in 1988.[4,28] The clinical and pathologic staging of Hodgkin's disease is described in Table 9–10.

At the time of diagnosis approximately 60% of children with Hodgkin's disease have pathologic stage I or II disease.[21,27,33,46] Pathologic stage III disease is diagnosed in approximately 30% of the children, and 10% have pathologic stage IV disease.[27,46]

Laparotomy with splenectomy was initially used to validate the LAG findings and to search for other sites of disease in the abdomen and pelvis. In children clinically staged before laparotomy, the laparotomy findings have resulted in a change in stage in one third of the children, allowing the administration of more appropriate therapy.[7,14,33,46] Laparotomy with splenectomy may be deferred in children with obvious advanced disease or if the choice of treatment will not be altered by the findings. Some centers now use clinical staging alone and omit the laparotomy with splenectomy.

The staging laparotomy includes a splenectomy and multiple biopsies. Because splenic involvement is usually focal, beginning with small nodular infiltrates only a few millimeters in diameter, the entire spleen and any accessory spleens are removed. The spleen is divided into sections and is examined at 1 to 3 mm intervals to determine the presence or absence of tumor.[27] Lymph nodes are taken at the splenic hilum, celiac axis, portal area, right and left para-aortic sites at the level of the kidneys, bifurcation of the aorta, right and left common iliac chain, and the mesentery of the superior mesenteric artery.[14] Liver biopsies include a wedge biopsy of the left lobe and needle biopsies of each lobe. A bone marrow biopsy is obtained from the iliac crest. Oophoropexy may be performed in girls, repositioning the ovaries to a midline location to minimize exposure from abdomi-

TABLE 9–10. *Staging of Hodgkin's Disease*

STAGING NOTATION	CRITERIA
Clinical or Pathological Stage*	
I	Involvement of a single lymph node region or lymphoid structure† (I) or a single extralymphatic site (I$_E$)
II	Involvement of two or more lymph node regions or lymphoid structures on the same side of the diaphragm; number of anatomic regions involved indicated by a subscript (e.g., II$_3$)
III	Involvement of lymph node regions or lymphoid structures on both sides of the diaphragm; may be subdivided into stage III$_1$ (spleen or splenic, hilar, celiac, or portal node involvement) or stage III$_2$, (para-aortic, iliac, or mesenteric node involvement)
IV	Diffuse or disseminated involvement of one or more extralymphatic sites with or without associated lymph node enlargement‡
Symptoms	
A	Asymptomatic
B	Symptoms include:
	Unexplained weight loss of more than 10% of body weight in 6 mo before initial staging
	Unexplained, persistent, or recurrent fever with temperatures above 38° C during previous month
	Recurrent drenching night sweats during previous month
Subscripts	
X	Bulky disease: ≥10 cm at maximal dimension
E	Extranodal extension: involvement of extralymphatic tissue by limited direct extension from an adjacent nodal site or a single extranodal deposit consistent with extension from a regionally involved node
PS sites	PS at a given site is indicated by a subscript: M = bone marrow; H = liver; L = lung; O = bone; P = pleura; D = skin

Data from references 4 and 28.
*Stages are designated as *clinical stage (CS)* when the extent of disease is determined by history, physical examination, radiologic and other imaging studies, laboratory tests, and initial biopsy results. *Pathologic stage (PS)* is designated when there is histologic confirmation of the presence or absence of involvement of specific sites.
†Lymphoid structures are the spleen, thymus, Waldeyer's ring (nasopharynx, tonsil, base of tongue), appendix, and Peyer's patches.
‡Liver involvement is always considered diffuse and therefore stage IV disease. Multiple extranodal disease is designated stage IV disease.

nal radiotherapy. If a LAG was done, an abdominal radiograph obtained during surgery can verify that all suspicious lymph nodes have been removed. Silver clips are left to mark the splenic pedicle and sites of lymph node biopsies. Postoperatively the clips assist in planning radiotherapy fields and evaluating possible recurrence.

TREATMENT

The goal of treatment is the cure of disease with minimal treatment-related toxicities and sequelae. Children who present with localized disease may be treated with radiotherapy alone. Most children are treated with a combined modality therapy using radiotherapy and chemotherapy.

Children with stage I disease in the upper neck or inguinal lymph nodes may be treated with involved-field radiotherapy alone.[10,21] In other patients with stage I and stage II or III disease, a decrease in the relapse rate has been observed with the use of extended-field (EF) radiotherapy.[7,10] In EF radiotherapy treatment is given to lymph nodes with known disease and adjacent uninvolved lymph node regions. Radiotherapy treatment fields used for Hodgkin's disease are shown in Figure 9–2. In more unfavorable situations such as

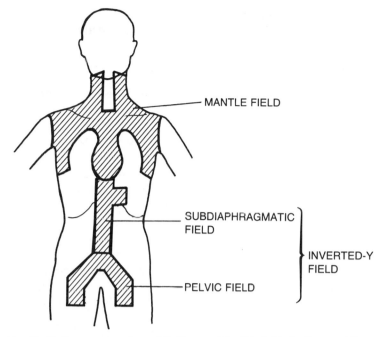

MANTLE FIELD

SUBDIAPHRAGMATIC
FIELD

INVERTED-Y
FIELD

PELVIC FIELD

FIGURE 9–2. Radiotherapy treatment fields used for Hodgkin's disease. The mantle field consists of the submandibular, submental, cervical, supraclavicular, infraclavicular, axillary, mediastinal, and hilar lymph nodes. Irradiation to the subdiaphragmatic field includes the para-aortic lymph nodes and the splenic pedicle or spleen. The pelvic field consists of the common iliac, external iliac, and inguinal-femoral lymph nodes. The inverted-Y field combines the subdiaphragmatic and pelvic fields. Total nodal irradiation includes the mantle field plus the inverted-Y field.

stage IIB and IIIB disease, total nodal irradiation (TNI) has been given. TNI treats the mantle field plus the inverted-Y field. In stage IV disease radiotherapy to areas of bulky or residual disease is optional. Radiotherapy is delayed until 8 years of age if possible to prevent retardation of bone growth and soft tissue development.

When a single field (e.g., mantle) is irradiated, a tumor dose of 3500 to 4400 cGy is given at a rate of 150 to 200 cGy per day five times a week.[12,27] When multiple fields will be irradiated such as the mantle and inverted-Y fields, the fields are usually treated sequentially, with a rest of approximately 4 weeks between each group of treatments. A booster dose of 500 to 1500 cGy may be given to very restricted fields to treat residual disease. Tumor dosages depend on the extent of involvement and whether chemotherapy will also be used. Dosages may be reduced in young children to minimize the effect on bone and soft tissue growth.[12]

The traditional mechlorethamine (nitrogen mustard), vincristine, procarbazine, and prednisone (MOPP) chemotherapy regimen has produced effective disease control but has the possible adverse effects of sterility in males and the development of leukemia. This regimen is given in 14-day courses at 28-day intervals or as tolerated for six cycles.

Other chemotherapy regimens have been developed for children with Hodgkin's disease. These regimens may include an alkylating agent, vinca alkaloid, adrenocorticosteroid, and anthracycline antibiotic. The number of chemotherapy cycles given in these regimens varies between series and protocols. Children with advanced disease receive chemotherapy as their primary treatment. The doxorubicin, bleomycin, vinblastine, and dacarbazine (ABVD) regimen was originally developed for the treatment of MOPP-resistant disease. The effectiveness of achieving dose reductions by alternating non-cross-resistant regimens (e.g., MOPP and ABVD) is being studied.[25,27] Single-agent chemotherapy is generally less effective and is given infrequently.

Radiotherapy may be administered before chemotherapy or alternated with courses of chemotherapy. The administration of chemotherapy before radiotherapy can reduce bulky disease, permitting the use of smaller radiotherapy fields and lower radiation doses.[10] Receiving radiotherapy limits the amount of chemotherapy that can be given and vice versa.[10,32] Studies are investigating the efficacy of limiting chemotherapy to three or four cycles when given with low-dose radiotherapy.[10,32]

Relapses historically have occurred within the first 3 years after treatment; however, the risk of relapse is present at least 10 years after diagnosis. The response to salvage therapy is very good with Hodgkin's disease. Patients with stage I and II disease who relapse in the previously treated radiotherapy field may be treated with chemotherapy alone. Radiotherapy may be used for recurrent disease outside the previous radiotherapy fields. Although there are fewer relapses in stage I and II patients treated with combined modality therapy, their response rate to salvage therapy is lower than that of patients who received radiotherapy alone.[10,12,26] Both chemotherapy and radiotherapy are used for new or recurrent disease in stages III and IV.[12,48]

Salvage chemotherapy has been administered using MOPP, ABVD, and chemotherapy regimens with agents non-cross-resistant to MOPP and ABVD such as the cytosine arabinoside, cisplatinum, and etoposide (APE) regimen.[27,51] Complete response rates in the range of 25% to 50% have been obtained in patients with relapsed disease.[51] Studies are investigating the effectiveness of intensive chemotherapy with allogeneic or autologous bone marrow transplantation for patients with multiple relapses. Prolonged clinical remissions have been obtained in 15% to 25% of these patients.[51]

The remission status is unclear in some patients. Patients are classified as having an "unconfirmed, uncertain complete remission" when they have no clinical evidence of disease but radiologic abnormalities inconsistent with the effects of therapy persist at the site of previous disease.[28] The significance of these abnormalities is presently unknown.

Young children whose spleens have been removed are at increased risk for fulminating bacterial infections, especially by encapsulated organisms such as *Streptococcus pneumoniae* and *Haemophilus influenzae*. Splenectomy may be deferred in children less than 5 years of age because of the immaturity of their immune systems. Lacking previous exposure, the young child has low levels of specific antibodies and cannot phagocytize bacterial pathogens at extrasplenic sites. Children with Hodgkin's disease are at further risk because of their underlying immunodeficiency. Treatment with chemotherapy and radiotherapy potentiates the risk of infection by reducing specific antibody activity. Functional hyposplenia has been observed after high-dose splenic irradiation.[5] The risk of infection after splenectomy or splenic irradiation apparently is lifelong. Use of a polyvalent pneumococcal vaccine in children with Hodgkin's disease has been discouraging; the level of antibody achieved or the duration of response may be inadequate for protection.[9] All children whose spleen has been removed should receive lifelong antibiotic prophylaxis with penicillin or erythromycin given orally twice daily.

PROGNOSTIC FACTORS

Clinical presentation with an advanced stage of disease (stage III or IV) and the presence of systemic symptoms (B symptoms) at the time of diagnosis are adverse prognostic indicators. Extralymphatic disease that is localized and can be treated definitively with radiotherapy does not adversely affect survival rates.[4,6]

Tumor bulk is an adverse factor. A lymph node or nodal mass is described as "bulky" when the largest dimension is 10 cm or greater.[28] A mediastinal mass is described as bulky when the maximal width seen on a chest radiograph is one third of the internal chest diameter at the level of T5-6.[28] Patients with stage I or II disease with a large mediastinal mass have an increased incidence of relapse when treated with radiotherapy alone.[6]

Certain clinical presentations have a very favorable prognosis in children. They include stage I nonbulky upper neck disease of any histologic type except LD, stage I nonbulky inguinal disease of any type, and stage I massive mediastinal disease of NS type.[10,12]

The prognostic significance of histology has declined with continued overall improvement in survival rates. The LP and NS types reportedly have a slightly more favorable prognosis than the MC and LD types.[10,13] The NS type has been classified into two grades; NS grade 2 contains areas of lymphocytic depletion and has a less favorable prognosis than NS grade 1, which does not have such areas.[13,19]

Test results may be closely associated with the stage of disease. Studies have shown that patients who present with an ESR greater than 50 mm/hour have a higher chance of relapse.[19,33,49] The presence of a WBC abnormality (either leukopenia or leukocytosis) at diagnosis is usually associated with an unfavorable course. High serum ferritin and low serum transferrin levels have been significantly associated with poor disease-free survival rates.[17]

Studies of serum copper level (SCL) in children have reported conflicting results. Some institutions have found a reliable correlation between SCL and disease activity in their pediatric populations.[47,48] In another study the SCL was frequently increased at the time of diagnosis and relapse; but elevated SCLs also occurred in children without active disease, and an increase was rarely the first sign of relapse. This study suggested that SCL determinations are not reliable predictors of disease activity.[50]

The soluble form of CD8 antigen (a surface membrane component of suppressor or cytotoxic T cells) has been measured in children with newly diagnosed Hodgkin's disease. Higher serum CD8 levels have been found in children with advanced disease (stage III or IV), B symptoms, and MC type. Having higher serum CD8 levels at diagnosis was significantly associated with an increased probability of treatment failure.[39]

PROGNOSIS

High survival rates have been obtained in children with Hodgkin's disease using different treatment strategies. Children with stage I or II disease have 10-year survival rates of over 90% with relapse-free survival rates of 70% to 90%.[10,27,46] More than 80% of children with stage III disease treated with combined modality therapy have attained 5-year survival rates.[27,46] The prognosis in stage IV disease continues to improve, and some children have complete, prolonged remissions consistent with a cure; a 70% 5-year survival rate has been reported.[27] Generally, children with systemic symptoms do less well than those without symptoms.

Aggressive treatment has increased long-term survival rates but also carries the inherent risk of long-term sequelae. A dose-related thyroid dysfunction, usually hypothyroidism, develops in up to 80% of patients treated with neck irradiation.[10,24] Cardiac dysfunctions, including pericardial effusion, constrictive pericarditis with tamponade, valvular heart disease, and coronary artery disease, can be induced by radiotherapy.[1,24,27] Pulmonary dysfunctions such as fibrosis or pneumonitis can occur in patients who received pulmonary radiotherapy or chemotherapy, especially bleomycin.[1,24] MOPP therapy can cause ovarian dysfunction in females and sterility in males.

The Late Effects Study Group has followed nearly 1000 children for a median of 7 years after treatment for Hodgkin's disease.[34] The cumulative probability of developing a second malignant neoplasm (SMN) was calculated at 2% at 5 years, 5% at 10 years, 9% at 15 years, and 20% at 20 years. Acute nonlymphocytic leukemia (ANLL) and non-Hodgkin's lymphoma occurred within a median time of 5 years after chemotherapy. The risk of developing an SMN was significantly greater if the patient received alkylating agents. All patients who developed ANLL received at least two alkylating agents for 6 months or longer. Solid tumors usually occurred within the radiation treatment field at a median time of 12 years after radiotherapy. The most common solid tumors were thyroid carcinoma and basal cell carcinoma. Adult-type cancers (breast and colon carcinoma), osteosarcomas, and soft tissue sarcomas have also been reported.[23,34]

Children treated for Hodgkin's disease will require continued observation for adverse late effects. The development of clinical trials with equivalent or better survival rates and reduced potential for late effects will further improve the prognosis for children with Hodgkin's disease.

REFERENCES

1. Blatt J, Copeland DR, Bleyer WA. Late effects of childhood cancer and its treatment. In Pizzo PA, Poplack DG (eds): Principles and Practice of Pediatric Oncology, 2nd ed. Philadelphia: JB Lippincott, 1993, pp 1091–1114.
2. Boren HA, Sullivan MP. Hodgkin's disease. In Hockenberry MJ, Coody DK (eds): Pediatric Oncology and Hematology: Perspectives on Care. St. Louis: CV Mosby, 1986, pp 54–80.
3. Boring CC, Squires TS, Tong T. Cancer statistics, 1993. Ca 1993; 43:7–26.
4. Carbone PP, Kaplan HS, Musshoff K, et al. Report of the committee on Hodgkin's disease staging classification. Cancer Res 1971; 31:1860–1861.
5. Coleman CN, McDougall IR, Dailey MO, et al. Functional hyposplenia after splenic irradiation for Hodgkin's disease. Ann Intern Med 1982; 96:44–47.
6. Donaldson SS. Current management and controversies: A radiotherapist's view. In Kamps WA, Humphrey GB, Poppema S (eds): Hodgkin's Disease in Children: Controversies and Current Practice. Boston: Kluwer Academic Publishers, 1989, pp 145–165.
7. Donaldson SS, Link MP. Combined modality treatment with low-dose radiation and MOPP chemotherapy for children with Hodgkin's disease. J Clin Oncol 1987; 5:742–749.
8. Donaldson SS, Link MP. Hodgkin's disease: Treatment of the young child. Pediatr Clin North Am 1991; 38:457–473.
9. Donaldson SS, Vosti KL, Berberich FR, et al. Response to pneumococcal vaccine among children with Hodgkin's disease. Rev Infect Dis 1981; 3(suppl 2):S133–S143.
10. Donaldson SS, Whitaker SJ, Plowman PN, et al. Stage I-II pediatric Hodgkin's disease: Long-term follow-up demonstrates equivalent survival rates following different management schemes. J Clin Oncol 1990; 8:1128–1137.
11. Dudgeon DL, Kelly R, Ghory MJ, et al. The efficacy of lymphangiography in the staging of pediatric Hodgkin's disease. J Pediatr Surg 1986; 21:233–235.
12. Gehan EA, Sullivan MP, Fuller LM, et al. The Intergroup Hodgkin's disease in children: A study of stages I and II. Cancer 1990; 65:1429–1437.
13. Glimelius B. Prognostic factors including clinical markers. In Kamps WA, Humphrey GB, Poppema S (eds): Hodgkin's Disease in Children: Controversies and Current Practice. Boston: Kluwer Academic Publishers, 1989, pp. 89–96.
14. Green DM, Ghoorah J, Douglass HO Jr, et al. Staging laparotomy with splenectomy in children and adolescents with Hodgkin's disease. Cancer Treat Rev 1983; 10:23–38.
15. Grufferman S, Cole P, Smith PG, et al. Hodgkin's disease in siblings. N Engl J Med 1977; 296:248–250.
16. Gutensohn NM, Shapiro DS. Social class risk factors among children with Hodgkin's disease. Int J Cancer 1982; 30:433–435.
17. Hann HW, Lange B, Stahlhut MW, et al. Prognostic importance of serum transferrin and ferritin in childhood Hodgkin's disease. Cancer 1990; 66:313–316.
18. Hardell L, Bengtsson NO. Epidemiological study of socioeconomic factors and clinical findings in Hodgkin's disease, and reanalysis of previous data regarding chemical exposure. Br J Cancer 1983; 48:217–225.
19. Haybittle JL, Easterling MJ, Bennett MH, et al. Review of British National Lymphoma Investigation studies of Hodgkin's disease and development of prognostic index. Lancet 1985; 1:967–972.
20. Hors J, Dausset J. HLA and susceptibility to Hodgkin's disease. Immunol Rev 1983; 70:167–191.
21. Jenkin D, Doyle J, Berry M, et al. Hodgkin's disease in children: Treatment with MOPP and low-dose, extended field irradiation without laparotomy late results and toxicity. Med Pediatr Oncol 1990; 18:265–272.
22. Kung FH. Hodgkin's disease in children 4 years of age or younger. Cancer 1991; 67:1428–1430.
23. Kushner BH, Zauber A, Tan CTC. Second malignancies after childhood Hodgkin's disease. The Memorial Sloan-Kettering Cancer Center experience. Cancer 1988; 62:1364–1370.
24. Lange BJ, Meadows AT. Late effects of Hodgkin's disease treatment in children. In Kamps WA, Humphrey GB, Poppema S (eds): Hodgkin's Disease in Children: Controversies and Current Practice. Boston: Kluwer Academic Publishers, 1989, pp 195–220.
25. Leventhal BG. The Pediatric Oncology Group: Studies in Hodgkin's disease. In Kamps WA, Humphrey GB, Poppema S (eds): Hodgkin's Disease in Children: Controversies and Current Practice. Boston: Kluwer Academic Publishers, 1989, pp 257–262.
26. Leventhal BG. Management of stage I-II Hodgkin's disease in children. J Clin Oncol 1990; 8:1123–1124. (Editorial.)
27. Leventhal BG, Donaldson SS. Hodgkin's disease. In Pizzo PA, Poplack DG (eds): Principles and Practice of Pediatric Oncology, 2nd ed. Philadelphia: JB Lippincott, 1993, pp 577–594.
28. Lister TA, Crowther D, Sutcliffe SB, et al. Report of a committee convened to discuss the evaluation and staging of patients with Hodgkin's disease: Cotswolds meeting. J Clin Oncol 1989; 7:1630–1636.
29. Lukes RJ. Criteria for involvement of lymph node, bone marrow, spleen, and liver in Hodgkin's disease. Cancer Res 1971; 31:1755–1767.
30. Lukes RJ, Craver LF, Hall TC, et al. Report of the Nomenclature Committee. Cancer Res 1966; 26(part 1):1311.
31. MacMahon B. Epidemiology of Hodgkin's disease. Cancer Res 1966; 26(part 1):1189–1200.
32. Maity A, Goldwein JW, Lange B, et al. Comparison of high-dose and low-dose radiation with and without chemotherapy for children with Hodgkin's disease: An analysis of the experience at the Children's Hospital of Philadelphia and the Hospital of the Uni-

versity of Pennsylvania. J Clin Oncol 1992; 10:929–935.

33. McClain KL, Heise R, Day DL, et al. Hodgkin's disease in children: Correlation of clinical characteristics, staging procedures, and treatment at the University of Minnesota. Am J Pediatr Hematol Oncol 1990; 12:147–154.

34. Meadows AT, Obringer AC, Marrero O, et al. Second malignant neoplasms following childhood Hodgkin's disease: Treatment and splenectomy as risk factors. Med Pediatr Oncol 1989; 17:477–484.

35. Mueller NE. The epidemiology of Hodgkin's disease. In Selby P, McElwain TJ (eds): Hodgkin's Disease. Boston: Blackwell Scientific Publications, 1987, pp 68–93.

36. Osoba D. The major histocompatibility complex and lymphomas. In Sutcliffe SB (ed): Immunology of the Lymphomas. Boca Raton, Fla.: CRC Press, 1985, pp 167–193.

37. Parkin DM, Stiller CA, Draper GJ, et al. The international incidence of childhood cancer. Int J Cancer 1988; 42:511–520.

38. Poppema S, Brinker MGL, Visser L. Evidence for a B-cell origin of the proliferating cells. In Kamps WA, Humphrey GB, Poppema S (eds): Hodgkin's Disease in Children: Controversies and Current Practice. Boston: Kluwer Academic Publishers, 1989, pp 5–27.

39. Pui CH, Ip SH, Thompson E, et al. Increased serum CD8 antigen level in childhood Hodgkin's disease relates to advanced stage and poor treatment outcome. Blood 1989; 73:209–213.

40. Riyat MS. Hodgkin's disease in Kenya. Cancer 1992; 69:1047–1051.

41. Romagnani S, Maggi E, Parronchi P. The immune derangement and strategies for immunotherapy. In Kamps WA, Humphrey GB, Poppema S (eds): Hodgkin's Disease in Children: Controversies and Current Practice. Boston: Kluwer Academic Publishers, 1989, pp 53–88.

42. Safai B, Diaz B, Schwartz J. Malignant neoplasms associated with human immunodeficiency virus infection. CA 1992; 42:74–95.

43. Spitz MR, Sider JF, Johnson CC, et al. Ethnic patterns of Hodgkin's disease incidence among children and adolescents in the United States, 1973-1982. J Nat Cancer Inst 1986; 76:235–239.

44. Strum SB, Rappaport H. Consistency of histologic subtypes in Hodgkin's disease in simultaneous and sequential biopsy specimens. Natl Cancer Inst Monogr 1973; 36:253–260.

45. Sullivan MP, Fuller LM. Hodgkin's disease in children. In Fuller LM, Hagemeister FB, Sullivan MP, et al. (eds): Hodgkin's Disease and Non-Hodgkin's Lymphomas in Adults and Children. New York: Raven Press, 1988, pp 247–269.

46. Tan CTC. Hodgkin's disease in children and adolescents: Experiences from the Memorial Sloan-Kettering Cancer Center, New York. In Kamps WA, Humphrey GB, Poppema S (eds): Hodgkin's Disease in Children: Controversies and Current Practice. Boston: Kluwer Academic Publishers, 1989, pp 291–302.

47. Tessmer CF, Hrgovcic M, Wilbur J. Serum copper in Hodgkin's disease in children. Cancer 1973; 31:303–315.

48. Thompson EI. Hodgkin's disease. In Fernbach DJ, Vietti TJ (eds): Clinical Pediatric Oncology, 4th ed. St. Louis: Mosby–Year Book, 1991, pp 355–375.

49. Tubiana M, Henry-Amar M, Burgers MV, et al. Prognostic significance of erythrocyte sedimentation rate in clinical stages I-II of Hodgkin's disease. J Clin Oncol 1984; 2:194–200.

50. Wilimas J, Thompson E, Smith KL. Value of serum copper levels and erythrocyte sedimentation rates as indicators of disease activity in children with Hodgkin's disease. Cancer 1978; 42:1929–1935.

51. Wimmer RS. Salvage treatment for patients with multiply relapsed Hodgkin's disease. In Kamps WA, Humphrey GB, Poppema S (eds): Hodgkin's Disease in Children: Controversies and Current Practice. Boston: Kluwer Academic Publishers, 1989, pp 187–194.

52. Young JL Jr, Ries LG, Silverberg E, et al. Cancer incidence, survival, and mortality for children younger than age 15 years. Cancer 1986; 58(suppl 2):598–602.

■ Non-Hodgkin's Lymphoma

Noreen McGowan Quinlan

Non-Hodgkin's lymphoma (NHL), the third most common childhood malignancy, is approximately 1½ times as prevalent as Hodgkin's disease in childhood. NHL occurs from infancy through adolescence, with a peak incidence between the ages of 7 and 11 years.[27,36] Boys are affected more than girls, with a 3:1 occurrence ratio.[8]

The origin and spread of NHL differ from the patterns of other neoplasms.[18] Most cancers originate in an organ or tissue and spread from a point of origin, either by local extension or metastasis. Malignant lymphomas are neoplasms of the lymph system, which is widely distributed throughout the body, accounting for the fact that most lymphomas are generalized diseases from the onset. The patterns of spread often mimic the migration pattern of the lymphomas' cells.[18,19]

Childhood NHL differs significantly from Hodgkin's disease in clinical behavior, pathology, mode of spread, and responsiveness to treatment. In childhood NHL the malignant cells appear undifferentiated, and the pattern of infiltration is diffuse. NHL tends to have a rapid onset, presents with widespread involvement at the time of diagnosis, and generally has a quick response to treatment; with Hodgkin's disease, on the other hand, the malignant cell is more differentiated, and the pattern of infiltration is more specific. The onset of Hodgkin's disease is typically subacute and prolonged, and a patient with it usually has localized disease at the time of diagnosis. Its response to therapy is typically slower than that of NHL.[27]

ETIOLOGY

The cause of NHL remains unknown. Genetic, immunologic, viral, and environmental factors may play important roles.[27]

A number of inherited and acquired conditions predispose the child to the development of lymphoma.[19] An increased incidence has been found in children with congenital immunodeficiency syndromes, including Wiskott-Aldrich syndrome, severe combined immunodeficiency syndrome, ataxia telangiectasia, common variable immunodeficiency, Bloom syndrome, and X-linked lymphoproliferative syndrome. Chronically immunosuppressed recipients of major organ transplants are also at high risk for development of NHL. It is hypothesized that an altered immune state provides the necessary susceptibility for this tumor induction.[8,15,19]

Patients with acquired immunodeficiency syndrome (AIDS) also have an increased risk of developing NHL, particularly primary lymphoma of the CNS.[3,37]

Some patients treated with chemotherapy and radiation for Hodgkin's disease and other neoplasms have developed NHL as a second malignancy.[27]

The Epstein-Barr virus (EBV) has been linked to the development of Burkitt's lymphoma in children in Africa where this type of NHL is endemic. These patients are clustered near the equator in various geographic regions that experience heavy rainfall. They often have tumor cells with the viral DNA and nuclear antigens and have high antibody titers against EBV. Jaw tumors are common in these patients.[12,18] This form of endemic NHL is associated with a break point on chromosome 8 that is usually some distance from the c-*myc* oncogene.[17] The form of Burkitt's lymphoma commonly seen in non-African children is sporadic, with neither clustering, obvious geographic distribution, nor climate influences. There has been only an occasional association with EBV in these non-African patients. They usually present with abdominal tumors rather than jaw disease.[12,18] This form of sporadic tumor is associated with a break point on chromosome 8 that is usually very close to or within the c-*myc* oncogene.[17] The reason for the differences between African and non-African Burkitt's lymphoma is unclear, although the possibility that they are etiologically separate entities has been raised.[27]

HISTOLOGY

The history of histopathologic classification in NHL is complex. Many classifications have been proposed for both adult and childhood NHL, resulting in difficulties in making comparisons among classification systems.[1] Two of these systems that can be applied to childhood NHL are a modified Rappaport classification schema and the Working Formulations for Clinical Uses.[26] They can be divided into three groups: lymphoblastic, small noncleaved cell, and large cell lymphomas.[4,18]

In individuals with lymphoblastic lymphoma the malignant cells have finely stippled nuclear chromatin, multiple nucleoli, nuclear convolutions, and only a small rim of cytoplasm. The lymphoblasts have a high mitotic index and an immature immunophenotype.[29] The majority of lymphoblastic lymphomas are of immature T-cell origin. The enzyme terminal deoxynucleotidyl transferase (TdT) is expressed in these cells.[17,18] Chromosomal translocations involving break points at either 14q11.2 (site of the gene coding the alpha chain of the T-cell receptor gene) or 7q34 (site of the gene encoding the beta chain of the T-cell receptor gene) frequently occur with lymphoblastic lymphoma.[1,12,28] Patients with lymphoblastic lymphoma commonly present with mediastinal disease, with or without extra thoracic involvement and peripheral nodal disease.[28,29]

Pathologic review of small noncleaved cell (Burkitt's or non-Burkitt's) lymphoma shows cells that are round and have prominent nucleoli and a small amount of basophilic cytoplasm that may contain prominent vacuoles. A scattering of normal macrophages results in a "starry sky" appearance that is classic for small noncleaved cell lymphoma.[29] These cells lack TdT, have a variable mitotic index, and usually have a B-cell origin.[17,18] Recurring chromosomal translocations between 8q24 (site of c-*myc* proto-oncogene) and 14q32 (site of immunoglobulin heavy chain gene) are characteristic of these cells.[13,17,20] The proto-oncogene c-*myc* is deregulated by this translocation. This process is believed one of the important steps in malignant transformation. Patients with small noncleaved cell lymphoma commonly present with intra-abdominal disease.[20,29]

Large-cell lymphoma shows malignant cells with a nucleus larger than a macrophage nucleus, prominent nucleoli, and a low nuclear-cytoplasmic ratio.[29] These cells lack TdT, and a majority are of B-cell origin, although

TABLE 9–11. *Important Features of Non-Hodgkin's Lymphoma*

RAPPAPORT CLASSIFICATION	WORKING FORMULATION CLASSIFICATION	CASES (%)	PHENOTYPE	CYTOGENETIC MARKERS	COMMON CLINICAL PRESENTATION
Diffuse lymphoblastic (convoluted or nonconvoluted)	ML, lymphoblastic	30–40	T cell TdT +	14q11 7q34	Mediastinal mass, pleural effusion, lymphadenopathy; superior vena cava syndrome; respiratory distress; propensity for rapid spread to bone marrow, CNS, and gonads
Diffuse undifferentiated (Burkitt's or non-Burkitt's)	ML, small noncleaved cell (Burkitt's or non-Burkitt's)	40–50	B cell NonT-nonB	8q24 14q32	Abdominal primary; tumor lysis syndrome; jaw tumor (African); propensity for spread to CNS and bone marrow
Diffuse histiocytic	ML, large cell	15	B cell T cell	t(2;5) (p23; q35)	Extranodal site common (lung, face, brain, skin, bone)

Data from references 1, 12, 18, and 29.
ML = malignant lymphoma; TdT = terminal deoxynucleotidyl transferase.

a small portion are of T-cell origin.[17,18] Chromosomal translocation t(2;5)(p23;q35) has been seen with large cell lymphoma. Waldeyer's ring and extranodal sites such as skin, lung, bone, and brain are common locations for large cell lymphoma.[12,29]

Some investigators for practical purposes have divided childhood NHL into two groups: lymphoblastic and nonlymphoblastic (undifferentiated lymphoma, Burkitt's and non-Burkitt's, large cell, or histiocytic).[22,25,27] Table 9–11 simplifies this complex classification and correlates other important factors of NHL such as phenotype, cytogenetic markers, and clinical presentation.

STAGING

Stages I, II, and III are relatively easy to define as seen in Table 9–12. Stage IV is more complex to define because of the controversy surrounding the distinction between lymphoma with bone marrow involvement and leukemia, an area often debated among investigators.[15,18] Stage IV NHL is most commonly defined as bulky disease with less than 25% blasts in the bone marrow. If the extent of bone marrow involvement is greater than 25%, this condition is classified as acute lymphoblastic leukemia (ALL) rather than lymphoma.[15,23] It is thought that these tumors have invaded the bone marrow and thereby have undergone leukemic transformation. The clinical behavior of this malignancy, which many refer to as *leukemia/lymphoma*, is more like that of lymphoma rather than leukemia (i.e., rapid onset, need for aggressive treatment, and quick response to therapy).[8]

Other investigators maintain that only with the evaluation of the total clinical picture and the primary site and histologic classification of biopsy sites can the differential diagnosis be made.[33] They believe that bone marrow involvement in NHL can be partial (<25% blasts or stage IV A) or total (>25% blasts or stage IV B) replacement, with or without peripheral blood involvement.[6,35]

Whether one refers to this disease as ALL, leukemia/lymphoma, or NHL stage IV, it is important to recognize that it is a rapidly progressing disease requiring aggressive treatment.

CLINICAL PRESENTATIONS

The majority of patients have stage III or IV disease at the time of diagnosis.[33] The time from onset of symptoms to diagnosis is usually from a few days to a few weeks.[8] Signs and symptoms vary considerably, depending on the specific organs involved.[12]

The most common site of disease in NHL is intra-abdominal, with mediastinal, peripheral nodal, and nasopharyngeal sites following in frequency of occurrence.[8,33] Intra-abdominal disease accounts for approximately one third of childhood NHL. Signs and symptoms associated with abdominal lymphoma may mimic those of appendicitis (i.e., pain, intestinal obstruction, right lower quadrant tenderness, with or without presence of fever). These acute findings are due to the involvement of the distal ileum, appendix, or cecum. Intussusception may also be caused by lymphoma. In fact, symptoms of intussusception in children over the age of 5 years should be highly suspicious for NHL. Other patients may present with ovarian, pelvic, or retroperitoneal masses and ascites. These patients often show signs of massive tumor burden such as increased levels of serum uric acid and lactate dehydrogenase (LDH) and are prone to tumor lysis syndrome, particularly during the initial phases of therapy. Patients with intra-abdominal NHL also tend to have bone marrow and CNS involvement.[8,18,27]

Primary mediastinal disease occurs in approximately one fourth of the children with NHL. Asymptomatic mediastinal involvement is possible. However, the usual presentation of mediastinal adenopathy is with acute respiratory symptoms; therefore close observation of respiratory status is essential. These patients have pleural effusion or tracheal compression, causing pain, tachypnea, cough, wheezing, dyspnea, or respiratory distress. The superior vena caval obstruction may cause plethora of the neck and face, edema of the upper extremities and face, conjunctivitis, or mental status changes. Patients with primary mediastinal disease can also have extensive disease outside the thoracic cavity such as abdominal, bone marrow, and CNS involvement. This disease tends to grow rapidly, causing severe respiratory compro-

TABLE 9–12. *Clinical Staging Systems for Childhood Lymphomas*

STAGE	MEMORIAL SLOAN-KETTERING CANCER CENTER	ST. JUDE CHILDREN'S RESEARCH HOSPITAL	STAGE	NATIONAL CANCER INSTITUTE
I	One single site	Single tumor (extranodal) or single anatomic area (nodal) with the exclusion of mediastinum or abdomen	A	Single solitary extra-abdominal site
II	Two or more sites on same side of diaphragm	Single tumor (extranodal) with regional node involvement Two or more nodal areas on the same side of the diaphragm Two single (extranodal) tumors, with or without regional node involvement, on the same side of the diaphragm Primary GI tract tumor, usually in the ileocecal area, with or without involvement of associated mesenteric nodes only	B	Multiple extra-abdominal sites
III	Disseminated disease without marrow or CNS involvement	Two single tumors (extranodal) on opposite sides of the diaphragm Two or more nodal areas above and below the diaphragm All the primary intrathoracic tumors (mediastinal, pleural, thymic) All extensive primary intra-abdominal disease All paraspinal or epidural tumors, regardless of other tumor site(s)	C	Intra-abdominal tumor
IV	Any of above with bone marrow and/or CNS involvement	Any of the above, with initial CNS or bone marrow involvement (<25% blasts)	D	Intra-abdominal tumor with involvement of one or more extra-abdominal sites
IVA	Bone marrow with <25% blasts		AR	Intra-abdominal tumor with more than 90% of tumor surgically resected
IVB	Bone marrow with >25% blasts			

Data from references 18, 22, 33, and 35.

mise. Therefore clinical and laboratory studies needed to establish a diagnosis should be done at once and appropriate therapy started as soon as possible.[8,22,27]

In addition to the obvious lymph node enlargement, peripheral nodal involvement can produce the following symptoms: fever, malaise, anorexia, sore throat, cough, weight loss, earache, night sweats, and bone and joint pain. Usually these patients have a history of no improvement in lymph node enlargement or progression of the enlargement despite antibiotic therapy.[33]

Primary nasal, paranasal, oral, and pharyngeal lymphoma (sometimes referred to as *nasopharyngeal lymphoma*) involves sites such as Waldeyer's ring, paranasal sinuses, maxilla, mandible, orbital cavity, and parotid or salivary glands. The most common symptoms include pain, nasal stuffiness, anorexia, rhinorrhea, epistaxis, headache, proptosis, irritability, and weight loss.[27,35]

Primary lymphoma of the CNS is relatively rare but is increasing in incidence in association with AIDS.[3,14] CNS involvement can affect either a primary site or a site of disseminated disease. It may include meningeal infiltration, cranial nerve infiltration, intracerebral disease, paraspinal disease, or some combination of these conditions, most often meningeal infiltration with cranial nerve involvement.[17] Meningeal involvement is associated with headache, vomiting, irritability, and papilledema. It is usually confirmed by lumbar puncture, which shows increased opening pressure, CSF pleocytosis in various degrees with positive cytology, and normal or abnormal sugar and protein levels.[33] Any cranial nerve can be involved, but the ophthalmic nerve and the facial nerves are most frequently affected. Paraspinal and epidural disease can lead to cord compression by extranodal involvement; therefore the neurologic status of these patients must be monitored closely.[18]

In other primary sites such as bone, skin, ovary, and testes the symptoms usually correlate with the sites involved and may also include fever, anorexia, weight loss, or pain.[5,12]

DIAGNOSIS

The diagnostic evaluation is planned carefully to ensure accuracy and to avoid delay in treatment. All samples (i.e., tissues, bone marrow, and CSF) are evaluated at a facility capable of performing histopathology, immunophenotyping, and cytogenetic studies.[12] Since approximately 20% of patients with NHL have bone marrow involvement at initial presentation, bone marrow aspirates and biopsies should be performed as initial evaluations on all patients, especially those with respiratory difficulties, before resorting to a thoracotomy. In other cases fluid from pleural effusions or ascites can be used for diagnostic examination without the need for tissue biopsy. A lumbar puncture is also performed on all patients to rule out the presence of malignant cells in the CNS. The diagnosis of NHL is never made solely on the basis of clinical symptoms.[8,14]

The workup also involves a history and physical examination and appropriate radiographic studies. Laboratory studies include CBC with differential, liver and renal function studies, electrolyte, calcium, phosphorus, magnesium, lactate dehydrogenase (LDH), and uric acid determinations, EBV titers, and urinalysis.[15,27]

PROGNOSTIC FACTORS

Many investigators believe that the most important prognostic factor in childhood NHL is the tumor burden at presentation. However, this is difficult to quantify since many staging systems do not accurately reflect tumor burden. Elevated levels of molecules secreted or shed by the tumor cells or those that accumulate as a consequence of tumor breakdown suggest the extent of tumor burden. These levels include those for LDH, uric acid, lactic acid, and polyamines. These levels may also provide tumor markers of value in assessing the progress of therapy.[18,29]

Age, sex, and race are not major prognostic factors.[24,34] Histology may have prognostic significance, especially in patients with advanced disease.[2,10,16] However, the prognostic significance of localized versus advanced disease may be the more important factor. The presence of CNS disease usually indicates a poor prognosis.[12,29] Patients with AIDS have a generally poor prognosis, attributed in part to the underlying immunosuppression and to intolerance to optimal chemotherapy.[37]

TREATMENT

Assessment of the patient's metabolic status before the initiation of therapy is important because one of the serious complications of NHL and its treatment is tumor lysis syndrome, which may occur in patients with advanced disease, especially Burkitt's and lymphoblastic types. It may be present before the start of therapy and often worsens once therapy is started. It results from rapid lysis of tumor cells, either by intrinsic cell death or in response to chemotherapy, for these cells release various electrolytes and metabolites into the circulation.[12] Hyperuricemia, hyperkalemia, hyperphosphatemia, and hypocalcemia are the primary metabolic consequences. The sudden alteration in serum chemistries may produce an electrolyte imbalance that can result in renal failure or cardiac arrest. It is essential these patients receive intensive hydration (3 L/m²/day), receive urinary alkalinization, and start allopurinol therapy before the initiation of treatment. Serum chemistries and urinary output must be closely monitored. Dialysis may be necessary if renal failure occurs before or during therapy.[14,27] In many centers patients who present with a high risk of tumor lysis (i.e., high tumor burden, high LDH level, or metabolic disturbances) often are admitted to a critical care unit for management.

Current treatment for NHL is multiagent chemotherapy to eradicate disease and to prevent further dissemination.[15] A number of different protocol regimens are used that consider disease stage, immunophenotype, and histology. Patients with localized disease (stages I and II) require therapy that is less intensive and of shorter duration, whereas patients with advanced disease (stages III and IV) require more aggressive therapy. The differentiation between lymphoblastic, small noncleaved cell, or large-cell lymphoma is widely used as a means of determining treatment protocols.[2,16,29]

In general, chemotherapy for small noncleaved lymphoma includes cyclophosphamide and methotrexate (e.g., the COMP regimen). Treatment for lymphoblastic lymphoma consists of multidrug combinations of cyclophosphamide, vincristine, daunomycin or doxorubicin, L-asparaginase, cytosine arabinoside, and methotrexate (e.g., the LSA_2L_2 or APO regimens).[2,11,30,32] The optimal therapy for large-cell lymphoma is not clear, but it is treated effectively with regimens used for both lymphoblastic and small noncleaved lymphomas.[2,14,32]

The induction phase of treatment involves 4 to 6 weeks of combined intensive multiagent chemotherapy such as cyclophosphamide, prednisone, vincristine, L-asparaginase, daunomycin or doxorubicin, cytosine arabinoside, VP-16, and methotrexate.[8,18,27] Along with tumor lysis syndrome, the systemic side effects of treatment can be severe during this phase. The advances in multidisciplinary and supportive care (mainly blood banking, use of colony-stimulating factors, and advances in the management of infectious diseases) have allowed administration of these intensive multiagent protocols relatively safely. The patient must be observed closely during this time since infection is another primary threat. Hospitalizations may be frequent, but usually at least a portion of this phase can be administered on an outpatient basis.

CNS protection is given during induction and throughout treatment to prevent meningeal relapse. Intrathecal chemotherapy includes methotrexate, cytosine arabinoside, or a combination of the two with hydrocortisone (triple IT).[18,21,27] In the past CNS radiation has been given as prophylactic treatment, but it currently is used only in cases of demonstrable CNS disease.[14,15] Induction therapy alone is not adequate for treatment; therefore continuous therapy or maintenance treatments are necessary to eradicate all the residual microscopic disease and prevent the emergence of drug-resistant malignant clones.[10] These regimens differ according to the protocols but may include cyclophosphamide, vincristine, oral 6-MP and methotrexate, cytosine arabinoside, daunomycin, BCNU, thioguanine, and hydroxyurea.[18,27] During this phase the systemic side effects of chemotherapy are not as severe as with induction therapy, and most patients can return to school and participate in normal childhood activities.

The length of treatment also varies depending on the protocol.[23] Most investigators believe patients with localized disease (stages I and II) need less therapy than those with advanced disease (stages III and IV).[11] The duration of chemotherapy generally has been 1 to 2 years, but recent data suggest that with intensive regimens, treatment may be reduced to 6 months.[14,32]

In the past radiation therapy has played a major role in the treatment of NHL in combination with chemotherapy. However, the use of radiation therapy has been questioned because of the additive and long-term effects of combined therapy. Studies have demonstrated that radiation therapy can be omitted from treatment of NHL if intensive chemotherapy regimens are used; therefore no clear survival benefit is added with the use of radiation therapy.[5,9,16,17]

A partial response can be seen as early as 1 to 2 days after therapy is started. Complete remission should be obtained within 4 to 6 weeks from the initiation of treatment. Relapse, if it occurs, is often seen early in the course of the disease, although late relapse after completion of effective treatment can occur. Some investigators believe there is a strong correlation between histology and the timing of relapse. Relapse in patients with nonlymphoblastic lymphoma may occur as early as 3 to 4 months after diagnosis, whereas relapse in patients with lymphoblastic lymphoma tends to occur late in treatment or after therapy has been completed.[24,25,29] The most common sites of relapse are the site of original disease, bone marrow, and CNS.[33] Many investigators refer to relapse in the bone marrow with more than 25% blasts as *leukemic conversion* or *transformation of NHL.*[18,27]

The treatment of relapsed NHL is extremely difficult, and patients with relapse have a very low survival rate.[25] Autologous or allogeneic bone marrow transplantation (BMT) may be treatment options. BMT in NHL appears more successful when used early in the course of treatment.[12,31]

In addition to BMT, future trends in the treatment of NHL include the use of biologic response modifiers alone or in combination with other treatment modalities. It is hoped these agents will improve the response achieved with standard therapy and provide prolonged response duration.[7]

PROGNOSIS

The rise in the cure rate of childhood NHL has corresponded directly to the increase in the intensity of combined chemotherapy. In the early seventies the overall survival rate

for NHL was 11%.[33,34] With aggressive therapy, the survival rate for patients with localized disease currently is nearly 90%, and for those with advanced disease it is 60% to 70%.[14,18,27] The key to this success is aggressive therapy from the onset of treatment combined with attentive, supportive, and multidisciplinary care.

REFERENCES

1. Amylon MD, Link MP, Murphy SB. Malignant T-cell and other non-Hodgkin's lymphomas. In Voute PA, Barrett A, Bloom HJ, et al. (eds): Cancer in Children: Clinical Management, 2nd ed. New York: Springer-Verlag, 1986, pp 152–163.
2. Anderson JR, Wilson JF, Jenkins RDH, et al. Childhood non-Hodgkin's lymphoma. The results of a randomized therapeutic trial comparing a four drug regimen (COMP) with a ten drug regimen (LSA₂-L₂). N Engl J Med 1983; 308:559–565.
3. Beral V, Peterman T, Berkelman R, et al. AIDS-associated non-Hodgkin's lymphoma. Lancet 1991; 337:805–809.
4. Burke J. The histopathologic classification of non-Hodgkin's lymphomas: Ambiguities in the working formulation and two newly reported categories. Semin Oncol 1990; 17:3–10.
5. Coppes MJ, Patte C, Couanet D, et al. Childhood malignant lymphomas of bone. Med Pediatr Oncol 1991; 19:22–27.
6. Duque-Hammershaimb L, Wollner N, Miller DR. LSA₂-L₂ protocol treatment of stage IV non-Hodgkin's lymphoma in children with partial and extensive bone marrow involvement. Cancer 1983; 52:39–43.
7. Gilewski T, Richards J. Biologic response modifiers in non-Hodgkin's lymphoma. Semin Oncol 1990; 117:74–87.
8. Graham M. Non-Hodgkin's lymphoma. Pediatr Ann 1988; 17:192–203.
9. Grayson J, Glatstein E. Radiation therapy in the non-Hodgkin's lymphoma. In Magrath IT (ed): The Non-Hodgkin's Lymphoma. London: Edward Arnold, 1990, pp 214–226.
10. Huizdala EV, Bernard C, Callihan J, et al. Nonlymphoblastic lymphoma in children—Histology and stage-related response to therapy: A pediatric oncology group study. J Clin Oncol 1991; 9:1189–1195.
11. Jenkin RDT, Anderson RR, Chilcote RR, et al. The treatment of localized non-Hodgkin's lymphoma in children: A report from the Children's Cancer Study Group. J Clin Oncol 1984; 2:88–97.
12. Kurtzberg J, Graham M. Non-Hodgkin's lymphoma, biologic classification and implication for therapy. Pediatr Clin North Am 1991; 38:443–454.
13. Lemerle J, Bernard A, Patte C, et al. Malignant B-cell lymphoma of childhood. In Voute PA, Barrett A, Bloom HJ, et al. (eds): Cancer in Children: Clinical Management, 2nd ed. New York: Springer-Verlag, 1986, pp 137–151.
14. Leventhal B, Kato G. Childhood Hodgkin and non-Hodgkin lymphoma. Pediatr Rev 1990; 12:171–179.
15. Link M. Non-Hodgkin's lymphoma in children. Pediatr Clin North Am 1985; 32:699–719.

16. Link M, Donaldson S, Bernard C, et al. Results of treatment of childhood localized non-Hodgkin's lymphoma with combination chemotherapy with or without radiotherapy. N Engl J Med 1990; 322:1169–1174

17. Magrath IT. Malignant non-Hodgkin's lymphoma in children. Hematol Oncol Clin North Am 1987; 1:577–603.

18. Magrath IT. Malignant non-Hodgkin's lymphoma in children. In Pizzo PA, Poplack DG (eds): Principles and Practices of Pediatric Oncology, 2nd ed. Philadelphia: JB Lippincott, 1993, pp 537–575.

19. Magrath IT. Lymphocyte ontogeny: A conceptual basis for understanding neoplasia of the immune system. In Magrath IT (ed): The Non-Hodgkin's Lymphoma. London: Edward Arnold, 1990, pp 29–48.

20. Magrath IT. Small non-cleaved cell lymphoma. In Magrath IT (ed): The Non-Hodgkin's Lymphoma. London: Edward Arnold, 1990, pp 256–278.

21. Magrath IT, Janus BK, Spiegel ES, et al. An effective therapy for both undifferentiated (including Burkitt's) lymphomas and lymphoblastic lymphoma in children and young adults. Blood 1984; 63:1102–1111.

22. Murphy SB. Classification, staging and end results of treatment of childhood non-Hodgkin's lymphoma: Dissimilarities from lymphoma in adults. Semin Oncol 1980; 7:332–339.

23. Murphy SB. Childhood lymphomas in current perspective. In Gale RP, Golde DW (eds): Recent Advances in Leukemia and Lymphoma. New York: Alan R Liss, 1987, pp 513–520.

24. Murphy SB, Fairclough D, Hutchison R, et al. Non-Hodgkin's lymphoma of childhood. An analysis of histology, staging and response to treatment of 338 cases at a single institution. J Clin Oncol 1989; 7:186–193.

25. Nachman J. Therapy for childhood non-Hodgkin's lymphoma non-lymphoma-blastic type. Am J Pediatr Hematol Oncol 1990; 12:359–366.

26. Non-Hodgkin's Lymphoma Pathologic Classification Project. National Cancer Institute—sponsor study of classification non-Hodgkin's lymphoma: Summary and description of a working formulation for clinical use. Cancer 1982; 49:2112–2135.

27. Poplack DG, Kun LF, Cassady JR, et al. Leukemia and lymphoma in childhood. In DeVita VT Jr, Hellman S, Rosenberg SA (eds): Cancer: Principles and Practices of Oncology, vol 2, 3rd ed. Philadelphia: JB Lippincott, 1989, pp 1684–1692.

28. Sanlund JJ, Magrath IT. Lymphoblastic lymphoma. In Magrath IT (ed): The Non-Hodgkin's Lymphoma. London: Edward Arnold, 1990, pp 240–255.

29. Smith S, Rubin CM, Horvath A, et al. Non-Hodgkin's lymphoma in children. Semin Oncol 1990; 17:113–119.

30. Weinstein HJ, Cassidy JR, Levey R. Long-term results of APO protocol (vincristine, doxorubicin [Adriamycin] and prednisone) for treatment of mediastinal lymphoblastic lymphoma. J Clin Oncol 1983; 1:537–541.

31. Williams SF. The role of bone marrow transplantation in the non-Hodgkin's lymphomas. Semin Oncol 1990; 17:88–95.

32. Wilson W, Magrath IT. Principles of chemotherapy. In Magrath IT (ed): The Non-Hodgkin's Lymphoma. London: Edward Arnold, 1990, pp 200–213.

33. Wollner N. Non-Hodgkin's lymphoma in children. Pediatr Clin North Am 1976; 23:371–378.

34. Wollner N, Exelby PR, Lieberman PH. Non-Hodgkin's lymphoma in children: A progress report on the original patients treated with the LSA$_2$L$_2$ protocol. Cancer 1979; 44:1990–1999.

35. Wollner N, Mandell L, Filippa D, et al. Primary nasal-paranasal oropharyngeal lymphoma in the pediatric age group. Cancer 1990; 66:1438–1444.

36. Young J, Bloeckler L, Silverberg E, et al. Cancer incidence survival and modality for children under 15 years of age. Cancer 1986; 58:598.

37. Ziegler JJ. "Biologic" differences in acquired immune deficiency syndrome–associated non-Hodgkin's lymphoma, J Clin Oncol 1991; 9:1329–1331. (Editorial.)

■ Wilms' Tumor

Rosemary Drigan
Arlene L. Androkites

Wilms' tumor (nephroblastoma), a primary tumor of the kidney, is the most common renal neoplasm of childhood. In 1899 Max Wilms,[24] a German surgeon, definitively described the neoplasm and was the first to suggest that the tumor had an embryonic origin.

EPIDEMIOLOGY

Wilms' tumor accounts for 6% of childhood malignancies, with an annual incidence of 7.5 per million white children and 7.8 per million African-American children under 15 years of age.[14] There are approximately 400 new cases each year, and the median age at diagnosis is between 2 and 3 years.[4] The sex ratio is 1:1; however, the frequency among females in the United States may be slightly higher.[6,22]

GENETICS

Most Wilms' tumors are sporadic cases that occur in children who have no known genetic predisposition. A minority of cases, however, are familial, and they are usually inherited in an autosomal dominant manner. Genetic counseling and examination of other family members are offered to detect familial cases early and initiate treatment promptly. Many sporadic and familial Wilms' tumors appear to result from inactivation of tumor suppressor genes on the short arm of chromosome 11.[12] Each cell contains two copies of chromosome 11, and it is believed that the Wilms' tumor genes on both chromosomes must be inactivated or deleted before tumor growth ensues. Individuals with familial Wilms' are born with inactivation or deletion of one copy of a Wilms' tumor gene.[12] Loss of the remaining copy—leading to tumor growth—is a likely event in these individuals. Sporadic Wilms' disease, on the other hand, results from loss of both copies of a Wilms' gene in a previously normal individual.

A small number of Wilms' tumors are associated with aniridia (congenital absence of the iris). Children with this syndrome are generally born with large deletions of the short arm of chromosome 11, which presumably results in loss of a Wilms' tumor gene[12] and many other important genes. These children often have associated physical and mental handicaps such as hemihypertrophy (relative increase in the number of cells in a segment on one side of the body as compared to the other), microcephaly, mental retardation, and genitourinary tract anomalies. Wilms' tumor has also been noted in association with Beckwith-Wiedemann syndrome (characterized by a large tongue, omphalocele, and large viscera) and neurofibromatosis. Denys and Drash have described an association of Wilms' tumor with pseudohermaphroditism and gonadal dysgenesis, especially in males.[22]

Children with these syndromes are at high risk for developing Wilms' tumor. An appropriate early detection surveillance program might include abdominal examination and urinalysis every 6 months, with yearly renal ultrasound during the first 6 years of age when children usually develop Wilms' tumor.[22]

HISTOLOGY

Wilms' tumors are usually large, rapidly growing lesions that may reach considerable size before they are clinically detected. Although the tumor is encapsulated, the capsule may be very thin and easily torn. Because of their rapid growth, the lesions are often vascular, soft, gelatinous, and necrotic in the center.

Histologically, the tumors are of two general types: favorable and unfavorable histology types. Favorable histology Wilms' tumor is derived from or composed of blastemic tissue, which is undifferentiated and found in primitive development.[1] Blastemic tissue is a precursor of stromal and epithelial cells that are differentiated. These tumors often contain tissue found in smooth or striated muscle, cartilage, fat, or bone.[1] Unfavorable histology, or anaplasia, occurs in tumors composed of cells with little evidence of differentiation. Characteristically these cells are more rapidly dividing, with hyperchromasia of enlarged nuclei.[13,22]

Anaplasia is more frequently seen in African-American than white children and in children 5 years of age or older.[22] It is more aggressive in nature and is the single most important poor prognostic factor.[10,22]

Another pathologic entity related to Wilms' tumor is nephroblastomatosis. The lesions can occur as diffuse involvement in one or both kidneys.[13] They take the form of small, usually microscopic clusters of blastemic cells, tubes, or stromal cells.[22] There apparently is a relationship between the location and number of lesions within the kidney and the development of Wilms' tumor.[13] When multifocal lesions are found, it is likely that Wilms' tumor will develop.[22]

Not all primary kidney tumors found in children are Wilms' tumors. Rhabdoid tumors may arise from neuroectodermal tissue.[14] They are monomorphorous and are found in infants and younger children.[22] Often CNS involvement occurs. Rhabdoid tumors are associated with a poor prognosis and death rates in excess of 80%.

Clear-cell sarcoma of the kidney is also a type of kidney tumor with a poor prognosis. Histologically there are distinct varieties such as epithelioid and cystic patterns.[22] This type of tumor has a high relapse rate, with metastases to bone and brain.

PRESENTATION

The most common presenting sign of Wilms' tumor is an abdominal mass in an otherwise healthy appearing child. The child is often asymptomatic, and the mass is frequently first detected by a family member. Some children experience pain, either microscopic or gross hematuria, malaise, fever, and hypertension, which is attributed to an increase in renin activity.[23]

Wilms' tumor is felt as a firm flank mass, usually nontender and confined to one side of the abdomen. A tumor that crosses the midline more likely will be a neuroblastoma.[22] Distended abdominal veins may indicate occlusion of the inferior vena cava. Areas of bony tenderness or cerebral abnormalities indicate tumor metastases. Associated genitourinary abnormalities include ambiguous genitalia, cryptorchidism, or hypospadias.[23] As previously mentioned, the tumor is as-

sociated with congenital hemihypertrophy and Beckwith-Wiedemann syndrome.[22,23]

Wilms' tumors metastasize either by hematogenous or lymphatic spread. Direct extension through the renal capsule or involvement in the renal sinus or intrarenal blood and lymphatic vessels is a common route of extrarenal spread. Regional lymph nodes and vena cava may be involved. The most common site of distant metastasis is the lungs.[13] Lesions may also occur in the liver, contralateral kidney, brain, or bones.[22]

DIAGNOSTIC EVALUATION

Any child with a suspicious abdominal mass needs an immediate and thorough diagnostic evaluation. An abdominal ultrasound is generally the initial study done to detect solid intrarenal mass, a tumor thrombus in renal veins, or abnormalities of the inferior vena cava. Ultrasonography outlines the kidneys, their shapes, and whether tumor is present in the contralateral kidney.

An abdominal CT scan or MRI will reveal the existence of tumor thrombi, enlarged lymph nodes, and the tumor's relationship to adjoining structures. A chest x-ray study and a chest CT scan should be done preoperatively to reveal any existent lung metastases since the findings may affect the surgical approach. A bone marrow aspirate and biopsy are not necessary since bone marrow involvement is rare. However, if metastatic disease to bone is suspected, both, along with a bone scan, may be useful.

A CBC and urinalysis should be obtained. Blood chemistry determinations included in the diagnostic workup include renal function tests (BUN, creatinine) and liver function tests (SGOT, SGPT, bilirubin).

Since manipulation of the tumor may cause the spread of malignant cells, the child's abdomen should not be palpated when the diagnosis of Wilms' tumor is suspected. It may be necessary to post a sign on the bed, "Do not palpate abdomen." Parents should be instructed to handle and bathe the child carefully to prevent trauma to the tumor.

Before surgery it is important to monitor vital signs for hypertension. Most cases of hypertension respond to nephrectomy, but some children may require antihypertensive therapy during the early phases of treatment. Surgery is usually scheduled within 1 to 2 days of hospitalization. Parents need immediate preparation for diagnostic and surgical procedures. The family must be aware of the location and size of the surgical incision to alleviate anxiety related to the operation.

The definitive diagnosis is made at the time of surgery when the tumor mass is removed, usually along with the entire kidney. Wilms' tumor is staged according to surgical findings, pathology, and the presence or absence of metastatic disease.

The one major staging system in current use is the one recommended by the National Wilms' Tumor Study Group (Table 9–13). Other staging systems are consistent, although some variations do exist.[17]

PROGNOSTIC FACTORS

As a result of improvements in therapy and subsequent increased survival time, prognostic factors are constantly changing. Recent studies show the major and most reliable prognostic factors are histology (favorable versus unfavorable) and extent of disease (stage).[13] Minor factors include age and size of the primary tumor.

Overall, children with favorable histology and nonmetastatic disease have a 90% chance for long-term survival.[5,10] Patients with either metastatic disease or unfavorable histology have approximately an 80% survival rate.[10] Prognostic factors need further refinement to identify patients requiring intensive therapy and those requiring minimal treatment for cure.

With tumor recurrence, approximately 50% of patients with Wilms' tumor can be salvaged with chemotherapy and/or radiation therapy and with surgical treatment, depending on site of relapse, histology, initial therapy, and whether the relapse occurred while the patient was receiving therapy or after treatment ended.[13,16] Recurrent disease can develop in the lungs, liver, opposite kidney, and, less commonly, other intra-abdominal sites, bone, and brain. The majority of relapses occur in the lung.

TABLE 9–13. *Pathologic Staging of Wilm's Tumor**

STAGE	DESCRIPTION
I	Tumor is limited to the kidney and is completely excised. Surface of the renal capsule is intact. Tumor was not ruptured before or during removal, and there is no residual tumor apparent beyond the margins of excision.
II	Tumor extends beyond the kidney but is completely excised. There is regional extension of the tumor (i.e., penetration through the outer surface of the renal capsule into the perirenal soft tissues). Vessels outside the kidney substance are infiltrated or contain tumor thrombus. Tumor may have been biopsied, or local spillage of tumor has been confined to the flank. No residual tumor is apparent at or beyond the margins of excision.
III	Residual nonhematogenous tumor is confined to the abdomen. Any of the following may occur: Biopsy specimens of lymph nodes reveal involvement of the hilus, the periaortic chains, or beyond. There has been diffuse peritoneal contamination by the tumor (e.g., by spillage of tumor beyond the flank before or during surgery or by tumor growth that has penetrated through the peritoneal surface). Tumor implants are found on the peritoneal surfaces. Tumor extends beyond the surgical margins either microscopically or grossly. Tumor is not completely resectable because of local infiltration into vital structures.
IV	Hematogenous metastases have occurred, and deposits are beyond stage III (e.g., in lung, liver, bone, and brain).
V	There is bilateral renal involvment. An attempt should be made to stage each side according to the above criteria on the basis of extent of disease before biopsy.

*Staging is the same for patients with either favorable or unfavorable pathology.

PREOPERATIVE THERAPY

Preoperative therapy (chemotherapy, radiation therapy) is routinely done in many centers throughout Europe.[22] This modality is successful in reducing tumor burden, rendering unresectable tumors resectable, and sparing normal renal parenchyma.[3] There is no evidence that long-term survival is improved with preoperative therapy; therefore in the United States it is reserved for patients with bilateral disease and those with a large unresectable tumor.

OPERATIVE AND POSTOPERATIVE TREATMENT

Surgery plays an extremely important role in the treatment of Wilms' tumor. The objectives are (1) to remove the tumor without producing hematogenous spread; (2) to prevent rupture of the tumor capsule with subsequent spillage of tumor cells; and (3) to provide tissue for pathologic examination and accurate assessment of tumor spread for staging.

The recommended surgical approach in routine cases is through a wide transverse abdominal incision that allows nephrectomy, lymph node sampling, and examination of the contralateral kidney. Examination of the opposite kidney is imperative since approximately 5% of Wilms' tumors are bilateral at diagnosis.[2]

Lymph node involvement is a major prognostic predictor; therefore inspection and sampling of suspicious regional nodes are essential. Careful exploration of other infradiaphragmatic organs is done for staging purposes.[2] Although rare, second-look surgical procedures may be indicated for abdominal recurrence, initially unresectable tumor, and bilateral Wilms' tumor.

RADIATION TREATMENT

Wilms' tumor is highly radiosensitive. The purpose of radiotherapy is to treat cells that may have escaped locally from the tumor.

Historically all children received radiation. Today this effective treatment modality is used for children with large tumors, metastatic spread, residual disease at the primary site, unfavorable histology, or tumor recurrence. Successive National Wilms' Tumor Study (NWTS) trials have shown that patients with stage I or stage II favorable histology, stage II tumors, or stage I anaplastic tumors do not require radiotherapy when they receive actinomycin-D and vincristine postoperatively.[9]

NWTS-4 currently recommends no radiation to stage I or II patients with favorable histology or stage I anaplastic lesions. Children with stage III favorable histology Wilms' tumor are given 1000 cGy. Stage IV children with favorable histology Wilms' tumor and with lung metastases receive whole-lung radiotherapy (1200 cGy) and abdominal irradiation (1000 cGy). Stage II, III or IV children with anaplastic tumors receive radiotherapy based on their age.[9] This regimen was developed in hopes of reducing the need for radiotherapy because of the known adverse effects on growth and development and the oncogenic potential of ionizing radiation.

CHEMOTHERAPY

Adjuvant chemotherapy significantly improves the overall survival rate of children with Wilms' tumor. The objectives of chemotherapy are to destroy any metastatic lesions or tumor cells in the bloodstream. Active agents include vincristine, actinomycin-D, doxorubicin, cyclophosphamide, cisplatin, etoposide (VP-16), and ifosfamide.[10] In an effort to answer a number of questions about the effectiveness of treatment for Wilms' tumor, the NWTS group was founded in 1969. The group represents the major cooperative groups involved in research on the treatment of cancer in children and a number of individual investigators. All patients enrolled in the NWTS receive chemotherapy. The fourth NWTS is currently enrolling patients.[9]

The conclusions of NWTS-1, NWTS-2 and NWTS-3 were as follows:

1. Actinomycin-D and vincristine, used in combination, give better results than either agent used alone.[9]

2. Routine flank radiotherapy is not necessary for children with stage I favorable histology Wilms' tumor, stage I anaplastic tumors, or stage II favorable histology Wilms'

tumor who received actinomycin-D and vincristine after nephrectomy.

3. Children with stage III favorable histology Wilms' tumor did equally well with either actinomycin-D, vincristine, and adriamycin with 1000 cGy radiation therapy to the flank or actinomycin and vincristine with 2000 cGy radiation therapy to the flank.

4. Adding cyclophosphamide to actinomycin-D, vincristine, and doxorubicin did not improve the survival rate for children with stage IV favorable histology Wilms' tumor. However, this drug combination may benefit children with stage II, III, or IV anaplastic tumors.

These results suggest that stage II and stage III favorable histology Wilms' tumor patients can be successfully treated with less intensive regimens. Treatment must be refined for stage IV disease and for those patients with unfavorable histology.

Some investigators administer chemotherapy to all children except those less than 2 years of age who have favorable histology stage I tumors. Treatment for this group (approximately 10%) consists of nephrectomy alone.[14a,20]

BILATERAL DISEASE

The incidence of synchronous bilateral Wilms' tumor ranges from 4% to 7% and metachronous bilateral Wilms' tumor from 1% to 1.9%.[22] The traditional surgical approach includes nephrectomy of the more involved kidney, with excisional biopsy or partial nephrectomy of the lesion in the remaining kidney. Patients are then treated with chemotherapy and/or radiation therapy, followed by a second-look surgical procedure. These children have a survival rate of 87%.

LATE EFFECTS

In general, the majority of children with Wilms' tumor have an excellent prognosis. It is important to follow children for tumor recurrence, damage to tissue and organ systems after treatment, and the development of second malignancies.[11]

Issues affecting long-term survivors are described in Chapter 17. The status of the remaining kidney is of particular importance to Wilms' tumor survivors. Urinalysis and ultrasound examination ascertain the state of the remaining kidney. Tumor has occurred in the opposite kidney more than 5 years after the initial nephrectomy.[13] The abdomen should be carefully palpated for evidence of recurrent tumor at the primary site and in the remaining kidney and liver.[22] Hypertension, associated with either renal or cardiovascular sequelae, is not a common late complication of Wilms' tumor.[18]

Late effects of trunk irradiation include scoliosis and soft tissue underdevelopment. Children who receive lung irradiation may develop functional thyroid abnormalities, thyroid adenomas or carcinomas.[14a] Hypoplasia of the hemithorax has also been reported.[19]

Abdominal radiation can cause damage to blood vessels, resulting in coarctation of abdominal aorta and of renal vessels.[8] Abdominal radiation predisposes females to low-birth-weight pregnancies; therefore they should be counseled appropriately.[21] Possible explanations for this finding include uterine muscle damage from direct or scatter radiation, constraint of fetal development associated with fibrosis and scoliosis, and vascular damage with reduced blood supply to the developing fetus.[15] These complications are associated with high-dose or megavoltage radiation. Studies indicate that Wilms' tumor does not develop in the offspring of patients with unilateral, nonfamilial disease.

Secondary malignant neoplasms occur and are probably more common in previously irradiated patients. The majority of tumors arise within the radiation field. Sarcomas, myeloid leukemias, and lymphomas,[22] followed by carcinomas,[7] have been reported. NWTS reports 7% of patients developed a benign tumor and 1% a second malignant neoplasm after treatment for Wilms' tumor. Relapse-free children surviving 5 or more years were evaluated for second malignancies.[9]

FUTURE DIRECTION

Now that a cure has been achieved for most children with Wilms' tumor, the focus is shifting to refining the treatment. Therapy may be minimized for children with a good prognosis. Children with unfavorable histology and/or metastatic disease may benefit from a more intensive approach. Effective techniques for salvaging the few children with recurrent disease are being developed.

The progress that has been made in treating Wilms' tumor is the very essence of the hopeful story of childhood cancer. The great strides that have been made have resulted from an organized, thoughtful approach to cooperative research. Perhaps the most important question for the future pertains to the long-term effects of the disease and its treatment. Further investigation to identify children and families at risk and disease prevention, if possible, through research in epidemiology and molecular biology will provide not only a better understanding of the malignant process, but also potential directions for future clinical trials.[22]

REFERENCES

1. Beckwith JB. Wilms' tumor and other renal tumors of childhood. An update. J Urol 1986; 136:320.
2. Belasco J, D'Angio GJ. Wilms' tumor. CA 1981; 31:258.
3. Bracken BR, Sutow WW, Jaffe N, et al. Preoperative chemotherapy for Wilms' tumor. Urology 1982; 19:55–60.
4. Breslow N, Beckwith JB, Ciol M, et al. Age distribution of Wilms' tumor. Report from the National Wilms' Tumor Study. Cancer Res 1988; 48:1653.
5. Breslow NE, Churchill G, Beckwith JB, et al. Prognosis for Wilms' tumor patients with non-metastatic disease at diagnosis. J Clin Oncol 1985; 3:521.
6. Breslow NE, Langholz B. Childhood cancer incidence: Geographical and temporal variations. Int J Cancer 1983; 32:703–716.
7. Breslow NE, Norkool PA, Olshan A, et al. Second malignant neoplasms in survivors of Wilms' tumor. J Natl Cancer Inst 1988; 80:592.
8. D'Angio GJ. The child cured of cancer: A problem for the internist. Semin Oncol 1982; 9:143.
9. D'Angio GJ, Beckwith JB, Breslow N, et al. Wilms' tumor: Status report, 1990. J Clin Oncol 1991; 9:877–887.
10. D'Angio, GJ, Breslow NE, Beckwith JB, et al. Treatment of Wilms' tumor. Results of the Third National Wilms' Tumor Study. Cancer 1989; 64:349–360.
11. Evans AE, Norkool P, Evans I, et al. Late effects of treatment for Wilms' tumor. A report from the National Wilms' Tumor Study Group. Cancer 1991; 67:331.
12. Francke U, Holmes LB, Atkins L, et al. Aniridia—Wilms' tumor association: Evidence for specific deletion of 11p13. Cytogenet Cell Genet 1979; 24:185–192.
13. Ganick DJ. Wilms' tumor. Hematol Oncol Clin North Am 1987; 1:695.
14. Green DM. The diagnosis and management of Wilms' tumor. Pediatr Clin North Am 1985; 32:735.
14a. Green DM, D'Angio GJ, Beckwith JB, et al. Wilms' tumor (nephroblastoma, renal embryoma). In Pizzo PA, Poplack DG (eds): Principles and Practice of Pediatric Oncology, 2nd ed. Philadelphia: JB Lippincott, 1993, pp 713–738.
15. Green DM, Fine WE, Li FP. Offspring of patients treated for unilateral Wilms' tumor in childhood. Cancer 1982; 49:2285.
16. Grundy P, Breslow N, Green DM, et al. Prognostic factors for children with recurrent Wilms' tumor: Results from the Second and Third National Wilms' Tumor Study. J Clin Oncol 1989; 7:638.
17. Hockenberry MJ, Coody DK. Perspectives on care. In Pediatric Oncology and Hematology: Perspectives on Care. St. Louis: CV Mosby, 1986.
18. Kantor AF, Li FP, Janov AJ, et al. Hypertension in long-term survivors of childhood renal cancer. J Clin Oncol 1989; 7:912.
19. Kinsella JP, Brasch RC, Ablin AS. Unilateral hypoplasia of the hemithorax causing "pseudoscoliosis" after lung irradiation in a child with Wilms' tumor. Pediatr Radiol 1985; 15:340.
20. Larsen E, Perez-Atayde A, Green DM, et al. Surgery only for the treatment of patients with Stage I (Cassady) Wilms' tumor. Cancer 1990; 66:264–266.
21. Li FP, Gimbrere K, Gelber R, et al. Outcome of pregnancy in survivors of Wilms' tumor. JAMA 1987; 257:216.
22. See reference 14a.
23. Whaley LF, Wong DL, Nursing Care of Infants and Children, 3rd ed. St. Louis: CV Mosby, 1987.
24. Wilms M. Die Mischgeschwuelste der Niere. Leipzig: A Georgi, 1899.

NEUROBLASTOMA

Mary C. Sullivan

Neuroblastoma was first described in 1864 by Virchow.[60] Later, in 1910, the term *neurocytoma*, or *neuroblastoma*, was proposed by Wright.[61] Wright described a tumor that was found in young children and neonates rich in cells of varying shapes and sizes. These cells were present in many parts of the body and were morphologically similar to the cells of the embryonic sympathetic nervous system. Neuroblastomas originate from neural crest cells that are precursors of the adrenal medulla and sympathetic nervous system. Therefore the tumor can be present wherever sympathetic nervous tissue is found.[3,27]

INCIDENCE

Neuroblastoma is the fourth most common childhood malignancy, with approximately 500 new cases diagnosed each year in the United States.[18,64] It is the most common tumor in children less than 1 year of age.[64] Roughly 60% of cases are diagnosed at less than 2 years of age, 75% at less than 5 years, and 84% at less than 10 years.[16] In the United States neuroblastoma occurs slightly more frequently among males than females and more frequently in white children than in African-American children. The annual incidence among white children is 9.6 per million and among African-American children, 7 per million.[64]

The true incidence of neuroblastoma, however, remains unknown because of the phenomenon of spontaneous tumor regression and maturation. This phenomenon, common in neonates and infants, allows cases of neuroblastoma to go uncounted.[3,18]

Beckwith and Perrin[1] first described clusters of neuroblastoma cells found incidentally at autopsy in the adrenal glands of newborns and young infants who died from other causes. They called this *neuroblastoma in situ* and proposed that in some cases these tumor cells disappeared spontaneously before clinical symptoms appeared. Other research supports this theory that microscopic clusters of neuroblastoma cells present from birth to 3 months of age can be normal embryonal variants without malignant potential.[58]

Japan initiated mass screening efforts to identify infants with asymptomatic neuroblastoma in 1973. The catecholamine metabolites vanillylmandelic acid (VMA) and homovanillic acid (HVA), known to be elevated in children with neuroblastoma, were measured in the infants' urine at 6 months of age. Because of the significant number of oncologic false positive results and missed positive cases throughout the period of observation, the results from these studies thus far do not support mass screening efforts for diagnosis of neuroblastoma.[23,40,43,44]

Additional studies have been undertaken to ascertain the proportion of neuroblastoma that can be detected by mass screenings, if late-stage disease can be prevented, and whether the prognosis can be improved by early detection. Such data could help determine whether mass screening would be worthwhile and cost effective.[23,40,43,44]

HISTOPATHOLOGY

Grossly, primary neuroblastoma is a solid, soft mass. It is usually encapsulated, with varied colors depending on the degree of necrosis and hemorrhage. These tumors often impinge on adjacent tissues and organs. Cross sections of the tumor reveal neoplastic tissue interspersed with areas of calcification and hemorrhage.[17] Microscopically, primitive undifferentiated neuroblastoma consists of closely packed, small, round cells with scant cytoplasm. Occasionally neurofibrils are interspersed among the cells that often group in circular structures called *rosettes*[17] (Figure 9–3).

Ganglioneuroblastoma tumor samples have areas of mature or benign cells interspersed with areas of undifferentiated or malignant cells. The areas of maturation consist of large ganglion cells with abundant cytoplasm and increased fibrillar material. The completely differentiated end of the spectrum is a benign tumor called *ganglioneuroma*. It is

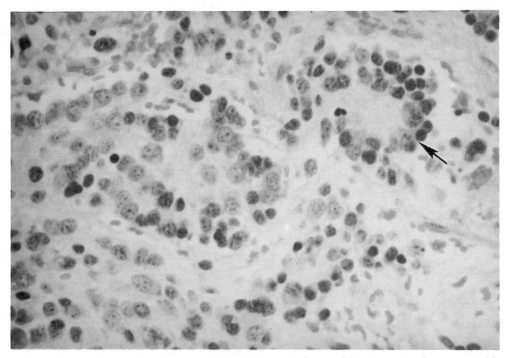

FIGURE 9–3. Neuroblastoma. Rosettes, composed of neuroblasts surrounding a central region of neurofibrillary stroma, are characteristic of the tumor (hematoxylin and eosin). *(Courtesy Dr. David Kelley, Children's Hospital, Birmingham, Alabama.)*

composed of ganglion cells, Schwann cells, and nerve bundles.[17,27] Such histopathologic variation may occur within the same tumor or between the primary site and its metastases.

ETIOLOGY

The etiology of neuroblastoma remains unknown. No specific pattern of congenital abnormalities has been associated with this tumor.[32,35,42,49] A matched case-control study in Minnesota of 97 patients with neuroblastoma showed no association between neuroblastoma and sex, race, parental age, parental education, complications of pregnancy, labor, delivery, birth weight, or gestational duration.[42] Neuroblastoma has, however, occasionally been found in patients with fetal hydantoin syndrome, neurofibromatosis, and Beckwith-Wiedemann syndrome.[49]

Genetic predisposition has been considered a possible cause, especially in the rare cases of patients with neuroblastoma who have a sibling with the same disease.[31,35] In 1972 Knudson and Strong[31] proposed that fa-

milial cases of neuroblastoma have an autosomal dominant pattern of inheritance. Early age at diagnosis and multiple primary sites further distinguished these patients from nonfamilial cases.

Another study of 23 aggregates of familial neuroblastoma by Kushner, Gilbert, and Helson[35] supported these findings. Nevertheless the calculated risk for siblings or offspring of neuroblastoma patients to develop the disease is less than 6%.[31,35]

GENETICS

In 1983 Schwab et al.[50] identified the N-*myc* oncogene as an amplified gene present in cell lines of human neuroblastomas. Further studies have shown an association between the number of N-*myc* copies present in neuroblastoma cells and the patient's prognosis. Many authors believe that amplification, or multiple copy numbers, of the N-*myc* oncogene correlates highly with rapid tumor progression and poor prognosis.[5,14,20,21,42,46,47]

Deletion of the short arm of chromosome 1 is another characteristic genetic feature of human neuroblastoma cells.[4] Brodeur first described this feature in 1975.[4,5] The region most commonly deleted is 1p and is thought to represent the loss of the neuroblastoma suppressor gene that prevents tumor development. At least 70% of karyotyped neuroblastomas have this abnormality. The relationship between the loss of this critical region on the short arm of chromosome 1 and the development or progression of neuroblastoma must be determined by further research. Yet some studies suggest the loss of the gene correlates with poor prognosis.[3–5]

A third intense area of genetic research centers on neuroblastoma DNA content and its relationships to prognosis. Several studies suggest that tumors with an abnormal or aneuploid DNA content respond better to treatment and have improved rates of survival. Conversely, patients with diploid neuroblastoma may have more aggressive disease and a poorer prognosis.[3,14,46,47]

The human multidrug resistance gene (MDR1) in patients with neuroblastoma may explain the frequent observation that disseminated neuroblastoma initially responds to chemotherapy but usually recurs and is resistant to subsequent chemotherapy regimens. Studies have found amplified MDR1 in some neuroblastoma cells, suggesting that high levels of MDR1 are associated with development of resistance to chemotherapy.[21,41]

The full clinical and prognostic significance of these genetic features is not fully understood. More studies are needed to show how each genetic rearrangement influences neuroblastoma development and progression. How these genetic events interrelate with each other is currently under investigation.

CLINICAL PRESENTATION

The signs and symptoms of neuroblastoma vary depending on the site of the primary tumor or metastatic disease. The most common primary site is the abdomen, either in the adrenal gland (40%) or paraspinal ganglia (25%). Less common primary sites are the paraspinal area of the thorax (15%), the neck (5%), and pelvis (5%).[27] Multiple primary sites can occur, and up to 10% of patients have no discernable primary sites.[33]

Metastases are found in approximately 70% of newly diagnosed patients. Metastatic sites are, in order of frequency, the bone marrow, bones, lymph nodes, liver, intracranial lesions (from direct extension of bony sites or orbits), skin, and testes.[3,27,33] Metastatic disease in the lung or parenchyma of the brain is very rare in patients with neuroblastoma.[3]

Frequently an abdominal mass is the first sign of disease. It is usually firm and irregular and may cross the midline of the abdomen. Masses in the thorax can be found on chest x-ray film and can, if large enough, cause respiratory symptoms or superior vena cava syndrome (congestion and edema of the face, neck, and upper torso, headache, visual changes). Upper thoracic or cervical neuroblastoma can cause Horner's syndrome (miosis, ptosis, exophthalmos, anhidrosis). Large retroperitoneal abdominal and pelvic tumors can cause vascular compression with edema of the lower extremities.

Paraspinal tumors in any site can grow into the spinal foramina, causing spinal cord compression (back pain, weakness of lower extremities, sensory loss, and loss of sphincter control). Bone and bone marrow involvement usually manifests as pain, causing limping or refusal to walk. Sphenoid bone and retro-orbital involvements characteristically cause ecchymosis of the eyelids and proptosis. Hepatic and subcutaneous spread is seen almost exclusively in infants.[3,27]

Rare symptoms in children with neuroblastoma include ataxia and opsomyoclonus, referred to as *acute cerebellar encephalopathy (ACE) syndrome* or "dancing eyes, dancing feet" syndrome. The prognosis for children with this syndrome is usually excellent. However, the symptoms can persist despite successful treatment of the tumor with chemotherapy and/or prednisone and adrenocorticotropic hormone (ACTH), often leaving neurologic sequelae such as learning disorders.[57]

Rarely, intractable diarrhea leading to hypokalemia and dehydration occurs. It is caused by a substance produced by tumor cells called *vasoactive intestinal peptide (VIP)*. The diarrhea resolves when therapy is successful. Return of diarrhea may signal a recurrence of neuroblastoma. Hypertension, another rare symptom, may be related to an overproduction of norepinephrine and epinephrine by the tumor.[3]

DIAGNOSIS

When neuroblastoma is suspected, obtaining a thorough history and performing a physical examination are required first. This initial workup should include a CBC, liver and kidney function tests, and a coagulation screen. Measurements of neuroblastoma tumor markers such as catecholamine metabolites (VMA and HVA), ferritin, neuron-specific enolase (NSE), and the ganglioside GD2 are useful in making the diagnosis and monitoring the disease.[3]

The measurement of VMA and HVA in urine is widely used as a diagnostic tool in determining the presence of neuroblastoma. More than 90% of all patients have increased urinary excretion of VMA and/or HVA at diagnosis, which may be due to overproduction by tumor cells or to defective storage within tumor cells. To obtain correct results, the 24-hour urine collection preceding surgery must take into account all drugs administered both on collection day and the previous day. Dietary restrictions of coffee, fruits, and foods containing vanilla are considered unnecessary for assay of VMA using gas chromatography or mass spectrometry or high-performance liquid chromatography (HPLC) methods of analysis.[2] Other technologies for assaying VMA may require dietary restrictions before collection.

Ferritin is a major iron-binding protein in blood and tissue. Elevations may be seen at diagnosis in patients with neuroblastoma and other malignancies without corresponding increases in iron storage. Increased serum ferritin levels correlate with poorer prognosis.[26,55]

The level of serum NSE, an enzyme produced by neuronal tissue, is usually elevated in patients with neuroblastoma. The level appears to correlate with the amount of active disease.[33]

Gangliosides are sugar-containing lipid molecules present on the surface of tumor cells. The ganglioside GD2 is present in large quantities on the surface of human neuroblastoma cells. It is also shed by tumor cells and can be measured in serum; therefore the detection of GD2 on the tumor cell surface or in the circulation can be a useful diagnostic tool in confirming neuroblastoma.[59]

DIAGNOSTIC EVALUATION

The results of bone marrow aspiration and biopsy can reveal marrow involvement and often confirm the diagnosis of neuroblastoma. Sampling multiple sites and screening the marrow cells using tumor-specific monoclonal antibodies can enhance the detection of metastatic neuroblastoma.[13,33]

A chest x-ray film can delineate primary thoracic neuroblastoma and vertebral or paravertebral involvements. An ultrasound of the abdomen can reveal the location of the mass and any impingement on other organs. The ultrasound does not use ionizing radiation and is not limited by the absence of fat.[56] These factors should be considered in choosing a study modality to evaluate abdominal masses in infants.

Computed tomography (CT) is currently the imaging study of choice to determine if the tumor is operable.[56] Magnetic resonance imaging (MRI) may also be useful and has the advantage of not exposing the patient to ionizing radiation.

New imaging studies, in addition to the routine bone scan, have greatly enhanced the identification of this tumor in children. Knowing the precise location of neuroblastoma at diagnosis helps in the selection of therapy. The following are nuclear medicine imaging studies used to identify neuroblastoma: bone scan, gallium scan, iodine 131-metaiodobenzylguanadine (^{131}I-MIBG) scan, and tumor-specific monoclonal antibody scan.

A radionuclide bone scan using technetium 99m-methylene diphosphonate (MDP) is part of the initial workup because more than half of all patients have bone metastases at diagnosis. The bone scan identifies 50% to 70% more bony sites than the conventional skeletal survey. The tracer localizes to bones in which repair is taking place. After treatment, bone scan results can remain positive for many months.[19]

Gallium 67 citrate scans can image osseous and nonosseous sites such as the primary tumor and lymph nodes. However, its use in diagnosing neuroblastoma is limited with the recent development of more sensitive imaging.[19]

The radiopharmaceutical agent ^{131}I-MIBG has been used to detect adrenergic tumors such as pheochromocytoma in patients for many years. MIBG is an analogue to norepinephrine and is highly specific for neuroendocrine tissue. It localizes in a variety of neuroendocrine tumors, including neuroblastoma.[54] The imaging process consists of radiolabeling MIBG with a relatively small dose of the radioisotope iodine 131, injecting it intravenously into the patient, and visualizing tumor sites 24, 48, and sometimes 72 hours later on nuclear medicine scans. The entire body is screened for primary and metastatic sites of neuroblastoma, both osseous and nonosseous.[28,29,54]

The use of ^{131}I-MIBG as a diagnostic agent does require some precaution despite the low dose of radioactive iodine used. Saturated solution of potassium iodide (SSKI) is administered to the patient orally to prevent thyroid uptake before the tracer is injected. Medical personnel should wear gloves when handling the patients's urine and feces for at least 48 hours after the injection or until a safe level is measured and always should observe good hand washing techniques.[30,54] The half-life of iodine 131 is 8 days; however, the bulk of the isotope is excreted in the first few days after injection. Parents should use good hand washing techniques and not allow their

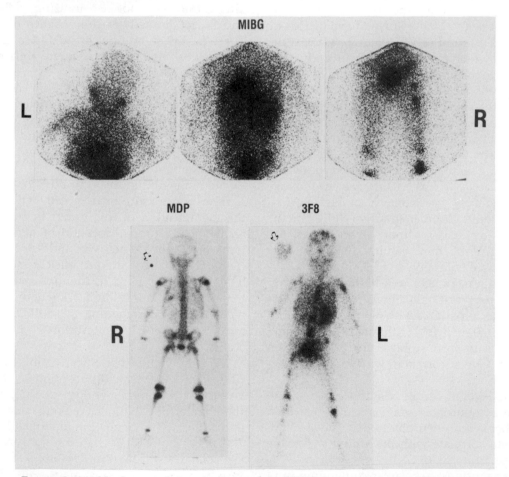

FIGURE 9–4. Nuclear medicine studies such as MIBG, bone scans, and 3F8 studies play an important role in imaging primary and distant metastatic tumor sites. *(From Yeh SDJ, Kushner BH, Sullivan MC, et al. Radioimmunodetection of neuroblastoma with iodine-131-3F8: Correlation with biopsy, iodine-131 metaiodobenzylguanidine and standard diagnostic modalities. J Nucl Med 1991; 32:769–776.)*

child to sleep with siblings. Additionally, some institutions recommend using disposable dishes and utensils until safe levels are reached in the child.

Current research focuses on radiolabeled monoclonal antibody imaging studies in patients with neuroblastoma. In recent studies the murine (mouse) monoclonal antibody 3F8, specific for the ganglioside GD2, was tagged with the radioisotope iodine 131 and administered intravenously to patients with neuroblastoma. Total body scans demonstrated localization in the mediastinum, abdomen, lymph nodes, bone marrow, and bone.[11] Comparisons between 3F8, MIBG, and bone scans suggest that the 3F8 scan may be more sensitive than the MIBG or bone scan in detecting metastatic sites of disease[62,63] (Fig. 9–4).

The 3F8's use in repeated imaging studies on the same patient may be limited, however, since 3F8 can stimulate the production of human neutralizing antibodies after initial exposure.[11,33] In other words, once exposed to the mouse monoclonal antibody 3F8, the patient's own immune system may recognize it as foreign and produce antibodies against it. For this reason, timing the exposure to the 3F8 when the patient is immunosuppressed and therefore less likely to develop antimouse antibodies is important.

STAGING

Four major staging systems are in use to estimate the prognosis of children with neuroblastoma: the systems used by the Children's Cancer Group (CCG), International Union Against Cancer (UICC), Pediatric Oncology Group (POG), and St. Jude Children's Research Hospital (SJCRH).[6,8]

In 1986 a group of internationally recognized experts in the field of neuroblastoma proposed a single staging system that incorporated the most important elements of the four current, but incompatible, systems. This system, ratified in 1987, is the International Staging System for Neuroblastoma (Table 9–14). It standardizes definitions for diagnosis, staging, and treatment and serves as a consistent reference for comparing data between

TABLE 9–14. *International Staging System for Neuroblastoma*

Stage 1	Localized tumor confined to the area of origin; complete gross excision, with or without microscopic residual disease, identifiable ipsilateral and contralateral lymph nodes negative microscopically.
Stage 2A	Unilateral tumor with incomplete gross excision; identifiable ipsilateral and contralateral lymph nodes negative microscopically.
Stage 2B	Unilateral tumor with complete or incomplete gross excision; with positive ipsilateral regional lymph nodes; identifiable contralateral lymph nodes negative microscopically.
Stage 3	Tumor infiltrating across the midline with or without regional lymph node involvement; or, unilateral tumor with contralateral regional lymph node involvement; or, midline tumor with bilateral regional lymph node involvement.
Stage 4	Dissemination of tumor to distant lymph nodes, bone, bone marrow, liver, and/or other organs (except as defined in stage 4S).
Stage 4S	Localized primary tumor as defined for stage 1 or 2 with dissemination limited to liver, skin, and/or bone marrow.

From Brodeur GM, Seeger RC, Barrett A, et al. International criteria for diagnosis, staging, and response to treatment in patients with neuroblastoma. J Clin Oncol 1988; 6:1874–1881.

institutions and as a foundation on which future advances can be built.[6,8]

PROGNOSTIC FACTORS

A major focus of neuroblastoma research is on the identification of factors that determine prognosis. Two well-known factors that predict a favorable prognosis are young age at diagnosis (<12 months) and stage of disease (stage I,II, or IVS).[3,7,27,34] Some authorities believe that patients with primary sites in the neck and thorax also have a favorable outlook.[15]

A feature at diagnosis associated with poor prognosis is a multiple N-*myc* oncogene copy number.[3–5,9,14,20,42,46,47]

Recent studies also suggest that the DNA content of tumor cells compared to that of normal cells (DNA index) is of prognostic significance in neuroblastoma. A DNA index is obtained through flow cytometry to designate a tumor as pseudodiploid, diploid, aneuploid, or hyperdiploid. DNA diploidy is associated with advanced-stage disease and poor prognosis.[3-5,9,14,46,47]

A histopathologic classification system developed by Shimada et al.[53] considers age, stage, and tumor morphology. It predicts prognosis based on the degree of cell differentiation present in the tumor. If the neuroblastoma cells appear primitive or poorly differentiated, the prognosis is poor. Conversely, the more highly differentiated end of the spectrum carries a better prognosis.[4,14,53,55]

Additionally, serum ferritin levels greater than 150 ng/ml and serum NSE levels greater than 100 ng/ml are associated with poor prognosis.[9,33,55] In contrast, VMA and HVA levels at diagnosis are not predictive of survival.[9] Prognostic research also focuses on how MDR1 influences therapy response in patients with neuroblastoma.[9,21,41]

TREATMENT AND PROGNOSIS

The current therapy for neuroblastoma is based on the stage and prognostic markers found at diagnosis.

Patients With Favorable Prognostic Features

Favorable prognostic features include less than 12 months of age and disease stages I, II, or IVS. Patients with favorable prognostic features usually require no treatment, minimal treatment, or surgical resection alone.

Surgery for neuroblastoma plays both a diagnostic and therapeutic role. Operations are either primary (before chemotherapy or radiotherapy) or secondary (after therapy). Primary surgery establishes the diagnosis, helps stage the disease, and completely resects or reduces the size of the tumor by partial excision. Secondary surgery assesses the results of therapy and excises any residual tumor.[27,52] Complete surgical resection is the only therapy required for the 10% to 15% of

patients who present with localized disease (stages I and II). Their disease-free survival rates range from 91% to 100%.[3,37,45]

Stage IVS (special) neuroblastomas occur almost exclusively in infants less than 1 year of age. These tumors have a high rate of spontaneous regression. Some oncologists elect to withhold all therapy while closely observing the infant and performing frequent physical examinations and diagnostic tests. Others treat with several cycles of low-dose chemotherapy and close observation. Survival rate differences between the untreated group and low-dose group are not significant. Disease-free survival rates in stage IVS range from 70% to 82%.[3,38]

Patients With Poor Prognostic Features

Poor prognostic features include disease stage IV, greater than 12 months of age, multiple N-*myc* copy number, DNA diploidy, undifferentiated histology, and high serum ferritin and NSE levels. Unfortunately, the majority of children with neuroblastoma are in this category. Intensive therapy is required for these patients with extensive, aggressive tumors and may include chemotherapy, radiation therapy, surgery, autologous or allogeneic bone marrow transplant, bone marrow rescue, and, more recently, MIBG and immunotherapy with monoclonal antibodies specific to neuroblastoma.

For stage III patients disease-free survival rates have improved with an intensive approach and range from 60% to 72%.[3,24] However, over the last two decades there has been little improvement in the cure rate (11% to 17%) for stage IV patients.[3,27]

Multiagent chemotherapy is the major treatment modality for children with advanced neuroblastoma. The agents most commonly used are cyclophosphamide, cisplatin, etoposide, VM26, doxorubicin, DTIC, and vincristine.[10] Although initial response rates to these agents remain high (86% to 100%), the disease eventually recurs, resuming its relentless course. Chemotherapy alone has not been curative in children with advanced stage disease.[10]

Once chemotherapy successfully shrinks

the tumor, a "second look" surgery is performed to remove any residual tumor tissue.[52] Complete tumor resection at the secondary surgery may improve survival rates in patients with stage III disease.[24,45,52]

Neuroblastoma is considered radiosensitive but radiation therapy is not curative when used alone. Painful bone metastases or unsightly soft tissue masses can be treated with low doses of radiation over a short period of time to achieve instant relief.[25] Local radiation to any residual disease in the context of a chemotherapy or bone marrow transplant protocol may be important for effective tumor control. In this setting the dose of radiation is higher, and its delivery is fractionated to allow for normal tissue repair.[22,25,51] Some bone marrow transplant protocols for patients with neuroblastoma use total body irradiation.[22,51]

An autologous or allogeneic bone marrow transplant may be used to consolidate remission after chemotherapy and/or surgery. Autologous transplants are more common in therapy for neuroblastoma, partly because of the lack of matched donors needed for allogeneic transplants.

INVESTIGATIONAL THERAPY

Children with neuroblastoma unresponsive to conventional therapy may be eligible for investigational treatment. Such treatment can include phase I or II chemotherapy, radiolabeled MIBG and 3F8, monoclonal antibody therapy, growth factors, and differentiating agents.

Ifosfamide, carboplatin, iproplatin, and epirubicin are new agents currently being evaluated. These new agents are analogues of common drugs such as cyclophosphamide, cisplatin, and doxorubicin. Their efficacy in preclinical trials is similar to that of their parent drugs. Thus far, side effects noted in phase I trials have often been less severe than with conventional agents.[10]

As described previously, MIBG and the monoclonal antibody 3F8 can be radiolabeled with a small dose of the radioisotope ^{131}I to locate tumor sites by nuclear medicine scans. When larger doses of ^{131}I are radiolabeled to MIBG or 3F8, therapeutic doses of radiation can be delivered to the tumor sites, using the MIBG and 3F8 as carriers of the radiation therapy. The acute side effects of ^{131}I-MIBG and [131]I 3F8 are minimal except for anorexia and mild nausea. Prolonged bone marrow suppression, particularly thrombocytopenia (low platelet count), is associated with these therapies.[11,29,54]

Parents and staff who come in contact with children receiving internal radiation must follow radiation safety precautions. The safety and nuclear medicine departments set time restrictions on patient care for each member of the treatment team. Parents must wear radiation safety badges to measure the amount of radiation exposure during their child's hospitalization.[29] Institutions differ on the amount of time parents are allowed in close contact with their child and whether the parents must take SSKI drops to protect their own thyroid glands. Differences in radiation safety precautions are partly explained by the larger dose of ^{131}I used in MIBG therapy (50 to 100 mCi) as compared with 3F8 therapy (20 mCi or less).

Targeted immunotherapy with monoclonal antibodies is yet another investigational treatment approach to neuroblastoma. The monoclonal antibody 3F8 binds to the GD2 present on most neuroblastoma cells and then signals various components of the immune system (e.g., leukocytes and complement) to attack tumor cells.[11,12,39] Side effects associated with this therapy (pain, urticaria, hypertension, and fever) are severe but temporary. A nurse must be present at the bedside throughout the intravenous injection to monitor the patient and administer medications (narcotics, antihistamines, acetaminophen) based on the patient's reaction to the antibody.[11,12]

Granulocyte-macrophage colony-stimulating factor (GM-CSF) and monocyte colony-stimulating factor (M-CSF) are being investigated in clinical trials of patients with neuroblastoma. GM-CSF stimulates the production of neutrophils, and M-CSF stimulates the proliferation and maturation of monocytes. They may reduce sequelae from myelosuppression and hasten recovery. In addition, GM-CSF and M-CSF may be able to amplify antibody 3F8 antitumor activity by stimulating the neutrophil and monocyte effector cells. Increased numbers of neutrophils and monocytes will in turn destroy more tumor cells.[11,34]

The observation that spontaneous regression and cell maturation frequently can occur with neuroblastoma has stimulated researchers to ask what factors influence neuroblastoma cells to mature. Several agents studied in the laboratory have induced maturation or differentiation of neuroblastoma cell lines in culture. However, few have reached the level of clinical trials in humans. *Cis*-retinoic acid (vitamin A) is one agent currently in phase I and II trials in the United States.[10]

Nurses and clinical oncologists who care for children with neuroblastoma are pioneers on the frontier of applying laboratory and biologic research to clinical practice. Nurses have always played a major role in the success of new cancer therapies. Neuroblastoma is fertile ground for the development of new therapies. Thus considerable challenges exist in the present and future care of children with this disease.

REFERENCES

1. Beckwith JB, Perrin EV. In situ neuroblastomas: A contribution to the natural history of neural crest tumors. Am J Path 1963; 43:1089–1100.
2. Bertani-Dziedzic L, Dziedzic SW, Gitlow SE. Catecholamine metabolism in neuroblastoma. In Pochedly C (ed): Neuroblastoma: Tumor Biology and Therapy. Boca Raton, Fla.: CRC Press, 1990, pp 69–91.
3. Berthold F. Overview: Biology of neuroblastoma. In Pochedly C (ed): Neuroblastoma: Tumor Biology and Therapy. Boca Raton, Fla.: CRC Press, 1990, pp 1–27.
4. Brodeur GM. Clinical significance of genetic rearrangements in human neuroblastomas. Clin Chem 1989; 35 7:B38–B42.
5. Brodeur GM. Molecular biology and genetics of human neuroblastoma. In Pochedly C (ed): Neuroblastoma: Tumor Biology and Therapy. Boca Raton, Fla.: CRC Press, 1990, pp 31–50.
5a. Brodeur GM, Castleberry RP. Neuroblastoma. In Pizzo PA, Poplack DG (eds): Principles and Practice of Pediatric Oncology, 2nd ed. Philadelphia: JB Lippincott, 1993, pp 739–767.
6. Brodeur GM, Seeger RC, Barrett A, et al. International criteria for diagnosis, staging, and response to treatment in patients with neuroblastoma. J Clin Oncol 1988; 6:1874–1881.
7. Carlsen NLT. Why age has independent prognostic significance in neuroblastomas. Evidence for intrauterine development and implications for the treatment of the disease. Anticancer Res 1988; 8:255–262.
8. Carlsen NLT. Clinical staging of neuroblastomas: Assessment of the various staging systems. In Pochedly

C (ed): Neuroblastoma: Tumor Biology and Therapy. Boca Raton, Fla.: CRC Press, 1990, pp 199–228.
9. Cassady Jr. Prognosis: Biological vagaries in neuroblastoma. In Pochedly C (ed): Neuroblastoma: Tumor Biology and Therapy. Boca Raton, Fla.: CRC Press, 1990, pp 369–380.
10. Castleberry RP. Chemotherapy for neuroblastoma. In Pochedly C (ed): Neuroblastoma: Tumor Biology and Therapy. Boca Raton, Fla.: CRC Press, 1990, pp 305–316.
11. Cheung NKV. Immunology and targeted immunotherapy of neuroblastoma. In Pochedly C (ed): Neuroblastoma: Tumor Biology and Therapy. Boca Raton, Fla.: CRC Press, 1990, pp 51–68.
12. Cheung NKV, Medof ME, Munn D. Immunotherapy with GD2 specific monoclonal antibodies. In Clinical and Biological Research, vol 271. New York: Alan R Liss, 1988, pp 619–632.
13. Cheung NKV, Von Hoff DD, Strandjord SE. Detection of neuroblastoma cells in bone marrow using GD2 specific monoclonal antibodies. J Clin Oncol 1986; 4:363–369.
14. Cohn SL, Rademaker AW, Salwen HR, et al. Analysis of DNA ploidy and proliferative activity in relation to histology and N-*myc* amplification in neuroblastoma. Am J Pathol 1990; 136:1043–1052.
15. Davis GF, Young DG, Neuroblastomas of the neck and chest. In Pochedly C (ed): Neuroblastoma: Tumor Biology and Therapy. Boca Raton, Fla.: CRC Press, 1990, pp 257–276.
16. Davis S, Rogers MAM, Pendergrass TW. The incidence and epidemiologic characteristics of neuroblastoma in the United States. Am J Epidemiol 1987; 126:1063–1074.
17. Dehner LP. Histiogenesis and histopathology of neuroblastoma. In Pochedly C (ed): Neuroblastoma: Tumor Biology and Therapy. Boca Raton, Fla.: CRC Press, 1990, pp 111–143.
18. Evans AE. Natural history of neuroblastoma. In Evans AE (ed): Advances in Neuroblastoma Research. New York: Raven Press, 1980, pp 3–12.
19. Garty I, Friedman A, Sandler MP, et al. Neuroblastoma: Imaging evaluation by sequential Tc-99m MDP, I-131 MIBG, and GA-67 Citrate studies. Clin Nuclear Med 1989; 14:515–521.
20. Garvin J, Bendit I, Nisen PD. N-*myc* oncogene expression and amplification in metastatic lesions of stage IV-S neuroblastoma. Cancer 1990; 65:2572–2575.
21. Goldstein LJ, Fojo AT, Ueda K, et al. Expression of the multidrug resistance, MDR1, gene in neuroblastoma. J Clin Oncol 1990; 8:128–136.
22. Graham-Pole J, Gee AP, Gross S, et al. Bone marrow transplantation (BMT) for advanced neuroblastoma (NBL). In Clinical and Biological Research, vol 271. New York: Alan R Liss, 1988, pp 215–224.
23. Gutjahr P. Editorial comment: Mass screening for early detection of neuroblastoma. Eur J Pediatr 1988; 147:312.
24. Haase GM, Wong KY, de Lorimier AA, et al. Improvement in survival after excision of primary tumor in stage III neuroblastoma. J Pediatr Surg 1989; 24:194–200.
25. Halperin EC. Radiotherapy for neuroblastoma. In Pochedly C (ed): Neuroblastoma: Tumor Biology and Therapy. Boca Raton, Fla.: CRC Press, 1990, pp 289–304.
26. Hann HL, Levy HM, Evans AE. Ferritin and cancer: Study of isoferritins in patients with neuroblastoma. In Evans AE (ed): Advances in Neuroblastoma Research. New York: Raven Press, 1980, pp 43–48.

27. See reference 5a.
28. Jacobs A, Delree M, Desprechins B, et al. Consolidating the role of I-MIBG-scintigraphy in childhood neuroblastoma: Five years of clinical experience. Pediatr Radiol 1990; 20:157–159.
29. Kelly JU. The use of an investigational radiopharmaceutical in neuroblastoma: A nursing perspective. J Pediatr Oncol Nurs 1989; 6:133–138.
30. Kemshead JT, Pizer BL, Patel K. Neuroblastoma: Perspectives for future research. In Pochedly C (ed): Neuroblastoma: Tumor Biology and Therapy. Boca Raton, Fla.: CRC Press, 1990, pp 381–395.
31. Knudson AG, Strong LC. Mutation and cancer: Neuroblastoma and pheochromocytoma. Am J Hum Genet 1972; 24:514–532.
32. Koren G, Demitrakoudis D, Weksberg R, et al. Neuroblastoma after prenatal exposure to phenytoin: Cause and effect? Teratology 1989; 40:157–162.
33. Kushner BH, Cheung NKV. Neuroblastoma. Pediatr Ann 1988; 17:269–284.
34. Kushner BH, Cheung NKV. GM-CSF enhances 3F8 monoclonal antibody-dependent cellular cytotoxicity against human melanoma and neuroblastoma. Blood 1989; 73:1936–1941.
35. Kushner BH, Gilbert F, Helson L. Familial neuroblastoma. Cancer 1986; 57:1887–1893.
36. Kushner BH, Helson L. Coordinated use of sequentially escalated cyclophosphamide and cell-cycle specific chemotherapy (N4SE Protocol) for advanced neuroblastoma: Experience with 100 patients. J Clin Oncol 1987; 5:1746–1751.
37. Matthay KK, Sathay HN, Seeger RC, et al. Excellent outcome of Stage II neuroblastoma is independent of residual disease and radiation therapy. J Clin Oncol 1989; 7:236–244.
38. McWilliams NB. Neuroblastoma of infancy. In Pochedly C (ed): Neuroblastoma: Tumor Biology and Therapy. Boca Raton, Fla.: CRC Press, 1990, pp 229–244.
39. Miraldi F. Monoclonal antibodies and neuroblastoma. Semin Nucl Med 1989; 19:282–294.
40. Murphy SB, Cohn SL, Craft AW, et al. Consensus statement from the American Cancer Society work on neuroblastoma screening. Do children benefit from mass screening for neuroblastoma? CA 1991; 41:227–230.
41. Nakagawara A, Kadomatsu K, Shin-iche S, et al. Inverse correlation between expression of multidrug resistance gene and N-*myc* oncogene in human neuroblastomas. Can Res 1990; 50:3043–3047.
42. Neglia JP, Smithson WA, Gundersen P, et al. Prenatal and perinatal risk factors for neuroblastoma. Cancer 1988; 61:2202–2206.
43. Nishi M, Miyake H, Takeda T, et al. Effects of the mass screenings for neuroblastoma in Japan. Eur J Pediatr 1988; 147:308–311.
44. Nishi M, Miyake H, Takeda T, et al. Cases of neuroblastoma missed by the mass screening programs. Pediatr Res 1989; 26:603–607.
45. Nitschke R, Smith EI, Shochat S, et al. Localized neuroblastoma treated by surgery: A pediatric oncology group study. J Clin Oncol 1988; 6:1271–1279.
46. Oppedal BR, Oien O, Jahnsen T, et al. N-*myc* amplification in neuroblastoma: Histopathological, DNA ploidy, and clinical variables. J Clin Pathol 1989; 49:1148–1152.
47. Oppedal BR, Storm-Matheson I, Lie SO, et al. Prognostic factors in neuroblastoma: Clinical, histopathologic and immunohistochemical features and DNA ploidy in relation to prognosis. Cancer 1988; 62:772–780.
48. Saarinen UM, Coccia PF, Gersen SL, et al. Eradication of neuroblastoma cells in vitro by monoclonal antibody and human complement: Method for purging autologous bone marrow. Cancer Res 1985; 45:5969–5975.
49. Schimke RN. The neurocristopathy concept: Fact or fiction? In Evans AE (ed): Advances in Neuroblastoma Research. New York: Raven Press, 1980, pp 13–24.
50. Schwab M, Alitalo K, Klempnauer KH, et al. Amplified DNA with limited homology to *myc* cellular oncogene is shared by human neuroblastoma cell lines and a neuroblastoma tumor. Nature 1983; 305:245–248.
51. Seeger RC, Moss TJ, Feig SA, et al. Bone marrow transplantation for poor prognosis neuroblastoma. In Clinical and Biological Research, vol 271. New York: Alan R Liss, 1988, pp 203–214.
52. Shaw A. Surgical management of neuroblastoma. In Pochedly C (ed): Neuroblastoma: Tumor Biology and Therapy. Boca Raton, Fla.: CRC Press, 1990, pp 277–288.
53. Shimada H, Chatten J, Newton WA, et al. Histopathologic prognostic factors in neuroblastic tumors: Definition of subtypes of ganglioneuroblastoma and an age-linked classification of neuroblastomas. J Natl Cancer Inst 1984; 73:405–413.
54. Shulkin BL, Shapiro B. Radioiodinated MIBG in management of neuroblastoma. In Pochedly C (ed): Neuroblastoma: Tumor Biology and Therapy. Boca Raton, Fla.: CRC Press, 1990, pp 171–198.
55. Silber JH, Evans AE, Fridman M. Models to predict outcome from childhood neuroblastoma: The role of serum ferritin and tumor histology. Cancer Res 1991; 51:1426–1433.
56. Sty JR, Wells RG. Radiographic imaging in neuroblastoma. In Pochedly C (ed): Neuroblastoma: Tumor Biology and Therapy. Boca Raton, Fla.: CRC Press, 1990, pp 147–170.
57. Telander RL, Smithson WA, Groover RV. Clinical outcome in children with acute cerebellar encephalopathy and neuroblastoma. J Pediatr Surgery 1989; 24:11–14.
58. Turkel SB, Itabashi HH. The natural history of neuroblastic cells in the fetal adrenal gland. Am J Pathol 1974; 76:225–235.
59. Valentino L, Ladisch S. Biochemical monitoring in neuroblastoma with serum ferritin and GD2 ganglioside. In Pochedly C (ed): Neuroblastoma: Tumor Biology and Therapy. Boca Raton, Fla.: CRC Press, 1990, pp 93–110.
60. Virchow R. Hyperplasie der zirbel und der nebennierin. In Die krankhaften Geschwulste, vol 2. Berlin: 1864–1865.
61. Wright JH. Neurocytoma or neuroblastoma, a kind of tumor not generally recognized. J Exp Med 1910; 12:556–561.
62. Yeh SDJ, Kushner BH, Sullivan MC, et al. Radio imaging of human neuroblastoma; A comparison between 131 I-3F8 and 131 I-MIBG. J Nucl Med 1988; 29:846.
63. Yeh SDJ, Larson SM, Burch L, et al. Radioimmunodetection of neuroblastoma with iodine-131-3F8: Correlation with biopsy, iodine-131 metaiodobenzylguanidine and standard diagnostic modalities. J Nucl Med 1991; 32:769–776.
64. Young JL, Miller RW. Incidence of malignant tumors in U.S. children. J Pediatr 1975; 86:254–258.

▇ RHABDOMYOSARCOMA

Geri VanWezel-Bolen

Soft tissue sarcomas are highly aggressive malignancies of childhood characterized by early infiltration and distant metastasis. All sarcomas originate in primitive mesenchymal cells. During embryonic growth, three germ layers, the endoderm, ectoderm, and mesoderm, differentiate and give rise to different organs. Mesoderm cells form tissue known as *mesenchyme*. The mesenchyme cells give rise to fibrous and adipose connective tissue, blood vessels, lymphatic structures, fasciae, synovial structures, and smooth and striated muscles.[62] Therefore sarcomas can arise in various sites throughout the body. Sarcomas differ and are identified by the mature cell type they most closely resemble. A sarcoma arising in the fibrous tissue contains tissue somewhat similar to mature fibrous tissue and therefore is called a *fibrosarcoma*. Rhabdomyosarcoma arises from tissue resembling striated muscle tissue, which contains rhabdomyoblasts, or primitive muscle cells.[49] Undifferentiated sarcoma also arises from mesenchymal cells but is so primitive that it does not resemble any mature tissue type.

Rhabdomyosarcoma and undifferentiated sarcoma account for 5% to 8% of childhood cancers and are the most common soft tissue sarcomas in children less than 21 years old.[44] The annual incidence of rhabdomyosarcoma in the United States is estimated as 4.3 per million white children and 3.3 per million African-American children under the age of 15 years.[8] Rhabdomyosarcoma and undifferentiated sarcoma occur throughout the world without predominance in any one specific geographic location. Sarcomas are slightly more common in males and are primarily a disease of people less than 21 years of age. An apparent bimodal age distribution occurs, with rhabdomyosarcoma evident at 2 to 6 years and again at 15 to 19 years.[33] Rhabdomyosarcoma of the bladder and vagina occurs most frequently in infants and is of a different histology than sarcomas of the trunk and extremities, which are more common in older children. The most frequent site of rhabdomyosarcoma is the head and neck region.

Head and neck rhabdomyosarcoma can occur throughout childhood but is most common in the first 8 years of life.[44]

The primary cause of rhabdomyosarcoma and undifferentiated sarcoma, like most childhood cancers, is still unknown. Rhabdomyosarcoma has been associated with familial cancer syndromes.[36] A study in 1969 first described an association between maternal breast cancer and soft tissue sarcoma in offspring.[37] A similar study in England demonstrated a 13½-fold increase in risk of developing breast cancer in mothers of children with soft tissue sarcoma.[3] Rhabdomyosarcoma has been associated with neurofibromatosis.[45] An increased incidence of adrenal cortical cancer and brain tumors has been reported in first-degree relatives of children with rhabdomyosarcoma.[37] At autopsy, 37 of 115 (32%) children with rhabdomyosarcoma had one or more congenital anomalies, with a majority of them minor ones such as bilateral hydroceles or ovarian cysts.[59] Molecular investigations of rhabdomyosarcoma, Wilms' tumor, and hepatoblastoma have demonstrated homozygocity for a mutant allele locus on chromosome 11.[32] This suggests that prenatal events may promote oncogenesis in the developing fetus. Epidemiologic studies of rhabdomyosarcoma have demonstrated an increased incidence of parental smoking and exposure to environmental chemicals and increased ingestion of animal organs in families of children with rhabdomyosarcoma.[18,19] Continued epidemiologic investigations are needed to clarify the importance of these findings and to identify other risk factors associated with the development of rhabdomyosarcoma and undifferentiated sarcoma.

CLINICAL PRESENTATION

The signs and symptoms of rhabdomyosarcoma vary according to the anatomic location of the tumor (Table 9–15) and the presence and extent of metastasis. Presenting symptoms may be caused by the primary tumor and/or by metastases.[44] Rhabdomyosarcoma

TABLE 9–15. *Histologic Classification of Rhabdomyosarcoma and Undifferentiated Sarcoma*

CLASSIFICATION	INCIDENCE (%)	CELL MORPHOLOGY	SITE AND AGE
Embryonal	56	Resembles fetal (7–10 wk) skeletal muscle Small round cells and spindle-shaped rhabdomyoblasts Longitudinal striations in spindle cells	Head and neck, orbit, genitourinary system (3–12 yr)
Botryoid (embryonal)	5	Polypoid "grapelike" mass: small round cells with myxoid stroma Inner layer of round and spindle-shaped rhabdomyoblasts	Nasopharynx (4–8 yr) Vagina, bladder (0–3 yr)
Alveolar	19	Firm mass Clusters of small round cells separated by bundles of connective tissue Cross striations more frequent	Trunk, extremities, perineal region (6–12 yr)
Pleomorphic	1	Multinucleated giant tumor cells Racket-shaped cells with cytoplasmic tails Cross striations present	Extremities, trunk (30–50 yr; rare in children)
Extraosseous	10	Uniform small round or oval anaplastic cells PAS-positive, diastase-sensitive rosette formations of cells	Extremities (adolescents)
Undifferentiated	9	Small round cell difficult to classify	Extremities, trunk (6–12 yr)

Data from references 33, 53, and 58.

and undifferentiated sarcoma metastasize by way of the blood and lymphatic systems. Frequent sites of metastases are lung, bone, bone marrow, brain, spinal cord, lymph nodes, liver, heart, and breast.[44] Early spread within the muscle of origin and to adjacent tissue is common.

Tumors in the orbital region grow rapidly and are usually detected early because of the obvious physical changes they produce. Approximately one fourth of head and neck rhabdomyosarcoma develops in the orbit.[53] Parents may note a developing ptosis, with or without lid swelling. Exophthalmos, or proptosis, may also occur. Occasionally orbital cellulitis is present because of tissue necrosis. Cranial nerves II, III, IV, and/or VI may be affected when inferior or posterior orbital rhabdomyosarcoma extends intracranially through the infraorbital fissure.[44]

Neoplasms originating in the paranasal sinuses can cause nasal obstruction, chronic sinusitis, epistaxis, swelling, or local pain. Signs and symptoms of tumors involving the nasopharynx include hypernasal speech, nasal obstruction and discharge, visible polypoid masses in the nasopharyngeal cavity, and serous otitis. Dysphagia and painful mastication are more characteristic of oropharyngeal tumors.

Signs and symptoms of chronic otitis media are common with rhabdomyosarcoma in the middle ear. Other possible symptoms include mucopurulent and sometimes sanguinous drainage from the affected ear, facial nerve palsy, and conduction types of hearing deficits. A polypoid mass may also protrude from the external ear canal.

Approximately one half of head and neck rhabdomyosarcoma and undifferentiated sarcoma arise in nonorbital parameningeal sites (paranasal sinuses, nasopharynx, middle ear, and pterygoid-infratemporal fossae) and have a high probability of direct extension into the meninges.[53] Multiple cranial nerve palsies may occur as the tumor invades the neurovascular sheath. The tumor may cross through multiple foramina and fissures and grow toward the epidural space. Intracranial spread can cause an increase in intracranial pressure (ICP), producing headache, morning vomiting, and/or diplopia.[58] Intracranial extension drastically reduces the overall survival rate.[57]

Tumors originating in the extremities are usually deep-seated, palpable masses with soft to firm consistency that may be mistaken for a traumatic hematoma, especially in school-age children.[17] The fact that injuries to the extremities are common in this age group often leads to a delay in correct diagnosis. Tumors are relatively fixed to the underlying musculature and occasionally involve the skin. Regional lymph node enlargement may be present, especially with alveolar rhabdomyosarcoma.[24]

Until tumor growth is extensive, tumors of the retroperitoneal area are usually asymptomatic. At diagnosis, the child may complain of vague abdominal pain and/or symptoms of bowel or genitourinary obstruction. A palpable mass may or may not be present. Metastasis to local lymph nodes is commonly observed. If the growing tumor impinges on the lumbosacral plexus, children may complain of weakness, parasthesia, and pain.[58]

Half of all cases of vaginal rhabdomyosarcoma is associated with abnormal vaginal bleeding, and the other half is associated with a protruding polypoid mass.[20,21] Pain is usually absent until the tumor is far advanced and has spread by direct extension to the pelvic structures, interfering with bowel and bladder functions.

A tumor arising low on the posterior wall of the bladder or in the prostate is the second most common rhabdomyosarcoma.[20] Presenting symptoms include urinary retention, straining to void, hematuria, or passage of tissue in the urine. Paratesticular tumors usually present as asymptomatic nontender masses in the scrotum, lying above and separate from the testes. They may be associated with pelvic or abdominal masses resulting from metastasis.

Involvement of the bone by rhabdomyosarcoma can produce symptoms similar to those of a bone tumor and/or leukemia (e.g., pain, swelling, and/or limping). Bone marrow metastasis can produce symptoms of pancytopenia, resulting in anemia, bleeding, and/or infection. Most children with bone marrow involvement have an extremity or trunk rhabdomyosarcoma and have concomitant metastases to bone, lung, and/or lymph nodes.[60] Primary lesions of the prostate and maxillary sinus are highly associated with bone marrow metastasis. Only 6% to 7% of children presenting with bone marrow involvement achieve long-term survival.[60]

DIAGNOSTIC EVALUATION

The diagnostic evaluation begins with a complete history and physical examination. Regional lymph node drainage areas are thoroughly examined and may be further evaluated by lymphangiograms, computed tomography (CT), or magnetic resonance imaging (MRI). Whenever possible, a wide excisional biopsy with sufficient margins of normal tissue is performed early. Wide excisional biopsies should be undertaken only in areas in which complete removal will not result in major cosmetic or functional impairment.[33] Biopsy results are important determinants of treatment and prognosis.

Evaluation also includes a complete blood count (CBC), platelet count, urinalysis, and renal and liver function studies. X-ray studies and/or CT and MRI scans of the primary site and chest, skeletal surveys, and bone and liver scans also aid in the determination of primary and metastatic tumor spread. Bone marrow aspiration and biopsy are necessary to assess the presence of bone marrow invasion by malignant cells.

Evaluation of children with tumors of the head and neck may include CT and/or MRI scans of the facial bones, skull, and nasopharynx and rarely cerebral angiography to determine the extent of tumor. Tumors of the middle ear, orbit, and nasopharynx have been known to extend through the adjacent bones into the cranial cavity.[44] A lumbar puncture is performed to examine the cerebrospinal fluid (CSF) for the presence of malignant cells, increased protein, and decreased glucose, which are signs of meningeal seeding.[54]

Other neoplasms such as neuroblastoma, Wilms' tumor, or lymphoma must be ruled out in children with abdominal disease. CT, MRI, ultrasound, and occasionally a voiding cystourethrogram (VCUG) are indicated for diagnostic evaluation.

ESTABLISHING THE DIAGNOSIS

Histologic and clinical staging is done after completion of diagnostic tests and excisional biopsy or surgical excision of the tumor. The histology of the tumor is an indicator of how the tumor will behave and respond to treatment. Clinical staging guides the choice of therapy and is an important determinant of prognosis. The use of uniform staging and classification systems enables institutions using different treatment regimens to compare results to determine more effective forms of treatment. Sixty institutions in the United States, Canada, and Western Europe formulated the first Intergroup Rhabdomyosarcoma Study (IRS) in 1972. Since that time, three successive studies—IRS-I (1972 to 1978), IRS-II (1978 to 1984), and IRS-III (1984 to 1991)—have generated data on approximately 2200 patients with rhabdomyosarcoma and undifferentiated sarcoma. Each study has demonstrated a statistically significant increase in the overall survival rate. The current IRS-IV (1991 to present) study is attempting to evaluate the effectiveness of chemotherapy combinations using ifosfamide, etoposide, melphalan, and doxorubicin in place of, or combined with, the standard vincristine/actinomycin/cyclophosphamide (VAC) and the role of hyperfractionated radiation therapy.[38]

PATHOLOGY

The history of the histologic classification of rhabdomyosarcoma is confusing, and there is no uniformly accepted classification scheme.[53] Historically, rhabdomyosarcoma was classified as embryonal, botryoid-embryonal, alveolar, pleomorphic, undifferentiated, and extraosseous Ewing's.[16] Characteristic cell morphology of each type and frequent sites for occurrence are included in Table 9–14. A classification system based on the cytologic features of the tumor has been proposed.[7,50] The presence of anaplastic changes or a uniform round cell pattern has been associated with poorer prognosis, regardless of clinical group. The IRS, National Cancer Institute (NCI), and International Society of Pediatric Oncology (SIOP) are evaluating data from IRS studies to identify and develop common histologic and clinical staging criteria for the classification of rhabdomyosarcoma.[7,34,56] Currently for treatment determinations, the IRS classifies rhabdomyosarcomas as *favorable histology* (mixed, undifferentiated, embryonal, botryoid, other) or *unfavorable histology* (alveolar).

In many cases tumor cells are classified as either embryonal or alveolar using conventional staining techniques and the light microscope. But because many rhabdomyosarcomas are primitive and poorly differentiated, it can be difficult to distinguish them from other primitive sarcomas such as extraosseous Ewing's sarcoma, primitive neuroectodermal tumors (PNETs) of soft tissue, or fibrosarcomas. Special stains such as phosphotungstic acid can accentuate the cross striations characteristic of rhabdomyoblasts.[53]

The increasing use of immunohistochemicals is not only important for making a diagnosis of rhabdomyosarcoma but also as prognostic indicators for subgroups of rhabdomyosarcoma. Antibodies specific to muscle protein such as desmin,[1] myoglobin,[6] and Z-band protein[12] are helpful in differentiating rhabdomyosarcoma from other primitive sarcomas. A study project of IRS-III confirmed the effectiveness of using a panel of immunohistochemical stains. Desmin and antimuscle-specific actin (MSA) were the most sensitive markers. Because positivity of muscle markers has been found in tissue from Wilms' tumors, ectomesenchyomas, and peripheral primitive neuroectodermal tumors, immunostaining must be combined with other techniques such as electron microscopy to determine the final diagnosis.[51]

The presence or absence of p-glycoprotein in tumor cells may be confirmed as prognostic indicator.[9] Increased levels of p-glycoprotein, thought to facilitate multidrug resistance (MDR) in rhabdomyosarcoma tumor cells, have been found in children with rhabdomyosarcoma who partially or fail to respond to chemotherapy.[9] P-glycoprotein screening may help explain why some children with favorable histology and clinical staging fail to respond to therapy.

The biology of the tumor may also be a contributing factor to treatment outcome. Abnormal cellular DNA content (ploidy) has been linked to tumor proliferation and subsequent prognosis. In one study of children with disseminated rhabdomyosarcoma, tumor-cell ploidy had a significant impact on survival.[61] Advanced rhabdomyosarcoma tumors with hyperdiploid DNA content had an increased likelihood to respond to conventional therapy, resulting in a prolonged survival time. Children with tumors with diploid DNA content appeared to respond poorly initially and had a worse overall survival rate.[61]

CLINICAL STAGING

Various clinical staging systems have been used in clinical studies of sarcomas, making comparisons among institutions extremely difficult. IRS-I devised a clinical staging system based on the extent of surgical tumor removal (Table 9–16). This clinical staging system has been used in IRS-I, IRS-II, and IRS-III. The tumor, node, metastasis (TNM) system, which is based on the presurgical extent of disease, has been used for adult cancers and pediatric sarcomas in Europe. One of the goals of IRS-III was to compare these two staging systems and possibly devise a modified system—tumor, grade or histology, node, metastasis (TGNM)—that incorporates aspects of the TNM and surgical-pathologic staging system. Continued analysis of the data from IRS-III will determine if a modified TNM staging system will be used in upcoming clinical studies of rhabdomyosarcoma and undifferentiated sarcoma.[44]

TABLE 9–16. *Rhabdomyosarcoma clinical Grouping System (IRS-I and IRS-II)*

GROUP	DESCRIPTION
I	A. Localized, completely resected, confined to site of origin
	B. Localized, completely resected, infiltrated beyond site of origin
II	A. Localized, grossly resected with microscopic residual
	B. Regional disease, involved lymph nodes, completely resected
	C. Regional disease, involved lymph nodes, grossly resected with microscopic residual
III	A. Local or regional grossly visible disease after biopsy only
	B. Grossly visible disease after greater than 50% resection of primary tumor
IV	Distant metastases present at diagnosis

Data from references 43 and 53.

TREATMENT

Before the combined use of radiation and chemotherapy, the overall prognosis for children with rhabdomyosarcoma and undifferentiated sarcoma was poor. Complete surgical excision of the tumor was the most successful treatment available. For most pediatric patients this was not an option since as many as 18% had metastasis at the time of diagnosis and tumors were often nonresectable.[35,43] The addition of radiation therapy in the 1950s and chemotherapy in the 1960s, first as a single agent (actinomycin D) and then as combination drug therapy for treatment of metastasis and prophylactic treatment for micrometastasis after excision, greatly improved the overall prognosis for children with rhabdomyosarcoma.[14,40,42]

The goal of surgical management is complete tumor excision while preserving vital and/or functionally useful organs. In many children this is not feasible, and only approximately one in six tumors can be completely removed because of tumor location, metastasis, or infiltration of adjacent organs.[44] Preoperative radiation therapy and chemotherapy can often decrease the necessity for radical surgical excision such as orbital or pelvic exenteration or amputation. Moreover, tumors inoperable at the time of diagnosis may become operable through preoperative therapy. In European protocols designed by the SIOP, chemotherapy and, if necessary, radiation therapy are used as primary therapy for rhabdomyosarcoma in the bladder, prostate, vagina, and uterus to prevent the use of radical surgery.[13]

The role of second-look surgery either to confirm tumor response or to attempt complete excision of the tumor is being explored. The second-look surgery is performed after 20 weeks of chemotherapy and/or radiation therapy to evaluate clinical response. The role of second-look surgery for children in clinical groups III and IV was evaluated by IRS-III.[53] Preliminary results suggest that complete response rates have increased for those children having second-look surgery.[52]

The primary purpose of radiation therapy is to control tumor growth by eradication of gross or microscopic disease. For some tumors (e.g., those of the middle ear and nasopharynx) that are unresectable, radiation therapy combined with chemotherapy may be the primary form of treatment.

Results of IRS-I indicated that postoperative radiation to the tumor bed after complete resection of the primary lesion (except for alveolar tumors) does not enhance disease control achieved by chemotherapy.[40] Currently children with group I disease (except alveolar histology) receive no radiation therapy after primary tumor removal and chemotherapy.[42] Because alveolar rhabdomyosarcoma has an increased risk of local recurrence, radiation therapy is used regardless of group. Children with group II to IV disease receive radiation with chemotherapy.[44] The current recommended dosage is 4000 to 5040 cGy to the primary tumor over 5 to 6 weeks.[53] The radiation dose is determined by tumor size (≥ 5 cm) and the child's age (≥ 6 years of age).

To minimize systemic toxicity and injury to normal tissue, the dosage and dose-time relationship may vary. Two important chemotherapeutic drugs used in the treatment of rhabdomyosarcoma, actinomycin D and doxorubicin, potentiate the effects of radiation. Appropriately scheduling the chemotherapy and radiation is important so that adverse side effects from both therapies are minimized.

The rate of local relapse remains high in children with group III and group IV rhabdomyosarcoma.[53] Hyperfractionated radiation therapy and brachytherapy (continuous low-dose irradiation) are being used in some children with small residual lesions or tumors in difficult to irradiate areas such as the retroperitoneum and pelvis in an attempt to avoid radical surgery yet obtain tumor control.[13,38]

The use of adjuvant chemotherapy has increased the overall survival rate for children with operable and inoperable rhabdomyosarcoma.[40,42] Chemotherapy is now recommended for all children with or without evidence of metastasis at the time of diagnosis. The four most effective drugs, actinomycin D, vincristine, cyclophosphamide, and doxorubicin, are currently used in varying two-, three-, and four-drug combinations.[40,42] Additional drugs such as cisplatin, ifosfamide, etoposide, or carboplatin are added when the disease is more extensive (groups III and IV) or has unfavorable histology, regardless of the clinical group.[44,53] Chemotherapy for groups I and II is usually continued for 1 year if there is no disease recurrence. Groups III and IV receive chemotherapy along with radiation therapy for 2 years.[41]

In IRS-III, children with group I disease, favorable histology, received vincristine and actinomycin D for 1 year. Cisplatin, doxorubicin, and cyclophosphamide were added to the vincristine-actinomycin combination, along with radiation for the treatment of stage I (unfavorable histology) and stage II (unfavorable histology) disease.[44,53]

Children with group II disease (favorable histology) received radiation therapy with chemotherapy consisting of vincristine, actinomycin, and doxorubicin for 1 year in IRS-III. Preliminary results of the IRS-III data suggest that overall survival rates for these groups did not differ much from those of IRS-II.[52]

The addition of other chemotherapeutic agents (DTIC, etoposide, or cisplatin), the role of second-look surgery, and the effectiveness of salvage chemotherapy for partial responses after initial chemotherapy are strategies still being evaluated in IRS-III to obtain better disease control for children with group III and IV disease.[41] The intensification of therapy for group III disease has resulted in improved outcome based on the preliminary results of IRS-III.[52] Children with group IV disease still did poorly in IRS-III despite the addition of different chemotherapeutic agents.[52]

For children with disease resistant to conventional therapy or with recurrent rhabdomyosarcoma or undifferentiated sarcoma, ifosfamide with mesna (a uroprotective agent), either as a single agent or in combination with carboplatin and/or etoposide, has been used.[47,48] In IRS-IV regimens consisting of vincristine and melphalan, ifosfamide and etoposide, or ifosfamide and doxorubicin as initial therapy and combined with VAC for maintenance are being investigated to improve the survival rate for children with metastatic disease.[55] Because of the severe myelosuppression with regimens containing ifosfamide, carboplatin, and/or etoposide, the concurrent administration of granulocyte-macrophage colony-stimulating factor (GM-CSF) is being studied.[2,46] Other therapies under investigation include melphalan (in previously untreated patients),[28] continuous (42-hour) infusion of high-dose methotrexate,[5] and autologous bone marrow transplantation for group IV disease.[31]

TREATMENT AND SURVIVAL RATES FOR SPECIFIC SITES OF RHABDOMYOSARCOMA AND UNDIFFERENTIATED SARCOMA
Head and Neck

Approximately 40% of childhood rhabdomyosarcoma occurs in the head and neck region: 10% in the orbit; 20% in cranial or parameningeal area; and 10% in areas such as the nasal sinuses, nasal cavity, cheek, middle ear–mastoid region, larynx, and tongue.[44] Biopsy (most are unresectable because of loca-

tion), radiation, and chemotherapy (four- or five-drug combinations) are the primary forms of treatment. Head and neck lesions usually are of a favorable histology (embryonal) but involve adjacent structures and nodes and are classified as clinical group III. Based on data from IRS-I and IRS-II, the overall 3-year survival rate for children with head and neck primary lesions, regardless of histology or site, was approximately 80%. Those with orbital lesions had a higher survival rate, whereas children with group III disease and age younger than 5 years tended to have lower survival rates.[44]

Tumors of the nasopharynx, nasal cavity, paranasal sinuses, and middle ear–mastoid and ptergopalatine and infratemporal fossae (termed *cranial parameningeal sites*) are likely to have CNS involvement at diagnosis or soon thereafter. Children with intracranial extension, tumor cells in the CSF, cranial nerve palsy, or bone erosion at the base of the skull have a high mortality rate and are treated with cranial radiation and intrathecal (IT) chemotherapy.[44]

For treating positive CSF cytology, IT chemotherapy consists of methotrexate (15 mg/m² [maximum, 15 mg]) with leucovorin rescue, cytosine arabinoside (60 mg/m²), and hydrocortisone (30 mg/m²). IT medications are given weekly until the CSF clears and then less frequently for 18 months. With the use of wider fields of craniomeningeal radiation and IT chemotherapy, the meningeal relapse rate was reduced from 28% in IRS-I to 6% in IRS-II.[44] The 5-year survival rate for children with cranial parameningeal rhabdomyosarcoma and undifferentiated sarcoma increased from 45% in IRS-I to 65% in IRS-II.[10]

Orbit

Treatment of orbital rhabdomyosarcoma consists of biopsy, chemotherapy, and radiation. Orbital exenteration is rarely indicated because local control can be achieved in 94% of cases with radiation and chemotherapy.[63] Most tumors are of embryonal histology and have a good prognosis. For children in groups I through III in the IRS-I and IRS-II studies, the 3-year survival rate was 93%.[44]

Genitourinary Tract

Genitourinary tract tumors account for 20% of rhabdomyosarcomas, with 12% in the bladder or prostate, 2% in the vagina or uterus, and 6% paratesticular in origin.[53] Most genitourinary tumors are of the embryonal type and are botryoid or "grapelike" in appearance. Tumors of the bladder arise posteriorly at the trigone or at the dome of the bladder, with a better prognosis for the latter location. Prostatic rhabdomyosarcoma tends to disseminate early to the lungs and is often resistant to treatment as evidenced by residual disease after chemotherapy or radiation. The role of prostatectomy for children with residual disease is unclear at this time.[44]

Pelvic exenteration, with ileal conduits and/or colostomies, followed by radiation and chemotherapy was associated with high rates of long-term survival in IRS-I.[40] The desire to produce the same long-term survival rates with less radical surgery led IRS-II investigators to use an approach of biopsy, chemotherapy for 4 or 5 months, and then surgical confirmation of response or residual disease. Those with residual disease, some still requiring exenteration, received radiation. Almost all of the children studied required surgery and radiation to achieve complete remission.[44] Because more effective therapy was needed, IRS-III added cisplatin and doxorubicin to the standard VAC therapy, and radiation was administered at 6 weeks.

Paratesticular rhabdomyosarcoma frequently spreads by the lymphatic system to the para-aortic nodes in the retroperitoneal space. Most lesions are of embryonal histology, and 90% are clinical group I or II.[44] Use of radical orchiectomy with high ligation of the cord, radiation, and chemotherapy resulted in 3-year survival rates of approximately 98% (group I), 90% (group II), and 67% (group III) in IRS-I and IRS-II.[44] Children with retroperitoneal rhabdomyosarcoma frequently have metastases at diagnosis and a less favorable prognosis. The 5-year survival rate was approximately 50% in IRS-II.[10]

Extremities

Rhabdomyosarcoma of the extremities accounts for 20% of diagnosed tumors and has a high relapse rate and low survival rate, regardless of clinical group.[23,41] Most tumors are of alveolar histology, and long-term survival is improved by total gross excision, usually amputation.[44] Postsurgical management should include intensive chemotherapy and radiation to involved sites.

Trunk

Rhabdomyosarcoma of the trunk is initially seen as lesions of the chest wall, paraspinal region, and abdominal wall. Trunk lesions comprise 10% of the diagnosed rhabdomyosarcoma and are associated with a poor prognosis. Most lesions are not completely resectable and are of alveolar or undifferentiated histology. In IRS-II the 5-year survival rate was less than 50%.[42]

Extraosseous Ewing's Sarcoma

The most common sites for extraosseous Ewing's sarcoma are the trunk, extremities and retroperitoneum. These tumors are histologically similar to Ewing's sarcoma of the bone but arise adjacent to the bone in soft tissue. The majority of lesions are localized at diagnosis and have a 3-year survival rate of 75% for all clinical groups.[44] Treatment is the same as that for rhabdomyosarcoma and undifferentiated sarcoma.

LATE EFFECTS

Children with genitourinary rhabdomyosarcoma who have had diversionary surgery (ileal conduit, colostomy) can develop stomal stenosis, ureteroileostenosis, ileoconduit stasis, or intestinal obstruction.[29] Radical lymph node dissections done for treatment of rhabdomyosarcoma of the prostate and paratesticular area can result in retrograde ejaculation and an increased incidence of bowel obstruction.[27,29,44] Ejaculatory dysfunction and decreased spermatogenesis secondary to alkylating agents have become important concerns for young patients who survive into adolescence and young adulthood. These children must be followed in a late-effects clinic in which their concerns about sexual function are appropriately and accurately addressed.

Radiation of the abdomen and pelvis that exceeds 2300 cGy has been associated with the development of chronic nephritis.[4] Chronic nephritis can result in fatigue, anemia, abnormal urinary sediment, hypertension, salt-wasting hyperuricemia with or without gout, and progressive renal failure. These symptoms occur within months or as long as 13 years after therapy.[29] Radiation of the abdomen can also cause retroperitoneal fibrosis with ureteral obstruction, possibly contributing to renal failure.[4]

Radiation therapy for orbital rhabdomyosarcoma can result in the development of cataracts, photophobia, keratoconjunctivitis, bone hypoplasia and facial asymmetry, delayed dentition, and growth hormone deficiency.[22,26] The development of second malignancies in previously irradiated fields is especially disturbing.[11] IRS-I and IRS-II reported the development of osteosarcoma, chondroblastic sarcoma, and thyroid carcinoma as radiation-related second malignancies.[25]

Changes in CT brain scans similar to those seen with leukoencephalopathy have been reported in children receiving cranial radiation and IT medication for parameningeal rhabdomyosarcoma.[15]

PROGNOSIS

The use of multimodal therapy for the treatment of rhabdomyosarcoma and undifferentiated sarcoma has improved the survival rate for children significantly.[14,40,42,53] In the 1960s the 5-year survival rate was less than 20%. It now exceeds 70% for children with nonmetastatic disease treated with combined therapy.[44] Approximately 1688 children were registered on IRS-I and IRS-II and followed for a median time of 9 + years for IRS-I and 5+ years for IRS-II. For these children there was a strong relationship between survival and clinical group in both IRS studies (Table 9–17). Survival at 5 years was 82% for those with group I disease (surgically resectable) and 24% for those with group IV disease (widespread metastasis). Children in group III showed the most significant improvement in 5-year survival rate (52% in IRS-I versus 65% in IRS-II) as the result of the addition of radiation and IT chemotherapy for parameningeal tumors.[10]

The importance of certain clinical features as related to prognosis varied among the dif-

TABLE 9–17. *Five-Year Survival Rates by Site and Clinical Stage—Comparison of IRS-I and IRS-II*

SITE	GROUP I		GROUP II		GROUP III		GROUP IV	
	IRS-I	IRS-II	IRS-I	IRS-II	IRS-I	IRS-II	IRS-I	IRS-II
TOTAL	83%	81%	71%	80%	52%	65%	21%	27%
	N = 101	N = 126	N = 175	N = 171	N = 281	N = 533	N = 129	N = 172
Orbit	100%	100%	95%	91%	88%	90%	50%	0%
	n = 3	n = 2	n = 19	n = 11	n = 41	n = 67	n = 2	n = 4
Head and neck (nonparameningeal)	100%	86%	73%	84%	64%	76%	25%	40%
	n = 8	n = 7	n = 26	n = 27	n = 25	n = 41	n = 8	n = 5
Parameningeal	100%	0%	70%	92%	45%	66%	11%	29%
	n = 1	n = 0	n = 10	n = 13	n = 88	n = 144	n = 19	n = 21
Genitourinary (include special pelvic sites)	93%	91%	79%	83%	64%	68%	47%	46%
	n = 44	n = 54	n = 38	n = 23	n = 40	n = 128	n = 25	n = 27
Extremity	68%	77%	74%	72%	33%	55%	3%	17%
	n = 34	n = 35	n = 46	n = 60	n = 24	n = 29	n = 34	n = 49
Other	82%	63%	42%	70%	35%	45%	24%	27%
	n = 11	n = 28	n = 36	n = 35	n = 63	n = 124	n = 41	n = 66

Data from reference 10.
N = number of all patients in group; n = number of patients in individual samples.

ferent clinical groups. For children with group I disease, histology and primary site were important variables. Those with tumors of alveolar histology had lower 5-year survival rates (47% in IRS-I and 57% in IRS-II) than those with botryoid-embryonal histology (95% in IRS-I and 92% in IRS-II). With the addition of more aggressive therapy for group I alveolar tumors in IRS-III, the 5-year survival rates hopefully will improve. Children with group I lesions of the extremities, most of which have alveolar histology, had relatively poor survival rates in both IRS studies.

No patient characteristics were significant indicators of prognosis for children with group II disease. Primary site was the most significant indicator of prognosis for children with clinical group III disease. Children with orbital primary sites had a better prognosis than those with parameningeal or extremity primary sites. Children with metastatic disease, clinical group IV, had a poorer prognosis in both IRS-I and IRS-II studies. Those with genitourinary sites in group IV had a better 5-year survival rate (50%) than did those with other primary sites.

Clinical grouping, anatomic sites, and histology have been used to design therapy for children with rhabdomyosarcoma, yet the cure rate remains at 50%. The use of a more specific pretreatment staging system combined with an improved understanding of the genetics and biology of rhabdomyosarcoma may more clearly identify subcategories of patients with increased risk for poor tumor response and/or relapse. This knowledge will aid in the development of better treatment programs with fewer late effects that will improve the survival rates for all children with rhabdomyosarcoma and undifferentiated sarcoma.

REFERENCES

1. Altmannsberger M, Weber K, Droste R, et al. Desmin is a specific marker for rhabdomyosarcoma of human and rat origin. Am J Pathol 1985; 118:85–95.
2. Antman KH, Griffin JD, Elias A, et al. Effect of recombinate human granulocyte-macrophage colony-stimulating factor on chemotherapy induced myelosuppression. N Engl J Med 1988; 319:593–598.
3. Birch JM, Hartley AL, Marsden HB, et al. Excess risk of breast cancer in the mothers of children with soft tissue sarcomas. Br J Cancer 1984; 49:325–331.
4. Blatt J, Copeland D, Bleyer WA. Late effects of childhood cancer and its treatment. In Pizzo PA, Poplack DG (eds): Principles and Practice of Pediatric Oncology, 2nd ed. Philadelphia: JB Lippincott, 1990, pp 1091–1114.
5. Bode U. Methotrexate as relapse therapy for rhabdomyosarcoma. Am J Pediatr Hematol Oncol 1986; 8:70–72.
6. Brooks JJ. Immunohistochemistry of soft tissue tumors: Myoglobin as a tumor marker for rhabdomyosarcoma. Cancer 1982; 50:1757–1763.
7. Caillaud JM, Gerard-Marchant R, Marsden HB, et al. Histopathological classification of childhood rhabdomyosarcoma: A report from the International Society of Pediatric Oncology Pathology panel. Med Pediatr Oncol 1989; 17:391–400.
8. Cancer Statistics Review, 1973–1986. NIH publication 89-2789. Bethesda, Md.: National Cancer Institute, May 1989.
9. Chan SL, Thorner PS, Haddad B, et al. Immunohistochemical detection of p-glycoprotein: Prognostic correlation in soft tissue sarcoma of childhood. J Clin Oncol 1990; 8:689–704.
10. Crist WM, Garnsey L, Beltangady MS, et al. Prognosis in children with rhabdomyosarcoma: A report of the Intergroup Rhabdomyosarcoma Studies I and II. J Clin Oncol 1990; 8:443–452.
11. Davidson T, Westbury G, Harmer CI. Radiation-induced soft-tissue sarcomas. Br J Surg 1986; 73:308–309.
12. Dickman PS. Electron microscopy for diagnosis of tumors in children. Perspect Pediatr Pathol 1987; 9:171–213.
13. Flamant F, Gerbaulet A, Nihoul-Fekete C, et al. Long-term sequelae of conservative treatment by surgery, brachytherapy and chemotherapy for vulvar and vaginal rhabdomyosarcoma in children. J Clin Oncol 1990; 8:1847–1853.
14. Flamant F, Hill C. The improvement in survival associated with combined chemotherapy in childhood rhabdomyosarcoma. A historical comparison of 345 patients in the same center. Cancer 1984; 53:2417.
15. Fusner JE, Poplack DG, Pizzo PA, et al. Leukoencephalopathy following chemotherapy for rhabdomyosarcoma: Reversibility of cerebral changes demonstrated by computed tomography. J Pediatr 1977; 91:77–79.
16. Gaiger AM, Soule EH, Newton WA Jr (for the IRS Committee). Pathology of the rhabdomyosarcoma experience of the Intergroup Rhabdomyosarcoma Study, 1972–1978. Natl Cancer Inst Monogr 1981; 56:19–27.
17. Ghavimi F, Mandell LR, Heller G, et al. Prognosis in childhood rhabdomyosarcoma of the extremity. Cancer 1989; 64:2233–2237.
18. Grufferman S, Wang HH, Delong ER, et al. Environmental factors in the etiology of rhabdomyosarcoma in childhood. J Natl Cancer Inst 1982; 68:107–113.
19. Hardell L, Sandstrom A. Case-control study: Soft-tissue sarcomas and exposure to phenoxyacetic acids or chlorophenols. Br J Cancer 1979; 39:711–717.
20. Hays DM. Pelvic rhabdomyosarcoma in childhood: Diagnosis and concepts of management reviewed. Cancer 1980; 45:1810–1814.
21. Hays D, Shimada H, Raney RB, et al. Clinical staging and treatment results in rhabdomyosarcoma of the female genital tract among children and adolescents. Cancer 1988; 61:1893.

22. Heyn RM. Late effects of therapy in rhabdomyosarcoma. Clin Oncol 1985; 4:287–297.

23. Heyn RM, Beltangady M, Hays D, et al. Results of intensive therapy in children with localized alveolar extremity rhabdomyosarcoma: A report from the Intergroup Rhabdomyosarcoma Study. J Clin Oncol 1989; 7:200–207.

24. Heyn R, Hays DM, Lawrence W, et al. Extremity alveolar rhabdomyosarcoma and lymph node spread: A preliminary report from the Intergroup Rhabdomyosarcoma Study (IRS)-II. Proc Am Soc Clin Oncol 1984; 3:80. (Abstract.)

25. Heyn RM, Newton WA, Ragab A, et al. Second malignant neoplasm in patients treated on the Intergroup Rhabdomyosarcoma Study I-II. Proc Assoc Soc Clin Oncol 1986; 5:215. (Abstract.)

26. Heyn R, Ragab A, Raney RB Jr, et al. Late effects of therapy in orbital rhabdomyosarcoma in children: A report from the Intergroup Rhabdomyosarcoma Study. Cancer 1986; 57:1738–1743.

27. Heyn R, Raney B, Hays D, et al. Late effects of therapy in patients with paratesticular rhabdomyosarcoma. J Clin Oncol 1992; 10:614–623.

28. Horowitz ME, Etcubanas E, Christensen ML, et al. Phase II testing of melphalan in children with newly diagnosed rhabdomyosarcoma: A model for anticancer development. J Clin Oncol 1988; 6:308.

29. Jaffe N. The sequelae of cancer and cancer therapy. In Fernbach DJ, Vietti TJ (eds): Clinical Pediatric Oncology, 4th ed. St. Louis: CV Mosby, 1991.

30. Jayalakshmamma B, Pinkel D. Urinary-bladder toxicity following pelvic irradiation and simultaneous cyclophosphamide therapy. Cancer 1976; 38:701–707.

31. Kinsella TJ, Miser JS, Triche TJ. Treatment of high-risk sarcomas in children and young adults: Analysis of local control using intensive combined-modality therapy. NCI Monogr 1988; 6:291.

32. Koufos A, Hansen M, Copeland NG, et al. Loss of heterozygosity in three embryonal tumors suggest a common pathogenetic mechanism. Nature 1985; 316:330–334.

33. Lankowsky P. Manual of Pediatric Hematology and Oncology. New York: Churchill Livingstone, 1989.

34. Lawrence W Jr, Gehan EA, Hays DM, et al. Prognostic significance of staging factors of the UICC staging system in childhood rhabdomyosarcoma: A report from the Intergroup Rhabdomyosarcoma Study (IRS-II). J Clin Oncol 1986; 5:46–54.

35. Lawrence W Jr, Jegge G, Foote FW Jr. Embryonal rhabdomyosarcoma: A clinicopathological study. Cancer 1974; 17:361.

36. Li FP, Fraumeni JF Jr. Prospective study of a family cancer syndrome. JAMA 1982; 247:2692–2694.

37. Li FP, Fraumeni JF. Rhabdomyosarcoma in children: Epidemiologic study and identification of familial cancer syndrome. J Natl Cancer Inst 1969; 43:1365–1373.

38. Mandell L, Ghavimi F, Exelby P. Alternating split course combination chemotherapy (CT) and hyperfractionated accelerated radiotherapy (HART) in the treatment of pediatric rhabdomyosarcoma (RMS) and Ewing's sarcoma (ES): Combined modality treatment revisited. Proc Am Soc Clin Oncol 1986; 5:212. (Abstract.)

39. Maurer HM. The Intergroup Rhabdomyosarcoma Study (NIH): Objectives and clinical staging. J Pediatr Surg 1975; 10:977–978.

40. Maurer HM, Beltangady MS, Gehan E, et al. The Intergroup Rhabdomyosarcoma Study I: A final report. Cancer 1988; 61:209–220.

41. Maurer HM, Gehan E, Crist W, et al. Intergroup Rhabdomyosarcoma Study III: A preliminary report of overall outcome. Proc Am Soc Clin Oncol 1989; 8:296.

42. Maurer HM, Gehan E, Beltangady M, et al. The Intergroup Rhabdomyosarcoma Study II: A final report. Cancer. (In press.)

43. Maurer HM, Moon T, Donaldson M, et al. The Intergroup Rhabdomyosarcoma: A preliminary report. Cancer 1977; 40:2015–2026.

44. Maurer HM, Ragab AH. Rhabdomyosarcoma. In Fernbach DJ, Vietti TJ (eds): Clinical Pediatric Oncology, 4th ed. St Louis: CV Mosby, 1991.

45. McKeen EA, Bordutha J, Meadows AT, et al. Rhabdomyosarcoma complicating multiple neurofibromatosis. J Pediatr 1978; 93:992–993.

46. Metcalf D. The colony stimulating factors: Discovery, development and clinical application. Cancer 1990; 65:2185–2194.

47. Miser J, Kinsella TJ, Triche T, et al. Ifosfamide with mesna uroprotection and etoposide: An effective regimen in the treatment of recurrent sarcomas and other tumors of young adults. J Clin Oncol 1987; 5:1191–1198.

48. Miser J, Kinsella M. High response rate of recurrent childhood tumors to etoposide (VP16), ifosfamide (IFOS) and mesna (MEU) uroprotection. Proc Am Soc Clin Oncol 1988; 5:206. (Abstract.)

49. Pack GT, Eberhart WF. Rhabdomyosarcoma of skeletal muscle: A report of 100 cases. Surgery 1954; 32:675–686.

50. Palmer N, Foulkes M. Histopathology and prognosis in the second Intergroup Rhabdomyosarcoma Study (IRS-II). Proc Am Soc Clin Oncol 1983; 2:229. (Abstract.)

51. Parham D, Webber B, Holt H, et al. Immunohistochemical study of childhood rhabdomyosarcoma and related neoplasms. Cancer 1991; 67:3072–3080.

52. Ragab A, Gehan E, Maurer H, et al. Intergroup Rhabdomyosarcoma Study (IRS): Preliminary report of major results. Proc Am Soc Clin Oncol 1992; 11:363. (Abstract.)

53. Raney RB, Hays DM, Tefft M, et al. Rhabdomyosarcoma and the undifferentiated sarcomas. In Pizzo PA, Poplack DG (eds): Principles and Practice of Pediatric Oncology, 2nd ed. Philadelphia: JB Lippincott, 1993, pp 769–791.

54. Raney RB, Tefft M, Newton WA, et al. Improved prognosis with intensive treatment of children with cranial soft tissue sarcomas arising in nonorbital parameningeal sites: A report from the Intergroup Rhabdomyosarcoma Study. Cancer 1987; 59:147–155.

55. Raney R, Crist WM, Donaldson SS, et al. A pilot study of ifosfamide, mesna and doxorubicin (Ifos/Dox) and followed by vincristine, actinomycin, cyclophosphamide (VAC) and hyperfractionated radiation therapy (HFRT) for children with metastatic soft tissue sarcoma: A report for the Intergroup Rhabdomyosarcoma Study (IRS). Proc Am Soc Clin Oncol 1991; 10:313.

56. Rodary C, Flamant F, Donaldson SS. An attempt to use a common staging system in rhabdomyosarcoma: A report of an international workshop initiated by the International Society of Pediatric Oncology (SIOP). Med Pediatr Oncol 1989; 17:210–215.

57. Rodary C, Rey A, Olive D, et al. Prognostic factors in 281 children with nonmetastatic rhabdomyosarcoma at diagnosis. Med Pediatr Oncol 1988; 16:71–77.
58. Ruymann FB. Rhabdomyosarcoma in children and adolescents: A review. Hematol Oncol Clin North Am 1987; 1:621–654.
59. Ruymann FB, Maddux HR, Ragab A, et al. Congenital anomalies associated with rhabdomyosarcoma: An autopsy study of 115 cases. A report from the Intergroup Rhabdomyosarcoma Study committee. Med Pediatr Oncol 1988; 16:33–39.
60. Ruymann FB, Newton WA, Ragab A, et al. Bone marrow metastasis at diagnosis in children and adolescents with rhabdomyosarcoma: A report from the Intergroup Rhabdomyosarcoma Study. Cancer 1984; 53:368–373.
61. Shapiro DN, Parham D, Douglass E, et al. Relationship of tumor cell ploidy to histologic subtype and treatment outcome in children and adolescents with unresectable rhabdomyosarcoma. J Clin Oncol 1991; 9:159–166.
62. Snell R. Clinical Embryology for Medical Students. Boston: Little Brown & Co, 1972.
63. Wharam M, Beltangady M, Reyn R, et al. Localized orbital rhabdomyosarcoma: An interim report of the Intergroup Rhabdomyosarcoma Study Committee. Ophthalmology 1987; 94:251.

■ BONE TUMORS

Donna Betcher

Malignant bone tumors account for approximately 5% of all childhood malignancies, with the majority occurring in adolescents. The major bone tumors are osteogenic sarcoma, which accounts for 60% of the cases, and Ewing's sarcoma, which comprises 30%, and 10% are a variety of miscellaneous tumors.[15]

The cause of most bone sarcomas is unknown.

OSTEOGENIC SARCOMA

Osteogenic sarcoma is a malignant tumor of the bone derived from bone-forming mesenchyme. It is characterized by the production of osteoid tissue or immature bone by the malignant proliferating spindle cell stroma.[17,20,34] The most common primary sites are the long bones (usually their metaphyses), although diaphyseal primary sites are well described.[5]

Epidemiology

Osteogenic sarcoma accounts for approximately 60% of malignant bone tumors in children and has a peak incidence during the second decade of life.[5,6] This suggests a causative relationship between the adolescent growth spurt and rapid bone growth and the development of this malignancy[5,6] (Fig. 9–5). Evidence supports this causative relationship concept. Children with osteogenic sarcoma are taller than their age peers and taller than patients with nonosseous malignancies.[10] In 1966 it was reported that large breeds of dogs have a much greater chance of developing osteogenic sarcoma than do small breeds.[38] Osteogenic sarcoma occurs at an earlier age in females, corresponding to the more advanced skeletal age and earlier adolescent growth spurt in females than males.[30] Before the adolescent years, the incidence of osteogenic sarcoma in boys and girls is equal. After this age the incidence for males continues to increase, but a plateau is reached in girls. The increased risk of osteogenic sarcoma in males among teenagers and adults may be related to the larger volume of bone formation during a longer growth spurt.[5] Osteogenic sarcoma occurs most often in the rapidly growing bones of adolescents—the distal femur, proximal tibia, and proximal humerus—where the greatest increase in length and size of bone occurs (see Fig. 9–5).

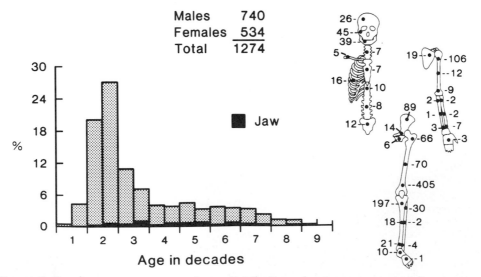

FIGURE 9–5. Age, sex, and skeletal site distribution of osteosarcomas in a large series of patients from the Mayo Clinic. *(From Dahlin DC, Unni KK. Osteosarcoma. In Fourth Edition Bone Tumors. Rochester, Minn.: Mayo Foundation, 1986.)*

Paget's disease is a precursor to osteogenic sarcoma in older patients. Paget's disease, also known as *osteitis deformans*, is the reverse of osteoporosis. Paget's disease of bone initially occurs when too much bone tissue is broken down, causing the body to increase the rate at which new bone is formed. The new bone is laid down in a disordered fashion and is sometimes weaker and softer than normal bone. Almost all osteogenic sarcoma patients older than 40 years have an association with this premalignant condition.[17] The osteogenic sarcoma lesions appear in the bones involved with Paget's disease and occur in axial locations in which Paget's disease is most common.

Trauma has often been associated with the development of bone tumors, but rather than causing the tumor, the injury simply brings the patient to a medical facility where radiographs coincidentally reveal the neoplasm. Trauma draws attention to an existing malignant lesion and does not play a role in its cause.

Genetics

Families have been described in which multiple members have developed osteogenic sarcoma, suggesting a genetic predisposition for this tumor. Children with the hereditary form of retinoblastoma have an increased risk of developing osteosarcoma. These osteosarcomas develop in the irradiation field, outside the radiation field, and in multiple sites.[20] DNA markers for chromosome 13 reveal deletion of genetic material at band 13q14 in patients with hereditary retinoblastoma, sporadic osteosarcomas, and osteosarcomas associated with retinoblastoma. A tumor-suppressing gene on chromosome 13 is involved in tumor development.[4] Additional conditions associated with osteosarcomas are multiple hereditary exostoses, Ollier's disease, osteogenesis imperfecta, polyostotic fibrous dysplasia, Paget's disease, and exposure to ionizing irradiation.[4,20]

Clinical Presentation

The patient with osteogenic sarcoma frequently presents with pain over the affected area, with or without an associated soft tissue mass. Activity often increases the pain, and weight bearing may cause a limp. In young children irritability, crying, decreased movement, limping, or refusing to walk may indicate pain. Local edema, tenderness, decreased range of motion, redness, and occasionally a pulsation or bruit are found on examination. Older children are usually able to pinpoint the source of pain accurately. The duration of signs or symptoms may be short, although 6 months or longer is not uncommon.

Ten to 20% of the patients will have metastases at diagnosis.[20] By far, the most common site of metastatic disease is the lung, although a small fraction of patients present with bone, pleural, kidney, adrenal gland, brain, and pericardial metastases.

Histology

A number of distinct histologic subtypes have been noted. The largest subtype and its variants are conventional osteogenic sarcomas, which are seen most often in children and adolescents[5,6,20] (Table 9–18). This type has three subclassifications based on the predominant differentiation of tumor cells: osteoblastic, chondroblastic, and fibroblastic.[6,7] The second group of osteogenic sarcomas is an unusual variant, called *telangiectatic,* which accounts for approximately 3% of all osteogenic sarcomas. This type almost always is lytic on radiographs and histologically demonstrates dilated spaces filled with blood and necrotic tissues within the tumor. The third group of osteogenic sarcomas is the less common parosteal and periosteal osteogenic sar-

TABLE 9–18. *Histologic Subtypes of Osteogenic Sarcoma*

Conventional
Osteoblastic
Chondroblastic
Fibroblastic
Telangiectatic
Parosteal and periosteal
Multifocal
Miscellaneous

comas, which arise on the surface of the bone without involvement of the marrow cavity.[7] The fourth is the rare entity called *multifocal osteogenic sarcoma*. Multiple skeletal lesions present at diagnosis apparently are separate primary tumors. In the fifth type of osteogenic sarcoma several different variants are distinguished because of differences in biologic behavior.[20] They include osteogenic sarcomas of the jaw, those occurring in patients with Paget's disease, and extraosseous osteogenic sarcomas. Osteogenic sarcoma of the jaw occurs most often in older patients and is associated with an indolent course, with a tendency to local recurrence rather than distant metastases.[20] Osteogenic sarcoma arising in patients with Paget's disease is always a fully malignant spindle cell sarcoma.[17] These patients have a very aggressive clinical course, and few survive. An uncommon variant, extraosseous osteogenic sarcoma, occurs outside the bone and is seen as a late complication of radiotherapy. Local recurrences and distant metastases invariably follow limited surgery.[20]

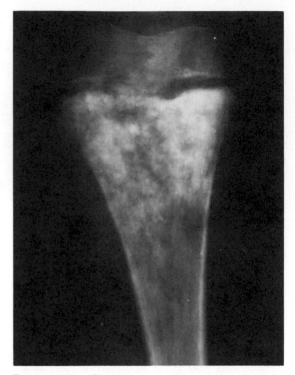

FIGURE 9–6. Osteogenic sarcoma of the distal femur involving the distal shaft, metaphysis, and the epiphysis. There is a mixed lytic and sclerotic lesion with destruction of the cortex in the metaphyseal region. *(Courtesy the Mayo Clinic.)*

Diagnosis and Stages

In a child with a suspected bone tumor, the evaluation begins with a history, physical examination, and radiographic evaluations. Plain films of the primary site and the chest are useful. Characteristic radiographic features, clinical information, and tumor location predict the histologic diagnosis in the majority of osteogenic sarcomas.[20] Further studies such as CT scans and MRI are needed to determine the extent of local and systemic disease before definitive surgery. Although the history, physical examination, and radiographic evaluations suggest osteogenic sarcoma, a biopsy is required to confirm the diagnosis.

Because the presence of metastases at diagnosis is an important prognostic variable, a CT scan of the chest and a radionuclide bone scan are indicated at diagnosis to help define the extent of the primary tumor and to detect skip and metastatic lesions. Skip lesions are tumor deposits in the affected bone that are separated from the primary tumor by several centimeters of normal bone. These tests are also important for surveillance of further metastatic lesions.

Before initiation of treatment, the following evaluations should be undertaken: chest x-ray studies, CT chest scan, bone scan, and a CT or MRI of the primary lesion. Specific serum examinations are needed before initiation of therapy to document the patient's beginning levels and prognostic factors and for evaluation of toxicities associated with therapy. These examinations include complete blood count, blood chemistries, and serum alkaline phosphatase and lactic dehydrogenase determinations.

Surgical Treatment

Surgery is a very important component in the treatment of osteogenic sarcoma. To prevent local recurrences, all gross and microscopic tumors must be removed. In the past amputation was considered the treatment of choice, but today the use of primary amputation has decreased, and many patients can be safely treated with limb-salvage procedures. Relative contraindications to limb-salvage procedures include a displaced pathologic fracture and skeletal immaturity.[9,22,33]

Both limb-salvage and amputation procedures incorporate the basic principle of en bloc excision of the tumor and biopsy site through normal tissue planes with a safety margin of 6 to 7 cm. Knowing the extent of the primary tumor is essential when planning the level of amputation or the resection margins when a limb-salvage procedure is an option. Whether an amputation or a limb-salvage procedure is planned, the goals are to control the primary lesion and to ensure long-term survival while maintaining as much function as possible.[23] Other procedures such as marginal resection and intralesional curettage, which are successful for benign lesions, are inadequate for local control of osteogenic sarcoma.

The dramatic change in surgical management was stimulated by a number of factors. Improved radiographic imaging allows more accurate planning and execution of surgical procedures. Neoadjuvant chemotherapy is begun before surgical resection to permit less radical surgery by reducing tumor size. While the patient is receiving preoperative chemotherapy, the individualized prosthetic device is designed and produced.

Limb-salvage procedures include rotationalplasties, autologous grafts, vascularized grafts, allografts, and endoprostheses. Rotationalplasty, as described by Van Nes, is essentially an intercalary amputation, with the distal portion of the limb rotated 180 degrees; after the resection of the distal femur, the ankle joint becomes the knee.[9] An endoprosthesis involves reconstructing the limb with a distal femoral knee prosthesis. Expandable endoprostheses allow periodic lengthening of the replaced segments.

The surgical procedure undertaken must be both oncologically and orthopedically sound. The health care team must consider at least two questions when determining the appropriate surgical procedure: (1) the safety of the procedure and (2) the functional restoration that will be achieved. For tumors that occur in the region of the knee, four types of procedures are most frequently used: custom-type prosthetic replacement, replacement with an allograft, rotationalplasty, and arthrodesis. Some of these prosthetic devices will fail as a function of time. The more biologic the reconstruction, the more likely it is to endure.

Limb-salvage procedures provide viable alternatives to amputation. Certain limb-salvage procedures are not feasible in the very young child or young adolescent because of the possibility of future leg length discrepancy, particularly if the resection involves one or more major growth plates in the lower extremity.

All limb-salvage surgery is done while acknowledging the potential for many serious risks and complications. Some of the complications can result in amputation. Early complications of limb-salvage surgeries include iatrogenic fractures, skin necrosis, wound infections, venous and arterial occlusions, neuropraxia, and joint dislocations. Delayed complications include local tumor recurrence, nonunion of osseous junctions, stress fractures of bone grafts, joint dysfunctions and arthritis, failure of fixation of prosthetic implants, and late hematogenous infections.[9,33]

Possible complications are related to psychologic adaptation. A full discussion of all appropriate methods of resection and reconstruction is carried out with each patient and family before a particular form of surgery is recommended. Patients and families must be educated about the advantages and disadvantages of the various surgical procedures so they can make informed decisions. The patient must understand the physical limitations of each proposed procedure. Opportunities for the patient to verbalize concerns about body image are provided. The importance of functional rehabilitation of the patient must be explained, and the patient must be an active participant in the planned rehabilitation program.

In summary, a majority of patients today can avoid amputation since there are many other surgical options. The selection of the appropriate procedure must be individualized to the needs of the patient. Local control must be adequate, and functional results must be continuously monitored.

Chemotherapy

Although surgery reliably controls the primary tumor, 80% of patients with osteogenic sarcoma treated with surgery alone develop metastatic disease and die.[20,24] Chemotherapy plays a very important role in the treatment of osteogenic sarcoma. With the advent of modern adjuvant chemotherapy, survival rates of 65% are common.[32,36] The use of adjuvant chemotherapy has an irrefutably positive impact on the natural history of osteogenic sarcoma and is now a component of treatment for all children with this bone tumor.[4,12,20,24] The adjuvant regimens contain various combinations of the following drugs: methotrexate, doxorubicin, bleomycin, cyclophosphamide, cisplatin, and ifosfamide.[4,12,20,23–25] In the past decade the role of neoadjuvant chemotherapy has been evaluated. It is possible that limb-salvage procedures are more successful if the tumor viability and extent are modified by chemotherapy. Tumor necrosis at time of definitive surgery is of prognostic significance and may influence dosages and length of postoperative chemotherapy.[14,24] With only 65% long-term survival, new approaches to administration of chemotherapy and new chemotherapeutic agents must be evaluated to make continued progress in the therapy of this disease.[32] After surgery it is important to delay chemotherapy temporarily to allow wound healing. Chemotherapy can usually be resumed 2 to 3 weeks after surgery.

Chemotherapy can be delivered intra-arterially directly to the tumor. This method of administration provides localized perfusion and produces maximal concentration of the drug to the tumor without the life-threatening side effects of intravenous chemotherapy. Intra-arterial therapy is most effective using drugs with a short half-life (e.g., doxorubicin and cisplatin). They may be used alone or in combination with intravenous adjuvant therapy.[2,37]

Osteogenic sarcoma is highly radioresistant and so is generally unresponsive to conventional-dose radiotherapy. High doses of radiation have been associated with only transient tumor control.[20] If the tumor is judged unresectable because of its location, radiation may become part of primary therapy, sometimes making resections possible in the future. Radiation therapy is particularly useful for palliation of pain from local recurrences or metastasis and to prevent the need for amputation in patients with unresponsive metastatic disease.

Prognosis

The prognosis for children with osteogenic sarcoma continues to improve. With effective neoadjuvant and postoperative chemotherapeutic regimens and advances in surgical and diagnostic imaging techniques, two thirds of patients who present without metastases can be cured. Less radical surgery is possible because of improved surgical techniques, thereby improving the quality of life of survivors.

The most significant prognostic factor in children with osteogenic sarcoma is the extent of disease at diagnosis.[20,24] The 10% to 20% of patients with metastatic diseases at diagnosis have an unfavorable outcome. Primary site of the osteogenic sarcoma is also an important variable. It has been suggested that tumors arising in certain axial skeletal sites (e.g., skull, vertebrae) have a poor prognosis because they are not amenable to curative surgery. In general, the more distal primary sites are associated with a more favorable prognosis.[20]

Elevated lactate dehydrogenase (LDH) is considered the single most powerful adverse prognostic factor for patients with nonmetastatic osteogenic sarcoma of the extremity. At 4 years from diagnosis, the projected disease-free survival rate for patients with an elevated LDH level at diagnosis was 32%, compared to 67% for patients with a normal LDH level at diagnosis.[20]

Other characteristics associated with prognosis are tumor size, age and sex of patient, alkaline phosphatase, and histology. The smaller the tumor is at diagnosis, the more favorable the prognosis, with size greater than 15 cm in diameter associated with a poorer prognosis.[4] It also appears that children less than 10 years of age fare worse and patients older than 20 years have a better prognosis. Females also have a more favorable outcome. Subsequent metastatic disease is associated with elevated serum and tumor tissue alkaline phosphatase.[20] Histologically the telangiectatic variant is associated with a worse outcome.

Metastases

Historically, most patients who developed metastases died within 2 years, with the lungs the most common site of metastasis. Because of the biology of osteogenic sarcoma, lung nodules can be resected successfully and the patients rendered disease free. When the lung is the only site of recurrence and the metastatic lesion(s) are resectable, children can be cured by pulmonary resection alone. Complete surgical resection of all overt metastatic disease is a prerequisite for long-term survival.[20] Patients who develop metastasis after initiation of chemotherapy have a significantly worse prognosis.

Patients with metastatic bone lesions have little hope of cure unless the bone lesion can be controlled with surgical removal. For patients with unresectable metastasis, the approach is palliative. Radiation and chemotherapy rarely produce complete responses; however, these treatments may shrink the tumor enough to allow surgical resection.

EWING'S SARCOMA

Ewing's sarcoma, a highly malignant tumor of the bone, occurs in any bone of the skeleton but often is seen in the extremities, with infiltration of soft tissue around the primary site. Ewing's sarcoma is rare in children less than 5 years of age and is uncommon in adults older than 30 years.[16,27] Ninety percent of all Ewing's sarcomas occur in patients less than 30 years of age, and 70% are diagnosed in patients less than 20 years of age (Fig. 9–7). In adolescence there is a slight preponderance in boys, whereas in prepubertal children there is no difference in incidence related to sex. In children the occurrence of Ewing's sarcoma represents approximately 1% of all cancers and 30% of pediatric malignant bone tumors. There is a very low incidence of Ewing's sarcoma in African-American and Chinese children. In the United States white children younger than 15 years of age have an incidence of 1.7 cases per million per year.[27]

There are no known pattern of hereditary transmission and no known karyotype ab-

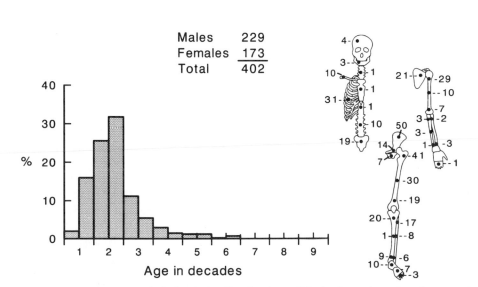

FIGURE 9–7. Age, sex, and skeletal site distribution of Ewing's sarcoma in a large series of patients from the Mayo Clinic. (*From Dahlin DC, Unni KK. Ewing's tumor. In Fourth Edition Bone Tumors. Rochester, Minn.: Mayo Foundation, 1986.*)

normality in patients with Ewing's sarcoma.[27] Other than a possible association with skeletal and genitourinary anomalies, no clearly predisposing process underlies the development of Ewing's sarcoma. There may be a history of trauma, but the bone injury is associated only with the event that brings attention to the malignant lesion.

Histology

The differential diagnosis of Ewing's sarcoma includes all the common solid tumors of childhood when they present in their primitive or undifferentiated form.[27] Small, round blue cell tumors of childhood include Ewing's sarcoma, primary bone sarcomas, rhabdomyosarcoma, lymphoma, metastatic neuroblastoma, and primitive neuroectodermal tumors.[22,27]

Ewing's sarcoma is a diagnosis of exclusion. No unique morphologic markers allow reliable distinction of Ewing's sarcoma from the other round cell tumors. The diagnosis of Ewing's sarcoma is made after exclusion of all the other common solid tumors of childhood when they present in their primitive or undifferentiated forms. Since no unique morphologic markers are evident in a patient with Ewing's sarcoma, the diagnosis depends on the absence of any specific features that would exclude it.[1,16,22,27]

Clinical Presentation

Although it can arise in any bone, Ewing's sarcoma most commonly affects bones of the pelvis, the tibia and fibula, and the femur. For example, in one series of Ewing's sarcoma, the primary site was the pelvis in 18%, the tibia and fibula in 17%, and the femur in 27%.[22] Unlike osteogenic sarcoma, which most commonly arises in the long bones of the extremities, Ewing's sarcoma most frequently involves the axial skeleton.[26] Symptoms are often present for several months before diagnosis.

The most common presentation is pain with increasing intensity and a soft tissue mass around the affected bone. Patients with metastatic disease may exhibit systemic symptoms such as anorexia, fever, malaise, fatigue, and weight loss. Other presenting symptoms are related to the site of the sarcoma. For example, patients with vertebral lesions may exhibit nerve root symptoms, and those with sacral lesions may exhibit a neurogenic bladder.

Staging

The initial diagnostic biopsy is a crucial component in the evaluation of Ewing's sarcoma. Because 10% to 30% of patients have metastatic disease at the time of diagnosis, initial workup includes evaluation for metastasis. Clinical evaluation also includes CT scan or MRI imaging of the primary tumor, chest x-ray films, CT chest scan, bone scan, and a bone marrow aspirate and biopsy.[22] Metastases may be found in the lung, other bones, or the bone marrow. Bone scans are sensitive tools to exclude the presence of distant bony metastases. When performing bone marrow examinations, the site must be distant from the primary tumor.

Prognostic Factors

The extent of disease at diagnosis is the most important prognostic factor.[27] The presence of disseminated disease is an adverse prognostic factor, regardless of the site of the primary lesions.[29] The type and extent of metastatic disease correlate with survival. For example, patients with metastatic bone or bone marrow disease have a poor prognosis. Patients with surgically resectable metastatic disease to the lung may fare better than those with unresectable metastasis.[27]

The Intergroup Ewing's Sarcoma Study (IESS) found that in patients with localized disease, the primary site was of prognostic significance, with pelvic and sacral lesions having the least favorable prognosis.[10,11,28,29] The most favorable sites were the bones of distal extremities. Others have documented that size, not site, of the primary tumor influences survival, with larger tumors faring worse.[14,15] Data from one study stated that a primary tumor size greater than 8 cm in maximal diameter is an adverse prognostic factor.[21,29]

Histologic response to chemotherapy correlates with prognosis. Patients with less than 10% viable tumor during histologic examination of surgical specimens have a better prognosis than those with more than 10% viable tumor.[29]

Other possible prognostic factors for patients with localized disease include age, leukocyte count, sedimentation rate, and serum LDH level.[1,15,16,29] IESS-I found that younger patients had a more favorable prognosis.[29] Elevation of the serum LDH level at diagnosis is associated with metastatic disease and a poorer prognosis.[34]

Treatment

Multimodal treatment of Ewing's sarcoma has significantly improved disease control and survival.[30,31] Surgery and radiation therapy are sufficient to control the primary lesion but not metastatic disease. Thus with radiotherapy or surgery alone, survival rates are from 0% to 25%.[13,22] In the 1960s and 1970s a variety of chemotherapeutic agents was used alone or in combination.[18] IESS protocols have documented the effectiveness of combination chemotherapy with the following agents: vincristine, dactinomycin, cyclophosphamide, and doxorubicin.[22] These studies have evaluated both "high-dose intermittent" and "low-dose continuous" chemotherapy and have focused on innovative ways of delivering the same drugs.[3] Two other drugs, ifosfamide and etoposide, have also shown positive activity in patients with Ewing's sarcoma, even in those with recurrent disease.[25,26,29]

Other studies have classified patients into high-risk and standard-risk categories.[21,29] High-risk patients are those with either pri-

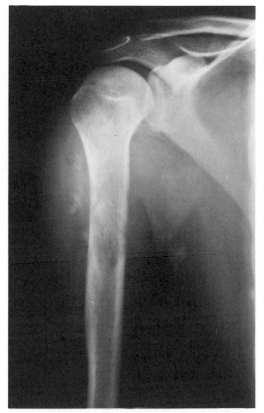

FIGURE 9–8. 1986: 18-year-old male with Ewing's tumor involving the proximal shaft of the right humerus. There is a permeative process in the proximal shaft with calcification in the soft tissues. (*Courtesy the Mayo Clinic.*)

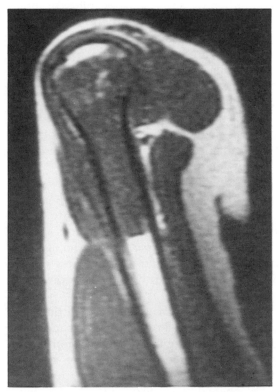

FIGURE 9–9. 1987: Same patient after chemotherapy and radiation therapy. The MRI with T1 weighting shows involvement from the midproximal portion of the humerus up to and including the epiphysis. (T2-weighted images are used to evaluate soft tissue involvement.) (*Courtesy the Mayo Clinic.*)

mary lesions greater than 8 cm in diameter or metastatic disease, and standard-risk patients have nonmetastatic disease and a primary lesion less than or equal to 8 cm. The standard-risk patients received treatment consisting of a four-drug chemotherapy regimen and radiation or surgery. These patients had a 2-year disease-free survival rate of 70%.[18,29] The high-risk patients received an intense 3-day chemotherapy regimen, radiotherapy, total body irradiation, intensification with vincristine, cyclophosphamide, and doxorubicin, and autologous bone marrow transplantation. Two-year disease-free survival rate was 80%.[21,29]

Surgical excision of a primary Ewing's sarcoma is considered whenever feasible. Most current protocols use initial intensive chemotherapy followed by surgery and/or radiation.[29] The timing of surgery and/or radiation is dependent on the radiographic response to chemotherapy and the accessibility of the lesion. Surgery is the treatment of choice for local control in easily accessible lesions when the procedure will not result in functional compromise. Lesions readily resectable include the ribs, proximal fibula, and other expendable bones. Pelvic tumors are the most difficult in which to obtain local control. Experience suggests that pelvic tumors treated with radiation therapy after initial chemotherapy fail to respond completely.[15,29] When these previously irradiated lesions were excised, viable tumor was found.

Surgery is sometimes necessary to correct complications of previous nonsurgical treatment. Patients can experience pathologic fractures through previous biopsy sites or irradiated bone. Frequently an orthopedic reconstructive procedure is required.[15,29]

Dramatic advances continue in the treatment of Ewing's sarcoma. Combination chemotherapeutic regimens are superior to single-agent therapies in controlling systemic disease. Local control of primary tumors is accomplished by surgery, radiation, or a combination of both.

Late Effects

With treatment advances and improved survival rates, the development of secondary ma-

lignancies has become an issue, even though the actual incidence of secondary neoplasms is unknown.[27] The phenomenon of radiation-induced malignancies in Ewing's sarcoma patients is apparent. It has been speculated that the risk of radiation-induced sarcoma is increased in patients who have also received multiagent chemotherapy.[26,35] Because of the risk of second malignancies, long-term follow-up of these patients is essential.

REFERENCES

1. Bacci G, Capanna R, Orlandi M, et al. Prognostic significance of serum lactic dehydrogenase in Ewing's tumor of the bone. Ric Clin Lab 1985; 15:89–96.
2. Benjamin RS. Regional chemotherapy for osteosarcoma. Semin Oncol 1989; 16:323–327.
3. Burgert EO, Nesbit M, Vietti T, et al. Ewing's sarcoma of the bone non-metastatic, non-pelvic primary, and Intergroup Ewing's Sarcoma Study II (IESS-II). Proc ASCO 1988; 7:264. (Abstract.)
4. Ching-Hou P, Crist W. Pediatric solid tumors. In Holleb AI, Fink D, Murphy G (eds): American Cancer Society Textbook of Clinical Oncology. American Cancer Society, 1991, pp 453–480.
5. Dahlin D. Bone Tumors: General Aspects and Data on 6221 Cases, 3rd ed. Springfield, Ill.: Charles C Thomas, 1978.
6. Dahlin D, Coventry M. Osteogenic sarcoma: A study of six-hundred cases. J Bone Joint Surg (Am) 1967; 49:101–110.
7. Dahlin D, Unni K. Osteosarcoma of bone and its important recognizable varieties. Am J Surg Pathol 1977; 1:61–72.
8. Eilber FR, Rosen G. Adjuvant chemotherapy for osteosarcoma. Semin Oncol 1989; 16:312–322.
9. Finn HA, Simon MA. Limb-salvage surgery in the treatment of osteosarcoma in skeletally immature individuals. Clin Orthop Related Res 1991; 262:108–118.
10. Fraumeni JF. Stature and malignant tumors of bone in childhood and adolescence. Cancer 1967; 20:967–973.
11. Gehan EA, Nesbit ME, Burgert EO, et al. Prognostic factors in children with Ewing's sarcoma. Natl Cancer Inst Monogr 1981; 56:273–278.
12. Gill M, McCarthy M, Murrells T, et al. Chemotherapy for the primary treatment of osteogenic sarcoma: Population effectiveness over 20 years. Lancet 1988; 1:689–692.
13. Green DM. Diagnosis and management of malignant solid tumors in infants and children. Boston: Martinus Nijhoff, 1985.
14. Grice B, Armen T, Raymond AK, et al. Osteosarcoma chemotherapy effect: A prognostic factor. Semin Diagn Pathol 1987; 4:212–236.
15. Hayes FA, Thompson ET, Meyer WH, et al. Therapy for localized Ewing's sarcoma of bone. J Clin Oncol 1989; 7:208–213.
16. Horowitz ME. Ewing's sarcoma: Current status of diagnosis and treatment. Oncology 1989; 3:101–106.
16a. Horowitz ME, DeLaney TF, Malawer MM, et al. Ewing's sarcoma family of tumors: Ewing's sarcoma

of bone and soft tissue and the peripheral primitive neuroectodermal tumors. In Pizzo PA, Poplack DG (eds): Principles and Practice of Pediatric Oncology, 2nd ed. Philadelphia: JB Lippincott, 1993, pp 795–822.

17. Huvos A. Tumors: Diagnosis, Treatment and Prognosis. Philadelphia: WB Saunders, 1979.

18. Jaffe N, Traggis D, Sallan S, et al. Improved outlook for Ewing's sarcoma with combination chemotherapy and radiation therapy. Cancer 1976; 38:1925–1930.

19. Kane M. Chemotherapy of advanced soft tissue and osteosarcoma. Semin Oncol 1989; 16:297–307.

20. Link M, Eilber F. Osteosarcoma. In Pizzo P, Poplack DG (eds): Principles and Practice of Pediatric Oncology, 2nd ed. Philadelphia: JB Lippincott, 1993, pp 841–866.

21. Marcus RB, Graham-Pole JR, Springfield DS, et al. High risk Ewing's sarcoma. End intensification using autologous bone marrow transplantation. J Radiol Oncol Biol Phys 1988; 15:53–59.

22. Meyers P. Malignant bone tumors in children: Ewing's sarcoma. Hematol Oncol Clin North Am 1987; 1:667–673.

23. Meyers P. Malignant bone tumors in children: Osteosarcoma. Hematol Oncol Clin North Am 1987; 1:655–665.

24. Meyers P, Heller TG, Healey J, et al. Chemotherapy for non-metastatic osteogenic sarcoma: The Memorial Sloan-Kettering experience. J Clin Oncol 1992; 10:5–15.

25. Miser JS, Kinsella TJ, Triche TJ, et al. Ifosfamide with mesna uroprotection and etoposide: An effective regimen in the treatment of recurrent sarcomas and other tumors of children and young adults. J Clin Oncol 1987; 5:1191–1198.

26. Miser JS, Kinsella TJ, Triche TJ, et al. Preliminary results of treatment of Ewing's sarcoma of bone in children and young adults. J Clin Oncol 1984; 6:484–490.

27. See reference 16a.

28. Nachman J. Controversies in the treatment of osteosarcoma. Med J Aust 1988; 148:405–415.

29. O'Connor MI, Pritchard DJ. Ewing's sarcoma: Prognostic factors, disease control, and the reemerging role of surgical treatment. Clin Orthop Related Res 1991; 262:78–87.

30. Price C. Primary bone forming tumors and their relationship to skeletal growth. J Bone Joint Surg (Br) 1958; 40:574–593.

31. Rosen G, Capurros B, Mosende C, et al. Curability of Ewing's sarcoma and consideration for future therapeutic trials. Cancer 1978; 41:888–899.

32. Santoro A, Bonadonna G. Soft tissue and bone sarcomas. Cancer Chemother Biol Response Modif 1988; 10:344–354.

33. Sim F, Ivins J, Taylor W, et al. Limb-sparing surgery for osteosarcoma: Mayo Clinic experience. Cancer Treat Symp 1985; 3:139–154.

34. Sissons H. The WHO classification of bone tumors. Recent Results Cancer Res 1976; 54:104–108.

35. Smith M, Ungerleider, Horowitz M, et al. Influence of doxorubicin dose intensity on response and outcome for patients with osteogenic sarcoma and Ewing's sarcoma. J Natl Cancer Inst 1991; 83:1460–1470.

36. Souham RI. Chemotherapy for osteosarcoma. Br J Cancer 1989; 59:147–148.

37. Tebbi C, Gaeta J. Osteosarcoma. Pediatr Ann 1988; 17:285–300.

38. Tjalma RA. Canine bone sarcoma: Estimation of relative risk as a function of body size. J Natl Cancer Inst 1966; 36:1137–1150.

■ RETINOBLASTOMA

Elizabeth A. Berro

Retinoblastoma is a malignant embryonic tumor arising from the retina of one or both eyes (unilateral or bilateral). Although retinoblastoma is a relatively rare tumor, it is the most common intraocular tumor, occurring in 1 of 20,000 live births, and is the eighth most common type of cancer in children.[16] Every year in the United States approximately 200 children are diagnosed with retinoblastoma. Retinoblastoma occurs without sex or race preference, although there is an unexplained increase in incidence in some African countries and in Haiti.[3,5]

GENETIC MECHANISMS

The role of genetics in cancer development has been the focus of research and dramatic advances in recent years. Retinoblastoma has become the prototype for such research, leading to the identification of a new classification of genes, the tumor suppressor genes. Inactivation of the retinoblastoma gene plays a critical role in the pathogenesis of retinoblastoma and possibly other malignancies.

Retinoblastoma occurs in two major forms: hereditary (familial), which includes 40% of retinoblastomas,[7] and sporadic (no family history), which accounts for 60% of all cases and typically involves unilateral disease. Hereditary retinoblastoma includes all of the bilateral cases and 15% of the unilateral cases. The rare instance of a "new," sporadic case of bilateral retinoblastoma (with no family history) occurs because of new mutation in genetic material transmitted to the gamete. It should be regarded as the hereditary form of retinoblastoma and not the sporadic form.

In 1971 Knudson[12] proposed his two-hit or two-mutation hypothesis to explain the genetic mechanism of retinoblastoma involved with both hereditary and sporadic cases. The theory proposed that retinoblastoma results from two separate, independent events or mutations. In children with sporadic retinoblastoma both mutations occur in the somatic line; in other words, they occur after the ovum is fertilized. The first mutation inactivates one allele of the retinoblastoma gene; the next mutation inactivates the second. The loss of both alleles in the somatic line results in the sporadic type of retinoblastoma. Because the mutation must occur in the somatic line of the same retinal cell for tumor growth to begin, sporadic retinoblastoma generally occurs unilaterally and at a later age (2 to 3 years).

In the hereditary form of retinoblastoma the first mutation is germinal, inherited from either parent, and present in all body cells, therefore in all retinal cells. The second mutation occurs after the egg is fertilized in the somatic line. All retinal cells experiencing this second mutation are involved with tumor formation. A germinal plus somatic mutation results in hereditary retinoblastoma. Clinical manifestation of multiple tumors in both eyes reflects a somatic second mutation occurring in several retinal cells.

The locus of the retinoblastoma gene defect is on chromosome 13, band q14, which is located on the long arm of the chromosome. During the development of retinal cells, mutations result in the loss of both copies of the retinoblastoma gene. As a result, a protein growth regulator that controls retinal cell growth is not produced. In the absence of this protein, normal barriers to cell growth are absent, leading to unregulated cell proliferation and tumor development. This unique pathogenesis has lead researchers to classify the retinoblastoma gene as a tumor suppressor gene.[23]

Other abnormalities have been associated with chromosomal 13q14 defects, including mental retardation, cardiovascular defects, Bloch-Sulzberger syndrome, extra digits, cataracts, imperforate anus, and failure to thrive.[8,24] In theory these defects could occur in a child with retinoblastoma; in fact, virtually all children with retinoblastoma (>99%) are without abnormalities.[10]

GENETIC COUNSELING

The unique hereditary nature of retinoblastoma places extreme importance on genetic counseling. Unilateral cases with a positive family history and all bilateral cases are autosomal dominant genetic disorders. As with all other autosomal dominant disorders, male or female carriers of the gene have an equal chance of transmitting the defective or mutated gene to offspring of either sex. Every child of an affected parent has a 50% chance of inheriting the mutated gene. Of the children inheriting the defective gene, 60% to 98% will develop the malignant tumors of the disease.[17] In genetic terminology the discrepancy between those with the gene and those with the disease is labeled *penetrance.* The penetrance is clearly comprehendible in light of Knudson's theory. Even if a child inherits the mutated gene, a somatic mutation still is required to develop the actual disease. Based on these genetic principles, a parent with hereditary retinoblastoma has a 40% chance of passing on the disease to an offspring.[9]

In unilateral cases of retinoblastoma without a family history the overall transmission rate is 6%. However, 10% to 20% of these cases result from a germinal mutation and are therefore heritable at a 40% chance of disease transmission as previously described. Therefore difficulty in genetic counseling and prediction arises because of the large discrepancy between the 6% and 40% occurrences.

If unaffected parents have a child with retinoblastoma, the risk to subsequent offspring depends on the type of retinoblastoma the child has. If the affected child has bilateral retinoblastoma, the risk to later children is 8%. The risk to later offspring is lowered to 1.6% if the earlier child has unilateral disease.[9]

In the case of unaffected parents bearing children with either type of retinoblastoma, there is a very small chance that a parent has the disease, which either is undiagnosed or has spontaneously regressed. Either scenario can be detected during an ophthalmic examination. Despite the minimal chance of this type of occurrence, an evaluation is warranted in this situation.

The risks mentioned are only statistical averages and should be used as general guidelines. Any individual with a positive family history should undergo genetic testing and counseling to identify his or her unique transmission pattern.

PATHOLOGY

Typically a child with retinoblastoma has multiple independent tumors of two main types. The first type is composed of highly undifferentiated cells. The second type has more differentiated large cells in a rosette formation. The presence of these different tumor types indicates independent tumors and not intraocular spread of disease.

Retinoblastoma, like other tumors, can extend locally or spread distantly. With local

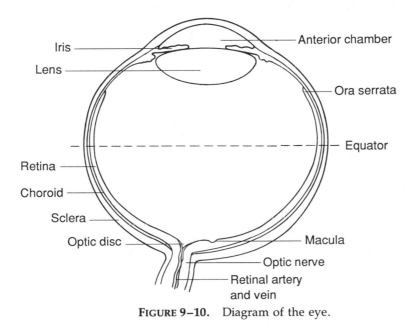

FIGURE 9–10. Diagram of the eye.

extension, the tumors generally grow within the intraocular space before invading the structures surrounding the globe (Fig. 9–10). Metastasis, or distant spread, occurs when tumor cells grow along the optic nerve, enter the subarachnoid space, and spread to the central nervous system. Tumor dissemination is more likely if the tumor extends to the retinal artery or vein. Cancer cells rarely spread to the bone marrow, liver, lymph nodes, or other parts of the body.

Approximately 1% of retinoblastoma cases undergo spontaneous regression, leaving a white scar.[17] Because of the rareness of spontaneous regression and the high mortality rate associated with metastatic disease, all retinoblastomas are treated immediately.

DIAGNOSTIC EVALUATION

The definitive diagnosis of retinoblastoma most often is made during a complete fundoscopic examination. With the patient under general anesthesia or sedation, the pupils are fully dilated so the entire retina can be visualized. The tumors appear as creamy pink or white masses but may be obscured by retinal detachment, hemorrhage, or cloudy fluid in the anterior chamber (Fig. 9–11).

Examinations other than the fundoscopic examination may be needed to assist in the differential diagnosis, identification of the tumor, and determination of the extent of intraocular disease. Additional examinations are particularly helpful if the tumors are obscured by retinal detachments and vitreous hemorrhage. Differential diagnoses include Coats' disease, congenital cataract, coloboma, retinopathy of prematurity, astrocytic hamartomas, and granulomas of *Toxocara canis*. Computed tomography (CT), ultrasound, magnetic resonance imaging (MRI), and x-ray studies permit accurate diagnosis. (Fig. 9–12). Results from biochemical tests of the aqueous humor for lactic acid dehydrogenase (LDH), serum levels of carcinoembryonic antigen (CEA), and alpha-fetoproteins (AFPs) may be elevated in the presence of retinoblastoma.

Because of the hereditary nature of the disease, children with a positive family history of retinoblastoma undergo a full eye examination a few days after birth, at 6 weeks of life, every 2 to 3 months until 2 years of age, and then every 4 months until 3 years of age. Hereditary retinoblastoma usually is diagnosed by age 2½ months.[1]

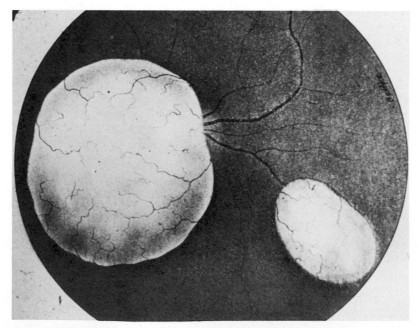

FIGURE 9–11.   Diagram of retinoblastoma tumors. *(Courtesy Dr. R.M. Ellsworth, The New York Hospital-Cornell Medical Center.)*

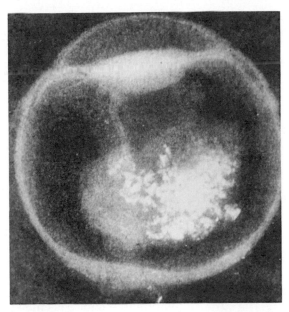

FIGURE 9–12. X-ray film revealing retinoblastoma tumor. *(Courtesy Dr. R.M. Ellsworth, The New York Hospital-Cornell Medical Center.)*

CLINICAL PRESENTATION

In children with a positive family history diagnosis is made and treatment begun before the development of clinical symptoms. In a child without a positive family history of dis-

ease diagnosis is not made until after clinical symptoms arise, generally between 1 and 2 years of age. Symptoms may occur at a later age but rarely after age 6 years. The symptoms of retinoblastoma, in order of frequency of occurrence, include the following:

1. Leukocoria, a white pupillary or "cat's eye" reflex seen as a white light in the pupil. It occurs only at certain angles when a light source, the pupil, and the tumor are aligned. Leukocoria is present in 60% of patients[13] (Fig. 9–13).

2. Strabismus (either exotropia or esotropia) of the involved eye can occur because of poor vision as a result of macular involvement by the tumors.

3. A red painful eye is a late symptom, resulting from inflammation, uveitis, or vitreous hemorrhage.

STAGING

In 1958 Ellsworth developed a classification system for the staging of retinoblastoma. It has since been modified by Reese and today is known as the Reese-Ellsworth classification system. Treatment modalities and prognostic evaluations are based on this classification system (Table 9–19).

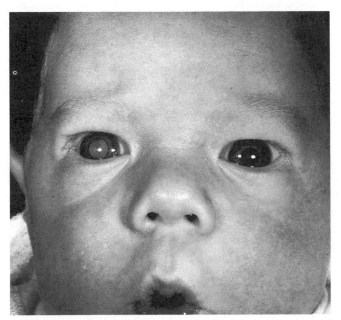

FIGURE 9–13. Leukocoria as a presenting sign of retinoblastoma. *(From Char DH. Clinical Ocular Oncology. New York: Churchill Livingstone, 1989, p 190.)*

TABLE 9–19. *Reese-Ellsworth Staging for Retinoblastoma*

Group I: Very Favorable Prognosis

A. Solitary tumor; <4 disc diameters (dd) in size at or behind the equator
B. Multiple tumors; no tumor >4 dd in size or behind the equator

Group II: Favorable Prognosis

A. Solitary tumor; 4 to 10 dd in size or behind the equator
B. Multiple tumors; 4 to 10 dd in size behind the equator

Group III: Doubtful Prognosis

A. Any lesion anterior to the equator
B. Solitary tumors >10 dd in size behind the equator

Group IV: Unfavorable Prognosis

A. Multiple tumors; some >10 dd in size
B. Any lesion extending anterior

Tumors are visualized by an indirect ophthalmic examination with the child under general anesthesia to determine tumor size in disc diameters (dd; 1 dd equals 1.5 mm) and their location relative to the equator of the eye. The equator divides the orbit equally into anterior and posterior sections. Both eyes always are examined, and any tumors are mapped out for later comparison (Fig. 9–14). Additionally, the presence or absence of orbital extension is noted. Further diagnostic examinations may be needed to determine the degree of orbital extension and/or the presence of metastatic disease. Tests may include an ultrasound of the eye, x-ray films of the eye and skull, and CT of the eye, head, and abdomen. Cerebrospinal fluid obtained through a lumbar puncture and aspirated bone marrow are tested for the presence of metastasized tumor cells. If indicated by suspected metastatic disease, a bone scan, liver and spleen scan, or biopsy of the tumor is performed.

Based on the information obtained in these examinations, the disease is staged from group I to group V. Group I includes disease initially seen as small tumors located on the posterior aspect of the retina. The prognosis for children diagnosed with group I disease is very favorable and worsens in the higher group classifications. In group V disease are many large tumors and/or vitreous seeding, which is the presence of tumor cells "floating" in the vitreous humor. The criteria for the Reese-Ellsworth staging are found in Table 9–19. There is no accepted system for staging retinoblastoma that has extended beyond the orbit.

TREATMENT

Treatment plans for retinoblastoma are individualized and are based on the extent of the disease while maintaining the goal of preserving useful vision. The treatment of intraocular (nonmetastatic) retinoblastoma includes surgery, radiotherapy, phototherapy, and/or cryotherapy.

The surgical treatment of choice is enucleation. Enucleation is indicated in the following situations: (1) severe retinal disruption with no possibility of restoration of vision; (2) extension of the tumor into the anterior chamber; (3) painful glaucoma with permanent loss of vision; and (4) unresponsiveness to other forms of treatment.

Although enucleation is the conventional treatment of retinoblastoma, its use is declining. One retrospective study found enucleations were used 97% of the time during the 5-year interval from 1974 through 1978. However, only 75% of patients received enucleations in the period from 1984 through 1988. Earlier diagnosis and refinement of nonsurgical treatment modalities are the main reasons for this trend away from enucleation.[22]

After the enucleation, the socket is cleansed with saline solution and an antibiotic ointment applied. A patch is used for up to 1 week postoperatively to keep the area clean. The socket can be fitted for an artificial plastic eye, usually in 3 to 6 weeks when healing is complete and swelling has subsided. The eye is sized for proper fit and the color matched with the remaining eye. The artificial eye and socket require minimal care and no special equipment. The artificial eye remains in place overnight and is cleansed while in the socket during normal face washing with a gentle soap and water. A patient generally visits the ophthalmologist every 6 months. The artificial eye can be "built up" to improve the fit

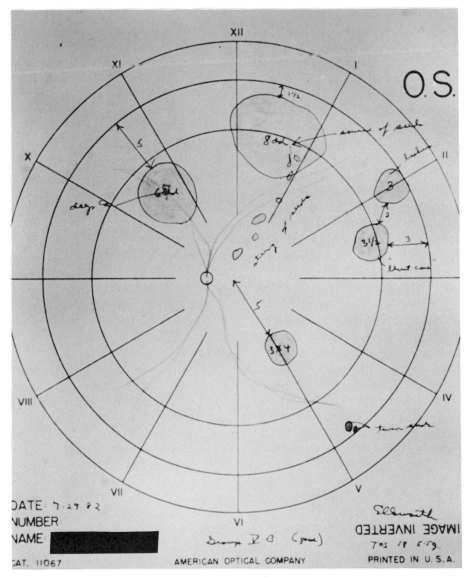

FIGURE 9–14. Mapping of retinoblastoma; used for later comparison. *(Courtesy Dr. R.M. Ellsworth, The New York Hospital-Cornell Medical Center.)*

in a growing child. A new artificial eye is needed approximately every 5 years.

After enucleations in children under 3 years of age, the socket does not grow normally. Loss of the orbit combined with the effect of external beam radiation results in local growth retardation, leaving the socket with a sunken appearance.

Special attention must be paid to educating the child about his or her enucleation and the artificial eye. It is reassuring to the parent and child that the empty socket, once healed, will not be tender or sensitive. Enucleation is

a technically simple surgery that is not physically painful. In discussion of the artificial eye, the nurse must be sensitive to the family's psychosocial concerns, be thorough in explaining care of the prosthesis, and be sure the child and family understand that the prosthesis, although cosmetically functional, does not restore vision. Use of safety glasses for sporting activities to protect the remaining eye should be emphasized.

Radiotherapy is helpful in controlling disease while preserving useful vision. Retinoblastoma is highly radiosensitive. Radiation therapy is administered by either external beam or application of radioactive applicators. External beam therapy is always used if there is a chance of restoring useful vision. Abramson has demonstrated a 75% cure in cases of intraocular tumors treated with radiation. Radiation doses vary with the Reese-Ellsworth staging and range from 3500 cGy to 4500 cGy in 9 to 12 fractions over 3 to 4 weeks.[6] New techniques in external beam therapy have made the precise delivery of radiation to the tumor sites possible and safer. To accomplish this therapy successfully, cooperation of the child is essential. Play therapy, practice sessions, and contact with consistent hospital personnel can help elicit cooperation from the child. Sedatives or anesthesia may also be used to assure accurate and safe delivery of the radiation therapy. Since the introduction of these radiotherapy techniques, complications are rare but may include vitreous hemorrhage, glaucoma, cataracts, and atrophy of surrounding bones. Tumor regression is followed by serial eye examinations throughout the treatment period. Several typical regression patterns have been identified. Differentiating these patterns requires experience but is valuable in monitoring patient response to treatment.

Use of radioactive surface applicators (plaques) is indicated if recurring small tumors remain after external beam therapy or as initial therapy for small solitary tumors. A surgical procedure is necessary to suture the radioactive device to the sclera. The device is left in place for 7 days, delivering 4000 cGy to the tumor. Both application and removal of the device are done with the child under general anesthesia. While this device is in place, the child must be in a single room to prevent unnecessary radioactive exposure of other patients and staff. Staff members wear radiation-sensitive badges to assure that their exposure is minimal and within safe limits set by the National Council on Radiation Protection and Measurement.

The care of these young patients and their families is a nursing challenge. Special attention must be given to the child and family to dispel the feeling of isolation. Collaboration with a play therapist can help in selecting activities to alleviate loneliness and boredom. Parents must be reassured that their child will receive appropriate care despite the isolation. The staff may need education about safety concerns related to radioactive applicators. Potential complications associated with radioactive applicators include hemorrhage and cataract formation.

Photocoagulation is a process that destroys the blood vessels surrounding and supplying the tumor. This therapy is generally used in conjunction with external beam radiation in tumors that fail to regress after 4 to 6 weeks of radiation therapy or recur after radiation therapy. Photocoagulation is performed under direct visualization and is the appropriate treatment for tumors located posterior to the equator. It also is used as initial therapy if the tumors are small and situated away from the optic nerve and macula. Complications include retinal edema, retinal detachment, or hemorrhage.

Cryotherapy destroys the tumor cells by forming intracellular ice crystals that disrupt the microcirculation of the tumor and cause cell death. Cryotherapy is generally used in conjunction with external beam therapy, and its indications are the same as for photocoagulation. It is performed by using a small probe on the sclera through an incision in the conjunctiva. Cryotherapy is most suitable for tumors anterior to the equator since the procedure does not require direct visualization. Potential complications include retinal edema, retinal detachment, or hemorrhage. Patients may experience nausea and vomiting after the procedure.[21]

Intravenous and/or intrathecal chemotherapy is administered if metastatic disease is present.[11] Methotrexate, cisplatin, and vincristine are the primary agents. Despite chemotherapeutic treatment, prognosis is poor in the presence of metastatic disease.

PROGNOSIS

The overall 5-year survival rate for children with retinoblastoma is 90%.[16] The 10% mortality rate is associated with metastatic disease.[14] Survival with useful vision varies with the staging of the disease. Of the children with group I retinoblastoma, 95% to 100% survive with useful vision; with group II, 87% to 100%; with group III, 67% to 86%; with group IV, 69% to 75%; with group V, 34% to 75%; and with extraorbital disease, 30% to 75%.[1]

Although overall recovery of visual acuity is encouraging, it is dependent on tumor location. Visual acuity is reduced if the tumors involve the macula. There is a greater risk of cataract development with tumors involving the ora serrata. Children are seen every 6 months to a year by their ophthalmologist for evaluation of remaining tumor scars and for consistent evaluation of the socket if enucleation has been performed.

Because of the high potential for a cure, particularly in cases of early diagnosis, careful screening is essential. Any child born with a familial history of retinoblastomas must be examined in infancy and seen regularly by an ophthalmologist knowledgeable about the disease.

Despite the encouraging high survival rates associated with early diagnosis of retinoblastoma, numerous studies have identified an increased incidence of secondary malignant tumors. These tumors are not metastases from the ocular disease but are primary cancers of other organs. Although osteosarcoma is the most common secondary tumor, there are also increased incidences of other types of cancer, including small cell lung carcinoma and cancer of the breast, prostate, and bladder.[2,22a] A study done in the Netherlands identified a 10% risk of secondary cancers in the survivors of hereditary retinoblastoma at age 35.[4] This increased susceptibility to cancer is most closely associated with survivors of bilateral retinoblastoma. It is postulated that the defective retinoblastoma gene plays an important role in the development of osteosarcomas and possibly other cancers such as aggressive ovarian cancers and soft tissue sarcomas.[19,20] These secondary tumors develop in the second and third decades of life and are often resistant to therapy.[18] Therefore children surviving retinoblastoma require extensive follow-up care, with frequent screening for the presence of secondary tumors.

ACKNOWLEDGMENT

The author extends special thanks to Dr. Robert M. Ellsworth, Director of the Ophthalmic Oncology Center, and Betty Ann Kirchhoffer, RN, at The New York Hospital–Cornell Medical Center.

REFERENCES

1. Abramson DH. Retinoblastoma: Diagnosis and Management. New York: American Cancer Society, 1982.
2. Abramson DH, Ronner HJ, Ellsworth RM. Second tumors in non-irradiated bilateral retinoblastoma. Am J Ophthamol 1979; 87:624–627.
3. Bishop JO. Retinoblastoma. Pediatr Ann 1979; 8:12.
4. Derkinderen DJ, Koten JW, Wolterbeek R, et al. Non-ocular cancer in hereditary retinoblastoma survivors and relatives. Ophthalmic Paediatr Genet 1987; 8:23–25.
5. Devesa SS. The incidence of retinoblastoma. Am J Ophthalmol 1975; 80:263–265.
6. Donaldson SS, Egbert PR, Lee WH. Retinoblastoma. In Pizzo PA, Poplack DG (eds): Principles and Practice of Pediatric Oncology, 2nd ed. Philadelphia: JB Lippincott, 1993, pp 683–696.
7. Gallie BL, Dunn JM, Chan HS, et al. The genetics of retinoblastoma. Pediatr Clin North Am 1991; 38:299–315.
8. Green DM. Retinoblastoma. In Green DM (ed): Diagnosis and Management of Malignant Solid Tumors in Infants and Children. Boston: Martinus Nijhoff, 1985, pp 90–128.
9. Harper PS. Practical Genetic Counseling, 3rd ed. London: John Wright, 1988.
10. Jensen RD, Miller RW. Retinoblastoma: Epidemiologic characteristics. N Engl J Med 1971; 285:307–311.
11. Kingston JE, Hungerford JL, Plowman PN. Chemotherapy in metastatic retinoblastoma. Ophthalmic Pediatr Genet 1987; 8:69–72.
12. Knudson AG. Mutation and cancer: A statistical study of retinoblastoma. Proc Natl Acad Sci U S A 1971; 68:620–623.
13. Lanzkowsky P. Manual of Pediatric Hematology and Oncology. New York: Churchill Livingstone, 1989.
14. Magramm I, Abramson D, Ellsworth RM. Optic nerve involvement in retinoblastoma. Ophthalmology 1989; 96:217–223.
15. Deleted.
16. Neglia JP, Robinson LL. Epidemiology of childhood acute leukemias. Pediatr Clin North Am 1988; 35:675–692.
17. Roberts DF, Aherne GES. Retinoblastoma. In Emery AEH, Rimoin D (eds): Principles and Practice of Medical Genetics. New York: Churchill Livingstone, 1990, pp 705–721.
18. Sanders BM, Draper GJ, Kingston JE. Retinoblastoma in Great Britain 1969–1980 incidence, treatment and survival. Br J Ophthalmol 1988; 72:576–583.
19. Sansano H, Comerford J, Silverberg SG. An analysis of abnormalities of the retinoblastoma gene in human ovarian and endometrial carcinoma. Cancer 1990; 66:2150–2154.
20. Scheffener M, Münger K, Byrne JC, et al. The state

of the retinoblastoma genes in human cervical carcinoma cell lines. Proc Natl Acad Sci U S A 1991; 88:5523–5527.

21. Servodidio CA, Abramson DH, Romanella A. Retinoblastoma. Cancer Nurs 1991; 14:117–123.

22. Shields JA, Shields CL, Sivalingam V. Decreasing frequency of enucleation in patients with retinoblastoma. Am J Ophthalmol 1989; 108:185–188.

22a. Smith JLS, Bedford MA. In Marsden HB, Steward JK (eds): Recent Results in Cancer Research, Tumors in Children, 2nd ed. New York: Springer-Verlag, 1976.

23. Vile R. Tumor suppressor genes. Br Med J 1989; 298:1335–1336.

24. Wong DL, Doran LR. Nursing care in childhood cancer: Retinoblastoma. Am J Nurs 1982; 82:425–431.

■ UNUSUAL TUMORS

Mary J. Waskerwitz

Children diagnosed with uncommon malignancies pose particularly challenging problems to nurses and all members of the pediatric oncology team. Because of their rarity, these diseases usually are not the focus of clinical trials. A patient's individual treatment may be based solely on anecdotal references to patients with similar diagnoses and clinical presentations. Even making the diagnosis may represent a very long, difficult process.

Nurses caring for children with less common malignancies are dealing with many unknowns as they themselves try to understand fully the child's probable course and treatment. In addition, educating parents about their child's diagnosis and treatment likely will be frustrating, with many unanswered questions, no long-range course description, and the availability of little, if any, written teaching materials. Meeting a family's support needs can be challenging because it is difficult to find another family within the area whose child has the same diagnosis. A possible resource is the *Candlelighters Newsletter*, which often contains open letters from parents seeking contact with other parents whose child has the same rare tumor.

LIVER TUMORS
Hepatoblastoma

Hepatoblastoma is the third most common intra-abdominal neoplasm of childhood[4] and the most common pediatric liver tumor, although it represents only 1% to 2% of all cancers in children. Eighty percent of children with hepatoblastoma are less than 3 years of age at diagnosis.[9]

Most often hepatoblastoma is initially seen as a large abdominal mass in a child who is otherwise well; thus some of these tumors are detected during routine physical examinations. Other signs and symptoms include weight loss, pallor, anorexia, hepatomegaly, pain, vomiting, and jaundice. Weakness, lethargy, diarrhea, pruritus, fever, splenomegaly, and right hemihypertrophy are much less common. Severe osteopenia (reduced bone mass) with vertebral compression fractures is caused in theory by a protein deficit resulting from hepatic dysfunction. It can result in back pain or refusal to walk.[56]

The right lobe of the liver, approximately 70% of the total hepatic cell mass, is most often the site of hepatoblastoma, which is seen as a unifocal lesion. The left lobe of the liver includes a medial and lateral segment, each containing approximately 15% of the hepatic cell mass (Fig. 9–15). Thirty percent of hepatoblastomas involve both lobes.[9] Twenty percent of patients have metastasis at diagnosis, usually to lungs or through intra-abdominal spread and rarely to bone, the central nervous system (CNS), and bone marrow.

The diagnosis of hepatoblastoma is made through imaging studies and laboratory evaluations. Abdominal radiographs will show the presence of a right upper quadrant mass. Ultrasonography will reveal diffuse hyperechoic patterns and can be used during and after treatment to follow tumor response and normal liver regeneration. Computerized tomography (CT) is the most accurate non-invasive diagnostic procedure to depict these large solitary lesions with low density areas. When enhanced by intravenous contrast medium, CT scans can outline vascular anatomy to aid in subsequent surgical resection. The accuracy of magnetic resonance imaging seems comparable to that of the CT scan.

Production of alpha-fetoprotein (AFP), a fetal antigen globulin, begins in the 1-month-old fetus, peaks at 14 weeks' gestation and achieves normal AFP levels (20 to 120 ng/ml) at birth. By 1 year of age, a healthy infant has the same level of AFP as an adult (3 to 15 ng/ml). AFP is also a biologic marker used to diagnose and follow hepatoblastoma. It is elevated in two thirds of patients with the disease to levels greater than 100 ng/ml and even as high as 500,000 ng/ml.[9,20] Serum AFP levels usually decrease with tumor resection and effective therapy. An elevation signals disease recurrence or metastases. Three percent of patients with hepatoblastoma are boys who se-

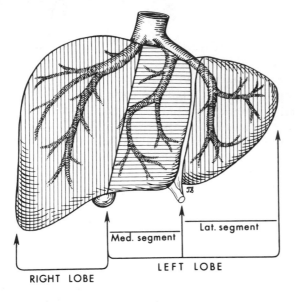

RIGHT LOBE   Med. segment   Lat. segment   LEFT LOBE

Figure 9–15. The liver consists of right and left lobes, which are divided by an imaginary line between inferior vena cava and gallbladder. Left lobe has a medial segment and a lateral segment, which are divided by the falciform ligament. The right lobe of the liver contains 70% of the liver's cell mass; each segment of the left lobe contains 15%. Most hepatoblastomas involve the right lobe of the liver. *(From Greenberg M, Filler R. Hepatic tumors. In Pizzo P, Poplack D (eds): Principles and Practice of Pediatric Oncology, 2nd ed. Philadelphia: JB Lippincott, 1993, pp 697–712.*

crete beta-human chorionic gonadotropin (β-HCG), resulting in precocious puberty with penile and testicular enlargement and pubic hair.[20] Complete blood counts (CBCs) can show anemia with moderate leukocytosis; thrombocytosis is common. Serum biochemical analysis of liver function (bilirubin, transaminases, and alkaline phosphatase) likely will be normal. Levels of serum ferritin, a form of iron stored in the liver, frequently are elevated.

The different histologic subtypes of hepatoblastoma are epithelial, containing fetal or embryonal cells or both, and mixed, with mesenchymal and epithelial elements. Fetal histology is associated with a good prognosis in patients whose tumors can be completely resected.

The primary goal of successful hepatoblastoma treatment is to achieve tumor resection surgically. Liver tissue is capable of regeneration. As much as 85% of the liver can be removed, and it will completely regenerate within 1 to 3 months.[20] A hepatectomy is performed if to do so appears feasible from CT scan. That surgical procedure, however, has significant risk of hemorrhage, resulting in a greater than 10% operative mortality. Recent advances in the use of hemodilution anesthesia, rapid blood transfusion, and profound hypothermia with circulatory arrest have increased the safety of the surgical excision necessary to achieve cure for these patients.[9,50] If

the tumor is not resectable, a wedge biopsy with gross inspection of the liver or a needle biopsy, which avoids the use of general anesthesia and significant tumor spill and is associated with less bleeding, is performed. Liver transplantation may be a viable option in the future for patients with nonmetastatic disease.

Chemotherapy is used as adjunct therapy for patients who undergo complete tumor resection and as preoperative therapy for patients whose tumors are initially considered unresectable. Courses of chemotherapy should not be instituted postoperatively until there is evidence of significant liver regeneration on follow-up studies, usually by 1 month. Cisplatin and/or doxorubicin used as a continuous intravenous infusion to avoid significant cardiotoxicity is the primary drug used for treatment of hepatoblastoma. Vincristine, cyclophosphamide, bleomycin, and 5-fluorouracil are also effective agents. Intraarterial chemotherapy, which delivers high concentrations of drug directly to tumor cells with reduction of systemic toxicity, may also be used in the future.[36,37]

The Childrens Cancer Group (CCG) and Pediatric Oncology Group (POG) have developed a staging classification for patients with hepatoblastoma,[9] on which the prognosis is based. The overall survival rate for children with hepatoblastoma is 35% to 45%.[21,55] The best results are achieved in children whose tumors are completely removed and of pure fetal histology.

Hepatocellular Carcinoma

Hepatocellular carcinoma is rarer than hepatoblastoma. Both tumors are treated with similar protocols, although each has certain unique features. Hepatocellular carcinoma tends to occur in older children and adolescents. The average age at diagnosis is 9 years.[9] It can occur in livers damaged by cirrhosis or chronic hepatitis B, among other conditions.[9] Abdominal pain and jaundice are often present at the onset of disease. Serum AFP is not often elevated, although serum ferritin levels usually are. Only one third of children with hepatocellular carcinoma have resectable lesions, primarily because both lobes of the liver usually are involved. Only one third of these children are long-term survivors.[20,39]

GERM CELL TUMORS

Germ cells develop in the human embryo yolk sac at approximately 4 weeks gestation, migrate to the gonadal ridge by 6 weeks, and then descend into the pelvis or scrotal sac, populating the developing ovary or testis. Germ cell tumors represent 3% of all childhood malignancies. They typically occur in the gonads or in tissues found along the midline migration path; thus they are intracranial, mediastinal, retroperitoneal, or sacrococcygeal. Two thirds of all germ cell tumors in children are located in those extragonadal sites.[39] Large numbers of germ cell tumors are benign. Table 9–20 shows the distribution of childhood germ cell tumors by site, age, and pathology.

Several cytogenetic changes have been associated with germ cell tumors. They include duplication or deletions of genes on the short arm of chromosome 1 and an isochromosome on the short arm of chromosome 12.[26a] The isochromosome is a chromosome abnormality in which the short arm of chromosome 12 has been duplicated and the long arm deleted. Also reported are abnormalities of the sex chromosomes, including 46 XY aneuploidy with an extra X chromosome. This has been associated with some extragonadal germ cell tumors. Also there is an association of certain germ cell tumors with phenotypic females (having all the characteristics of a female) who actually have the XY male chromosome rather than the XX female pattern.[26a] In addition to these genetic abnormalities, a number of congenital defects are associated with germ cell tumors, including CNS and genitourinary tract malformations and major malformations of the lower spine.[26a,45]

The common histologic classifications of germ cell tumors of infants, children, and adolescents include teratomas, germinomas (dysgerminomas, seminomas), endodermal sinus tumors (yolk sac tumors), choriocarcinomas, and embryonal carcinomas. It is not unusual for one tumor to include more than one cell type. Metastasis can occur to lungs, liver, regional nodes, and CNS or less often to bone, bone marrow, or other distant areas.

Levels of AFP, the main fetal serum protein, which is replaced by albumin at birth, and β-HCG, a glycoprotein produced by placental cells to promote implantation of fertilized eggs, frequently are elevated in patients with germ cell tumors. Secretion of β-HCG can cause early breast enlargement, pubic hair, and menarche. The level of lactic dehydrogenase (LDH) also often is elevated in these patients, although it is not specific for tumors of germ cell origin.

Local disease control is achieved with surgical excision of germ cell tumors. Historically, most patients with malignant germ cell tumors died without adjuvant therapy.[2] Many patients require treatment with chemotherapy such as cisplatin, actinomycin, doxorubicin, cyclophosphamide, and etoposide.[1,2] Some germ cell tumors are radiosensitive, although radiation therapy is reserved as salvage therapy.

Sacrococcygeal Teratomas

The most common germ cell tumor in children is the teratoma, a tumor composed of tissue from the germinal layers of the embryo. Within teratomas, both solid and cystic components can coexist with mature well-differentiated, immature, and malignant cells. More than half of all childhood teratomas are sacrococcygeal, 90% are diagnosed in new-

TABLE 9–20. *Distribution of Childhood Germ Cell Tumors*

CHILDHOOD GERM CELL TUMORS	RELATIVE FREQUENCY (%)	MOST COMMON AGE AT DIAGNOSIS	PATHOLOGY
Extragonadal, 63%			
Sacrococcygeal	41	Infancy (70% females)	65%, benign teratoma 5%, immature 30%, malignant
Mediastinal (anterior, superior; posterior)	6		Teratoma Embryonal carcinoma (pure and endodermal sinus tumors)
Abdominal (retroperitoneum; stomach, omentum, liver)	5	Under 2 yr	Benign or malignant
Intracranial (pineal; suprasellar, infrasellar)	6	Children	Any type
Head and neck (oral cavity, pharynx, orbit, neck, upper jaw)	4	Infants	Usually benign
Vaginal	1	Under 3 yr	Usually malignant
Gonadal, 36%			
Ovarian	29	10–14 yr	65%, benign teratoma 5%, immature teratoma 30%, malignant (dysgerminomas and endodermal sinus tumors)
Testicular	7	Infancy and after puberty	82%, malignant (endodermal tumors; adenocarcinoma) 18%, benign (teratoma)

Modified from Ablin A, Isaacs H. Germ cell tumors. In Pizzo P, Poplack D (eds): Principles and Practice of Pediatric Oncology, 2nd ed. Philadelphia: JB Lippincott, 1993, pp 867–888.

borns, and three fourths occur in girls.[39] Other primary sites include the cervical neck, upper jaw, nasopharynx, intracranium, retroperitoneum, mediastinum, and gonads. Most sacrococcygeal teratomas are benign; less than 10% contain malignant components.[2] Early diagnosis and prompt treatments are imperative because with time the tumor cells are capable of malignant degeneration.

Most newborns with sacrococcygeal teratomas have large external masses. The Altman classification is used to describe the precise location of these tumors.[9] Almost one half of infants have masses that are predominantly external, and another one third have predominantly external masses with some intrapelvic extension.[9] Infants with internal, presacral masses often present with constipation, urinary frequency, or leg weakness. A discrete posterior mass is palpable on rectal examination. A significant number of these newborns (18%) have other congenital anomalies, often related to the musculoskeletal system or CNS.[9]

Complete surgical excision of sacrococcygeal teratomas, including removal of the coccyx, results in a 95% cure rate.[9] Exenterative measures, which would include radical excision of pelvic content, are not necessary. Chemotherapy with cisplatin, bleomycin, vinblastine, etoposide, vincristine, actinomycin, cyclophosphamide, and/or doxorubicin is given if the tumor is not completely resected or contains malignant elements. Radiotherapy may be combined with the chemotherapy.[9,42] Recurrences can be successfully treated with similar therapy. Because of the possibility of malignant recurrence in patients with initially benign disease, these infants should have regular follow-up examinations.

Ovarian Tumors

Ovarian tumors are very rare before 5 years of age, and only 20% of girls with ovarian tumors are premenarchal at diagnosis.[2] The age distribution of ovarian cancers has led some researchers and physicians to theorize that the increased ovarian activity at puberty stimulates the cancer's growth since most patients are adolescents.[2] In general, younger girls have a less hopeful prognosis.[29]

Two thirds of pediatric ovarian tumors are of germ cell origin,[9] and most often are benign teratomas, followed by dysgerminomas, endodermal sinus tumors, immature teratomas, mixed cell tumors, and embryonal carcinomas.[2] Patients usually are seen initially with abdominal swelling and a palpable mass associated with pain, nausea, vomiting, constipation, or other genitourinary symptoms. If ovarian torsion occurs, pain escalates rapidly. The tumor mass can be identified on abdominal CT scan and ultrasound. Unlike most other solid tumors, the presence of radiographic calcifications usually indicates benign tumors.[2] A chest CT scan, chest x-ray studies, and bone scan are obtained to assess for metastasis. Assessment of the tumor markers AFP and β-HCG is necessary preoperatively, and they are followed postoperatively since they are reliable markers except for dysgerminomas.[29]

A laparotomy is performed to remove the tumor and determine the histology and staging. The surgery includes an oophorectomy, examination of the contralateral ovary and peritoneal surfaces, and lymph node sampling. The International Federation of Gynecology and Obstetrics (FIGO) has established a staging system for ovarian tumors (Table 9–21).[6]

Most malignant ovarian tumors are stage I dysgerminomas, which are cured with surgical excision alone, even though the tumor mass can measure up to 20 cm in diameter.[2] Dysgerminomas are very radiosensitive.[29] Emergent radiotherapy is given at presentation when a large tumor mass is impeding vital function.[30] Chemotherapy is used for in-

TABLE 9–21. *FIGO Staging System for Ovarian Tumors*

Stage I	Tumor growth is limited to ovaries.
Stage II	Tumor has pelvic extension.
Stage III	Tumor has widespread abdominal metastases.
Stage IV	Tumor has distant metastases.

Data from reference 6.
FIGO = Federation of Gynecology and Obstetrics.

operable, advanced, or recurrent disease and results in a nearly 100% cure rate.[2]

Endodermal sinus tumors are very aggressive neoplasms that spread rapidly from the ovaries to adjoining tissues and carry a poor prognosis. Almost 75% of patients have stage III or IV disease at diagnosis.[33] The best prognosis is for patients with less advanced disease and smaller tumors. Since complete surgical excision is necessary for cure, the definitive surgical procedure may be delayed while neoadjuvant chemotherapy is given preoperatively. Recurrent disease or metastasis often occurs within 2 years. Chemotherapy is always given. The commonly used agents include vincristine, actinomycin, cyclophosphamide, cisplatin, vinblastine, bleomycin, etoposide, doxorubicin, and ifosfamide. Radiotherapy is not very successful in these patients.[2,33,43]

Testicular Tumors

Ninety percent of all testicular tumors are of germ cell origin. Two thirds of them are endodermal sinus tumors,[9] and only 25% are benign.[39] Other neoplasms include teratomas, seminomas, and embryonal carcinomas. The peak incidences for these rare tumors occur in infancy and in postpubertal boys.[39]

Testicular tumors present as slow-growing, painless, irregular scrotal masses often associated with reactive hydroceles or inguinal hernias. Differential diagnosis includes simple hydrocele, epididymitis, testicular torsion, and orchitis.

The incidence of testicular malignancies is 20 to 50 times higher in males who have a history of cryptorchidism (undescended testes). An increased incidence of tumors in

TABLE 9–22. *Testicular Tumors Classification*

Stage I	Tumor confined to scrotum
Stage II	Metastasis present but below the diaphragm only
Stage III	Metastasis present above the diaphragm

Data from reference 14.

the contralateral descended testis suggests that orchioplexy to descend surgically the previously undescended testis may not influence the development of malignancy.[2] For all fully developed males the American Cancer Society recommends monthly testicular self-examination for which it provides related professional and lay literature. This is especially important for males with the aforementioned history.[44]

Evaluation for testicular malignancy includes ultrasonography to localize the mass and a CT scan of the pelvis, abdomen, and chest to determine the extent of disease. Serum AFP and β-HCG may be helpful tumor markers. A universal staging system for testicular tumors is not available; however, Evans, D'Angio, and Schneider[14] use the classification criteria presented in Table 9–22.

Initial treatment includes radical orchiectomy through an inguinal approach with high ligation of the spermatic cord at the inguinal ring.[52] Retroperitoneal lymph node dissection is not performed because of a significant risk of associated postoperative ejaculatory dysfunction.[9] Boys with stages II and III disease or recurrent stage I disease may receive neoadjuvant chemotherapy to allow for less extensive debulking procedures. Postoperative chemotherapy is also used. Agents used include cisplatin, vinblastine, bleomycin, ifosfamide, and etoposide. Radiotherapy is of questionable benefit. With current therapies, the survival rate for boys with an endodermal sinus tumor of the testes is 70% overall and 85% for stage I disease.[9]

THYROID CANCER

The thyroid gland, an endocrine gland situated in the lower anterior neck, consists of two lobes, one on either side of the trachea. It secretes, stores, and liberates the thyroid hormones thyroxine (T_4) and triiodothyronine (T_3), which require iodine for their elaboration in order to regulate the body's metabolic rate. The thyroid gland also secretes thyrocalcitonin. Although cancer of the thyroid gland is more common in adults, it represents at least 1% of childhood malignancies. Adult thyroid nodules more likely will be benign than those in children. Two thirds of all children with thyroid cancer are girls; the peak incidence occurs between 7 and 12 years of age.[12]

The cause of thyroid cancer often is linked to previous exposure to radiation: atomic, nuclear, or therapeutic. Currently radiation is used only as treatment for malignancies. In the past therapeutic radiation was used somewhat indiscriminately to treat benign conditions such as enlarged tonsils, adenoids, or thymus and even skin diseases such as acne vulgaris and tinea capitis. Any radiation to the neck area can later result in thyroid cancer, which is often reported as a second malignant neoplasm in survivors of childhood cancer. Radiation doses between 120 cGy and 2000 cGy are associated with the development of thyroid cancer. Doses higher than that are less often oncogenic, probably because they cause ablation of the thyroid.[23] Some genetic basis may exist for the development of thyroid cancer since more than one third of medullary carcinomas of the thyroid are familial.[12]

Most children with thyroid cancer present with anterior cervical adenopathy. Careful physical examination often reveals a hard, firm, fixed thyroid nodule. Hoarseness and laryngeal nerve paralysis or palsy are signs of advanced disease. Laboratory test results of thyroid function will likely be normal. An important test is the scintiscan, which is performed in the nuclear medicine department. Scintiscan produces a two-dimensional representation of the gamma rays emitted by an injected radiopharmaceutical radioisotope, revealing varying concentrations in specific body parts. "Cold" areas on the scan are those that do not take up much of the radioisotope. Patients with thyroid cancer demonstrate cold nodules on scintiscan. If results from the scintiscan are "positive," quantification of antithyroid antibodies in the serum should be obtained. These antibodies counteract the synthesis of thyroid hormone. High or elevated antibody levels are suggestive of Hashimoto's thyroiditis, an autoimmune disease involving the thyroid. If antithyroid antibody levels are low or normal, needle or excisional biopsy of the nodule is warranted. The workup must also include a chest x-ray study since many children with thyroid cancer have nodular or diffuse lung metastases. Metastases to brain or bone occur rarely. The histopathology of most childhood thyroid cancer is differentiated: papillary (70% to 80%) or follicular (20%). A small percentage is undifferentiated medullary (5% to 10%). Medullary carcinomas are often familial and secrete high levels of serum calcitonin. An anaplastic tumor is highly aggressive and is associated with hypercalcemia.[12]

Definitive surgical intervention is the mainstay of treatment for thyroid cancer. All thyroid tissue that takes up radioisotope should be removed with a lobectomy on the positive side and a subtotal lobectomy on the contralateral side. The procedure includes lymph node dissection on the involved side and superior mediastinum. Total thyroidectomy is avoided because of the potential for damage to the laryngeal nerve and parathyroid glands.

Postoperatively, patients are given T_4 replacement to suppress thyroid-stimulating hormone (TSH), which could potentiate tumor regrowth. Subsequently the T_4 and T_3 levels are monitored and thyroid hormone replacement doses adjusted to ensure hormone levels above normal to continue the TSH suppression.

If the postoperative scans 6 weeks after diagnosis suggest the presence of pulmonary or residual disease, radioactive iodine is given. Before receiving radioactive iodine, the patient should avoid iodine-containing foods, salt, and x-ray contrast material. Any thyroid hormone replacement therapy is stopped several weeks before the procedure. The radioactive iodine is taken up by most thyroid tumors, targeting high levels of radiation to the tumor cells. One or two doses of the radiation given at 3-month intervals is usually curative. Potential side effects of the radioiodine include transient bone marrow suppression,

nausea and vomiting, gastritis, inflammation of the salivary gland with teeth deterioration, xerostomia, pain at metastatic sites, pulmonary fibrosis, infertility, and very rarely, leukemia. External beam radiation and chemotherapy are seldom used to treat thyroid cancer in children.

Long-term follow-up of children with a history of thyroid cancer should include regular monitoring of T_4 and T_3, physical examination of the neck area, and chest x-ray examinations. The 10-year survival rate for children with thyroid cancer is 98%, decreasing to 78% at 25 years.[26] Since late relapses do occur, the follow-up period should be indefinite. Because children who have been treated with radiation for other head and neck cancers have a high incidence of thyroid cancer and other thyroid abnormalities, they should be monitored closely for the development of thyroid cancer.

FIBROSARCOMA

Ten percent of soft tissue sarcomas in children are fibrosarcomas,[16] which represent more than 1% of all childhood cancers.[32] This tumor can occur in adults, but in children the two peak ages of incidence are from birth to 5 years and from 10 to 15 years.[32] More than one third of these cases are discovered at birth.[16] Ionizing radiation has been implicated as a causative agent for some patients, with a median latency period to the development of fibrosarcoma of 14½ years.[24,40]

Fibrosarcomas are malignant tumors that arise within any fibrous tissue, especially skeletal muscle, and extend to surrounding tissues. This tumor has a propensity to recur locally rather than to metastasize. A pathologic grading system consisting of grades 1 to 4 describes cellular differentiation from well-differentiated to poorly differentiated.[16]

Children with fibrosarcoma initially are seen with firm, solitary, painless soft tissue masses. Nearly three fourths of primary tumors are located in the extremities, especially the lower ones.[24] Others occur in the trunk, head, and neck regions (orbit, eyelid, brain, larynx, pharynx, or jaw). Metastases are especially rare in infants and younger children.[24] One review of 52 cases of childhood fibrosarcomas showed an 8% metastatic rate and 27% local recurrence rate for children with extremity primaries and a 20% metastatic rate and 13% local recurrence rate for truncal primaries.[32]

Complete wide local excision of the tumor mass is curative in most cases. Local recurrences can also be treated successfully with surgery. Regional lymph node dissections are unnecessary because the disease does not spread to lymph nodes.

Radiotherapy and chemotherapy are used preoperatively for unresectable tumors. Radiotherapy doses are 6000 to 6500 cGy.[16] Effective chemotherapy can also be used to treat metastatic disease. Fibrosarcomas are sensitive to vincristine, doxorubicin, cyclophosphamide, actinomycin, DTIC, ifosfamide, and etoposide.[24,32,39]

Survival rates for infants and children with fibrosarcoma vary from nearly 100% for those with extremity lesions to almost 75% for patients with truncal lesions. Overall, the prognosis for fibrosarcoma is better in infants and children (84%) than in adults (60%).[24,32]

SYNOVIAL SARCOMA

Synovial sarcoma, although rare, is one of the more common nonrhabdomyosarcoma soft tissue sarcomas in children.[15] The median age of occurrence is in the third decade of life, although almost one third of cases are found in persons less than 20 years of age.[32]

Synovial sarcoma is initially seen as a deep mass that is often painful and tender. The onset of disease is insidious, with reported duration of symptoms up to 2½ years.[24] Most lesions are located at the thigh or in the knee. Others occur in the foot, upper extremity, hand, trunk, and head and neck regions. Most tumors seem to originate within muscles, tendons, or subcutaneous tissue. Adjacent bones may be involved. Up to one third or more of cases show radiographic signs of calcifications.[24,51] Distant metastasis is usually to lungs and less likely to regional lymph nodes and bone. Evaluation should include karyotyping because a specific translocation between the X chromosome and chromosome 18 has been identified in patients with synovial sarcoma.[24]

Synovial sarcoma is a highly malignant tumor that requires aggressive multimodal treatment. Primary therapy consists of wide local or radical excision of the tumor. Amputation does not seem to offer any survival advantage over extensive excisional procedures.[7,24]

Postoperative radiotherapy enhances local control of microscopic disease and modifies the reported 30% to 70% local recurrence rate.[7,24,48]

Adjunctive chemotherapy likewise has some benefit. The tumor is responsive to combinations of agents such as cyclophosphamide and doxorubicin and to vincristine, actinomycin, DTIC, ifosfamide, and etoposide.[24,32]

The reported overall historical 5-year survival rate for patients with synovial sarcoma is 25% to 64%.[7,19,24,51,57] The rate decreases over time to historical 10-year survival rates of 11% to 38%,[24,59] although 10 months is the median time for occurrence of metastasis. Late metastases have been discovered up to 20 years after the initial diagnosis.[22] Young children seem to have the best prognosis, with one study reporting a 59% survival rate for children less than 14 years of age versus a 40% survival rate for all age patients.[7,24] Currently all studies seem to conclude that small tumor size (<5 cm in diameter) is the best prognostic indicator.[24,46,51]

MALIGNANT MELANOMA

Malignant melanoma is the most common skin cancer in children, although it represents only slightly more than 1% of all childhood cancers.[41] The disease is rare before adolescence and is extremely rare in African-American children.[8] It is far more common in adults in whom the incidence is rapidly escalating. *Time* magazine highlighted the problem of skin cancers in a cover article, "Vanishing Ozone: The Danger Moves Closer to Home," stressing that as the earth's protective ozone layer is depleted, the incidence of skin cancer could rise even higher.[31]

Certain conditions predispose individuals to the development of melanomas, most notably excess cumulative exposure to ultraviolet light from the sun or tanning salons and ionizing radiation. Immunodeficiency and immunosuppression may also increase the risk. Melanomas have been reported to arise within burn scars. Blue-eyed blondes or redheads with fair skin who sunburn easily have a propensity to develop melanomas.[28] Such persons and those with outdoor jobs in particular must take steps to prevent sunburn and cumulative ultraviolet light exposure.

Case reports of melanomas in close relatives of children with various malignancies indicate the likelihood of a genetic and familial predisposition to melanoma.[8] Persons with dysplastic nevi (a circumscribed malformation of the skin that develops abnormally) comprise another group at high risk for development of melanoma.[41] Ten percent of all large congenital nevi will develop into malignant melanomas unless they are removed.[28]

Most malignant melanomas consist of painless, slow-growing peripheral enlargement of existing skin lesions. These flat lesions can undergo radial changes in diameter or vertical changes in depth. Malignant changes in a skin lesion can include changes in color and irregularity of its border or surface elevation. These changes can take place over several years.[28] Spitz nevi are juvenile or prepubertal benign lesions that are very similar in appearance and histology to malignant melanoma, although they exhibit indolent behavior.[3,54]

There are four major growth patterns of melanoma lesions. The aforementioned superficial spreading melanomas represent 70% of all cases. Others are aggressive nodular melanomas not associated with preexisting lesions (15% to 30% of cases); lentigo maligna melanomas typically located on the face of older Caucasians (4% to 10% of cases); and acral-lentiginous melanomas occurring on palms, soles, or beneath nailbeds (2% to 8% of cases in Caucasians; 35% to 60% of cases in dark-skinned persons).[53]

Primary lesions are usually found on the extremities and less often in the head and neck area or trunk. Metastasis occurs to regional lymph nodes, then to abdominal viscera, lungs, bone, and brain. Metastatic evaluation should include chest x-ray studies, chest CT scan, enhanced CT scan of the brain, a liver-spleen radionuclide scan, and an abdominal ultrasound.

Clark and Breslow noted the correlation of the increasing thickness of melanoma lesions with poorer prognosis, so they devised classification systems to reflect that phenomenon. The Clark classification defines the depth of the lesion's skin invasion as levels I to V. Breslow divides thickness of lesions from less than 0.85 mm to greater than 3.6 mm into four categories. Persons with lesions less than 0.85 mm have a greater than 95% survival. Persons with lesions greater than 3.6 mm have less than 40% survival.[10,41] Malignant melanomas are staged by extent of disease (Table 9–23).[8] The American Joint Committee on Cancer uses yet another staging system based on microstaging and metastases.[53]

Treatment is based on disease stage. Stage I disease requires only wide local excision, which may require extensive skin grafting. Treatment for stage II disease also includes regional lymph node dissection and chemotherapy. Children with stage III disease have a grim prognosis, and chemotherapy must be given.[8] Single-agent chemotherapy with DTIC is as effective as multiagent programs using vincristine, actinomycin, and cyclophosphamide.[8] The response rates for metastatic disease are less than 20%.[53] New chemotherapeutic approaches include the use of other agents such as cisplatin and nitrosourea, autologous bone marrow transplantation procedures, and regional perfusion of drugs for extremity lesions.[27,58] Preoperative topical 5-fluorouracil has been used experimentally to improve surgical results for patients with a poor prognosis.[49]

Many cases of malignant melanoma are treatable if detected early and are preventable if measures are taken, starting at an early age, by individuals to protect themselves from

TABLE 9–23. *Malignant Melanoma Staging*

Stage I	Disease confined to primary skin lesion
Stage II	Regional lymph node involvement
Stage III	Involvement of other organs

Data from reference 8.

damaging exposure to ultraviolet rays of the sun. Although malignant melanoma may not affect many children, children represent the generation that can be protected from the ravages of this disease.

NASOPHARYNGEAL CARCINOMA

Nasopharyngeal carcinoma is much more common in adults than in children. Only 9% of all reported cases of nasopharyngeal carcinoma in the United States occur in children less than 15 years of age, and 90% of those cases are in children 10 to 15 years of age. It is the second most common pediatric tumor of the upper respiratory tract, following rhabdomyosarcomas of the head and neck region.[8] One third of all pediatric nasopharyngeal neoplasms are nasopharyngeal carcinoma, although it represents less than 1% of all childhood malignancies.[41] Environmental factors such as smoking and air pollution have been implicated as causative factors in adults. There is an apparent geographic distribution of nasopharyngeal carcinoma in adults, with especially high incidence of the disease in the Far East and North Africa. In the United States an increased incidence of the disease occurs among African-American teenagers in the South.[8,41] A significant male predominance among adults with nasopharyngeal carcinoma is not found among children.[8]

In children this tumor is associated with the Epstein-Barr virus (EBV), with DNA from EBV found in biopsy specimens. Children with certain types of nasopharyngeal carcinoma have significantly elevated levels of EBV antibody titers, which can be used as tumor markers to follow the course of disease.[8,17,22,35,41]

The World Health Organization has classified three histologic subtypes of nasopharyngeal carcinoma: type 1, squamous cell carcinoma; type 2, nonkeratinizing carcinoma; and type 3, undifferentiated carcinoma with lymphocytic infiltration prominent or minimal. Children usually have type 3 pathology, with lymphocytic infiltration historically termed *lymphoepithelioma*.[8] Types 2 and 3 are associated with high EBV titers.[41]

Nasopharyngeal carcinoma arises in the pharyngeal recess and initially spreads to cervical lymph nodes. Signs and symptoms are related to the presence of tumor mass and its extension. Cervical lymphadenopathy is usually the initial finding. Nasal obstruction, epistaxis, trismus or lockjaw, hearing loss, earache, headache, and chronic otitis media can occur. Tumor erosion of the base of the skull causes cranial nerve palsies involving the oculomotor (III), trigeminal (V), and abducens (VI) cranial nerves, with hoarseness, dysphagia, sternocleidomastoid weakness, nasal regurgitation, and strabismus. Half of all children have cranial nerve involvement.[8] Distant metastases to lungs, vertebrae, long bones, or liver can occur. An odd syndrome of noticeable osteoarthropathy, with joint swelling, clubbing and pain, is associated with advanced systemic disease.[41]

Adequate examination of the nasopharynx may be difficult. Pharyngoscopy can be performed indirectly with a special mirror or directly through the nares when the area is premedicated with a local anesthetic spray. The examination of children usually requires their sedation. A head and neck CT is used to assess the tumor's dimensions.

Metastatic evaluation includes chest and abdominal CT, skull films, skeletal survey, chest x-ray films, radionuclide bone, liver, and spleen scans, and lumbar puncture for cerebrospinal fluid examination. Special EBV serologic studies include determining IgA and IgG antibodies to viral capsid antigen (anti-VCA).[41] Baseline endocrine hormone levels for pituitary and thyroid function are also obtained and used to monitor future changes.

No staging system is universally accepted for pediatric nasopharyngeal carcinoma. The American Joint Committee on Cancer uses the tumor, node, metastasis (TNM) classification to describe nasopharyngeal carcinoma. T1 delineates visible tumor or tumor confined to one site, T2 involves two sites (posterosuperior and lateral walls), T3 extends into the nasal cavity or oropharynx, and T4 invades the skull or is associated with cranial nerve involvement.[41]

The diagnosis of nasopharyngeal carcinoma is usually made with a cervical lymph node biopsy. Exenterative procedures are not performed, although surgical resections may be considered after radiotherapy for accessible resistant disease.

All children receive large-volume radiotherapy to the nasopharynx, posterior nasal cavity, posterior maxillary sinus, base of the skull, sphenoid and cavernous sinuses, and cervical lymphatics, including supraclavicular nodes. A total of 6000 to 7000 cGy is given, resulting in significant acute and long-term toxicity.[41] Xerostomia, dry mouth, begins during treatment and is permanent. Fibrosis of the neck tissue and trismus with potential for cranial muscle atrophy are other late effects. Fifty percent of patients develop endocrine dysfunction.[5,8] Second malignancies have also been reported within the radiotherapy fields.[8,11]

Chemotherapy seems to influence favorably the course of the disease, although no large, randomized clinical trials have been performed because of small patient numbers. Tumors are responsive to drug combinations of cisplatin, 5-fluorouracil, methotrexate, bleomycin, vincristine, cyclophosphamide, doxorubicin, and etoposide.[13,18,25,41,47] Because of the tumor's association with EBV, future investigation may focus on the use of interferon, acyclovir, and other biologic response modifiers.[41]

Survival for children with localized stage T1 or T2 disease is 75% or more.[19,41] More advanced stage T3 or T4 disease carries a much less favorable prognosis, with 8% to 37% survival rates.[41] One review of 18 cases showed 0% survival for nine children treated with radiotherapy alone and 78% survival for nine children who received both radiotherapy and chemotherapy.[47]

REFERENCES

1. Ablin A. Malignant germ cell tumors in children. Front Radiat Ther Oncol 1982; 16:141–149.
2. Ablin A, Isaacs H. Germ cell tumors. In Pizzo P, Poplack D (eds): Principles and Practice of Pediatric Oncology, 2nd ed. Philadelphia: JB Lippincott, 1993, pp 867–888.
3. Allen A. Introduction to "Melanoma of Childhood" by Spitz. CA 1991; 41:37–39.
4. Amendola M, Blane C, Amendola B, et al. CT findings in hepatoblastoma. J Comput Assist Tomogr 1984; 8:1105–1109.
5. Bajorunas D, Ghavimi F, Jereb B, et al. Endocrine sequelae of antineoplastic therapy in childhood head

and neck malignancies. J Clin Endocrinol Metab 1980; 50:329–335.
6. Breen J, Bonamo J, Maxson W. Genital tract tumors in children. Pediatr Clin North Am 1981; 28:355–367.
7. Buck P, Mickelson M, Bonfiglio M. Synovial sarcoma: A review of 33 cases. Clin Orthop 1981; 156:211–215.
8. Cangir A. Miscellaneous childhood tumors. In Fernbach D, Vietti T (eds): Clinical Pediatric Oncology, 4th ed. St. Louis: Mosby–Year Book, 1991, pp 627–646.
9. Castleberry R, Kelly D, Joseph D, et al. Gonadal and extragonadal germ cell tumors. In Fernbach D, Vietti T (eds): Clinical Pediatric Oncology, 4th ed. St. Louis: Mosby–Year Book, 1991, pp 577–594.
10. Conti C, Slaga T, Klein-Szanto A. Skin tumors: Experimental and clinical aspects. In Hansen R, Schachner L (eds): Pediatric Dermatology. New York: Churchill Livingstone, 1988, p 553.
11. Cooper J, Scott C, Marcial V, et al. The relationship of nasopharyngeal carcinomas and second independent malignancies based on the radiation therapy oncology group experience. Cancer 1991; 67:1673–1677.
12. Chrousos GP. Endocrine tumors. In Pizzo P, Poplack D (eds): Principles and Practice of Pediatric Oncology, 2nd ed. Philadelphia: JB Lippincott, 1993, pp 889–912.
13. Daghistani D, Davis J, Toledano S. Case report of successful use of VP-16 in nasopharyngeal carcinoma. Med Pediatr Oncol 1989; 17:168–169.
14. Evans AE, D'Angio JG, Schneider H. Selecting initial therapy for pediatric genito-urinary cancers. Cancer 1987; 60:480.
15. Exelby P. Surgery of soft tissue sarcomas in children. Natl Cancer Inst Monogr 1981; 56:153–157.
16. Festa R. Soft tissue sarcomas. In Lanzkowsky P (ed): Pediatric Oncology: A Treatise for the Clinician. New York: McGraw-Hill, 1983, pp 267–292.
17. Fu K. Prognostic factors of carcinoma of the nasopharynx. Int J Radiat Oncol Biol Phys 1980; 6:523–526.
18. Gasparini M, Lombardi F, Rottoli L, et al. Combined radiotherapy and chemotherapy in stage T3 and T4 nasopharyngeal carcinoma in children. J Clin Oncol 1988; 6:491–494.
19. Golough R, Vuzevski V, Bracko M, et al. Synovial sarcoma: A clinicopathological study of 36 cases. J Surg Oncol 1990; 45:20–28.
20. Greenberg M, Filler R. Hepatic tumors. In Pizzo P, Poplack D (eds): Principles and Practice of Pediatric Oncology, 2nd ed. Philadelphia: JB Lippincott, 1993, pp 697–712.
21. Hata Y. The clinical features and prognosis of hepatoblastoma: Follow-up studies done on pediatric tumors enrolled in the Japanese Pediatric Tumor Registry between 1971 and 1980. Jpn J Surg 1990; 20:498–502.
22. Hawkins E, Krischer J, Smith B, et al. Nasopharyngeal carcinoma in children—A retrospective review and demonstration of Epstein-Barr viral genomes in tumor cell cytoplasm: A report of the Pediatric Oncology Group. Hum Pathol 1990; 21:805–810.
23. Jaffe N. Late sequelae of cancer and cancer therapy. In Fernbach D, Vietti T (eds): Clinical Pediatric Oncology, 4th ed. St. Louis: Mosby–Year Book, 1991, pp 647–674.
24. Kim T, Bell B, Maurer H, et al. Sarcomas of the soft tissues and their benign counterparts. In Fernbach

D, Vietti T (eds): Clinical Pediatric Oncology, 4th ed. St. Louis: Mosby–Year Book, 1991, pp 517–544.

25. Kim T, McLaren J, Alvarado C, et al. Adjuvant chemotherapy for advanced nasopharyngeal carcinoma in childhood. Cancer 1989; 63:1922–1926.

26. Kirkland J, Kirkland R. Tumors of the endocrine glands. In Fernbach D, Vietti T (eds): Clinical Pediatric Oncology, 4th ed. St. Louis: Mosby–Year Book, 1991, pp 595–610.

26a. Kirsch IR. Genetics of pediatric tumors: The causes and consequences of chromosomal aberrations. In Pizzo P, Poplack D (eds): Principles and Practice of Pediatric Oncology, 2nd ed. Philadelphia: JB Lippincott, 1993, pp 29–56.

27. Kleeberg V, Rumke P, Kirkwood J. Systemic chemotherapy of advanced melanoma. Pigment Cell Res 1990; 10:91–104.

28. Koh H. Cutaneous melanoma. N Engl J Med 1991; 325:171–182.

29. Kurman R, Petrilli E. Germ cell tumors of the ovary: Pathology, behavior and treatment. In Griffiths C, Fuller A (eds): Gynecologic Oncology. Boston: Martinus Nijhoff, 1983, pp 103–153.

30. Lange B, D'Angio G, Ross A, et al. Oncologic emergencies. In Pizzo P, Poplack D (eds): Principles and Practice of Pediatric Oncology, 2nd ed. Philadelphia: JB Lippincott, 1993, pp 951–972.

31. Lemonick M. The ozone vanishes. Time, Feb 17, 1992, pp 60–63.

32. Miser J, Triche T, Pritchard D, et al. The other soft tissue sarcomas of childhood. In Pizzo P, Poplack D (eds): Principles and Practice of Pediatric Oncology, 2nd ed. Philadelphia: JB Lippincott, 1993, pp 823–840.

33. Morris H, LaVecchia C, Draper G. Endodermal sinus tumor and embryonal carcinoma of the ovary in children. Gynecol Oncol 1985; 21:7–17.

34. Mulvihill J. Childhood cancer, the environment and heredity. In Pizzo P, Poplack D (eds): Principles and Practice of Pediatric Oncology, 2nd ed. Philadelphia: JB Lippincott, 1993, pp 11–28.

35. Norris C, Cady B. Head, neck, and thyroid cancer. In Holleb A, Fink D, Murphy G (eds): American Cancer Society Textbook of Clinical Oncology. Atlanta: American Cancer Society, 1991, pp 306–328.

36. Ogita S, Tokiwa K, Taniguchi H, et al. Intraarterial chemotherapy with lipid contrast medium for hepatic malignancies in infants. Cancer 1987; 15:60:2886–2890.

37. Ogita S, Tokiwa K, Taniguchi H, et al. Intraarterial injection of anti-tumor drugs dispersed in lipid contrast medium: A choice for initially unresectable hepatoblastoma in infants. J Pediatr Surg 1987; 22:412–414.

38. Ortega J, Malogolowkin M. Epithelial and neuroectodermal tumors of the gastrointestinal, genitourinary, and gynecological tracts. In Fernbach D, Vietti T (eds): Clinical Pediatric Oncology, 4th ed. St. Louis: Mosby–Year Book, 1991, pp 611–626.

39. Pizzo P, Horowitz M, Poplack D, et al. Solid tumors of childhood. In DeVita V, Hellman S, Rosenberg S (eds): Cancer Principles and Practice of Oncology, vol 2, 3rd ed. Philadelphia: JB Lippincott, 1989, pp 1612–1670.

40. Prasad M, Hagapatra A, Dinda A, et al. Fibrosarcoma of the scalp following postoperative radiotherapy for medulloblastoma. Acta Neuro Chir 1991; 109:145–149.

41. Pratt C, Douglass E. Management of less common cancers of childhood. In Pizzo P, Poplack D (eds): Principles and Practice of Pediatric Oncology, 2nd ed. Philadelphia: JB Lippincott, 1993, pp 913–938.

42. Raney RB, Chatten J, Lutman P, et al. Treatment strategies for infants with malignant sacrococcygeal teratoma. J Pediatr Surg 1981; 16:573–577.

43. Raney RB, Sinclair L, Uri A, et al. Malignant ovarian tumors in children and adolescents. Cancer 1987; 59:1214–1220.

44. Redmond M. Cancers of the male genital organs. In Baird S (ed): A Cancer Source Book for Nurses, 6th ed. Atlanta: American Cancer Society, 1991, pp 242–251.

45. Robison L, Mertens A, Neglia J. Epidemiology and etiology of childhood cancer. In Fernbach D, Vietti T (eds): Clinical Pediatric Oncology, 4th ed. St. Louis: Mosby–Year Book, 1991, pp 11–28.

46. Rooser B, Willen H, Hugoson A, et al. Prognostic factors in synovial sarcoma. Cancer 1989; 63:2182–2185.

47. Roper H, Essex-Cater A, Marsden H, et al. Nasopharyngeal carcinoma in children. Pediatr Hematol Oncol 1986; 3:143–152.

48. Ryan J, Baker L, Benjamin R. The natural history of metastatic synovial sarcoma: Experience of the Southwest Oncology Group. Clin Orthop 1982; 164:257–260.

49. Ryan R, Krementz E, Litwin M. A role for topical 5-fluorouracil therapy in melanoma. J Surg Oncol 1988; 38:250–256.

50. Schaller R, Schaller J, Furman E. The disadvantages of hemodilution anesthesia for major liver resection in children. J Pediatr Surg 1984; 19:705–710.

51. Scialabba F, DeLuca S. Synovial cell sarcoma. Am Fam Physician 1990; 41:1211–1212.

52. Shende A, Valderama E. Miscellaneous childhood tumors. In Fernbach D, Vietti T (eds): Clinical Pediatric Oncology, 4th ed. St. Louis: Mosby–Year Book, 1991, pp 360–385.

53. Singletary S, Balch C. Malignant melanoma. In Holleb A, Fink D, Murphy G (eds): American Cancer Society Textbook of Clinical Oncology. Atlanta: American Cancer Society, 1991, pp 263–270.

54. Spitz S. Melanomas of childhood. CA 1991; 40–51.

55. Tan A, Tan C, Phua K, et al. Chemotherapy for hepatoblastoma in children. Ann Acad Med Singapore 1990; 19:286–289.

56. Teng C, Daeschner W, Singleton E, et al. Liver diseases and osteoporosis in children. J Pediatr 1961; 59:684–702.

57. Tsuneyoshi M, Yokoyama K, Enjoji M. Synovial sarcoma: A clinicopathologic and ultrastructural study of 42 cases. Acta Pathol Jpn 1983; 33:23–36.

58. Wanebo H, Litle V, Muchmore J. Regional perfusion of extremity lesions. In Yokich JJ (ed): Cancer Chemotherapy by Infusion, 2nd ed. Chicago: Precept Press, 1990, pp 599–618.

59. Wright P, Sim F, Soule E, et al. Synovial sarcoma. J Bone Joint Surg 1982; 64:112–122.

■ HISTIOCYTOSIS

Jacquie Toia-Marino

Langerhans cell histiocytosis (LCH) is a benign, rare disease of unknown cause that has presented great difficulties related to diagnosis and treatment. It is an incompletely understood condition that is initially seen clinically in patients with a wide array of symptoms ranging from mild skin lesions to organ dysfunction. Because the disease is not well known, there may be considerable delay and possibly misdiagnosis before a definitive diagnosis is made. In spite of these difficulties, major advances have been made in the evaluation and treatment of LCH since it was first described in 1893.[1]

The true incidence of LCH is unknown, but approximately 1200 new cases are diagnosed each year in adults and children in the United States.[3] Calculating disease incidence is complicated because many patients with mild cases recover spontaneously.[5] Other patients with single-system involvement (e.g., only skin lesions or single bone lesions) are treated by dermatologists or orthopedic surgeons rather than oncologists. Children who require treatment for this benign disease are often referred to a hematologist-oncologist because chemotherapy is the recommended treatment.

The term *Langerhans cell histiocytosis* replaces the older terms *histiocytosis X* (in which X represented the unknown), *eosinophilic granuloma*, *Letterer-Siwe disease*, and *Hand-Schüller-Christian syndrome* because the Langerhans cell is involved in all of these syndromes. Although not a neoplasm, LCH is considered a proliferative disorder, possibly secondary to a defect in immunoregulation in which multiplication of normal cells causes destruction or impairment of various organ systems.[4] Nomenclature changes for disease involving the proliferation of histiocytic cell types result from improvement in identifying and categorizing the various cells involved. The Histiocytosis Society, established in 1985, has played an important role in facilitating the development of standardized criteria and an international staging system (Table 9–24). This staging system aids in classification of

TABLE 9–24. *Clinical Staging System for Histiocytosis X*

VARIABLE	NO. OF POINTS
Age at Presentation	
<2 yr	0
>2 yr	1
Number of Organs Involved	
<4	0
4 or more	1
Presence of Organ Dysfunction*	
No	0
Yes	1
Stage†	TOTAL
I	0
II	1
III	2
IV	3

From Lavin P, Osband M. Evaluating the role of therapy in histiocytosis-x. Hematol-Oncol Clin North Am 1987; 1:40.
*Hepatic, pulmonary, or hematopoietic.
†Stage is determined by addition of points for the three variables.

disease and determining a prognosis. It is hoped that additional advances will result from widespread implementation of the staging system.

The diagnosis of LCH is confirmed by the presence of the dendritic histiocyte, also called the Langerhans cell, which contains characteristic Birbeck granules made visible by electron microscopy. Additional criteria for pathologic diagnosis of LCH established by the Histiocytosis Society include the presence of two or more of the following: positive immunostaining for S100 protein (α-D-mannosidase), characteristic binding of peanut lecithin, or positive stain for adenosine triphosphatase (ATPase).[7]

Any organ system can be involved with LCH. The organs most commonly involved are skin, bone, ears, maxilla, mandible, lymph nodes, endocrine system, lung, liver, spleen, bone marrow, and brain. The kidneys, thymus, thyroid, and intestinal tract are less frequent sites of involvement. The signs and symptoms are directly related to the infiltration of Langerhans histiocytes, which compress, displace, or destroy normal tissues. The number of organ systems involved and any coexisting functional impairment of certain vital systems at the time of diagnosis correlate with the subsequent clinical response and prognosis.[5]

SITES OF INVOLVEMENT
Skin

Skin is a common site of involvement, with skin rashes the most frequently identified problems for a child with LCH. Skin involvement appears in a variety of ways, usually with an oily, seborrheic type of rash. Maculopapular rashes may also appear and can be mistaken for chickenpox. A diaper rash may be diagnosed when in fact LCH is the cause of the skin breakdown. Skin presentations can also include nonthrombocytopenic petechial or purpuric rashes, xanthomas, and mucocutaneous granulomas. Skin lesions are commonly noted on the scalp, neck, axillae, and inguinal regions. Management of skin involvement includes the use of steroids. Often a superimposed fungal infection is present. If fungal infection does not respond to treatment, a skin biopsy may be indicated.

Skin involvement, although often benign, is very frustrating for the child and family because of the discomfort from the rash and/or itching. Teaching families proper handwashing skills and adequate hygiene techniques is important to decrease the possibility of infection or spread of the infection.

Bone

The skeleton is the most consistently involved major organ system.[5] Lytic bone lesions can be single or multiple. Often children present with a soft tissue mass over the involved area, dull aching pain, limitation of movement, or inability to bear weight.[5] Single lesions are often treated with curettage. Multiple bone lesions often require short courses of steroids. If any of the lesions are large and in a weight-bearing bone, 800 to 1000 rads of radiation therapy over 5 days are indicated. Nursing responsibility includes patient and family

teaching about pain control and accurate assessment and analgesic administration. It may help to include teaching that relates to improving comfort measures.

Ears

Recurrent otitis media, with or without mastoid involvement, is a common problem in patients with LCH. Drainage from the external auditory canal or an aural polyp can provide tissue for confirmation of the diagnosis.[5] It is often necessary to use the expertise of an ear, nose, and throat specialist. Children with chronic otitis media require special attention to alleviate their discomfort and to evaluate their hearing routinely.

Mandible

Premature eruption of teeth, loss of teeth, and gingival problems are associated with involvement of the mandible or maxilla. Oral hygiene is an important aspect of care with these children. Routine dental follow-up is also recommended, as are periodic panorex films to assess for "floating teeth."

Lymph Nodes

A child with LCH can present with lymphadenopathy. If a single node is involved, total excision is the treatment of choice. Multiple node involvement may require radiation therapy (800 to 1000 rads) or chemotherapy.

Endocrine System

LCH in children can involve the endocrine system. Presenting symptoms can result from panhypopituitarism caused by histiocytic involvement of the pituitary gland. Results from an MRI scan will be either normal or show a destructive lesion of the sella turcica or a pituitary mass. A serious complication associated with endocrine involvement is diabetes insipidus (DI). The presenting symptoms include polydipsia and polyuria. Parents report that these children are not able to quench their thirst. DI is a physical complication of LCH that presents challenges to family functioning. It can occur at anytime; thus parents must know its signs and symptoms. Nursing plays an important role in providing support and education to those families.

DI is controlled with intranasal desmopressin acetate (DDAVP) and thyroid and cortisone replacement when indicated. Radiation is administered only if the pituitary lesions are of sufficient size to produce symptoms of increased intracranial pressure. Since the pituitary gland is destroyed by disease before the diagnosis is made, treatment with radiation therapy and/or chemotherapy will not cure the condition.

Growth impairment from pituitary involvement is also a concern for children with LCH. Follow-up care of the endocrine system is essential to ensure proper growth or to institute necessary growth hormone, for DI usually is a lifelong complication; however, symptoms can be controlled with therapy.

Lung

Lung involvement is manifested clinically by dyspnea, cough, and tachypnea. Radiographic findings may include a bilateral, generalized, interstitial, and focally granulomatous process that begins centrally and spreads peripherally.[5]

Liver and Spleen

Hepatosplenomegaly, either with or without nodules, can be present in children with LCH. Nodules are identified by ultrasound. This presentation is not a poor prognostic sign, although these patients require treatment with chemotherapy. If abnormal liver functions are noted, the prognosis is less favorable.

Bone Marrow

Bone marrow involvement causes changes in the peripheral blood count, with a decrease in the white blood cell count and hemoglobin or platelet level. A bone marrow aspirate reveals histiocytic cells. Bone marrow involvement indicates poor prognosis. The effects of progressive bone marrow involvement include a bleeding diathesis secondary to thrombocytopenia or, rarely, disseminated intravascular coagulation, progressive anemia, and increased susceptibility to infection.[5]

TREATMENT

Treatment modalities vary, depending on the extent of LCH involvement. Management of each case is individualized, taking into consideration the patient's age and the extent and severity of organ system involvement.[5] Chemotherapy is the treatment of choice. Various chemotherapeutic agents and multidrug combinations have been used, including alkylating agents, antimetabolites, vinca alkaloids, and corticosteroids. Duration of therapy varies according to the extent of involvement at diagnosis and the individual response to therapy.

Radiation therapy in low doses is also useful in the management of LCH. Responses have been obtained in localized LCH bone lesions.[6] If LCH is widespread, combination therapy with both chemotherapy and radiation is indicated. Radiation doses from 800 to 1000 cGy are effective in producing local control.

LCH is not a congenital, hereditary, or infectious disease. It is not a thoroughly understood disease; therefore it leaves patients, families, and professionals sometimes frustrated in seeking to obtain and provide quality care. When more than one site is involved, the disease course can be either chronic or acute. The chronic form tends to evolve over the years, causing significant morbidity and disability, but not death. The acute form involves significant morbidity and mortality.[3] One of the most frequent areas of confusion concerns the question of whether LCH is a cancer, for children with LCH receive treatment similar to that for children with cancer. This is often very confusing and sometimes frightening for the families. Quality teaching for these families is crucial so that they can understand the disease. Additional teaching materials must be developed for this population. Most importantly, resources must be made available for families affected by LCH.

An available resource is the Histiocytosis Association of America, a parent-run organization that provides information and support for families. Its address is as follows:

Histiocytosis Association of America, Inc.
609 New York Road
Glassboro, NJ 08028

CLASS II HISTIOCYTOSIS OF MONONUCLEAR PHAGOCYTES OTHER THAN LANGERHANS CELLS

Other types of histiocytosis are seen less frequently but require more aggressive treatment and have a less favorable prognosis. The class II histiocytoses are disorders that include the nonmalignant, non-Langerhans histiocytoses in which the histiocytic proliferation is associated with phagocytosis. The predominant cell is the normal monocyte or macrophage frequently seen in a mixed lymphohistiocytic infiltrate.[4]

The proliferating histiocytes in class II disease are morphologically normal and do not have the cellular atypia of malignant histiocytes, but their uncontrolled growth can cause morbidity and mortality. These histiocytes proliferate in lymph nodes, liver, spleen, bone marrow, and the central nervous system. The confusion about class II histiocytoses results from the overlap in clinical characteristics of several syndromes, including familial erythrophagocytic lymphohistiocytosis (FEL), hemophagocytic lymphohistiocytosis (HL), virus-associated hemophagocytic syndrome (VAHS), and sinus histiocytosis with massive lymphadenopathy (SHML).[4]

CLASS III MALIGNANT HISTIOCYTIC DISORDERS

Malignant histiocytic disorders are distinct neoplastic diseases—acute monocytic leukemia, malignant histiocytoses, and true histiocytic lymphomas.[7] Malignant histiocytosis is a nonfamilial, rapidly fatal disorder characterized by fever, generalized tender lymphadenopathy, hepatosplenomegaly, subcutaneous inflammatory infiltration, pancytopenia, and a Coombs-positive hemolytic anemia. Malignant histiocytosis is a systemic malignancy involving the entire reticuloendothelial system.[4] A characteristic finding is erythrophagocytosis in the bone marrow, liver, and spleen, along with histiocytic infiltration of the subcapsular and medullary regions of lymph nodes.

Note there are significant differences in LCH and class II and III disorders pertaining to diagnosis, treatment and prognosis.

REFERENCES

1. Berry D, Becton D. Natural history of histiocytosis-X. Hematol Oncol Clin North Am 1987; 1:23–34.
2. Ladisch S, Jaffe E. The histiocytoses. In Pizzo P, Poplack D (eds): Principles and Practice of Pediatric Oncology, 2nd ed. Philadelphia: JB Lippincott, 1993, pp 617–632.
3. Lavin P, Osband M. Evaluating the role of therapy in histiocytosis-X. Hematol Oncol Clin North Am 1987; 1:35–47.
4. McClain KL. Histiocytic proliferative diseases. In Fernbach DJ, Vietti T (eds): Clinical Pediatric Oncology, 4th ed. St. Louis: CV Mosby, 1991, pp 397–408.
5. Murphy S, Ranson L. Histiocytosis X. Pract Pediatr 1977; 31:1–10.
6. Richter MP, D'Angio G. The role of radiation therapy in the management of children with histiocytosis X. Am J Pediatr Hematol Oncol 1981; 3:161–163.
7. Writing Group of the Histiocyte Society. Histiocytosis syndromes in children. Lancet 1987; 1:208–209.

NURSING MANAGEMENT OF PHYSICAL CARE NEEDS

Cheryl Panzarella
Janet Duncan

Specific nursing care problems related to physical care most often result from the disease process or the complications and side effects of treatment. Because the various systems of the body are interrelated, involvement of one system may affect others. When performing patient assessments and planning for care, the nurse must have a thorough understanding of anatomy, pathophysiology, and principles of therapy and how they are manifested or altered in the child with cancer. Knowledge of the possible side effects of treatment aids in the prevention and early detection of many problems.

NEUROLOGIC SYSTEM
Increased Intracranial Pressure

Etiology. Children with primary or metastatic central nervous system (CNS) tumors can have increased intracranial pressure (ICP) as a result of tumor mass, edema, bleeding, or obstruction of cerebrospinal fluid (CSF) flow. Symptoms of increased ICP include headaches that may be focal or generalized and often are more severe in the morning. Vomiting, usually unaccompanied by nausea, behavior changes, lethargy, irritability, pupillary changes, and increased head circumference or bulging fontanelle in the infant are all potential manifestations of increased ICP.[35]

Nursing Assessment. Nursing assessment includes monitoring for signs and symptoms of increased ICP. When assessing level of consciousness (LOC), obtaining baseline data about the child's normal behavior and activities is important. Parents can be very helpful in identifying behavioral changes, and their input is incorporated into the assessment when possible. The child is monitored for lethargy or undue irritability. With increased ICP, pupils are dilated and have a decreased response to light. Ptosis may also be present as a result of nerve compression. Papilledema can cause hemorrhaging in the optic discs, and the child may complain of blurred vision or diplopia. Infants may have poor visual tracking. If the child is old enough, the presence of headaches is assessed. The presence of vomiting is also assessed, including time of day and related activities. Although vomiting is more common in the morning, it may occur at night and when the child moves from a reclining to an upright position.

Nursing Interventions. Nursing management of the child with increased ICP includes careful monitoring of intake and output. Fluids are restricted as ordered. The head of the bed is elevated to avoid cerebral venous congestion. Dexamethasone is administered as ordered to decrease or prevent swelling.

Seizures

Etiology. The causes of seizures in children with cancer vary and include tumors, bleeding, metabolic imbalance, and infection. Primary tumors, metastatic lesions, or CNS leukemia can cause seizures as can intracranial hemorrhage resulting from thrombocytopenia. Spontaneous cranial hemorrhage can occur with a platelet count of less than 10,000. Children who receive cyclophosphamide or vincristine may develop syndrome of inappropriate secretion of antidiuretic hormone (SIADH), which can lead to serum sodium deficiency and subsequently seizures. Infections of a viral, fungal, or bacterial nature can also cause seizures.

Nursing Assessment. Seizures can occur with little warning. It is important to assess behavior before the seizure, the type of movements observed, the time the seizure began and ended, body areas involved, LOC, pupils, respiratory changes, and behavior after the seizure.

Nursing Interventions. The airway is the first concern. Position the child to ensure a patent airway and protect the child from aspiration. A supplemental airway, suctioning equipment, and oxygen may be needed. Remain with the child and notify the physician immediately. Anticonvulsant drugs such as diazepam and phenytoin (Dilantin) are administered as ordered. Blood is sent for immediate analysis of serum electrolytes and glucose values to determine if the cause was metabolic. A head computed tomography (CT) scan and electroencephalogram (EEG) may also be ordered to determine the cause of the seizure.

Spinal Cord Compression

Etiology. Spinal cord compression is an oncologic emergency. Prompt assessment and early intervention are critical in preventing permanent damage. Spinal cord compression can result from a primary tumor of the spine or from spinal metastases.

Nursing Assessment. Signs and symptoms of spinal cord compression are similar for all types of tumor. The most common finding is motor weakness. Weight bearing may be difficult, or the child may develop a limp. The child may complain of paresthesias. Shooting back pain may be present and is accentuated by coughing, sneezing, or movements that stretch the nerve roots. Changes in bowel and bladder function, including loss of control or severe constipation, may indicate spinal cord compression.

Nursing Interventions. The child at risk is closely monitored for signs and symptoms. Symptoms of cord compression may be the first indication of tumor growth or metastases. Magnetic resonance imaging (MRI) or myelography is usually performed immediately if cord compression is suspected. In acute situations emergency surgery or radiation therapy is needed to relieve the compression. Spinal cord compression can be very frightening for the child and family. They must be kept informed about changes in patient status, and their fears about loss of function require supportive attention.

CARDIOPULMONARY SYSTEM

A number of factors related to the disease or treatment can compromise the cardiopulmonary status of the child with cancer.

Etiology. The lungs or the heart can be directly affected by tumor or leukemic infiltrates. Surgery for tumor removal or lung biopsy will result in cardiopulmonary compromise. Anemia may lead to shortness of breath as a result of decreased oxygenation of the blood. The administration of intravenous (IV) fluids and blood products can stress the cardiovascular system. Radiation to the lungs can cause pneumonitis or pulmonary fibrosis. Radiation toxicity to the heart can result in pericardial effusion or constrictive pericarditis. Busulfan, bleomycin, and methotrexate can cause pulmonary toxicity. Anthracyclines in cumulative amounts and cyclophosphamide in high doses are potentially cardiotoxic. Steroids can cause fluid and sodium retention, which can lead to hypertension. Sedative drugs and narcotics potentially can cause respiratory depression. Anaphylactic reactions, although rare, sometimes occur after the administration of some drugs. Antibiotics and some chemotherapeutic agents can cause hypersensitivity reactions, which can lead to anaphylaxis. Hives and itching may develop first, followed by respiratory difficulty such as wheezing. Circulatory failure may follow.

Nursing Assessment. The baseline cardiopulmonary status of the child must be established to allow the prompt recognition of changes. Tachycardia can be caused by fever, hypoxia, or shock. Tachypnea may indicate hypoxia or respiratory infection. Hypertension may be the result of fluid overload, whereas hypotension may be a sign of shock.

Auscultation of the chest is done regularly to assess for abnormal or decreased breath sounds, arrhythmias, a gallop, or a friction rub.

Respiratory distress may indicate an infection. The child may have a cough, dyspnea, nasal flaring, grunting, substernal or intercostal retractions, cyanosis, or decreased activity tolerance. Pulse oximetry may be used to monitor and detect changes in oxygenation levels. A chest x-ray film helps detect an infection, and sputum cultures may also be obtained. Oxygen support may be necessary; if oxygen demand continues to increase, ventilatory assistance also may be needed.

Nursing Interventions. If a child is short of breath, measures should be taken to decrease the body's demand for oxygen and increase tissue perfusion. The head of the bed is elevated, particularly if the tumor is directly causing respiratory compromise, for optimal lung expansion and air exchange occur in an upright position. Activities are spaced to avoid dyspnea and fatigue. Measures are taken to decrease anxiety. The child's blood counts are monitored, and anemia is treated with transfusions.

Baseline echocardiograms are obtained and repeated intermittently during and after treatment with anthracyclines to monitor for any changes. Signs and symptoms of conges-

tive heart failure include congestion in the lungs, cough, dyspnea, orthopnea, tachycardia, fatigue, weight gain, edema, and distended neck veins. On auscultation a gallop may be heard. Close monitoring of the cardiopulmonary system is necessary if boluses of IV fluids are required.

Central Venous Access Devices

Central venous access devices play a vital role in the treatment and supportive care necessary for the child with cancer. They can be used to draw blood and to administer total parenteral nutrition (TPN), blood products, IV antibiotics, and chemotherapy infusions. They also ensure safe access for vesicant chemotherapy administration.

There are two major types of devices: partially implanted and totally implanted. Partially implanted devices are catheters whose proximal end is threaded internally through a major blood vessel. The catheter is advanced until the tip reaches the superior vena cava just above the right atrium. The proximal end is then tunneled from the entrance site— the subclavian vein or internal jugular vein— through the subcutaneous fascia of the chest and is brought out through an exit site on the chest.[42] Single-lumen or multiple-lumen catheters are available. Venous access ports are totally implantable, and placement is similar to that for partially implanted devices. Instead of the catheter's exiting through the skin, it is connected to a port placed in a subcutaneous pocket on the chest or the abdomen (Fig. 10–1). Dual-port systems are available for patients who require multiple access.

Nursing Implications. There are advantages and disadvantages to both types of central venous access devices. Totally implanted venous access ports require no home maintenance or limitations on activity and produce only minimal change in body appearance; however, the skin must be pierced with a special noncoring needle each time the port is used. Partially implanted devices produce no discomfort to the child; however, they require regular flushing and care of the exit site. The

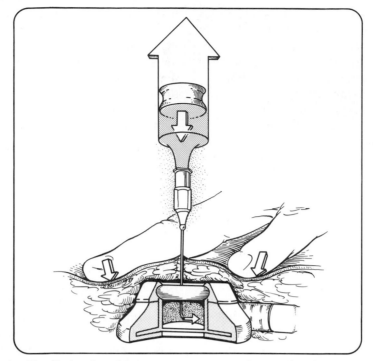

FIGURE 10–1.   Totally implantable venous access port shown placed in the subcutaneous tissue. A noncoring needle is used to access the port. *(Courtesy BARD Access Systems, Salt Lake City, Utah.)*

child and family must learn catheter care, which can be fairly complicated.

The type of dressing varies with the type of device and the particular institutional policy. Central venous catheters require regular injection cap changes and a regular flushing schedule. The strength of the heparin solution usually depends on institutional policy. Some choose to use only normal saline solution for flushing. Groshong catheters do not require the use of heparin and are routinely flushed with normal saline solution.

Because venous access ports have a self-sealing material, only a noncoring needle is used. During long-term continuous use, the needle is changed on a regular basis to avoid the risk of infection.

Complications of venous access devices include infection, occlusion, displacement, and cardiac tamponade. For central venous catheters, patient and family education is very important to ensure meticulous catheter care at home.

Sepsis is the most common serious complication of venous access devices. Research studies indicate a slightly lower incidence of infection in totally implanted ports compared to that of partially implanted catheters.[3,33]

All venous access devices must be considered a potential portal of entry for infection and assessed routinely for signs and symptoms. If a child develops a fever, the central venous access device must be considered as a potential source. Many catheter-related infections can be successfully treated with antibiotics while the catheter is left in place. At times removal of the catheter is necessary to control infection, particularly with tunnel infections and persistent positive blood culture results.

Thrombotic occlusion is a frequent complication of central venous access devices. Usually urokinase or streptokinase is effective in dissolving clots; but sometimes continuous infusions of low-dose urokinase are necessary to dissolve a clot completely. A radiographic dye study is usually done before starting the continuous infusion of urokinase to verify thrombotic occlusion. The child receiving continuous-infusion urokinase must have daily coagulation studies, close monitoring for bleeding, and protection from injury that may lead to bleeding. The child is also monitored for signs and symptoms of pulmonary embolism should the clot dislodge.

If occlusion is due to mineral precipitates, 0.1 N hydrochloric acid can be instilled into the catheter to dissolve the precipitate.[32] Urokinase is not effective for mineral precipitates.

Displacement of the catheter can occur as a result of tugging on the catheter. Implanted ports can become separated from their catheters, allowing the catheter to migrate. The nurse must be alert to complaints of chest pain and difficulty with flushing or blood drawing, which may be the only symptoms indicating catheter displacement. Concerns about displacement must be evaluated by x-ray examination or radiographic dye study. Displacement usually necessitates catheter removal.

Cardiac tamponade can result when a catheter tip in the right atrium causes cardiac perforation or erosion. This is a life-threatening event that can be prevented by awareness of proper catheter tip placement. The catheter tip is placed between the junction of the superior vena cava and the right atrium. Position of the catheter tip is always confirmed by a chest x-ray film immediately after placement and before use. Placement is clearly documented in the patient's record, and verification continues with each subsequent chest x-ray film.

For the child with a partially implanted catheter, knowledge deficit related to catheter care is a major patient problem. The child and/or the parents must be given extensive education about dressing changes, flushing, cap changes, and safety measures. Before discharge the child and/or parents must demonstrate competent catheter care. It is helpful to enlist both the support of a visiting nurse who can follow-up with the family at home and that of the clinic nurses who can follow-up on patient education.

Children with totally implantable ports routinely do not need to do daily care at home. However, if they receive home TPN, antibiotics, or chemotherapy, they also require the same intensive teaching as patients with external catheters. Additionally they will have to learn to access the port.

SKIN AND SENSE ORGANS

Since the skin is the body's natural barrier against infection, breaking this barrier creates a portal of entry for infection. Good hygiene is extremely important since the child's own body flora is the primary source of infection.

Nursing Assessment. All the areas of the skin should be examined daily in a systematic manner from head to foot for signs of infection or skin breakdown. An opportune time to make a thorough assessment is when bathing the child. All injection sites are closely monitored for signs of infection.

It is critical to remember that the child with cancer may not manifest an inflammatory response or the response may be decreased, particularly if the child is neutropenic. Therefore signs of redness or pus formation may be missing at the site of infection.

Nursing Interventions. To protect the integrity of the skin, keep the child clean and dry. Frequent bathing and immediate washing of urine and stool from the skin are important. Protect the skin from dryness. Bath oil can be added to the water during bathing to help seal in moisture. Creams or lotions can be applied after bathing. However, if a child is receiving radiation therapy, the use of creams and lotions is avoided in the radiation field. The child is discouraged from nail biting and picking of the cuticles, lips, and nose. Fingernails are kept clean and trimmed.

Some chemotherapeutic agents cause photosensitivity, which can result in a severe sunburn. The child must avoid prolonged exposure in the sun, wear protective clothing, and use maximal protection sunscreen.

Intramuscular injections are avoided whenever possible. If an injection is required, the skin is prepared with povidone-iodine, allowed to dry, and then wiped with alcohol. If a tourniquet is necessary for blood drawing or IV line insertion, padding is placed under the tourniquet to lessen trauma to the skin. When using adhesive tape to secure IV tubing, double-back it to prevent undue irritation. Padded armboards are used for IV lines. The tape and the armboards are changed at regular intervals, and the area of the child's skin that rests on the armboard is cleaned. Dressings for central venous access devices are changed according to institutional protocol, and specific assessment of the site is documented.

The IV site is observed frequently for signs of infection, infiltration, or phlebitis. If these complications arise, the IV line should be discontinued.

Impaired Skin Integrity

Healing of any lesion, incision, or wound may be more prolonged in children receiving chemotherapy or radiation because of the interference with cell replication that is necessary for wound healing. In some instances postponing the chemotherapy or radiation treatment may be necessary until wound healing has occurred.

Nursing Implications. To promote healing and prevent infection, strict aseptic technique must be observed when cleaning wounds or changing dressings. Good hand washing still remains the key element to infection control.

Research findings suggest that use of full-strength povidone-iodine and hydrogen peroxide to cleanse wounds has adverse effects on healing tissue.[7,9] Physiologic solutions such as isotonic saline and lactated Ringer's can be used to irrigate wounds without harm. A moist environment is recognized as the most effective for the promotion of wound healing.[9] Moisture enables the epidermal cells to migrate across the wound surface to promote healing. It has also been suggested that a moist environment enhances the synthesis of collagen in dermal repair.[9]

Occlusive dressing materials maintain a moist environment and protect the wound from external bacterial recontamination. Studies have shown that neutrophils in the fluid beneath the occlusive dressing actively phagocytize and destroy bacteria during the first 24 hours after placement of the dressing.[9]

No specific dressing can provide the optimal microenvironment for all wounds or for all healing stages.[9] When selecting a dressing, the wound size, location, and depth and the exudate must be considered. A large array of dressings are available that range from thin transparent films to hydrating gels.

The systems of the body are interrelated, especially when considering the complex process of wound healing. In addition to providing the proper environment and dressing to promote wound healing, other body systems must be considered. Successful wound healing relies on adequate nutritional stores and intake of protein, carbohydrate, fat, vitamins, and minerals.[16] Blood volume must be adequate and well oxygenated to deliver optimal tissue oxygenation.

If a patient receives radiation therapy, special skin problems may arise. Erythema, dryness, itchiness, increased pigmentation, and dry desquamation may require several interventions. Irradiated skin is cleansed with warm water and patted dry. A mild soap may be used. It is important not to wash off the skin markings used for treatment. Skin irritation and reactions to radiation can be decreased by eliminating the use of perfumes, cosmetics, creams, lotions, and deodorants.[10] The area should not be massaged, rubbed, or exposed to the sun. The use of hot packs, ice packs, and heat lamps is contraindicated. Loose-fitting cotton clothes over the irradiated skin are best. To treat dry skin, mild water-based topical ointments such as Eucerin, Aquaphor, or Lubriderm may be used sparingly. Cornstarch can relieve pruritus but should be used only on dry skin.[10] The use of topical steroid medications is not recommended because of vasoconstriction and the increased susceptibility to skin injury.

Treatment of moist desquamation necessitates other interventions. For reactions in perineal or groin folds, the skin is kept clean and free of drainage. An antibiotic ointment may be used, but a dressing is usually impractical to maintain. Whirlpool baths or showers may help promote comfort and healing. For other areas, dressings may be used after gentle cleansing with normal saline solution. To debride necrotic tissue, a wet to dry dressing is used. Once the necrotic tissue has been removed, a nonadherent dressing can be placed. Avoid putting tape directly on the irradiated skin.

MUSCULOSKETAL SYSTEM
Pain and Fractures

Etiology. Musculoskeletal problems are caused by the disease process itself or as a result of therapy. Children with leukemia often have bone and joint pain caused by leukemic infiltration. Infiltration of the bone by malignant cells can cause thinning of the bone's cortex, fractures, and pain because of inflammation or compression of other tissues. Primary bone tumors can cause pain and fractures. Stress fractures may also be a complication after radiation therapy. Young children particularly develop deformities since radiation can limit their potential growth. Osteoporosis can occur as a consequence of steroid treatment.

Nursing Implications. Complaints of pain are monitored carefully. Changes in gait or activity are closely assessed. X-ray studies and a bone scan may be necessary. If a child has a fracture, activity is restricted accordingly. Bone pain from tumor and malignant infiltrates can be very debilitating. The child should receive the appropriate amount of medication to control pain. Nonsteroidal medications act at the site of the bone pain to reduce the release of prostaglandins. Nonsteroidal medications that are platelet sparing such as trilisate are available. At times systemic narcotics or radiation is needed to control the pain effectively.

Sensory Alterations

Vinca alkaloids and cisplatin can affect the musculoskeletal system because of their neurotoxic effects on the peripheral nervous system, which result in sensory alterations.

Nursing Implications. Before administering vinca alkaloids or cisplatin, assess for signs of neurotoxicity. Early signs of neural irritation include numbness and tingling of the extremities, weakness of the hands, legs, and feet, and jaw pain. Another possible consequence is loss of deep tendon reflexes, most commonly the Achilles tendon or ankle jerk reflex. Approximately 50% of patients experience one or more of these symptoms.[45] The very young child may refuse to walk, or parents will report gait disturbances. For children old enough to follow simple instructions, request that they button and unbutton a button and take five steps on their heels and then on their toes to assess for neurotoxicity. Documentation and communication of the assessment are important since changes in the dose or frequency of administration may be needed.

Impaired Physical Mobility

There are times when a child becomes so debilitated by disease or treatment that immobility becomes a problem. Care must be taken to maintain skin integrity, promote circulation, and prevent muscle wasting and contractures.

Nursing Implications. A child predominantly confined to bed will benefit from mattress overlays or specialty beds. A number of foam or inflatable pressure-relieving mattress overlays are effective in preventing pressure sores.[43] The use of specialty beds is indicated when overlays do not adequately relieve pressure or when turning is problematic or contraindicated.

Sheepskin also helps minimize harm to the skin. Range-of-motion exercises to all joints every 4 hours prevent contractures. Using footboards and wearing high-top sneakers can prevent footdrop. Collaboration with the physical therapist can meet the child's need and prevent the further debilitation that can occur with immobility.

GASTROINTESTINAL SYSTEM
Nutrition

Adequate nutrition is extremely important because children who are well nourished are better able to resist infection and tolerate treatment.[41] The nurse has a special role in helping the child maintain an optimal nutritional status. Unfortunately, maintaining this status becomes difficult because of the heavy demand cancer cells place on the body's nutrient stores. Since protein is needed for cell division, the body's amino acid reserves are reduced. In addition, the anorexia, nausea, vomiting, stomatitis, and diarrhea that some children experience as a result of their therapy can further compromise their nutritional status. Malabsorption or enteropathy can occur from abdominal radiation, chemotherapy, abdominal surgery, or frequent antibiotic use.[1a]

Before treatment begins, the nurse carefully assesses the child's baseline nutritional status. This involves history taking, physical assessment, and consultation with the dietician. Together the nurse and dietician consider the child's likes and dislikes, number of meals and snacks eaten in an average day, and the family's ability to supplement or provide adequate nutrition. The nurse measures the child's height and weight and assesses skin turgor, muscle tone, the presence of fat, the presence of dental caries, and the general appearance of the child's hair and skin. This baseline assessment allows the team to evaluate the child's progress or deterioration throughout the course of therapy.

Anorexia

Appetite suppression and decreased food intake may result from anorexia-inducing substances secreted by the tumor cells, pain, nausea, vomiting, metabolic disturbances, and alterations in taste and from psychologic and sociocultural factors.[18]

Nursing Assessment. Assessment of anorexia is difficult because it includes both the subjective experience of appetite loss and the objective decrease of food intake. Ongoing assessment of nutritional status is necessary, including regular monitoring of height and weight, vital signs, laboratory tests, and intake and output records. Inquire about the child's food preferences and patterns and encourage that favorite foods be brought from home. Nutrition support services can assist by calculating caloric and protein intake, taking a variety of body measurements, consulting with families, and making recommendations for food selection, supplements, and alternate feeding methods.

Taste alterations contribute to anorexia and occur because of the pathology of cancer, the treatment, and other related social and emotional factors. Certain chemotherapy

drugs have been reported to cause constant or intermittent metallic or bitter tastes and an increased threshold for sweet tastes that can result in an aversion to sweet foods. Radiation can cause alterations because of destruction of microvilli of the taste buds and of the epithelial cells lining the salivary glands. Xerostomia, or dryness of the mouth, may be irreversible, depending on the radiation dose and tissue exposed.[34] It affects taste since food must be in solution to stimulate taste buds. Finally, surgery to the oral cavity or surrounding areas may cause absence or decrease in the taste sensation.[45]

Crisis and confrontation can occur between parent and child over food. Often the parents believe this is one of the few areas in which they can affect the outcome and have some control. Likewise the child may pick this domain to control.

Nursing Interventions. The nurse, dietician, oncologist, and family together develop a nutritional care plan. First, it is necessary to manage treatment toxicities. Pharmacologic interventions for anorexia include using antiemetics to control nausea and vomiting, analgesics to relieve pain, steroids to increase appetite, and replacement of depleted trace elements that may play a part in taste and smell sensations.[18] Altered taste sensations are improved by keeping the oral mucosa moist by drinking liquids, decreasing obnoxious odors in the environment, and maintaining excellent oral hygiene.[40]

Patient and family teaching can allay anxieties and myths and provide practical strategies. Supplementing the child's diet with high-calorie milkshakes or concentrated formula with added carbohydrate, fat, and/or protein is possible. Offering frequent small meals or snacks may be helpful.

When control issues are a problem, minimal coercion is recommended. Explanations and mutual goals may lead to understanding and compliance by older children. For younger children, offering frequent small meals and allowing them to feed themselves may be beneficial. For the child and family, it is important to provide an environment conducive to eating while in the hospital or at home.

If these attempts to promote adequate oral intake do not result in sufficient caloric intake, alternate feeding methods such as parenteral nutrition or tube feedings may be necessary.

Cachexia

Despite efforts to promote adequate nutrition, nausea, vomiting, anorexia, diarrhea, and stomatitis may be so severe that weight loss, cachexia, and debilitation result. The progressive wasting of cachexia is thought to result from an imbalance in the energy needed by the body versus the energy available because of inadequate intake and biochemical alterations. One theory is that regardless of intake, alterations in host metabolism are the real cause of cancer cachexia. Therefore nutritional support cannot reverse cachexia without successful treatment of the malignancy.[29]

Nursing Assessment. Assess the child for weight loss, anorexia, weakness, muscle atrophy, easy fatigue, impaired immune function, decreased motor and mental skills, shorter attention span, and reduced concentration. The treatment team must devise a plan of care to reverse the cachexia while continuing to treat the cancer. Consulting nutritional, developmental, and behavioral experts assists the primary care team's planning. Certain groups of children are at high nutritional risk. They include the children who at diagnosis are nutritionally depleted, those with a large abdominal tumor, or those with diseases requiring intense chemotherapy and radiation to the abdomen, neck, or pharynx. A suggested working definition of nutritional depletion for children is weight for height less than the fifth percentile, a weight loss greater than 10%, or a serum albumin level less than or equal to 3.2 g/dl.[6]

Nursing Interventions. Three ways to meet the minimal caloric and protein requirements are by oral intake, IV nutritional support, or enteral tube feedings. These methods are used alone or in combination during the child's therapy. The goals are (1) to prevent nutritional depletion and treat existing deficits; (2) to meet increased need for nutrients during treatment; and (3) to maintain or improve the patient's quality of life.[77] Liquid supplements can be used when the child is unable to eat regular meals.

When oral intake is insufficient to correct the nutritional depletion, IV nutrition is frequently used. A 10% dextrose solution can be given through a peripheral vein. This high-glucose solution has a high osmolality, which can be irritating to the vein; therefore lipids generally also are infused piggyback since they are isotonic and can provide nonprotein calories.

Multilumen central venous catheters, right atrial catheters, and implantable ports can be used to deliver TPN. TPN sepsis largely is caused by contamination of the catheter at the exit site and migration of bacteria along the line.[44] Dressing change procedures vary greatly among institutions, but the goal always is to prevent infection.

All TPN solutions contain water, protein, carbohydrate (10% to 30% dextrose), fat (10% to 20%), electrolytes, vitamins, and trace elements, which are carefully calculated to each child's needs.[44] Fat, in the form of lipid emulsions, can be administrated daily or several times a week.

TPN solutions are initiated slowly and advanced only as the patient can tolerate the fluid and dextrose infusion. Infusion pumps are used to ensure a constant rate. Blood glucose, electrolytes, and urinary glucose levels and weights are checked regularly. Eventually TPN is infused over 12 to 14 hours to facilitate home care or allow hospitalized patients greater mobility and is cycled for ½ to 1 hour before and after an infusion to prevent hypoglycemia or hyperglycemia. The solution is refrigerated until shortly before its use, and the bag is changed every 24 hours because of the possibility of bacterial growth in the high-dextrose solution. The use of filters is controversial because they often will not accommodate the fat emulsion; therefore the lipid infusion is piggybacked below the filter. Ideally the line for TPN is used solely for that purpose, thereby decreasing repeated entry and the risk of contamination.

Although the use of TPN may have little impact on the outcome of cancer, its use can affect the treatment course by preventing the development of adverse effects of protein malnutrition, thereby improving tolerance to therapy, increasing energy for daily activities, and improving the child's sense of well being.[6,41] Through coordination of inpatient and outpatient services, an increasing number of children can receive supplemental TPN at home, greatly enhancing the child's quality of life.

The third method of supplementation is by tube feedings into a functional gastrointestinal (GI) tract. A variety of gastrostomy tubes are available for this purpose.

Care of gastrostomy tubes and devices varies with institutions and home care companies. Keeping the skin clean and dry is important. Daily cleansing with soap and water may be sufficient, with no dressing or with a split gauze around the tube, depending on patient comfort.

Feeding may be continuous or intermittent or progress gradually to determine the tolerance of the individual to the type of formula and rate. Intermittent feeding is desirable because it allows the child freedom from the feeding equipment and mimics the normal stomach functioning. Consultation with the dietician is beneficial to determine the feeding schedule, type of formula, and sufficient nutrient intake.

With gastrostomy tube feeding, the nurse ensures correct placement of the tube, checks residuals, ensures optimal patient position during and immediately after feedings with the head of the bed elevated at least 30 degrees, avoids tube obstruction by flushing frequently, and monitors for undesirable complications such as aspiration, hyperglycemia, diarrhea, abdominal distension, and fecal impaction.[38] Discharge teaching is of prime importance, providing both information about the care of the tube and feeding regimen and emotional support to the family and patient.

Weight Gain

Steroids can cause increased appetite, fluid retention, and weight gain. The child with cancer often must take steroids as part of the treatment.

Nursing Implications. The child receiving steroid therapy often develops a ravenous appetite. To prevent fluid retention and to limit weight gain, some dietary changes are necessary. Encourage intake of foods low in sodium and adherence to a no-added-salt diet. Since the child will feel hungry more often than usual, plan meals and snacks that are satisfying but not overly high in calories. The appetite changes and fluid retention are temporary and will resolve after completion of steroid therapy.

Nausea and Vomiting

Nausea and vomiting often are a problem for the child undergoing chemotherapy or radiation therapy to sites such as the head or GI tract. In some cases nausea and vomiting persist for weeks after the treatment stops. Persistent vomiting can result in fluid and electrolyte imbalances and can also be disturbing to the child and family. Therefore it is crucial to manage this problem with foresight and achieve control with minimal side effects.

Etiology. Nausea and vomiting are controlled by the CNS. The actual act of vomiting is controlled by the vomiting center, which is located in the medulla. The vomiting center receives input from a variety of sources, including the chemoreceptor trigger zone (CTZ), the cerebral cortex, and peripheral efferent pathways, which include the vagus nerve. The CTZ detects noxious substances in the blood and CSF.[17] The cerebral cortex is affected by increased ICP, disagreeable tastes and smells, and psychogenic factors.[17] The vagus nerve receives input from the pharynx and GI tract. Because of the different stimuli that can affect the vomiting center, a combination of modalities is needed to prevent or control nausea and vomiting.

Nursing Implications. The child and parents must be informed that nausea and vomiting can occur with chemotherapy and radiation therapy. They also need reassurance and education about measures that can be used to limit the incidence. The child's first treatment is a critical time for many reasons. Control of nausea and vomiting is an important component from the first day because it can have lasting effects, for negative conditioning can begin with the first treatment if it is not managed properly.[21] The goal is to prevent chemotherapy- and/or radiation-induced nausea and vomiting.

A variety of techniques can be used to control nausea and vomiting. The most common is the administration of antiemetics selected to fit the emetogenic potential of the treatment. In addition to considering the type of chemotherapeutic agent, the nurse must also consider the dose and the route of administration since these two factors also influence the potential for nausea and vomiting.

Antiemetics are administered 30 minutes to 1 hour before the chemotherapy to block the pathways to the vomiting center. Some chemotherapy agents cause immediate nausea and vomiting, whereas others have a delayed effect, which can last several hours to days. Since most antiemetics are ordered on an as-needed basis, it is important to consider the emetogenicity of each chemotherapeutic agent when planning the child's care. If a chemotherapeutic agent has a known 24-hour emetogenic potential, schedule the antiemetics at regular intervals as opposed to as needed.

Potential side effects of intensive antiemetic therapy such as dystonic reactions and sedation must also be considered. The administration of IV phenothiazine derivatives or metaclopramide can potentially cause dystonic reactions. Slow IV administration (30 minutes to 1 hour) and concurrent administration of antihistamines can limit the incidence of dystonic reactions. Serotonin antagonists do not have the unpleasant side effect of dystonic reactions because their mechanism of action is different. Instead of affecting the dopamine receptors, which are responsible for dystonic reactions, serotonin receptors are affected. For patients who are highly sensitive to the side effects of the phenothiazine derivatives, there is a clear advantage to using serotonin antagonists. Another advantage of serotonin antagonists is that they do not cause sedation.

Sedation is still a problem caused by antiemetic therapies such as diphenhydramine and lorazepam. Some patients prefer to be sedated near the time of chemotherapy administration. Nursing assessment for the child who is sedated from antiemetic therapy should include close monitoring of respiratory rate, blood pressure, and LOC for up to several hours after completion until they are alert and able to tolerate oral intake. Dose adjustments may be necessary if the level of sedation is a concern. The child's safety is also a nursing concern, and the child is protected from falls when in bed or when ambulating. The infant or very young child is positioned on its side to prevent aspiration.

When an antiemetic regimen is effective for a particular child, it is reviewed with the parents and is documented in a place where it can easily be accessed for the next clinic visit or hospital admission. Parents must be informed about the delayed onset of nausea and vomiting related to particular chemotherapeutic agents since they will be managing this problem at home. The child should be sent home with antiemetic medications and specific instructions on their use. For home chemotherapy that is potentially emetogenic, nurses must educate parents further about the administration of antiemetics and the guidelines for maintaining their hydration status.

Manipulation of the environment may also help control nausea and vomiting. Sights, smells, and sounds that contribute to the child's feeling nauseated should be avoided. As a child's treatment progresses, he or she often becomes more sensitive to certain environmental stimuli. The nurse must continually reassess the child's preferred environment and reactions and make changes as necessary. Distraction, relaxation, and imagery are other methods that can help control nausea and vomiting.

Anticipatory nausea and vomiting are a major problem for some children. It occurs in 11% to 50% of pediatric patients.[21] Generally, anticipatory nausea and vomiting occur around the fourth or fifth treatment, and they are more common in adolescents than in younger children.[21] Children may feel nauseous from the moment they enter the clinic as a result of sights, smells, or colors. Psychogenic factors can stimulate the vomiting center just as noxious stimuli can, which is why it is particularly important to avoid negative conditioning with the first treatment. Relaxation, guided imagery, desensitization, self-hypnosis, and distraction can be very effective for a receptive child. Also antiemetics given at home the night before and again the morning of a clinic visit can be useful.

The child who suffers from vomiting must have accurate records of intake and output. Emesis should be measured and tested for blood. Guaiac materials are sensitive to gastric secretions and are used when testing for blood in emesis. Guaiac-positive results can be caused by irritation from vomiting and should be discussed with the physician. A more effective antiemetic regimen may be needed. For the child with persistent vomiting, IV fluids are needed, both for hydration maintenance and fluid replacement.

If the child is unable to tolerate oral medications because of vomiting, they are given intravenously if possible. If they can only be given orally, their administration should coincide with that for antiemetic therapy. If the medications are vomited, directions are determined about when and if the full dose should be repeated.

The decision to discontinue IV fluids is based on the child's ability to tolerate adequate amounts of fluids without vomiting. Oral intake should not be forced on the child. Small amounts of clear fluids or bland foods such as crackers can be offered when the child feels ready. Some children may have a specific food or drink they prefer to try after periods of nausea. As the child resumes oral intake, every effort is made to avoid potentially disturbing environmental stimuli such as strong smells.

Problems of the Oral Cavity

A healthy oral cavity is essential to maintain adequate nutrition and the prevention of infection. Many factors can cause changes in the oral mucosa of the child with cancer. Some chemotherapeutic drugs cause stomatitis and mucositis. Additionally, anorexia, lack of oral intake, and oral irradiation can cause changes in the oral mucosa such as decreased salivation. Oral problems occur in approximately 90% of children being treated for cancer.[4]

Nursing Assessment. A baseline assessment of the oral cavity is essential for the evaluation of changes. A systematic assessment of the lips, tongue, gingivae, mucous membranes, saliva, ability to swallow, and ability to eat should be performed at regular intervals. Numerical and descriptive rating scales are available that provide cues to ensure thorough and consistent assessment.[11,13] When possible, dental examinations are done before the start of treatment to treat preexisting problems and limit the risk of new problems.

Meticulous oral hygiene is a major patient goal. Patient education about oral hygiene techniques begins at diagnosis. The child's usual oral hygiene routine is assessed and changes made if needed. The use of soft-bristled toothbrushes is recommended, and flossing can continue if there are no mouth sores or bleeding. Four times a day is an appropriate schedule for preventive oral care.[28] Radiation to the oral cavity can cause decreased saliva production, and saliva constitutes part of the child's natural defenses against tooth decay.[28] Fluoride rinses are indicated when radiation treatments include the oral cavity. In addition to fluoride treatments, the use of saliva substitutes helps keep the mouth moist and maintains mucosal and hard tissue integrity.[34]

Stomatitis is likely to develop in children who receive radiation therapy that includes the oral cavity and intensive chemotherapy. The epithelial cells of the oral mucosa and GI tract are prime targets for toxicity because they rapidly proliferate. Mucosal deterioration can begin as early as 2 to 3 days after chemotherapy.

Three major nursing care problems are related to stomatitis: (1) impaired tissue integrity, (2) alteration in comfort, and (3) altered nutritional intake. The signs of impaired tissue integrity can range from reddened areas to ulcerations to white patches. Other characteristics include erythema, pain, difficulty swallowing, and drooling. Infections that are often associated with stomatitis are herpes simplex, candidiasis, and *Pseudomonas*.

Nursing Interventions. Early identification and prompt treatment can decrease the severity of stomatitis. Interventions focus on keeping the oral mucosa clean and free of debris. A variety of oral rinses can be used, including normal saline solution, baking soda solution, and chlorhexidine.

Whatever rinse is used, it should be swished and spit to loosen and remove debris. In some cases, toothettes are used to remove the debris loosened by the rinsing completely. For children less than 6 years old who may not be able to swish and spit, cleansing can be done with toothettes dipped in a solution. Rinses are done two to four times a day.[15]

Nystatin or special combination antifungal and antibacterial mouthwashes are commonly used after oral rinses to treat or prevent infection. Oral intake is restricted for approximately 30 minutes after using these agents to allow them time to penetrate the mucosa. For herpetic infections, acyclovir may be used topically for lip lesions or given orally or intravenously for severe infections.

The second problem for the child with stomatitis is alteration in comfort. Pain associated with stomatitis should not be underestimated. Pain assessment is as important as visual inspection of the child's oral mucosa. Stomatitis pain can be treated topically or systemically. Topical agents commonly used are dyclonine (Dyclone), diphenhydramine (Benadryl) and Kaopectate (1:1), and viscous lidocaine (viscous Xylocaine). These agents can be applied directly to the sore or swished and spit. The potential side effects of viscous lidocaine such as decreased gag reflux, tingling, and seizures must be considered. Swallowing the solutions is avoided, and the dosage should not exceed 15 ml every 3 hours.[15]

Often local pain relief methods are combined with centrally acting narcotics. For some children an IV bolus of narcotic before mouth care is helpful, but many children require continuous infusion narcotics to control the pain of severe stomatitis adequately. Even with continuous narcotic infusions, the child may need a bolus before mouth care or meal time. Patient-controlled analgesia may be useful.

The third patient problem is altered nutritional intake. The child's nutritional and fluid status is evaluated through accurate recordings of intake, output, and weight. Often chewing and swallowing become too difficult, and the child may tolerate only liquids such as ice chips, frozen fruit drinks, or milk shakes. If the child cannot maintain an adequate oral fluid intake, supplemental IV fluids are necessary. If the stomatitis persists and weight loss becomes a problem, the child may require TPN until the oral cavity heals.

As the white blood cell count rises or radiation therapy is discontinued, the oral mucosa regenerates new healthy tissue, a process that can take up to 2 to 3 weeks. For children who are able to receive granulocyte colony-stimulating factor, recovery from stomatitis may be much quicker since the period of neutropenia will be less severe and prolonged.[34] In the meantime it is a nursing challenge to provide appropriate supportive care to the child suffering from stomatitis.

Children who receive radiation therapy to the oral cavity are at risk for chronic dental problems, including delayed tooth eruption, shortening or thinning of dental roots, small teeth, and enamel grooves and pits. Children at risk for chronic dental problems must understand the importance of continuing meticulous oral hygiene and the need for consistent dental checkups after completion of cancer treatment.

Abdominal Pain

The causes of abdominal pain vary and include hepatomegaly and splenomegaly caused by leukemic infiltrates, GI ulcerations, ileus, pancreatitis, typhlitis (inflammation of the cecum), constipation, or bowel obstruction.

Nursing Assessment. All complaints of abdominal pain must be carefully assessed. Ascertain the location and severity of the pain and whether it is constant or intermittent. Hepatomegaly and splenomegaly can be determined by palpation. GI ulcerations secondary to an infectious process can be associated with pain when eating and can be relieved with medications that coat the GI tract. The child receiving L-asparaginase is at risk for developing pancreatitis, which is usually accompanied by complaints of tenderness in the epigastric region and is easily confirmed by an elevated serum amylase level. Typhlitis develops only in neutropenic patients and elicits complaints of abdominal pain localized to the right lower quadrant.[25]

Nursing Interventions. Both pancreatitis and typhlitis require aggressive supportive care aimed at GI rest, pain control, and nutritional support. Additionally, the child with typhlitis is at great risk for sepsis should necrosis of the cecum develop. Surgery is not indicated but sometimes is done secondary to concerns about appendicitis.

Diarrhea

Diarrhea in the child with cancer may be due to surgery, radiation, chemotherapy, increased stress, use of nutritional supplements, lactose intolerance, fecal impaction, tumor growth, infection, or antibiotics. This abnormal increase in quantity, frequency, and fluid content of stool can lead to fluid and electrolyte imbalance, dehydration, perianal discomfort, and change in life-style.

Nursing Assessment. Assessment includes keeping an accurate record of intake and output and noting the number, amount, consistency, and color of stools. Stools are tested for occult blood and may be sent for culture. Nutritional status, fluid and electrolyte imbalance, and skin integrity are monitored.

Nursing Interventions. A bland, low-residue, or lactose-free diet may be suggested. Fluid and electrolyte imbalance is corrected by diet alterations or administration of IV fluids, which may also be used to correct dehydration. Medications are used to thicken stools, decrease peristalsis, or treat infection. Skin excoriation frequently occurs; therefore careful attention to skin cleansing and drying is needed. Frequent sitz baths provide comfort, and exposing the area to air or applying topical ointments such as an antifungal or barrier-type cream is used for skin protection and to promote healing.

Constipation and Ulceration of the Lower GI Tract

Constipation occurs often as a result of the use of chemotherapy agents, particularly the vinca alkaloids, or the administration of narcotics. It also may result from tumor growth, decreased mobility, dehydration, or altered nutrition and patterns of elimination.[2] Constipation may aggravate rectal fissures or perineal abscesses. Constipation or an ileus can be very painful and serious. Aggressive interventions aimed at prevention are required.

Nursing Assessment. To prevent constipation or to plan interventions to treat it, keep an accurate record of the number and consistency of stools. The abdomen is examined and assessed for pain, swelling, and rigidity and is auscultated for bowel sounds. If increasing abdominal size is occurring, abdominal girths at the same place are measured every day. The genitalia and anal area are inspected regularly and kept clean and dry. Diet is assessed.

Nursing Interventions. A stool softener is started prophylactically when vinca alkaloids or narcotics are administered; if this treatment is ineffective, gentle cathartics are used. To prevent or minimize rectal fissures and perineal abscesses, manipulation of the rectum with enemas, suppositories, digital examination, or rectal thermometers is avoided except in extreme situations. Exercise and adequate fluid intake are important interventions, even for a weak or bedridden child. Perineal hygiene is important, particularly if a child develops an abscess or fissure. Sitz baths or perineal irrigations help heal the area, and 5% lidocaine jelly and/or IV pain medication may be necessary to control pain. After discharge the child is encouraged to continue good hygiene, diet, and the use of stool softeners to prevent exacerbation of problems.

GI Bleeding

GI bleeding caused by thrombocytopenia and mucosal damage from chemotherapy or radiotherapy may be a problem for the child with cancer. The use of steroids can also cause gastric disturbances and stress ulcers. Persistent vomiting can precipitate GI bleeding.

Nursing Implications. The side effects of steroid therapy can be minimized by giving the child milk, ice cream, or an antacid with the drug.

All emesis and stools are tested for blood, using guaiac material. Clear documentation of results is noted so changes can be promptly identified. Guaiac-positive stools could indicate bleeding anywhere in the GI tract. The color of the stool can help identify the possible location of the bleeding. Black, tarry stools usually indicate bleeding from the upper GI tract, whereas bleeding from the colon produces bright red blood in the stools. A stool that is blood streaked may indicate a rectal fissure or ulcer. Hemoptysis may also be a sign of GI bleeding. Vomited blood nearly always indicates bleeding above the duodeno-jejunal junction. The color of the emesis should be assessed. Fresh blood appears bright red, and old blood is dark red and resembles coffee grounds.

An acute GI bleed can be life threatening. A massive bleed is characterized by loss of more than 15% of intravascular blood volume within a few minutes to hours.[19] The child is monitored closely for signs of shock such as cool skin, decreased peripheral pulses, and oliguria.

Interventions for the child focus on stopping the bleeding and replacing the volume. If the patient is vomiting bright red blood, a nasogastric tube is inserted to provide iced saline solution lavages, which cause vasoconstriction of the blood vessels of the stomach. Additionally, if the child is thrombocytopenic, platelets are administered as soon as possible. If blood loss has been significant, the child needs volume expanders immediately with administration of saline or lactated Ringer's solution. The blood volume lost may be significant enough for the child to require a blood transfusion.

After the child has stabilized, attempts are made to determine the cause of the bleeding. The child's disease process and treatment should be considered, as should laboratory values, including platelet count and coagulation studies. Further blood product support may be necessary. Vitamin K may be ordered to promote the formation of prothrombin, which is necessary for clotting. Finally, cimetadine may be ordered to inhibit gastric acid secretion.

RENAL SYSTEM

A number of factors can adversely affect the functioning of the child's renal system. Alterations most commonly occur as a result of chemotherapy, radiation therapy, or tumor lysis syndrome.

Alterations Secondary to Cancer Treatment

Nursing Implications. The urine of children receiving cyclophosphamide or ifosfamide should be checked for blood with each void because the breakdown products of these drugs can irritate the bladder wall and cause bleeding. Patients receiving these drugs should be well hydrated and encouraged to void frequently to prevent urine stasis in the bladder for an extended period of time. Administration of the drug mesna helps reduce the risk of hemorrhagic cystitis. Mesna is only active in the urine. It binds with acrolein, the harmful by-product of cyclophosphamide and ifosfamide, to reduce the risk of bladder toxicity. A child who has received pelvic irradiation in addition to cyclophosphamide or ifosfamide is at high risk for developing hemorrhagic cystitis. If hemorrhagic cystitis develops, bladder irrigation may be needed to prevent further damage to the bladder wall. Hemorrhagic cystitis can occur months after the administration of cyclophosphamide or ifosfamide; therefore periodic urinalysis is required.

SIADH can also be a problem for the child with cancer. Vincristine and cyclophosphamide particularly can precipitate this syndrome. The symptoms include hyponatremia, low serum osmolarity, high urinary specific gravity and osmolarity, and decreased urinary output. Hyponatremia is commonly associated with thirst, headache, fatigue, and nausea. The goal is to increase the urinary output so that it is greater than input. The child is put on a regimen of fluid restriction to below maintenance levels. Careful monitoring of intake is required, with accurate recording of output and the specific gravity of each void. A decrease in specific gravity indicates that fluid balance is being restored.

Tumor Lysis Syndrome

Tumor lysis syndrome can cause renal problems in the child with cancer. The most common diseases associated with tumor lysis syndrome include Burkitt's lymphoma, T-cell lymphoma, and acute leukemia. These tumors are very sensitive to the effects of chemotherapy. With the initial treatment, they respond so rapidly that they can induce metabolic abnormalities. Children with large tumor burdens at diagnosis are especially at risk for tumor lysis syndrome.

The metabolic abnormalities of tumor lysis syndrome include hyperuricemia, hyperkalemia, hyperphosphatemia, and hypocalcemia. These serum laboratory values are closely monitored during periods of tumor lysis. If uric acid, phosphorus, and potassium are released by the cells in larger quantities than the kidney can excrete, the serum laboratory values will be elevated. Hypocalcemia is a part of the tumor lysis syndrome because of its interaction with phosphorus. If phosphorus is elevated, it reacts with extracellular calcium, causing the release of calcium salts with subsequent hypocalcemia.

Nursing Implications. Maintaining an alkaline urine during periods of tumor lysis helps prevent the development of uric acid crystals. Uric acid is more soluble in alkaline urine. Uric acid crystals are of concern because they can be deposited in the kidneys, ureters, or bladder. Obstruction can occur, with subsequent oliguric renal failure. If uric acid levels are very high, uric acid crystals are visible in the urine. If they are seen, the physician is notified immediately since renal damage may be impending. Sodium bicarbonate is commonly added to the IV solution to alkalinize the urine. Allopurinol is administered IV or by mouth (PO) to decrease the production of uric acid. The urine is tested for pH with each void. A pH of seven or greater is desirable. The physician is notified if the urine is not alkaline. Careful recording of intake and output is essential during expected periods of tumor lysis. Urinary output is maintained at 1 ml/kg/hour or greater. Careful and close assessment by the nurse will promote early detection of renal problems.

Fatigue

Fatigue is a major problem for the child with cancer before and during treatment, although no specific physiologic mechanism of cancer fatigue has been clearly identified. Fatigue includes both psychologic and physiologic components. The psychologic component may be due to knowledge deficit about the disease and treatment and to anxiety and depression about treatment. The physical components include inadequate nutrition, infection, anemia, pain, decreased pulmonary or cardiac reserves, sleep disturbances, and altered mobility. One theory is that prolonged stress causes chronic fatigue.[1] Another theory indicates that factors affecting skeletal muscle may induce cancer fatigue: first, cancer cachexia may result in skeletal muscle wasting; second, tumor necrosis factor, either exogenous or endogenous, may result in metabolic changes in skeletal muscle; and third, exercise may adversely alter the concentration of skeletal muscle metabolites.[39]

Nursing Assessment. Assessment of the psychologic and physiologic components of fatigue is essential to symptom management. Acknowledging parental input and noting the child's verbal and nonverbal cues are important. Assessing the child's nutritional status, the side effects of chemotherapeutic agents, the side effects of exercise regimens, and the need for activity limitations is the team's responsibility.

Nursing Interventions. Anxiety about the unknown is alleviated by family teaching about the disease and treatment. Helping a child understand procedures through play and written materials and helping the child discover new coping skills or build on existing ones decrease the child's fear and depression. Encourage parents and children to talk with others with similar diagnoses and challenges to learn appropriate ways of coping.

Nutritional status is enhanced by controlling nausea, vomiting, diarrhea, and constipation. Encouraging small meals, providing nutritional supplements, and obtaining a nutritional consult are helpful. Providing alternate methods of feeding (i.e., gastrostomy tube or nasogastric tube) or providing TPN also may be necessary. To control infections, preventive measures such as maintaining skin integrity, following good hand washing practices, and avoiding exposure to infection are taught and antibiotics administered as ordered. Monitoring sources of bleeding and transfusing red blood cells as ordered control anemia. Decreasing pain by using behavioral interventions and administering prescribed medications can greatly reduce fatigue. Interventions to promote sleep, rest periods, and adequate oxygenation all enhance the child's well being.[1] Although studies with adults have shown a benefit to individuals receiving treatment who participate in exercise programs, this area needs further research.[31] Given the many factors associated with fatigue, recommendations about exercise programs or limits must be made collaboratively.

SUMMARY

The child with cancer is vulnerable to a wide range of physical problems resulting from the disease itself and treatment. Knowledgeable and careful nursing assessment is paramount in identifying specific nursing care problems and providing appropriate interventions.

REFERENCES

1. Aistars J. Fatigue in the cancer patient: A conceptual approach to a clinical problem. Oncol Nurs Forum 1987; 14:25–30.
1a. Alexander HR, Norton JA. Nutritional supportive care. In Pizzo PA, Poplack DG (eds): Principles and Practice of Pediatric Oncology, 2nd ed. Philadelphia: JB Lippincott, 1993, pp 1021–1038.
2. Basch A. Changes in elimination. Semin Oncol Nurs 1987; 3:287–292.
3. Becton DL, Kletzel M, Golladay ES, et al. An experience with an implanted port system in 66 children with cancer. Cancer 1988; 61:376–378.
4. Campbell S. Spotlight on children: Mouthcare in cancer patients. Nurs Times 1987; 83:59–60.
5. Charuhas PM. Nutrition support of the cancer patient. Registered Dietician 1990; 10:1–12.
6. Coates TD, Rickland KA, Grossfeld JL, et al. Nutritional support of children with neoplastic diseases. Surg Clin North Am 1986; 66:1197–1209.
7. Cooper D. Optimizing wound healing: A practice within nursing's domain. Nurs Clin North Am 1990; 25:165–180.
8. Cornwell CM. The ommaya reservoir: Implications for pediatric oncology. Pediatr Nurs 1990; 16:249–252.
9. Cuzzell JZ, Stotts NA. Wound care: Trial and error yields to knowledge. Am J Nurs 1990; 90:53–63.
10. Dow KH, Hilderley LJ. Nursing Care in Radiation Oncology. Philadelphia: WB Saunders, 1992.
11. Dudjak L. Mouth care for mucositis due to radiation therapy. Cancer Nurs 1987; 10:131–140.
12. Edelstein S. Nutritional assessment in cancer cachexia. Pediatr Nurs 1991; 17:237–240.
13. Eilers J, Berger AM, Petersen MC. Development, testing, and application of the oral assessment guide. Oncol Nurs Forum 1987; 15:325–330.
14. Eisenberg P. Enteral nutrition. Nurs Clin North Am 1989; 24:315–337.
15. Galbraith LK, Bailey D, Kelly L, et al. Treatment for alteration in oral mucosa related to chemotherapy. Pediatr Nurs 1991; 17:233–236.
16. Garvin G. Wound healing in pediatrics. Nurs Clin North Am 1990; 25:181–192.
17. Goodman M. Management of nausea and vomiting induced by outpatient cisplatin (Planitol) therapy. Semin Oncol Nurs 1987; 3(suppl 1):23–35.
18. Grant M. Nausea, vomiting, and anorexia. Semin Oncol Nurs 1987; 3:277–286.
19. Happ M. Life threatening hemorrhage in children with cancer. J Pediatr Oncol Nurs 1987; 4:36–40.
20. Hockenberry M, Coody DK, Bennett BS. Childhood cancers: Incidence, etiology, diagnosis, and treatment. Pediatr Nurs 1990; 16:239–246.
21. Hockenberry-Eaton M, Benner A. Patterns of nausea and vomiting in children: Nursing assessment and intervention. Oncol Nurs Forum 1990; 17:575–584.
22. Hotter AN. Wound healing and immunocompromise. Nurs Clin North Am 1990; 25:193–203.
23. Huddleston KC, Ferraro AR. Preparing families of children with gastrostomies. Pediatr Nurs 1991; 17:153–158.
24. Huddleston KC, Palmer KL. A button for gastrostomy feedings. MCN 1990; 15:315–319.
25. Kinrade LC. Typhlitis: A complication of neutropenia. Pediatr Nurs 1988; 14:291–295.
26. Kohn C, Keithley J. Enteral nutrition. Nurs Clin North Am 1989; 24:339–353.
27. Knox LS. Maintaining nutritional status in persons with cancer. Selected papers from First National Conference on Cancer Nursing Research. American Cancer Society, 1989, pp 1–11.
28. Lilley LL. Side effects associated with pediatric chemotherapy: Management and patient education issues. Pediatr Nurs 1990; 16:252–255, 272.
29. Lindsey AM. Cancer cachexia: Effects of the disease and its treatment. Semin Oncol Nurs 1986; 2:19–29.
30. Lipshultz SE, Colan SD, Gelber RD, et al. Late cardiac effects of doxorubicin therapy for acute lymphoblastic leukemia in childhood. N Engl J Med 1991; 324:808–815.
31. MacVicar MG, Winningham ML, Nickel JL. Effects of aerobic interval training on cancer patients' functional capacity. Nurs Res 1989; 38:348–351.
32. Marcoux C, Fisher S, Wong D. Central venous access devices in children. Pediatr Nurs 1990; 16:123–133.
33. Mirro J, Rao BN, Stokes DC, et al. A prospective study of Hickman/Broviac catheters and implantable ports in pediatric oncology patients. J Clin Oncol 1989; 7:214–222.
34. National Institutes of Health Consensus Development Conference on oral complications of cancer therapies: Diagnosis, prevention, and treatment. 1990; 9:1–26.

35. Pack B, Maria B. Neurological emergencies in pediatric oncology. J Pediatr Oncol Nurs 1987; 4:8–18.
36. Deleted.
37. Shulman RJ, Smith EO, Rahman S, et al. Single- versus double-lumen central venous catheters in pediatric oncology patients. Am J Dis Child 1988; 142:893–895.
38. Starkey JF, Jefferson PA, Kirby DF. Taking care of PEG. Am J Nurs 1988; 88:42–45.
39. St. Pierre BA, Kasper CE, Lindsey AM. Fatigue mechanisms in patients with cancer: Effects of tumor necrosis factor and exercise on skeletal muscle. Oncol Nurs Forum 1992; 19:419–425.
40. Strohl R. Understanding taste changes. Oncol Nurs Forum 1984;11:81–84.
41. Van Eys J. Nutrition in the treatment of cancer in children. J Am Coll Nutr 1984; 3:159–168.
42. Viall CD. Your complete guide to central venous catheters. Nurs 90 1990; 20:34–41.
43. Willey T. High-tech beds and mattress overlays. Am J Nurs 1989; 89:1142–1145.
44. Worthington PH, Wagner BA. Total parenteral nutrition. Nurs Clin North Am 1989; 24:355–371.
45. Yasko JM (ed). Nursing Management of Symptoms Associated With Chemotherapy. Columbus, Ohio: Adria Laboratories, 1986.
46. Young SB. Nursing considerations in caring for the child with vincristine-induced neurotoxicities. J Pediatr Oncol Nurs 1990; 7:9–13.

Nursing Management of the Child or Adolescent in Pain

Elizabeth Hannigan Whittam

Exploring the concept of pain and the nurse's role in its management approaches the very essence of nursing care. The nurse, by virtue of all the time spent at the bedside with the child, is in an ideal situation to be the primary advocate, educator, and comforter of the child in pain. The nurse must be sensitive to and aware of the potential vulnerability, powerlessness, and dehumanization that pain brings to a child and family.

The World Health Organization (WHO) estimates that 30% to 50% of cancer patients, or approximately 4 million people, suffer daily from cancer pain, with or without satisfactory treatment. The prevalence of pain increases as the disease progresses, with significant variation according to the primary site of the cancer. Although WHO has made no predictions about the prevalence of pediatric pain, the potential for pain in pediatric cancer patients can be extrapolated.[70] In one study 50% of patients assessed in the hospital and 25% of the patients assessed in the outpatient clinic were experiencing some degree of pain at the time of assessment.[39]

Children with cancer experience pain from disease, from the diagnostic and monitoring procedures, and from the treatment. Children have historically suffered needlessly from undermedication, largely as a result of insufficient knowledge about the pharmacology of analgesics (i.e., route, dosage ranges, rate of administration, side effects). Little research has been conducted in the area of pediatric pain, and few pediatric assessment tools exist.[27,53] In addition, health care providers and parents alike have multiple misconceptions about narcotics, ranging from excessive fear of addiction to fear of overmedication. Furthermore, the "culture" of a particular nursing unit may not emphasize the importance of pain assessment and pain management.[18]

Many studies document the epidemic of undermedication of pain in children.[32,59] In one only 3% of nurses surveyed suggested that complete pain control after surgery was the goal of therapy, and 40% said that the goal was to relieve pain just enough to allow the child to function.[8] Other studies have shown that nurses tend to use less potent narcotics at lowered doses if given the chance.[59] Furthermore, when adults and children were matched for diagnosis, fewer and less potent analgesics were administered to the children.[3] Unfortunately, care may focus on prolonging life and achieving cure with inadequate attention to alleviating suffering.[5] The nurse must understand that pain control does not await the discovery of new drugs or approaches. Adequate treatment of cancer

353

pain can be achieved *now* if current knowledge is used.

Research in the area of pediatric pain has increased dramatically in the past 10 years and continues to grow—raising consciousness to the importance of proper pain management. For example, WHO has chosen some states in the United States to pilot multidisciplinary "Pain Initiatives" to bring together various health organizations statewide to develop comprehensive plans of action to improve pain management in people with cancer.[10] In addition, WHO, the American Academy of Pediatrics, and others held a consensus conference on cancer pain in children to organize available information into a usable format and to develop research directions and prioritize them for the future,[60] and the Oncology Nursing Society published a three-part position paper on cancer pain, which addressed pediatric pain.[62-64] It called attention to the problem of unrelieved cancer pain, defined responsibilities for the professional nurse, and gave directives for clinicians, educators, researchers, and administrators. The U.S. Department of Health and Human Services published clinical practice guidelines for pain management for use by both the public and professionals.[65,66]

DEFINITIONS OF CANCER PAIN

Despite the universal nature of pain, the actual pain experience remains highly individual and unique. As such, there is inherent difficulty in definition and identification. McCaffery's classic definition[29] describes pain as "whatever the experiencing person says it is, existing whenever he or she says it does." This is an excellent theoretic framework from which to practice because more is learned about pain if suspicions about its subjectivity are suspended. *The first step in comfort is believing a person's claim to his or her pain.*

Pain has been described in several other ways. The International Association for the Study of Pain[23] defines pain as an unpleasant *sensory* and *emotional* experience associated with actual or potential tissue damage or described in terms of such damage. The *experience* of pain is always subjective. Each individual learns the application of the word

TABLE 11–1. *Multidimensional Aspects of the Pain Experience*

Physical	**Behavioral**
Cause of cancer	Verbal expression
Side effects of treatment	Facial expression
Fatigue	Associated muscle tension
Insomnia	"Favoring" affected limb
Acute pain	Asking for attention
Chronic pain	
	Psychologic
Social	Helplessness
Change in body image	Fear of the meaning of the pain
Change in family system	Uncertainty about the future
Change in roles of family	Depression
Failure of peer group to understand	Guilt
Parental influence on child's perception of pain and acceptance of medication	Anxiety
	Change in self-concept
	Loss of control
Spiritual	**Developmental**
Who am I?	Child's cognitive level
Why am I here on Earth?	Inability to express pain
Will I die?	Magical thinking as cause of pain
Why do good people suffer?	
Where is God?	

Data from references 1 and 43.

through experiences related to injury in early life.

Others suggest the experience of pain must be viewed through a multidimensional mode.[1,43] Physical, social, developmental, cultural, behavioral, psychologic, and spiritual components exist. Each component represents potential pain and suffering to the body, mind, or spirit. Pain in this model is not simply a physical stimulus to the body but rather an experience with potential to affect a child and family in multiple ways (Table 11–1). In addition to understanding the multidimensional aspects of cancer pain, the nurse must clearly understand the physical sources of the pain.

SOURCES OF CANCER PAIN

Miser and Miser[40,41] identify the physiologic causes of cancer pain in children and note differences between childhood cancers and adult cancers. Several situations can produce pain: (1) the malignancy (i.e., bone or bone marrow invasion, soft tissue invasion, capsular distension, hollow viscous obstruction, invasion or compression of central or peripheral nervous systems); (2) the treatment (i.e., mucositis, postoperative pain, infection, radiation dermatitis, constipation, vomiting, postlumbar puncture headache, drug-induced neuropathy, phantom limb pain); and (3) the procedures (i.e., bone marrow aspirate, lumbar puncture, needle sticks for blood drawing). These pains can be acute or chronic and may take on much added meaning and intensity during the terminal phase of the disease.

Hester,[18] in a thorough review of pediatric pain nursing research, found that the most consistently reported cause of "worst pain" in children was invasive procedures. Needle sticks and injections ranked first, followed by lumbar punctures and bone marrow aspirations. Repeated invasive procedures are the most difficult to handle.

DEVELOPMENTAL CONSIDERATIONS OF CHILD IN PAIN

Children at different developmental ages possess different abilities to express and understand pain. An infant displays diffuse body movements, and parents often can distinguish pain by the nature of their child's cry. Other signs include wrinkling of the forehead, withdrawing the affected extremity, and moving the arms and legs.[44]

Toddlers and preschool children react both by withdrawing the affected body part and moving the body away from the painful stimulus.[44] Of importance for the nurse to remember is that egocentricity and magical thinking dominate this developmental level; thus toddlers and preschoolers may see themselves as responsible for the pain (i.e., punishment for a "bad thought" or misdeed). In addition, children at this age have poor temporal relationships. They cannot conceive of pain ending or that this current pain or treatment will lead to future healing. Using time frames familiar to the child such as length of a television cartoon may help provide concrete answers for the child. The presence of a parent during painful periods or procedures is critical for comfort of this age group.

School-age children display an ability to communicate effectively about their pain; however, knowledge and understanding of pain are low for their developmental level.[56] Hospitalized children less than 4 years old do not understand the word *pain,* and children 4 to 7 years old use words such as "owie" or "hurt" to express pain.[18] The majority of school-age children define pain as general discomfort ("pain is when it hurts").[56] These children have little understanding of the warning or diagnostic aspects of pain but do not attribute pain as punishment for misbehavior.

Adolescents show an increased ability to describe pain if the nurse can help with descriptive words and a thorough verbal assessment of the pain. Adolescents particularly suffer from changes in body image and are increasingly sensitive to changes in family functioning. They may experience decreased contact with their peer group as a result of their pain. Hallmark tasks of adolescents—independence and development of distinct identity—may be greatly affected by pain. With an understanding of developmental issues specific to pediatric pain, the nurse is more equipped to make accurate assessments and to plan proper pain relief measures.

NURSING ASSESSMENT
Self-Assessment

Assessment of pain must begin with the nurse's own self-assessment of his or her attitudes, knowledge, and beliefs about pain and pain relief. Unfortunately, many nurses still practice under some misguided myths (Table 11–2).[12] Information to refute these myths is available.[12,30,55]

Attitudes of society in general must be explored since they may erect barriers to proper assessment and management. Pain and suffering are strongly related to religious experiences and often are viewed as a consequence of moral failure.[59] Parallel to that is the attitude that tolerating pain is a sign of a strong character and that complaints about pain or requests for relief are signs of weakness. In addition, we live in an antidrug age of "Say No to Drugs," and as a society there may be a generalized belief that we are drug dependent and not self-reliant. Unfortunately, limited distinction is made between the use of narcotics for medical purposes versus their illicit use. Since narcotics are controlled substances and are associated with abuse and crime, their use, for whatever purpose, is suspect.[21,59]

Misconceptions and attitudes about pain in children still significantly affect nurses' decisions to medicate children in pain.[59] Nurses caring for children with cancer must determine what myths exist in their own practices and modify them so that the children experience optimal comfort.

Parental Assessment

Parental attitudes toward narcotics must be assessed. Frequently there is fear of addiction. Since parents are affected by societal influences, it is critical to assess and change, if necessary, their attitudes about their child's use of narcotics and to discuss more than once the concepts of addiction, physical dependence, and tolerance. *Tolerance* means that a larger dose of narcotic analgesic is required to maintain an original analgesic effect. *Physical dependence* is characterized by the onset of signs and symptoms of withdrawl if the narcotic is suddenly stopped or a narcotic antagonist is given. Unlike physical dependence, *addiction* is a behavioral pattern of compulsive drug abuse characterized by a craving for the drug and overwhelming involvement in obtaining and using it for effects other than pain relief.[5,25] The nurse should explain that, although tolerance and physical dependence occur commonly when using opioid analgesics, addiction (psychologic dependence) is rare and almost never occurs in the absence of drug abuse before cancer illness. Understanding these concepts and the role they play in pain management is very important to the proper use and compliance on the part of the child and family.

McCaffery and Beebe[30] have developed a parent interview regarding a child's pain, which serves to involve the parent in the assessment and relief of the child's pain (Fig. 11–1). Parental involvement is a critical component of assessment.

Patient Assessment

Proper assessment of pain includes "measuring the interplay of different factors on the experience of pain."[32] Factors could include

TABLE 11–2. *Myths About Pain Management in Children*

1. Children's nervous systems are not the same as adult's, and therefore children do not experience pain with the intensity that adults do.
2. Active children cannot be in pain.
3. It is unsafe to administer narcotics to children because they become addicted.
4. Narcotics always depress respirations in children.
5. Children always tell you if they have pain.
6. Children cannot tell you where they hurt.
7. The best way to administer analgesics is by IM injection.
8. Parents know the solution about their children's pain.
9. The child is crying because he is restrained, not because he hurts.

From Eland JM. The child who is hurting. Semin Oncol Nurs 1985; 1:116–122.

PARENT INTERVIEW REGARDING CHILD'S PAIN/HURT

Child: _____   Parent/caregiver: _____
Date: _____

I. Total Current Situation
   What are your major concerns (unrelated to pain), if any, about the current situation/hospitalization in general, e.g., finances, care of other children, cause or seriousness of illnesses?

   What are your child's major concerns (unrelated to pain), if any, about the current situation/hospitalization in general, e.g., being separated from parent, sleeping in a different bed or room, missing a birthday party, schoolwork?

II. Child's Previous Experience with Pain/Hurt
   What types of pain has your child had before? Include descriptions of cause, duration, severity, frequency, and other important aspects.

   What words, if any, does your child use for pain or hurt?

   How does your child usually act when he/she is suddenly hurt, e.g., falls down?

   How does your child usually act when he/she has been hurting for a long time, e.g., with a sore throat or earache?

III. Assessment of the Child's Current Pain
   Since no one but the child knows if he/she hurts, the health team needs your help in finding out when your child is hurting and whether efforts to relieve the pain are working. What behaviors indicate that your child is or is not in pain right now? For example, can you get your child to smile at you?

   A written record, called a "flow sheet," can be very helpful. What do you suggest be recorded on the flow sheet? List behaviors that probably indicate pain:

   List behaviors that probably indicate comfort:

IV. Comforting the Child and/or Relieving the Pain
   When your child hurts, what do you do to comfort your child or relieve the pain? Which works best? Which could you do now?

   When your child hurts, what does the child do for himself/herself that seems to help? How can we help the child help himself/herself?

   Considering the pain your child has now or will have, what are your concerns about being with your child while he/she is hurting or is undergoing a painful procedure?

FIGURE 11–1. Parent interview designed to involve parent in assessment and relief of the child's pain. (*From McCaffery M, Beebe A. Pain: A Clinical Manual for Nursing Practice. St. Louis: CV Mosby, 1989, pp 272–273.*)

Continued on the following page.

PARENT INTERVIEW REGARDING CHILD'S PAIN/HURT

What would you like to learn about how you can soothe or distract your child during pain?

If painful procedures are performed, do you wish to be with your child? If this wish varies, during which procedures do you wish to be present, and which procedures would you rather avoid?

Do you have any ideas about how far in advance your child would like to be informed about a painful procedure?

V. Other Comments

Is there anything special we should know about your child and pain? Is there anything the child finds disturbing that we should not do?

FIGURE 11–1. *Continued*

the emotional response to pain, the role of family styles on the perception of the pain, the impact on families of having a child in pain, and the meaning of the pain to the child and to the family. There are three primary components of pain assessment: (1) cognitive or self-report, (2) behavioral manifestations, and (3) physiologic responses. All must be examined in the context of the child's developmental level.

Self-Report.   Self-report relies on the skill of the interviewer and the child's developmental ability and willingness to express the location, intensity, duration, quality, and quantity of the pain. It is also influenced by the child's perception of the consequences of admitting pain is present. Children may deny pain when they are asked because they fear needle sticks.[13] In addition, shyness may inhibit a child's verbal expression, especially in the hospital setting. School-age children's responses vary greatly, depending on who asks them about their pain.[57] When explaining pain to their mothers, these children tend to give concise and unemotional responses. By contrast, their response to their peers emphasizes the discomfort aspects in a highly emotional way.

It is also essential to determine the child's understanding of the word *pain* and ascertain from the family what word the child uses for pain. For example, the nurse may ask, "What is hurting or ouching you now?" rather than,

"Do you have pain?" The former example lets the child know the nurse assumes there is pain, and the child is more likely to disclose the discomfort.

To assist children with self-report, the nurse should use words that help to describe pain (e.g., hurting like a knife, cold, cruel, tugging, tingling, cutting, pulling, horrible, tiring, like a sting, biting, hot, itching, unbearable).[58] Others have suggested words such as squeezing, burning, and scraping.[68] These words help clarify the descriptive component of pain.

To identify the intensity of pain, various tools have been developed to assist in its measurement and assessment. These tools should be taught to the child, preferably before he or she is in pain, and used to evaluate the effectiveness of the medication.

Hester's "poker chip" tool[17,20] is a type of numerical scale to assess acute pain.[31] Children are presented with four red poker chips. The children are asked to indicate how many pieces of hurt they feel (choosing zero to four chips). The concrete nature of this task enables children age 4 to 7 years to respond readily. The results are consistent with the behavioral distress the children demonstrate.

Visual Analogue Scales (VAS) can be used by children over 7 years old.[34] VAS consists of a line (usually 10 cm), either vertical or horizontal, with anchors such as "no pain" and "severe pain" at each end. Children are asked to indicate how much pain they are experiencing.

Beyer and Aradine's "Oucher" scale,[2] a type of visual analogue and facial scale, consists of six photographs of a child's face in different expressions of pain positioned at 20-unit intervals along a 0 to 100 vertical numerical rating scale.[4,32] It is considered a valid tool for the measurement of postsurgical pain. Children are asked to indicate the face that most closely approximates the pain they are feeling.

Happy-sad faces scales have been investigated by researchers.[34,49,69] In face scales, five to seven faces depicting different degrees of pain are presented to children, and the children choose the one that most closely approximates their pain. Face scales are easily understood by children (Fig. 11–2).

Varni/Thompson Pediatric Pain Questionnaire (PPQ) includes a visual analogue scale, color-coded rating scales, and verbal descriptors to provide information about the sensory, affective, and evaluative dimensions of children's chronic pain.[31,68] The PPQ provides information about the child's and the family's pain history, symptomatology, interventions, and socioenvironmental situations that may influence pain.

The Eland Color Tool[12] is an instrument that uses body outlines and markers or crayons for children to indicate where and how much they hurt. The child constructs a personal color scale from eight crayons, choosing which color represents different levels of hurt from "no hurt at all" to "worst hurt." Children then use the body outline to color the different areas of their body where they have pain (Fig. 11–3).

A child may prefer to make a scale, and to do so should be encouraged and the scale used (Fig. 11–4). Once it is determined to which scale the child responds best, it should be used consistently, particularly before and after receiving medications, to determine the effectiveness of the intervention. All the previously mentioned tools are accepted once the child becomes familiar with them. These scales can be used by any member of the health care team, including the parents.[14] Creating a comfortable psychologic climate and establishing rapport with the child are critical to developing trust and helping the child learn how to use the tools. Without rapport and trust, the nurse will not be able to assess the child's pain accurately.[57]

In addition to self-report tools, a pain experience history is important. Hester and

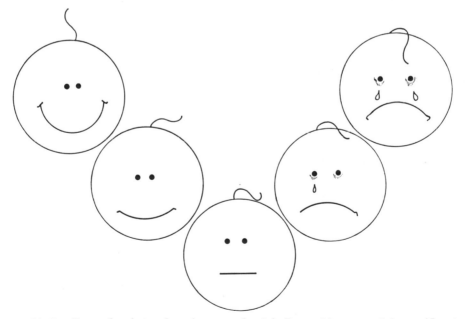

Figure 11–2. Example of visual analogue scale: Ada Rogers' happy-sad faces. *(Courtesy Ada Rogers.)*

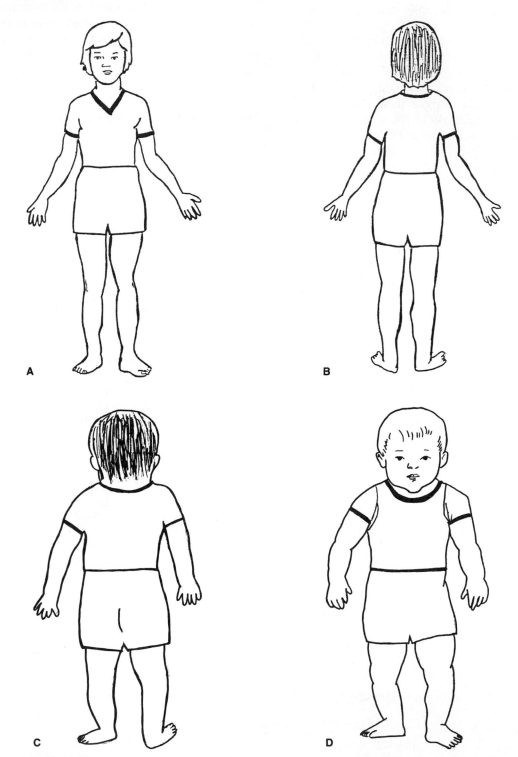

FIGURE 11–3. Eland Color Tool uses body outlines and markers or crayons selected by the child to indicate the location and intensity of hurt. *(Courtesy Joann M. Eland, University of Iowa.)*

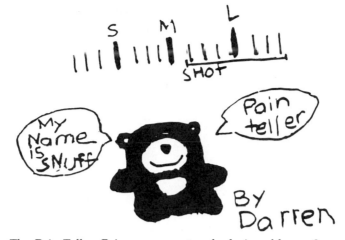

FIGURE 11–4. The Pain Teller. Pain assessment scale designed by an 8-year-old boy to help his mother with assessment of his pain. *(Courtesy Memorial Sloan-Kettering Cancer Center, New York.)*

Barcus[19] have developed a brief history, which when used, can add greatly to accurate assessment of the pain experience (Fig. 11–5).

Behavioral Manifestations. Behavioral manifestations of pain in children have been identified by several researchers.[27] Examples include crying, facial expression, muscle tension, screaming, pain verbalization, physical resistance, favoring affected body parts, asking for attention, and stalling. They are more likely demonstrated during procedural pain or acute episodes.

Chronic pain is more difficult to identify behaviorally. Children, especially those with end-stage disease, may become so accustomed to living with pain that they no longer expect relief and learn to live with the pain. Chronic pain is usually not characterized by specific behaviors at any one time but by the overall pattern of the behavior.[31] This pattern may include staying very still or moving around to create distraction. An example of not understanding this behavior pattern is the health care provider who states, "I was just in the child's room. He was watching TV and looks fine," or "Johnny is down in the playroom. He must be fine." Activity is appropriate for children and may serve as a distraction. The quality of the activity is also important to evaluate. Is it purposeful, or is the child moving in an undirected, distracted, or restless way? Irritability and restlessness are hallmark signs of pain, especially in young children.[11]

In addition, pain is very sensitive to environmental cues. It is critical to analyze situations in the environment that ameliorate or exacerbate pain but also to remember that just because pain becomes worse or better in a particular situation does not mean the pain is not real. For instance, a child may complain more about pain when the parent is present. This may be because the child actually does "feel" more pain in the safe presence of his or her mother or father. This should not be confused with fabricating about the nature of pain.[16]

Physiologic Responses. Physiologic responses consistent with stress arousal often occur with painful episodes. The problem lies in the interpretation of these physiologic responses as indicators of pain. Most of the research in the area of physiologic responses is in the area of procedure-related pain.[20] Physiologic signs are less reliable indicators of chronic pain. Children's responses to recurrent pain are usually not characterized by specific physiologic responses at any one time but by an overall pattern.[31] Evaluation of sweating palms, increased heart and respiratory rates, and increased blood pressure

Name of child: _____   Informant: _____

Age: _____   Sex: _____   Ethnicity: _____

PAIN EXPERIENCE HISTORY: CHILD INFORMANT

Tell me what pain is.

Tell me about the hurt you have had before.

Do you tell others when you hurt?

What do you want others to do for you when you hurt?

What don't you want others to do for you when you hurt?

What helps the most to take away your hurt?

Is there anything special that you want me to know about you when you hurt?
(If yes, have child describe.)

FIGURE 11–5. Example of a pain experience history to obtain from the child to help assess his or her pain experience. *(From Hester NO, Barcus CS. Assessment and management of pain in children. Pediatr Nurs Update, 1986; 1:2–8. © Continuing Professional Education Center, Inc., Skillman, N.J.)*

should be used in conjunction with thorough assessment of behavior and self-report using one of the aforementioned tools.

Even when an assessment has been performed and it is determined that pain is present, some nurses still do not take action to provide pain control.[18] The nurse must be an advocate for the patient and assure that relief is achieved. The nurse, the child, and the family mutually decide on appropriate pain relief goals. For instance, an adolescent trying to achieve autonomy may prefer having increased awareness to complete relief of the pain. Patient preference is critical in the assessment. Depending on the child's condition, these goals may differ.[41] For example, a child with severe mucositis may require an IV bolus of morphine before mouth care or even a continuous infusion of morphine. In this instance, the goal is complete removal of the pain. On the other hand, if the child is experiencing end-stage progressive disease, it may be more difficult to achieve complete relief of all pain. For instance, the child may be comfortable at rest but have some degree of pain on movement.

INTERVENTIONS

The best way to treat cancer pain in children is removal of its source. Chemotherapy, radiation therapy, and surgery, treatments to destroy tumors and disease, are the first line of attack against disease pain. However, while treatment is going on or if treatment to abolish the disease fails, the nurse must implement comfort measures pharmacologically and use adjunctive nonpharmacologic approaches.

Pharmacologic Interventions

Administration of opioid drugs is the main stay of pain control for childhood malignancy.[40] Opiates are a group of drugs whose action is "morphine like." *Opiate* refers to phenanthrene alkaloids such as morphine or codeine, which are derived from opium, an extract of the poppy seed. Opiates are generally thought to provide analgesia by binding to opioid receptors in the brain, brainstem, and spinal cord, mimicking the effects of endogenous opioid peptides.[61] These analgesics are used to relieve initial, intermittent, or procedural pain or as a long-term intervention for chronic pain.

Generally the physician or nurse practitioner should follow an analgesic ladder developed by WHO when prescribing medications to relieve pain (Fig. 11–6). Mild pain is controlled with nonopiates, whereas moderate to severe pain usually requires the use of weak or strong opioids either by the oral or parenteral route. Adjuvant drugs may be used at each step. The nurse must be familiar with the drugs prescribed. This knowledge will make him or her more comfortable with administering the drug and put him or her in

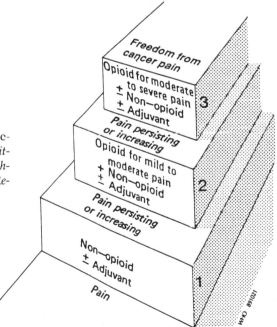

FIGURE 11–6. World Health Organization's three-step analgesic ladder. *(From WHO Expert Committee. Cancer pain relief and palliative care. WHO Technical Report Series No. 804. Geneva: WHO, 1990. Reproduced with permission.)*

an excellent position to advocate for the child who may be undermedicated.

Table 11–3 lists commonly used analgesics, both narcotic and nonnarcotic.[14] Dosages are calculated using 0.1 mg/kg/dose of morphine sulfate as a standard. Conversions to pediatric doses are based on milligrams per kilogram.[14] It must be emphasized, especially in the case of terminal malignant pain, that these are starting dosages. Opioid analgesics do not have a ceiling effect; therefore increasing the dose will provide increased analgesia. Unless the child is demonstrating signs of toxicity or unacceptable adverse side effects, *the dose should be increased until adequate pain relief is achieved.* In addition, dosing can be extremely individualized (i.e., there can be great variability in the dose needed for two children of similar weight to achieve a similar outcome). Because of its neurotoxic side effects, meperidine has intentionally been excluded from the table since it is not the drug of choice for long-term use in children.

Rogers[46-54] cites common prescribing errors in dealing with a child's pain:

1. Prescribing medications at too great an interval, not taking into consideration the faster biotransformation of the child
2. Assuming the "clock-watcher" is becoming addicted, rather than recognizing the development of tolerance
3. Assuming that increasing a dose will always cause respiratory depression

Severe pain often acts as an antagonist to the respiratory and sedative effect of the opioid analgesic. Increasing the dose for the child in

TABLE 11–3. *Narcotic and Nonnarcotic Agents Used for Analgesia*

DRUG	DOSE	PEAK	DURATION	PRECAUTIONS	COMMENTS
Narcotic					
Morphine sulfate	0.1 mg/kg/dose IV	15–30 min	2–4 hr	Nausea; constipation; in large doses may cause CNS excitation.	May cause oversedation, confusion, visual disturbances, and urinary retention.
	0.3 mg–0.6 mg/kg/dose orally	2 hr	4–5 hr		
Codeine	0.5–1.0 mg/kg/dose orally	2 hr	4–6 hr	Nausea, constipation; *not for IV use.*	Good for mild to moderate pain.
Hydromorphone HCl (Dilaudid)	0.015 mg/kg/dose IV	15 min	2–3 hr	Nausea; constipation; in large doses may cause CNS excitation.	Quick onset of action; available as high-potency solution (10 mg/ml) for tolerant patients.
	0.075 mg/kg/dose orally	1 hr	3–4 hr		
Levorphanol tartrate (Levo-Dromoran)	0.02 mg/kg/dose IV	15–30 min	3–4 hr	Contraindicated in patients with impaired ventilation, asthma, elevated intracranial pressure, and kidney and liver failure.	Begin as needed for 72 hr to establish dose frequency and adverse effects; may then be given around-the-clock.
	0.04 mg/kg/dose orally	2 hr	4–5 hr		
Methadone HCl	0.1 mg/kg/dose IV	15–30 min	3–4 hr	Contraindicated in patients with impaired ventilation, asthma, elevated intracranial pressure, and kidney and liver failure.	Begin as needed for 72 hr to establish dose frequency and adverse effects; may then be given around-the-clock.

Modified from Foley G, Whittam EH. CA 1990; 40:327–351, based on the work of Ada Rogers, RN.
*Recommended starting doses are calculated using 0.1 mg/kg/dose of morphine as standard.
IV = intravenous; IM = intramuscularly; CNS = central nervous system.

TABLE 11–3. *Narcotic and Nonnarcotic Agents Used for Analgesia* Continued

DRUG	DOSE	PEAK	DURATION	PRECAUTIONS	COMMENTS
Narcotic— cont'd					
Methadone HCl—cont'd	0.2 mg/kg/ dose orally	2 hr	4–5 hr	May cause oversedation, visual disturbances, urinary retention.	
Oxycodone (Percocet with acetaminophen) (Roxicodone 5 mg/5 ml solution)	0.3 mg/kg	1 hr	3 hr	May cause constipation; Percodan should not be used because of aspirin content.	Not available IM or IV. One tablet of Percocet contains 5 mg oxycodone and 325 mg acetaminophen. Oxycodone has quicker onset than codeine.
Oxymorphone (Numorphan)	0.01 mg/kg IV	15–30 min	3–4 hr	Similar to morphine.	Not available orally; suppositories available only in 5 mg.
	0.1 mg/kg rectally	2 hr	4–6 hr		
Nonnarcotic					
Acetaminophen	60 mg/yr of age/dose orally or rectally *or* 10 mg/ kg/dose orally or rectally	2 hr	4 hr	In large doses may cause liver toxicity.	Antipyretic; weak antiinflammatory action.
Hydroxyzine pamoate (Vistaril)	1 mg/kg/ dose IV 2 mg/kg/ dose orally	1 hr	4–6 hr	Sedation; *cannot be given IV push;* irritating to veins.	May potentiate barbiturates, meperidine, and other depressants. Has analgesic properties.
Dexamethasone (Decadron)	0.25–0.5 mg/kg/ day IV 0.25–0.5 mg/kg/ day orally		6 hr	With prolonged use, hypokalemic alkalosis, glycosuria, increased susceptibility to infection, exacerbation of peptic ulcers, and myopathy.	In dying child, liberal use of steroids can greatly reduce pain caused by tumor pressure or inflammation. Pain relief may outweigh increased risk of infection and other risk factors.

pain should not produce respiratory depression or oversedation.

It is critical that the nurse not feel "trapped" by a written pain regimen, and he or she should act as an advocate to inform the physician when pain relief is not being achieved. A statement such as "It's not time for your pain medicine yet" is counterproductive; however, it is appropriate to say, "It sounds like your pain medicine is not working right now, and we need to make some changes." If the child is asking for the medication before the prescribed time, it should be assumed that a change in the plan is needed. Table 11–4 outlines strategies to deal with specific problems of pain management.[14]

Under most circumstances, the oral route is preferable. Advantages include ease of administration (if severe nausea and vomiting are not an issue) and the gradual and longerlasting blood level of the drug. If taking oral medication becomes difficult or does not relieve the pain, intermittent parenteral injections of opioid narcotics provide the most

TABLE 11–4. *Strategies for Resolution of Problems Related to Pain Relief*

PROBLEM	STRATEGY
Less than 50% relief; child taking drug infrequently.	Change order from as-needed to around-the-clock.
Relief for only 2 hr; child taking medication but order is for every 4 hr.	Change order to every 3 hr and add acetaminophen if child is not receiving it in a combination drug.
Relief for only 2 hr on short-acting narcotic.	Change to longer-acting narcotic.
Relief for only 2 hr; child becoming tolerant to all routes of narcotic administration.	Increase dose until adequate relief obtained.
Child tolerant to narcotics; high doses give only slight relief.	Cross tolerance to narcotics is not complete; switch, but decrease to 50% of equivalent dose of an opioid analgesic with short half-life. *or* Switch to narcotic with longer half-life (e.g., methadone or levorphanol) but decrease equivalent dose by 75% to 80%. Give as needed for 72 hr.
Medication takes too long to work.	If child is already taking around-the-clock medications plus antipyretics, choose narcotic with quicker onset of action.
Child has incident pain; increase in oral narcotic caused oversedation.	Use enough oral narcotic to control pain at rest. Supplement with 20% to 40% equivalent intravenous dose.
Child complaining of sedation or drowsiness.	Frequently sedation and drowsiness subside in a few days as child becomes accustomed to the drug. If sedation persists, change to another opioid analgesic.
Child nauseated; does not like the way narcotic is making him or her feel.	Change drug; if receiving long-acting narcotic, switch to short-acting drug; if all narcotics cause nausea, add antiemetic.
Child is vomiting and unable to swallow; cannot take oral analgesics; platelet count 30,000; rectal suppository and intramuscular or subcutaneous injections contraindicated.	Intravenous narcotic indicated, especially if child has broviac central line catheter. Can be given as intermittent push or continuous infusion.
Child is depressed; depression thought caused by inadequate control of pain-causing anxiety.	Inadequate pain relief may cause anxiety and depression; therefore control pain adequately; if depression and anxiety persist, reassess need for anti-anxiety drugs or behavioral interventions.
Child complains of phantom-limb pain.	Give amitriptyline (Elavil) PO at bedtime, with dose dependent on age of child; begin at 5 mg for children 6 yr old, 10–25 mg for ages 6–12, and 25–150 mg for age 12.
Patient refusing pain medication because of fear of sedation.	Explore the meaning of sedation and narcotic use for the patient. Jointly develop a plan for pain management that keeps the patient at the desired level of alertness.
Pruritus from spontaneous histamine release related to narcotics.	Does not necessarily indicate allergic reaction. May give oral antihistamine in conjunction with narcotic or change to analgesic that does not release histamine (e.g., oxycodone, oxymorphone, or fentanyl).[67]
Child is constipated from opioid narcotics.	Give laxatives prophylactically during administration of opioid analgesics.

Modified from Foley G, Whittam EH. CA 1990; 40:327–351, based on the work of Ada Rodgers, RN.

common and effective way to relieve pain. Since fear of needles often prevents a child from acknowledging pain, many children have an indwelling central venous catheter; others have a peripheral intravenous line by which to administer the medication. Rectal administration of opioid narcotics yield similar analgesia to that of the oral route but should never be used in a child who is neutropenic because infection, perianal abscess, or bleeding may result.

Pain medicine should be given on an "around-the-clock" basis since it provides better pain relief than an "as needed" order for the following reasons: (1) adequate blood plasma levels are maintained; and (2) the child's fear that the pain medication will not arrive promptly when needed is prevented or decreased. It is critical to consider the paradoxic dynamic that may be set up between a nurse and a patient if proper dosing and scheduling do not exist. Consider the following scenario[16]:

> The child is experiencing repeated episodes of acute pain. The physician writes a PRN order for a pain medication. The child asks the nurse for medication because of pain. After assessing the child's pain, the nurse gets the medication but, despite all efforts, there is a time lapse in getting the medication back to the child. The child's anxiety and pain build as he waits for the medication and so the pain actually becomes more difficult to control. The medication is given and the child experiences some relief. However, the child has learned how long it takes to get the pain medication and that the pain got worse while waiting. The fear of not getting the pain medication may lead him to request it more frequently or complain more about the degree of pain. The next time he feels the pain coming back, even in the slightest way, there is a call for the medication. Again the nurse assesses the child and now recognizes that there does not seem to be as much distress as the first request. This may *incorrectly* lead the nurse to feel that the child is exaggerating the degree of pain and that abuse of the medication is occurring. The nurse may question the degree of the pain or even verbally state that she does not believe the child. This sets up a destructive cycle of mistrust between the nurse and the patient.

If an adequate dose is ordered on an around-the-clock basis, the question of when to medicate is no longer an issue. The nurse would be assessing the child's pain status throughout the day rather then awaiting notification of pain, which may actually encourage focus on pain and symptom complaints. In the rare case in which the child is oversedated, the decision to hold or decrease the medication may be made. Often the child requires less pain medication on an around-the-clock basis because the blood plasma level remains constant, avoiding large peaks and valleys. At any time during the treatment, if the dosage must be reduced, reduction should be done gradually since abruptly stopping the drug will bring on symptoms of withdrawal.

Unpredictability, lack of control, or lowered expectation for pain relief can affect children's pain reports. A specific charting system can be designed to enable them to follow the time course for their medication. Encourage children to make their own chart. This will provide them with a sense of control and higher expectations for pain relief.[31]

Some situations require special consideration. In the case of acute or rapidly changing pain, patients may require around-the-clock dosing *and* intermittent "break-through or rescue" dosages. Patients with renal or liver failure, in whom clearance of the narcotic may be difficult, should be monitored closely for signs of overmedication. Infrequent or intermittent pain may be treated on solely an as-needed basis. Close physician-nurse communication is necessary to reassess these changing clinical situations.

Continuous infusion of morphine sulfate delivered intravenously or subcutaneously in children with severe pain can provide adequate relief.[37,38,40,41] Advantages to using these routes include more consistent therapeutic blood levels of narcotic, no delay in medication administration, and the decreased burden of taking oral drugs, especially if nausea and vomiting are occurring. Coyle et al.[9] describe care of the subcutaneous infusion site and a care plan for treatment. Continuous infusion pumps or patient-controlled analgesia (PCA) pumps are set at a milligram-per-hour dosage, and a preset "rescue" or "bolus" dose is programmed into the pump. It allows the patient to give an extra push of pain medicine should a sudden severe episode of pain occur. The ability to give a bolus dosing during a continuous infusion provides the additional flexibility of increasing narcotic coverage for the child before activities expected to cause increased pain.

In the case of end-stage pain, many other emotions and fears are present as parents grieve the many losses in the child's life and begin to address the once unthinkable thought of their child's death. The use of narcotics may be seen as an indication of advancing disease or worsening condition. The parent's emotional pain should be explored patiently and compassionately, and adequate time should be given them to express their grief and sadness about losing their child. The family must understand that narcotics should not be withheld because of a concern of having enough drug in the future. Discussions about the concepts of addiction, tolerance, and physical dependence are critical patient and family education since there is often much confusion about the differences. Lack of information may result in undermedicating and needless anxiety.

Adjunctive, Nonpharmacologic Approaches

The literature on psychologic and nonpharmacologic interventions focuses mostly on acute treatment-related pain (i.e., injections, bone marrow aspirates, and lumbar punctures). This emphasis has likely evolved because of the severity of the distress consistently documented in children undergoing these procedures.[26] This does not mean, however, that nonpharmacologic means should be limited to acute pain and distress since the child with chronic pain also benefits from adjunctive nonpharmacologic approaches.

Breitbart[5] cautions that "behavioral techniques should not be used as a substitute for proper analgesic management but as part of a comprehensive approach to cancer pain. Successful use of cognitive-behavioral techniques should never lead to the erroneous conclusion that pain was psychogenic in origin and as such not real."

Nonpharmacologic or behavioral methods include reassurance, positioning, distraction with age-appropriate toys or books, deep breathing, minimization of environmental stimuli, listening to music, praying, progressive relaxation, imagery, therapeutic touch, or massage.[19] McCaffery and Beebe[30] provide an excellent patient and family education resource to assist the nurse in learning and teaching techniques such as imagery and relaxation. Hypnosis, which begins with relaxation but includes changes in cognition, memory, and perception, can add greatly to a child's sense of control and pain relief through a procedure or treatment.[67,72] In addition, some centers have well-developed child-life programs to aid in age-appropriate activities for children.

Distraction, focusing on stimuli other than pain (e.g., music, conversation, and counting), and relaxation in the form of deep breathing and imagery are used as preparatory methods before cancer treatments or procedures.[22] Imagery is concentrated, focusing on images formed in the mind and using all the senses. For instance, the nurse could say to the child, "Notice the flying elephant about to squirt water on us" and ask the child to describe what he or she sees.[71] Distraction, on the other hand, focuses on objects in the room rather than on something imagined. For instance, the child may squeeze his or her mother's hand, count, take deep breaths, or count the colors of the rainbow on the wall. All these techniques help distract the child from pain and help him or her gain control over the situation.

Adequate preparation is critical to a child's ability to cope with the stress of the procedure. Preparation involves giving the child information about what will be done, letting the child handle the equipment and practice on a doll or teddy bear, introducing the child to the person who will be performing the procedure, and allowing the child to ask questions and discuss fears and feelings.[71] Positive reinforcement for adaptive coping behaviors during procedures is critical. Children report that the "thing that helped most," regardless of type of pain experience, was to have a parent present.[57] On the other hand, an anxious parent may increase the distress and decrease positive coping skills in the child.[24] However, if parents have been taught how to help their child, less parental anxiety results.

Behavioral interventions should be taught to the parent and child to control distress and pain during invasive procedures. Parental and child distress can be significantly reduced with parental coaching, attentional distraction, and positive reinforcement.[28] Parental participation is thought to reduce parental anxiety additionally by increasing a sense of control and serving as attentional distraction. Rather than helplessly watching their child endure a painful procedure, parents are cooperating and contributing to the control of the pain, which leads to an increased sense of mastery.

Behavioral techniques are best taught to parents and the child at the beginning of treatment. Psychologists lament that referrals for behavioral techniques often are made too late when the child has already developed an inconsolable fear or aversion to procedures. This creates anticipatory dread of the next procedure and colors the child's attitude toward those who provide care.[60]

SUMMARY

Patients and parents must be educated that cancer pain *can* be relieved. For every message nurses give a patient and family, they are receiving a hundred others from family members, friends, and society. A particularly excellent resource for parents is *Making Cancer Less Painful: A Handbook for Parents* available from the authors.[33] Other excellent patient education booklets exist to assist in teaching and clearly explain answers to frequently asked questions by children and families.[7,36,42]

Pain control must be recognized as a priority. The question of accountability is ever present. The nurse must accept responsibility for accurate and successful assessment and management of pain. Pain as a problem, with established ways to assess, implement, and evaluate it, should appear in every nursing care plan. Implementation of quality assurance programs to monitor the pain is an excellent way to heighten awareness and maintain high standards for compassionate care.[6,22]

It has been said, "There is no profit in curing the body, if in the process we destroy the soul."[15] As health care providers frequently around people in distress and suffering, we must become increasingly sensitive to the pain around us and take appropriate steps to relieve the pain of our patients. Pain relief is, indeed, the very essence of nursing practice.

REFERENCES

1. Ahles TA, Blanchard EB, Ruckdeschel JC. The multidimensional nature of cancer related pain. Pain 1983; 17:277–288.
2. Beyer JE, Aradine CR. Content validity of an instrument to measure young children's perception of the intensity of their pain. J Pediatr Nurs 1986; 1:386–395.
3. Beyer JE, DeGood DE, Ashley LC, et al. Patterns of postoperative analgesia use with adults and children following cardiac surgery. Pain 1983; 17:71–81.
4. Beyer JE, Wells N. The assessments of pain in children. Pediatr Clin North Am 1989; 36:837–885.
5. Breitbart W. Psychiatric management of cancer pain. Cancer 1989; 63:2336–2342.
6. Bond MR, Charlton JE, Woolf CJ (eds). Proceedings of the 6th World Congress on Pain. New York: Elsevier Science Publishers, 1991; pp 185–189.
7. Children's Pain Can Be Relieved: A Guide for Parents and Families, 1989. Available from Wisconsin Cancer Pain Initiative, 3675 Medical Sciences Center, University of Wisconsin Medical School, 1300 University Avenue, Madison, WI 53706.
8. Cohen FL. Postsurgical pain relief: Patients' status and nurses' medication choices. Pain 1980; 9:165–174.
9. Coyle N, Mauskey A, Maggard J, et al. Continuous subcutaneous infusion of opiates in cancer patients with pain. Oncol Nurs Forum 1986; 13:53–57.
10. Diekmann JM, Engber D, Wassem R: Cancer pain control: One state's experience. Oncol Nurs Forum 1989; 16:219–223.
11. Dunlop J. Just Be Brave with Me. A guidebook for health professionals and volunteers caring for dying children and adolescents. Walnut Creek, Calif.: Medical Professional Pool, 1989, pp 34–40.
12. Eland JM. The child who is hurting. Semin Oncol Nurs 1985; 1:116–122.
13. Eland JM, Anderson JE. The experience of pain in children. In Jacox AK (ed): A Source Book for Nurses and Other Health Professionals. Boston: Little Brown & Co, 1977, pp 453–471.
14. Foley G, Whittam EH. Care of the child dying of cancer. CA 1990; 40:327–351.
15. Golter S, Executive Director, City of Hope Medical Center, 1926-1953. Quotation at entrance to City of Hope, Duarte, Calif.
16. Gorfinkle K, research fellow in psychology. New York: Psychiatry Service, Memorial Sloan-Kettering Cancer Center, December 1990. (Personal Communication.)
17. Hester NO. The preoperational child's reaction to immunization. Nurs Res 1979; 28:250–253.
18. Hester NO. Pain in Children. (In press.)

19. Hester NO, Barcus CS. Assessment and management of pain in children. Pediatr Nurs Update, 1986; 14:2–8.
20. Hester NO, Foster RL, Beyer JE. Clinical judgment in assessing children's pain. In Watt-Watson JH, Donovan M (eds): Nursing Perspective: St. Louis: CV Mosby, 1992, pp 236–294.
21. Hill S. Pain management in a drug-oriented society. Cancer 1989; 63:2383–2386.
22. Hockenberry MJ, Bologna-Vaughan S. Preparation for intrusive procedures using noninvasive techniques in children with cancer: State of the art vs. new trends. Cancer Nurs 1985; 8:97–102.
23. International Association for the Study of Pain, Subcommittee on Taxonomy. Pain terms: A list with definitions and notes on usage. Pain 1979; 6:249–252.
24. Jacobsen PB, Manne SL, Gorfinkle K, et al. Analysis of child and parent behavior during painful medical procedures. Health Psychol 1990; 9:559–576.
25. Jaffe JH. Drug addiction and drug abuse. In Goodman LS, Gillman A (eds.): The Pharmacological Basis of Therapeutics. New York: Macmillan, 1965, pp 285–311.
26. Jay S, Elliott C, Varni J. Acute and chronic pain in adults and children with cancer. J Consult Clin Psychol 1986; 54:601–607.
27. Jeans ME. The measurement of pain in children. In Melzack R (ed): Pain Measurement and Assessment. New York: Raven Press, 1983, p 183.
28. Manne SL, Redd WH, Jacobsen PB, et al. Behavioral intervention to reduce child and parent distress during venipuncture. J Consult Clin Psychol 1990; 58:565–572.
29. McCaffery M. Nursing Management of the Patient with Pain. Philadelphia: JB Lippincott, 1979.
30. McCaffery M, Beebe A. Pain. Clinical Manual for Nursing Practice. St. Louis: CV Mosby, 1989.
31. McGrath PA. An assessment of childrens' pain: A review of behavioral, physiological and direct scaling techniques. Pain 1987; 31:147–176.
32. McGrath PA. Pain in Children: Nature, Assessment and Treatment. New York: The Guilford Press, 1990.
33. McGrath PJ, Finley GA, Turner C. Making Cancer Less Painful: A Handbook for Parents. Available from P. McGrath, Department of Psychology, Clinical Psychology Program. Halifax, Nova Scotia. Canada B3H 4J1. Telephone: (902) 494-1580.
34. McGrath PJ, Unruh AM. Pain in Children and Adolescents. New York: Elsevier, 1987, pp 73–104.
35. McGuire DB. The perception and experience of pain. Semin Oncol Nurs 1985; 1:83–86.
36. Milch R, Freeman A, Clark E. Palliative Pain and Symptom Management for Children and Adolescents. Alexandria, Va.: Children's Hospice International, 1985.
37. Miser AW. Continuous intravenous infusion of morphine sulfate for control of severe pain in children with terminal malignancy. J Pediatr 1980; 96:930–932.
38. Miser AW. Continuous subcutaneous infusion of morphine in children with cancer. Am J Dis Child 1983; 137:383–385.
39. Miser AW, Dothage JA, Wesley RA. The prevalence of pain in a pediatric and young adult cancer population. Pain 1987; 29:73–83.
40. Miser A, Miser J. Management of childhood cancer pain. In Pizzo PA, Poplack DG (eds): Principles and Practice of Pediatric Oncology, 2nd ed. Philadelphia: JB Lippincott, 1993, pp 1039–1050.
41. Miser A, Miser J. The treatment of cancer pain in children. Pediatr Clin North Am 1989; 36:979–999.
42. Moldow D, Martinson I. Home Care for the Seriously Ill Child: A Manual for Parents. Alexandria, Va.: Children's Hospice International, 1990.
43. Multidimensional Aspects of the Pain Experience. Developed from contributions during week-long seminar on cancer pain management given by the Oncology Nursing Society. Keystone, Colo., August 1990.
44. Patterson KL, Klopovich PM. Pain in the pediatric oncology patient. In McQuire DB, Yarbro CH (eds): Cancer Pain Management. New York: Grune & Stratton, 1987, pp 259–272.
45. Deleted.
46. Rogers A. Narcotic drug therapy in children. In Management of Cancer Pain. New York: Memorial Sloan-Kettering Cancer Center, 1985, pp 169–174.
47. Rogers A. Changing route of administration in children. J Pain Symptom Manage 1986; 1:33.
48. Rogers A. Considering histamine release when prescribing opioid analgesics. J Pain Symptom Manage 1991; 1:44–45.
49. Rogers AG. The assessment of pain and pain relief in children with cancer. Pain 1981; 1 (suppl):S11.
50. Rogers AG. Analgesic consultation: How to manage incident pain. J Pain Symptom Manage 1987; 2:99.
51. Rogers AG. Analgesic consultation: Use of continuous infusion of narcotics in chronic cancer pain. J Pain Symptom Manage 1987; 2:167–168.
52. Rogers AG. Analgesic consultation: The use of methadone in opioid-tolerant patients. J Pain Symptom Manage 1988; 3:45.
53. Rogers AG. Analgesics: The physician's partner in effective pain management. Va Med 1989; 116:164–170.
54. Rogers AG. Pain Service. New York: Memorial Sloan-Kettering Cancer Center, 1992.
55. Ross DM, Ross SA. Childhood Pain. Current Issues, Research and Management. Baltimore: Urban & Schwarzenberg, 1988.
56. Ross DM, Ross SA. Childhood pain: The school-aged child's viewpoint. Pain 1984; 20:179–191.
57. Ross DM, Ross SA. The importance of type of question, psychological climate and subject set in interviewing children about pain. Pain 1984; 19:71–79.
58. Savedra M, Gibbons P, Tesler M, et al. How do children describe pain? A tentative assessment. Pain 1982; 14:95–104.
59. Schechter N. The undertreatment of pain in children: An overview. Pediatr Clin North Am 1989; 36:781–791.
60. Schechter N, Altman A, Weisman S (eds). Report on the consensus conference on the management of pain in childhood cancer. Pediatrics 1990; 86:814–834.
61. Shannon M, Berde CB. Pharmacologic management of pain in children and adolescents. Pediatr Clin North Am 1989; 36:855–871.
62. Spross J, McGuire D, Schmitt R. Oncology Nursing Society position paper on cancer pain. Part 1. Oncol Nurs Forum 1990; 17:596–612.
63. Spross J, McGuire D, Schmitt R. Oncology Nursing Society position paper on cancer pain. Part 2. Oncol Nurs Forum 1990; 17:751–760.
64. Spross J, McGuire D, Schmitt R. Oncology Nursing Society position paper on cancer pain. Part 3. Oncol Nurs Forum 1990; 17:943–955.
65. U.S. Department of Health and Human Services.

Clinical Practice Guideline. Acute Pain Management: Operative or Medical Procedures and Trauma. AHCPR Pub. No. 92–0032. Rockville, Md.: Agency for Health Care Policy and Research, Public Health Service, U.S. Dept. of Health and Human Services, February 1992.

66. U.S. Department of Health and Human Services. Clinical Practice Guideline. Acute Pain Management in Infants, Children, and Adolescents: Operative and Medical Procedures. AHCPR Pub. No. 92–0020. Rockville, Md.: Agency for Health Care Policy and Research, Public Health Service, U.S. Dept. of Health and Human Services, February 1992.

67. Valente S. Using hypnosis with children for pain management. Oncol Nurs Forum 1991; 18:699–704.

68. Varni J, Thompson K, Hanson V. The Varni/Thompson pediatric pain questionnaire. I. Chronic musculoskeletal pain in juvenile rheumatoid arthritis. Pain 1987; 28:27–38.

69. Wong D, Baker C. Pain in children: Comparison of assessment scales. Pediatr Nurs 1988; 14:9–14.

70. World Health Organization Expert Committee. Cancer pain relief and palliative care. WHO Technical Report Series, No. 804. Geneva: WHO, 1990.

71. Zeltzer LK, Jay SM, Fisher DM. The management of pain associated with pediatric procedures. Pediatr Clin North Am 1989; 36:941–964.

72. Zeltzer L, LeBaron S. The hypnotic treatment of children in pain. Adv Dev Behav Pediatr 1986; 7:197–234.

12

NURSING MANAGEMENT OF THE CHILD OR ADOLESCENT WITH INFECTION

Meredith Happ Weintraub

Children with cancer are at an increased risk for serious bacterial, viral, fungal, and protozoan infections secondary to multifactorial defects in immune function. In the terminal stages of malignant diseases, infection is often the final cause of death[3,8]; therefore proper nursing management of children with malignant diseases requires a broad understanding of host defenses, common infections, diagnostic approaches, and nursing and medical interventions.

RISK FACTORS

Risk factors that predispose children with cancer to serious infections include (1) neutropenia secondary to bone marrow invasion by the primary malignancy or secondary to chemotherapy; (2) primary or secondary defects in cell-mediated and/or humoral immunity; (3) loss of normal barriers to microbial invasion because of skin breakdown and mucosal ulceration; (4) presence of foreign bodies that serve as a nidus for infection; (5) obstruction to urinary, cerebrospinal fluid (CSF), or gastrointestinal (GI) drainage; and (6) nutritional deficits.

The single most important factor determining susceptibility to bacterial and fungal pathogens is the number of circulating neutrophils,[8] which are a specific type of white blood cell (WBC) that engulfs, digests, and removes foreign organisms, dead cells, and other debris.[5] In the child with cancer neutropenia, an inadequate number of neutrophils ($<500/mm^3$), may be present because of the effects of chemotherapy, radiation, or the malignant process. The risk of a serious infection is directly related to the length and severity of neutropenia.[12] The incidence of infection rises rapidly when the absolute neutrophil count (ANC) is less than $500/mm^3$, with the greatest risk occurring when the number of neutrophils is less than $100/mm^3$.[2] ANC is calculated by multiplying the percentage of neutrophils ("polys" or "segs" and "bands" or "stabs") by the total WBC. A value of 500 to $1000/mm^3$ represents moderate risk, whereas $500/mm^3$ or less represents severe risk for infection.

Immunosuppression also alters the patient's ability to resist infection, for neutropenia is only one factor that affects the child's immune status. The cellular and humoral components of the immune response undergo changes in the child with cancer. Cellular immunity is impaired in children with Hodgkin's disease and other lymphoid malignancies. Chemotherapy, especially steroids, and total body irradiation in preparation for bone marrow transplantation contribute to the impairment of the cellular immune system. Steroids inhibit inflammation by maintaining normal vascular responsiveness to circulating vasoconstrictor factors while opposing the increase in capillary permeability normally found in a patient with inflammation. Humoral immunity is adversely affected by cytotoxic chemotherapy. Both B and T lymphocytes are impaired, resulting in deficient production of antibodies and processing of antigens, thus reducing the body's ability to kill bacteria.[8] Splenectomy, which may be done for staging Hodgkin's disease, depresses humoral immunity because the spleen is the principle organ of the reticuloendothelial system. The reticuloendothelial system is reponsible for specific antibody production and filtering encapsulated organisms from the circulation.[12]

The type of neoplasm also influences the incidence of serious, often fatal infections. The lymphoproliferative malignancies, particularly leukemia, are associated with a higher number of infectious complications than are solid tumors.[21] This can result from deficiency in lymphocyte function caused by the disease process or treatment-induced abnormalities. As described previously, lymphocyte function is an important determinant of the child's immune status. In addition, steroids are commonly used to treat lymphocytic malignancies, and this class of drugs has a detrimental effect on immune response.

Disruption of the integumentary barrier also increases the risk of infection in the immunocompromised host. The skin is the first line of defense against microbial pathogens because it acts as a mechanical barrier and provides specialized cells that enhance defense against exogenous organisms. Disruption of the barrier can occur as a result of local tumor invasion, surgery, radiation, or chemotherapy. Invasive procedures such as bone marrow aspirations, venipunctures, or spinal taps or indwelling catheters can disrupt the skin barrier.[12]

A change in the level of consciousness can be associated with a diminished or absent gag reflex, which increases the risk for aspiration pneumonia. Pharyngeal organisms, usually gram-negative aerobes, can colonize, invade, and disseminate from a pulmonary source.[12]

Primary or metastatic tumors in the biliary tree, GI and genitourinary tracts, or respiratory passages can lead to obstruction of that area. GI obstruction may also be caused by severe constipation secondary to vincristine, a common chemotherapeutic agent. Obstruction in any area can promote infection by organisms' colonizing at the site of obstruction and thus is another risk factor.[12]

Malnutrition further compromises a patient's immune status. Poor nutrition leads to a negative nitrogen balance, which results in a decreased ability to form antibodies and enzymes. This loss of normal immune function gives every microbe a chance to become a pathogen, and even normal pathogens may become virulent.[12] In addition, an inadequate serum protein level is a known risk for certain infectious complications such as *Pneumocystis carinii* pneumonia.[6]

BACTERIAL INFECTIONS

The immunocompromised pediatric cancer patient is at risk for infection from a variety of pathogens (Table 12–1). Bacterial infection is the most frequent complication that contributes to mortality and morbidity.[8] Gram-negative enteric organisms are a common cause of systemic infections and generally occur when the child is neutropenic. Enteric organisms are those commonly found in the small intestine. Although the frequency of specific organisms vary in different institutions, *Escherichia coli*, *Klebsiella pneumoniae*, and *Pseudomonas aeruginosa* are the more common gram-negative organisms seen in this population.[8] Clinical manifestations of the gram-negative infections include septicemia, pneumonia, urinary tract infections, perianal cellulitis, and skin infections.[2]

Gram-positive organisms can also cause infections in the child with cancer. The most common bacteria in this class that affect the pediatric cancer patient are *Staphylococcus aureus* and *Staphylococcus epidermidis*.[8] *S. aureus* usually enters through the skin or through an indwelling catheter. Clinical signs of the infection are cellulitis, abscess, osteomyelitis, and septicemia. *S. epidermidis* can enter through an existing vascular or central nervous system (CNS) catheter.[8] Encapsulated

TABLE 12–1. *Predominant Pathogens in Pediatric Cancer Patients*

Bacteria—Gram Positive

Staphylococci (coagulase negative; coagulase positive)
Streptococci (hemolytic; group D)
Corynebacterium
Listeria

Bacteria—Gram Negative

Enterobacteriaceae
Pseudomonades (multiply resistant species)
Anaerobes

Fungi

Candida spp.
Aspergillus spp.
Phycomycetes
Cryptococcus

Viruses

Herpes simplex
Varicella-zoster
Cytomegalovirus
Epstein-Barr virus
Respiratory syncytial virus
Adenoviruses
Influenza
Rotavirus

Other

Pneumocystis carinii
Toxoplasma gondii
Strongyloides stercoralis
Cryptosporidium

From Freifeld AG, Hathorn JW, Pizzo PA. Infectious complications in the pediatric cancer patient. In Pizzo PA, Poplack DG (eds): Principles and Practice of Pediatric Oncology, 2nd ed. Philadelphia: JB Lippincott, 1993, pp 987–1020.

bacteria such as *Streptococcus pneumoniae*, *Haemophilus influenzae*, and *Neisseria meningitidis* are the principle organisms responsible for sepsis and meningitis in all children. The potential for serious infections from these organisms is even greater for children with defects in the humoral immune system such as the child whose spleen has been removed.[8]

Infections caused by anaerobic bacteria such as *Bacteroides*, *Clostridium*, and anaerobic cocci should be suspected in patients with a necrotic tumor or when there is evidence of intra-abdominal or pelvic infections.[8] Such an abdominal or pelvic infection may indicate typhlitis, a potentially life-threatening inflam-

matory cellulitis involving the cecum. It most commonly occurs in a child with chronic granulocytopenia and with the use of broad-spectrum antibiotic therapy in patients with acute leukemia, although, any neutropenic patient is at risk. Clinical presentation includes subacute or acute onset of right lower-quadrant abdominal pain along with fever and diarrhea.[12]

As discussed previously, children without a spleen are at high risk for infections from encapsulated organisms. To reduce this risk significantly, these patients should receive a pneumococcal vaccine before spleen removal, with repeat vaccinations at 5-year intervals. In addition, this group of patients should receive daily prophylactic doses of penicillin. The necessary duration for this preventive measure is not well documented in the literature; however, it is commonly prescribed at least through adolescence.

Assessment and Intervention

Because of the risk of overwhelming infection, prompt interventions must occur when the child with cancer develops a significant fever (>38.3° C or 101° F). Initially the ANC must be determined and a physical examination performed to determine appropriate interventions. The febrile patient with an ANC greater than 500/mm^3 often is managed as any other child with fever.[8] Cultures of, for example, urine, stool, the throat, or the rectum or a chest radiograph may be needed based on the individual assessment. If a specific source of infection such as otitis media is identified, appropriate oral antibiotic therapy is initiated. If no source of fever is identified, the child is monitored at home unless clinical symptoms change or blood cultures are positive. If fever persists, a repeat physical examination, appropriate cultures, and complete blood count are required.

Special consideration must be given to the febrile patient with an indwelling catheter, even when the ANC is adequate. Infection is a significant complication of indwelling vascular access devices. The non-neutropenic immunocompromised host must be examined for localized signs of infection and have peripheral and central venous line blood cultures obtained. In the event of a temperature greater than 38.3° C, blood cultures should be obtained from at least one peripheral site and from all lumens of the central catheter. Some clinicians recommend immediate initiation of intravenous antibiotics, even in the non-neutropenic patient, if an indwelling catheter is present. The antibiotic regimen includes vancomycin in combination with an aminoglycoside or a cephalosporin. This combination combats the most common catheter-related pathogens such as *S. aureus, S. epidermidis, Bacillus* species, and gram-negative aerobes. Antibiotics, if initiated, are stopped after 48 to 72 hours if all preantibiotic blood culture results remain negative. If the results are positive, a full therapeutic course is necessary. If results remain positive after 48 hours of therapy, the catheter is removed.[12] Some institutions initiate intravenous antibiotics in the febrile, non-neutropenic patient with an indwelling catheter only if blood cultures are positive unless the patient is clinically unstable.

Empiric antibiotic therapy must be started immediately in the child with neutropenia (ANC <500/mm³) and fever. Appropriate broad-spectrum antibiotics are started, even if there are no clinical findings that indicate a bacterial infection. The drug combination used must adequately combat potential gram-positive and gram-negative organisms, provide bactericidal drug levels, and be as nontoxic as possible. If the child has an indwelling central venous catheter, vancomycin is added.[12,20] The final decision about the appropriate empiric regimen must be individualized because each institution has different patterns of microbial isolates and antibiotic resistant organisms. Regardless of the regimen chosen, clinicians must monitor the patient's status to determine necessary modifications.[12]

How long to continue antibiotic therapy is a controversial issue. Children with a documented clinical or microbial infection who are responding to therapy (fever resolving) and show an upward trend in ANC should receive appropriate antibiotic therapy for 10 to 14 days. To complete the required treatment for a documented infection, home intravenous antibiotic therapy is an option for some children after fever and neutropenia have re-

solved. If no infection is documented and fever and neutropenia resolve, antibiotic therapy is discontinued.[12,20] Children without a documented infection who become afebrile but remain neutropenic present a more difficult problem. The benefits of continuing administration of antibiotics until neutropenia resolves must be weighed against the risk of bacterial or fungal suprainfections in children who continue to receive broad-spectrum antibiotics. Some clinicians recommend continuing antibiotic therapy until the neutropenia has resolved, but others treat until the patient remains afebrile for 24 to 48 hours. Discontinuing antibiotic therapy before resolution of neutropenia often is based on documentation of negative blood cultures, low risk factors for development of infection, and evidence that neutrophil recovery has begun.[20]

Prophylactic or therapeutic transfusion of granulocytes has been explored as an adjunct to antibiotic therapy for neutropenic patients.[25] In recent years, however, the benefits of these transfusions have been questioned because more effective antimicrobial regimens are available. No recent studies have documented that the use of granulocyte transfusions would further improve the short- or long-term survival rate of infected neutropenic patients. In addition, the cost and the potential for severe transfusion reactions do not support the use of granulocyte transfusions.[12]

The use of growth factors such as granulocyte-macrophage colony-stimulating factor (GM-CSF) or granulocyte colony-stimulating factor (G-CSF) to reduce the severity and duration of neutropenia decreases the chance of infection for some children undergoing myelosuppressive therapy. This supportive intervention is discussed in detail in Chapter 7.

Children with neutropenia and fever require a meticulous physical examination, blood and urine cultures, and chest x-ray studies to investigate sources of fever before the initiation of empiric antibiotics. The physical examination includes close attention to the skin, sites of intravenous devices, perioral and perirectal areas, and the lungs. Subtle signs of inflammation are considered signs of infection since, without adequate neutrophils, the inflammatory process is often diminished.[11]

The number of new active cases of tuberculosis, an infectious microbacterial disease, declined rapidly from 1974 until 1985 in the United States. Since 1985, however, the incidence of this disease has shown a sharp departure from this downward trend. Some reasons for the lack of continued progress toward control or eradication of tuberculosis in the United States include relaxed immigration laws, apathy among health care professionals, increased susceptibility in the population with human immunodeficiency virus, and the emergence of resistant strains. The implications of the rise in tuberculosis infections for the pediatric oncology patient remain unclear at this time but require future consideration.[15]

Nursing Assessment and Interventions

Nurses play an important role in both prevention and treatment of infections in the child with cancer. Physical assessment of the child with fever and neutropenia is an important nursing function. Close monitoring of vital signs around the clock is essential so that fever can be documented and changes in cardiovascular status detected. Close attention to peripheral pulses and capillary refill can determine the child's perfusion. Careful skin inspection is needed, especially in skinfold areas at high risk for infection such as the buttocks, axilla, and perineum, and sites of intravenous catheters. Daily inspection of the mouth is essential. Respiratory assessment is needed to detect any decrease in breath sounds, increase in respiratory rate, or other changes in the patient's pulmonary status. GI assessment includes auscultation for the presence of bowel sounds and palpation for any abdominal tenderness. Normal bowel function helps prevent the introduction of pathogens through altered GI mucosa. Abdominal tenderness may indicate an infectious or inflammatory process. The nurse should note frequency, dysuria, cloudy urine, or hematuria when assessing the urinary tract.[4]

Nursing interventions are an important component of health care for the neutropenic patient. Nearly 85% of organisms responsible for infection in cancer patients are derived from endogenous flora (i.e., organisms already present in the patient).[12] Nearly half of this flora is influenced by the hospital environment, and these hospital-acquired organisms, often gram-negative bacilli, may be more virulent or more resistant to standard antimicrobial regimens.[5] Inanimate objects within the hospital environment (e.g., faucets, pumps, floors) are reservoirs of pathogenic organisms but require a human vector for transmission; therefore the most important intervention in preventing infections is strict hand washing.[8] The best ways for nurses to enforce this policy are by example and by family education. Educating family members allows the parents and child to observe or question all those who come in close physical contact with the child about washing their hands.

Children with neutropenia and fever no longer are isolated in private rooms in every institution. The most important considerations are to place these patients with others who have noncontagious illnesses and to enforce strict hand washing. Protective or reverse isolation has not been shown to decrease infections in the neutropenic patient[8,20]; therefore it is not recommended because of its apparent lack of benefit in addition to the cost, inconvenience, and social isolation of the child and family. A total protective environment, including use of a laminar air flow room, reduces the incidence of severe bacterial infections in severely granulocytopenic patients[8]; however, the cost, inability to control infections, failure to maintain persistent gut sterility, and psychologic stress of continued isolation have limited its use in clinical practice. It sometimes is used for children undergoing bone marrow transplantation or intensive chemotherapy who likely will be granulocytopenic for 30 days or more.[8]

Teaching family members to monitor the child for infections while out of the hospital is an important nursing responsibility. The family must notify the health care team immediately if the child develops any localizing signs of infection or has a temperature greater than 38.3° C. When they are not hospitalized, the recommended activity for children with neutropenia varies among institutions. Some institutions allow children with a low ANC to maintain regular activity, including school attendance, whereas other institutions recommend keeping children home when the ANC is less than 500.

Good nutrition with a high-calorie, high-protein diet is recommended for the immunocompromised patient, for as discussed previously, malnutrition further compromises the child's immune status. A neutropenic diet is a regimen that limits food known to contain significant amounts of bacteria. Its use remains controversial for infection prevention. Some clinicians recommend avoiding raw fruits and vegetables and allowing only well-cooked foods so that the alimentary tract is not colonized with organisms from fresh fruits and vegetables.[5,20]

Stagnant water can be a source of *P. aeruginosa*. Drinking water in bedside pitchers should be changed several times a day and respiratory equipment maintained according to departmental infection control policies. Personal humidifiers cannot be allowed because of their potential for contamination and as a reservoir for bacteria. Other sources of stagnant water include plants and cut flowers. If flowers are in the room, the water should be changed daily.[2]

Scrupulous mouth and skin care is essential for the neutropenic patient. Mouth care is performed several times a day to keep the mouth as clean as possible. A washcloth or a soft brush such as a toothette is used for routine brushing. Use of a mouth rinse such as chlorhexidine helps prevent dental plaque and gingivitis and reduces the amount of oral bacteria present in the mouth. Mouth care, although important, does not prevent chemotherapy-induced stomatitis.[17]

Daily bathing is important, with close attention to the groin, axilla, and skin folds. Family education about hygiene allows the child and parents to participate in the care and teaches them the care to continue at home. Appropriate care of central venous lines is also essential and includes cleaning the site and changing the dressing at regular intervals. The family must be taught daily catheter care. Other interventions to prevent introduction of organisms through the integumentary system include double-prepping the skin with povidone-iodine and alcohol before all invasive procedures, taking no rectal temperatures, using no enemas or suppositories, and avoiding catheterization and tracheal suctioning when possible. Stool softeners may be needed to prevent straining that could lead to anal tearing.[5] Mobility of children hospitalized with fever and neutropenia is encouraged to prevent atelectasis. Maintaining adequate hydration helps prevent colonization of organisms in the urinary tract.

VIRAL INFECTIONS

Viral infections can cause problems for the immunocompromised pediatric patient. The number and severity of these infections are influenced by the patient's age, immunity from previous exposure, the underlying malignancy, and the degree of immunosuppression. Children with alterations in cellular immunity are predisposed to certain viral infections, especially those of the herpesvirus group. The most common viruses that affect the immunocompromised pediatric patient are herpes simplex (HSV), varicella-zoster (VZV), and cytomegalovirus (CMV).[8] General guidelines for management of viral infections are to diminish exposure to the viruses, administer postexposure prophylaxis when available, and administer antiviral drugs.

Primary infection with VZV can lead to chickenpox. After a primary infection with VZV has occurred, the virus becomes latent in the nerve tissue. Reactivation of this virus can occur, leading to the development of herpes zoster (shingles). The reactivated virus appears along dermatomes, with the thoracic and lumbar dermatomes the most common sites. The major concern in the immunocompromised host with shingles or chickenpox is the potential for dissemination of the virus.[24] Dissemination is more common in patients with an absolute lymphocyte count less than 500/mm³.[5] If dissemination does occur, life-threatening complications may develop such as varicella pneumonia, hepatitis, and CNS involvement.[24]

HSV in immunocompromised children can cause local infections such as stomatitis, conjunctivitis, keratitis, vesicular skin lesions, genital tract lesions, pneumonia, hepatitis, and encephalitis. However, even when local infection is severe, dissemination is rare.[2,18]

The Centers for Disease Control (CDC) estimates that half of the adult population in the United States has been infected with CMV and that in lower socioeconomic groups the prevalence is close to 80%.[26] The virus is transmitted through contact with body fluids, and pediatric oncology patients have traditionally had high CMV antibody levels, probably secondary to blood transfusions.[2] Active CMV infection in the immunocompromised host can result from reactivation of the patient's own latent infection or the acquisition of CMV from transfused blood products, from a donor organ or bone marrow, or less likely, from contacts with other people.[7] Acute CMV infections are characterized by fever, rash, hepatosplenomegaly, retinitis, pneumonia, colitis, and CNS symptoms.[2] CMV infection occurs more commonly in the immunosuppressed patient who does not have antibodies against this virus; however, with major immunosuppression such as during a bone marrow transplant, acute infection from CMV may develop, even if the CMV antibody is present. Pneumonitis is the most common clinical consequence of CMV infection in patients immunosuppressed secondary to treatment for a malignancy or undergoing bone marrow transplant.[7]

Treatment and Nursing Implications

Exposure to the varicella virus in the form of chickenpox or herpes zoster requires specific interventions for the pediatric cancer patient. *Exposure* is defined as close one-on-one contact with someone who has chickenpox or herpes zoster or who develops one of these illnesses within 24 to 48 hours of the contact. Varicella-zoster immunoglobulin (VZIG) is given, preferably within 72 hours but no more than 96 hours after exposure to the virus, at a dose of 125 U/10 kg, with a maximal dose of 625 U. If a second exposure should occur more than 3 weeks after VZIG is given, another dose is required.[12] When possible, severely immunosuppressive therapy such as prednisone is withheld during the 21-day incubation period. If VZIG is given, the incubation period is extended to 28 days because the passive immunity that VZIG provides may not prevent the development of herpes zoster but only slow its course and reduce the incidence of complications. In addition, if the child is hospitalized or would be seen in the outpatient clinic for any reason during the incubation period, he or she must be isolated. Isolation would start at day 10 after exposure and extend to day 21 or 28, depending on whether or not VZIG was administered. A person is contagious for 24 to 48 hours before the onset of symptoms, and transmission easily occurs by droplet spread from sneezing or coughing.[2]

Attempts to develop a vaccine for VZV are currently underway. The major obstacle to routine immunization of all children is whether vaccine-induced immunity is long lasting. In addition, there is concern about inducing a population of susceptible adults who were vaccinated as children. More research is needed to determine the role of varicella vaccine in both healthy and immunosuppressed children.[9,10]

If chickenpox or herpes zoster does occur, the patient is treated with intravenous acyclovir (500 mg/m^2 IV every 8 hours for 7 to 10 days or until no new lesions are documented).[18] The patient is considered contagious until all blisters have crusted. One major side effect of acyclovir is renal toxicity, which can be prevented by adequate hydration and infusion of the drug over at least 1 hour. Other potential complications from this drug include phlebitis, transient increase in creatinine level, and rash. Less common side effects include hematuria, hypotension, headache, nausea, and encephalopathy.[2]

Nurses must educate the family about exposure to varicella. The family should report immediately if the child has had contact with someone who has chickenpox or herpes zoster. The family or health team must also tell school officials to report such exposure because school often is where the child is exposed to the virus. Family members must be able to recognize varicella if the child develops suspicious lesions, especially since early lesions may appear very benign. In immunocompromised patients skin lesions may be more numerous and larger and have a hemorrhagic base.[20] To protect other patients, reporting any questionable lesions before the child is brought to the oncology clinic is particularly important.

HSV may also require treatment with intravenous acyclovir if the infection is severe. Mild herpetic lesions often resolve without treatment. Topical acyclovir may help speed the healing of mild to moderate skin lesions.[2] Gloves are necessary when providing direct patient care, for transmission can occur through direct contact with the lesions.

Effective antiviral treatment of CMV has been difficult to achieve. The virus has not been very responsive to acyclovir, transfer factor, adenine arabinoside, interferon alpha, or CMV immunoglobulin. Use of some investigational drugs is considered if the infection is severe and life threatening. Two drugs currently being studied for treatment of CMV in the immunocompromised host are gancyclovir and foscarnet.[7]

All patients who may receive very intensive immunosuppressive therapy such as allogeneic bone marrow transplantation should be evaluated for the presence of CMV antibodies. If a child receiving intensive immunosuppressive therapy is seronegative for CMV at the start of treatment, administration of CMV-negative blood products would be advisable. This practice is expensive, however, and may be logistically difficult, especially in areas where a large percent of blood donors are CMV positive. One alternative is to transfuse white cell–depleted blood products instead of selecting CMV-seronegative donors. Studies have shown that using a leukocyte filter to administer blood products is beneficial in preventing primary CMV infections from blood transfusions since WBCs are believed to carry CMV.[6]

FUNGAL INFECTIONS

Fungal infections are an increasing cause of morbidity and mortality in pediatric cancer patients. They account for fatal infections in 20% to 30% of patients with lymphoma and approximately 5% of patients with solid tumors.[2] The major risk factor for fungal infection is intensive use of broad-spectrum antibiotics during periods of prolonged neutropenia.[12] Another risk factor is the hospital environment, especially around construction areas where *Aspergillus* is often prevalent.[12]

The most common fungal organism found in neutropenic children is *Candida*. Other organisms include *Aspergillus, Mucor, Cryptococcus,* and *Histoplasma*. Common sites for fungal infections are the oral cavity, sinuses, lungs, bloodstream, and liver. Diagnosis is often difficult because of nonspecific clinical manifestations. Documentation of fungal infections requires biopsy of suspicious lesions if the patient's condition allows and monitoring of blood cultures for fungal growth.[12]

Treatment and Nursing Implications

Since early treatment of fungal infections often improves the prognosis, empiric treatment may be indicated in selected patients. With the empiric approach, therapeutic doses of antifungal therapy are given despite the lack of documentation of a systemic infection. This approach is used because fungal infections are hard to diagnose in the immunocompromised host. Withholding treatment until the diagnosis is confirmed may allow dissemination. Prolonged use of antibiotics increases the risk of fungal infections. In the neutropenic patient the addition of fungal therapy must be considered if fever persists after 5 to 7 days of antibiotic therapy.[8]

Local fungal infections such as oral candidiasis (thrush) are treated vigorously to reduce the chance of dissemination. Nystatin is the most common drug used in this clinical situation. It should be given four times a day, held in the mouth for 1 minute, and then swallowed. For documented fungal infections such as those in the lungs, liver, or bloodstream, amphotericin B is the drug of choice. Use of an oral antifungal agent, ketoconazole, may also be considered if no fungal infection has been documented but empiric treatment is clinically indicated. This agent is easier to administer and less toxic than amphotericin B.[12] Normal liver function should be documented before the initiation of oral ketoconazole since the major side effect of this drug is liver toxicity.[2]

In addition to ketoconazole, another azole

compound, fluconazole, has shown potential as an oral agent for treatment of systemic fungal infection. Fluconazole is absorbed well orally, penetrates the CSF better than other drugs in this class, and is less hepatotoxic. It is promising therapy for cryptococcal meningitis and urinary tract infection caused by *Candida* species and other fungi. Toxicity has been minimal and includes nausea and other mild GI symptoms and asymptomatic elevations of hepatic enzymes. More clinical trials are underway to define further the role of fluconazole as an antifungal agent.[19,23]

Although amphotericin B is a very active agent against fungal organisms, the side effects of this drug can complicate the care of the child. One major toxicity is renal damage, which may be manifested by an increased creatinine level, azotemia, and mild renal tubular acidosis. Other side effects include fever, chills, nausea and vomiting, anaphylaxis, hypotension, arrhythmias, seizures, and electrolyte imbalances (Table 12–2). Fever and severe chills are common and may be caused by changes in the hypothalamus or by induction of synthesis of prostaglandin E_2, a potent pyrogen.[21]

Amphotericin is usually initiated using a test dosage of 1 mg over 1 hour to assess for anaphylaxis or other adverse reactions. If tolerated, the dosage is escalated over 2 to 3 days until the therapeutic dose of 0.25 mg/kg is achieved. Some documented systemic fungal infections may require 6 to 12 weeks of therapy, whereas *Candida* esophagitis or empiric use during neutropenia and fever requires fewer infusions. Amphotericin B is administered in D_5W solution over several hours. Allowing the drug to infuse over several hours lessens the incidence of fever and chills without influencing efficacy.[21] Depending on the family situation and available resources, some long-term amphotericin treatments are given at home.

Nursing care is important in monitoring and managing the side effects of amphotericin B (see Table 12–2). Renal function is monitored, and if signs of renal damage occur, lowering the dosage or administering the drug on alternate days may reduce the toxicity. Hypokalemia is the major electrolyte imbalance caused by amphotericin B. Monitoring serum potassium levels, administering oral potassium, and encouraging foods high in potas-

TABLE 12–2. *Management of Side Effects of Amphotericin B*

SIDE EFFECT	INTERVENTION
Nephrotoxicity	Monitor blood urea nitrogen and creatinine levels.
	Maintain strict intake and output.
	Administer lower dosage if renal function is impaired.
	Give drug on alternate days if renal function is impaired.
Hypokalemia	Monitor serum potassium levels.
	Assess for cardiac changes.
	Administer oral or intravenous potassium supplements.
	Educate family about high-potassium diet.
Hypomagnesemia	Monitor serum magnesium levels.
	Assess for muscle tremors, tingling, and paresthesias.
	Administer oral or intravenous magnesium as indicated.
Fever and chills	Premedicate with acetaminophen and antihistamine as ordered.
	Monitor vital signs during infusion.
	Use comfort measures during chilling phase: warm, quiet environment, cover over extremities
	Administer narcotics as ordered during chilling phase.
	Apply cooling blankets and tepid sponge baths during febrile phase.
Anaphylaxis	Administer initial test dose to determine patient's response.
	Monitor vital signs during infusion as per institution's protocol.
	Stop infusion for signs of anaphylaxis such as sudden drop in blood pressure or shortness of breath.

sium such as bananas and oranges are necessary nursing functions.[21]

Several medications are commonly given before or during amphotericin B therapy to reduce fever and chills, including acetaminophen, antihistamines, and narcotics. Although their use remains controversial, steroids may be mixed with the continuous infusion to decrease the incidence but not the severity of fever and chills. Antihistamines prevent histamine release during allergic reactions, block the histamine receptors of the vomiting center, and relieve both the vasodilator and vasoconstrictor effects of histamine. In addition, the sedative properties of antihistamines reduce the heightened muscle tone and skin vasoconstriction that are part of shivering. Narcotics, primarily meperidine, are also used to suppress amphotericin B–induced shivering. Intravenous meperidine is most effective if it is administered as the chilling begins rather than as a premedication.[21] During chilling, cooling blankets and tepid sponging are ineffective in cooling the patient because vasoconstriction and shivering may actually drive the body temperature higher.[22]

PROTOZOAN

The most common protozoan infection in immunosuppressed children is *P. carinii*.[8] *Toxoplasma gondii*, although less common, is another protozoan infection affecting this population.[8] *P. carinii* causes severe pneumonitis in children with cancer. Clinical symptoms include abrupt onset of fever and cough followed by tachypnea. As the disease progresses, respiratory symptoms worsen. Manifestations include nasal flaring, cyanosis, increasing tachypnea, and intercostal retractions. The patient's oxygen saturation may decrease to between 80% to 90%. Radiographic findings show diffuse bilateral alveolar disease with hyperexpansion. In many cases diagnosis can be made by sputum analysis, or bronchoalveolar lavage can yield a diagnosis in 85% to 90% of patients with *Pneumocystis* pneumonia. Transbronchial biopsy or open-lung biopsy is necessary to diagnose the remaining patients.[27]

Toxoplasmosis, although a rare occurrence, is transmitted to humans by raw or inadequately cooked meat or by cat feces. In the immunocompromised patient it may be a new infection or reactivation of a latent infection. The most common clinical signs in immunocompromised patients are necrotizing encephalitis with CNS symptoms, myocarditis, or pneumonitis. Toxoplasmosis may also result in a mild infectious mononucleosis-like illness, maculopapular rash, or hepatosplenomegaly. Diagnosis is made by isolation of the organism from body fluids or tissue or characteristic lymph node histology.[1,6]

Treatment and Nursing Implications

Oral trimethoprim-sulfamethoxazole is given prophylactically to children at risk for the development of *Pneumocystis* infection. The current recommended prophylactic dose is 5 mg/kg/day of the trimethoprim component divided twice daily and given 3 consecutive days a week. Three-times-weekly prophylactic therapy has proved equally effective and less toxic to the bone marrow than previously recommended daily dosages. This prophylactic therapy should be continued until 3 to 6 months after immunosuppressive therapy is completed.[11]

Treatment of *Pneumocystis* infection requires supportive care and intravenous trimethoprim-sulfamethoxazole in therapeutic dosages. Supportive care consists of using continuous oximetry monitoring, providing oxygen by face mask or nasal cannula, placing the child in a semi-Fowler's position, and providing a calm, quiet environment. If these measures still do not allow adequate oxygenation, intubation may be required. Intravenous trimethoprim-sulfamethoxazole is given at a dose of 20 mg/kg/day divided into every 8 to 12 hours dosages. Potential side effects of this drug are neutropenia, skin rash, and nausea and vomiting.[8] For those children who do not respond to trimethoprim-sulfamethoxazole or who are allergic to this drug, pentamidine (4 mg/kg/day) may be given. This drug, however, has more severe side effects, including hypotension, tachycardia, vomiting, hypoglycemia, and mild renal or hepatic injury. Current trials are underway to investigate the use of aerosolized pentamidine for both therapeutic and prophylactic treatment of *Pneumocystis* infection in children.[14]

Treatment of patients with toxoplasmosis consists of administering oral pyrimethamine and sulfadiazine. In immunosuppressed patients the therapy should be continued for 4 to 6 weeks after the resolution of all clinical signs and symptoms of the infection.[12]

SEPTIC SHOCK

Septic shock is one of the most serious complications in the cancer patient. It is caused by overwhelming infection from microorganisms in the blood, with resultant circulatory failure, inadequate tissue perfusion, and hypotension. The highest percentage of deaths from sepsis occurs among patients with persistent neutropenia of less than $100/mm^3$.[16]

Although a variety of organisms can cause septic shock in neutropenic patients, most bacteremias are due to gram-negative organisms. The more common gram-negative organisms that can cause septic shock include *E. coli, K. pneumoniae, P. aeruginosa,* and *Proteus.*[16] As these bacteria die, they autolyze, split by their own enzyme, and release the endotoxins into the bloodstream. The endotoxins then interfere with the uptake and transport of oxygen.[13]

Exactly how endotoxins induce shock is not clear. It is believed that the immune system engages the endotoxins in an antibody-antigen reaction. Vasodilators are released, causing a decrease in vasomotor tone and peripheral resistance, and hypotension develops. Hypotension leads to impaired blood flow and decreased tissue perfusion. Tissue damage caused by endotoxins leads to disseminated intravascular coagulation (DIC) by activation of the coagulation sequence.[13]

The use of monoclonal antibodies has been investigated, and substantial therapeutic benefit in patients with gram-negative bacteremia, including those with septic shock reported. Although the clinical use of this technique remains controversial, exploration of the use of monoclonal antibodies in this setting will continue.[28]

The clinical course of shock may progress through three stages: hyperdynamic-compensated, hyperdynamic-uncompensated, and cardiogenic shock (Table 12–3). During compensated (warm) shock, the child appears flushed because of a maldistribution of blood flow. The child is tachycardic and tachypneic. After initially normal blood pressure measurements, the pulse pressure begins to widen. As symptoms continue to progress, the child develops uncompensated septic (cold) shock. The child becomes hypotensive. The diastolic pressure falls first; then the mean and systolic pressures fall. Metabolic acidosis occurs as a result of inadequate tissue perfusion. Increased capillary permeability produces systemic and pulmonary edema, which can lead to hypoxia and progressive tachypnea. After uncompensated shock, the child may demonstrate signs and symptoms of late septic shock (cardiogenic shock). Severe circulatory compromise is evident as progressive left ventricular dysfunction contributes to the fall in cardiac output. Extremities are cold, and hypotension and severe acidosis

TABLE 12–3. *Signs and Symptoms of Compensated, Uncompensated, and Cardiogenic Shock*

COMPENSATED SHOCK	UNCOMPENSATED SHOCK	CARDIOGENIC SHOCK
Elevated *or* subnormal temperature	Hypotension	Hypotension
Flushed, warm, dry skin	Tachycardia with thready peripheral pulses	Bradycardia
Widening pulse pressure	Progressive tachypnea	Cool trunk and cold extremities
Tachycardia	Cool, clammy extremities	Pulmonary edema
Tachypnea	Decreased urinary output	Oliguria
Change in mental status—irritability or restlessness		Deterioration of mental status

are present. Multisystem organ failure such as respiratory and renal failure occurs.[13]

Accurate assessment for clinical signs of shock and initiation of appropriate treatments are important nursing functions. The single most important observation that can be made about any potentially critically ill patient is the determination that a patient "looks good" or "looks bad" (Table 12–4).[13] This evaluation requires an experienced bedside clinician because the child may actually look bad before measurable changes in vital signs or laboratory data occur. To assess the child's general appearance, note the child's color, skin perfusion, general responsiveness, and feeding behavior. A well-appearing child has pink nailbeds and mucous membranes and a consistent skin color over the trunk and extremities. Poor systemic perfusion causes pallor and mottling of the skin. With good perfusion, the skin is warm, and capillary refill is brisk. If perfusion is compromised, the skin begins to cool, extremities cool in a peripheral-to-proximal direction as shock progresses, and capillary refill is delayed (>4 to 5 seconds). The child that looks good should be alert and playful and engage in age-appropriate play. The ill-appearing child may be irritable and uninterested in surroundings. As shock progresses, the patient becomes lethargic and difficult to arouse. When assessing infants, their feeding behavior helps determine their overall condition. A healthy infant has a strong suck, whereas the ill infant tires during feeding and has a poor suck.[13]

With the first signs of potential shock, an emergency cart should be made readily available. The intensive care setting may provide the most appropriate care for the child. Blood and other surveillance cultures are obtained, and broad-spectrum antibiotic therapy is started immediately. Adequate oxygenation and good venous access are quickly established. If arterial blood gas values indicate that supplemental oxygen by face mask or nasal cannula is not sufficient, mechanical ventilation is needed. Normal saline intravenous fluids and blood products correct plasma volume deficits and anemia. The patient's hemoglobin level must be within normal limits to maintain oxygen-carrying capacity. A central venous pressure (CVP) line is used to assess the adequacy of volume replacement. If normal blood pressure is not restored with a normal saline solution bolus, dopamine or other vasopressors are needed. Diuretics may be needed if urinary output is inadequate. Electrolyte abnormalities, metabolic acidosis, hypocalcemia, and hypophosphatemia are common during septic shock and require appropriate interventions. In addition, hypoglycemia or hyperglycemia, coagulopathies, and thrombocytopenia may occur. Correction of these abnormalities optimizes cardiac function and metabolic processes.

TABLE 12–4. *Characteristic Clinical Appearance Used to Determine That Child "Looks Good" Versus "Looks Bad"*

CHARACTERISTICS	LOOKS GOOD	LOOKS BAD
Color	Pink mucous membranes and nailbeds	Pale mucous membranes and nailbeds
	Consistent color over trunk and extremities	Mottled color over extremities, trunk
	Instantaneous capillary refill	Prolonged capillary refill
Temperature	Warm trunk, extremities	Cool extremities, then cool trunk (central fever may be present with cool extremities)
Activity, appearance	Alert, responds to parents and therapy (can be distracted with play)	Irritable, then lethargic, ultimately unresponsive even to pain
Infant feeding	Strong suck; eats well	Weak suck, tires easily
		Tires during or refuses feeding

From Hazinski MF. Cardiovascular disorders. In Hazinski MF (ed): Nursing Care of the Critically Ill Child, 2nd ed. St. Louis: Mosby–Year Book, 1992, pp 172–181.

Providing psychosocial support to the child and family is important during this critical time. Emotional support is provided by allowing the family members to verbalize their concerns and by offering frequent updated reports about the child's condition. Although much frantic activity is involved in caring for the child in shock, the emotional needs of the child cannot be overlooked. Major stresses for the child include separation anxiety, loss of control, physical restrictions, and fear of pain caused by invasive procedures. Developmentally appropriate explanations are given to the child. The child should be reassured at frequent intervals. Anxiety can place added stress on the body, with increased demands for oxygen. Patients may also need frequent orientation to day, time, and place because intensive care unit settings can cause disorientation.[16]

SUMMARY

Infection remains a major complication in the treatment of childhood cancer. Understanding the risk factors, assessing for this complication, and initiating appropriate interventions are important functions of the pediatric oncology nurse. In addition, the patient and family must be educated about the prevention of infections and identification of potential problems.

REFERENCES

1. Barry SA. Septic shock: Special needs of patients with cancer. Oncol Nurs Forum 1989; 17:31–35.
2. Barson WJ, Brady MT. Management of infections in children with cancer. Hematol Oncol Clin North Am 1987; 1:801–839.
3. Boggs DR, Wintrobe MM, Cartwright GE, et al. The acute leukemias. Medicine 1962; 41:163.
4. Brandt B. A nursing protocol for the client with neutropenia. Oncol Nurs Forum 1984; 11:24–28.
5. Carlson AC. Infection prophylaxis in the patient with cancer. Oncol Nurs Forum 1985; 12:56–63.
6. deGroan-Hentzen YCE, Gratana JW, Mudde GC, et al. Prevention of primary cytomegalovirus infection in patients with hematologic malignancies by intensive white cell depletion of blood products. Transfusions 1989; 29:757–760.
7. Falloon J, Masur H. Cytomegalovirus and the immunosuppressed patient. In Galasso GJ, Whitley RJ, Merigan TC (eds): Antiviral Agents and Viral Diseases of Man. New York: Raven Press, 1990, pp 669–689.
7a. Freifeld AG, Hathorn JW, Pizzo PA. Infectious complications in the pediatric cancer patient. In Pizzo PA, Poplack DG (eds): Principles and Practice of Pediatric Oncology, 2nd ed. Philadelphia: JB Lippincott, 1993, 987–1020.
8. Frenck R, Kohl S, Pickerin LK. Principles of total care: Infections in children with cancer. In Fernbach DS, Vietti TS (eds): Clinical Pediatric Oncology, 4th ed. St. Louis: Mosby–Year Book, 1991, pp 249–271.
9. Gershon AA. Live attenuated varicella vaccine. Annu Rev Med 1987; 38:41–50.
10. Gershon AA. Live attenuated varicella vaccine. J Pediatr 1987; 110:154–158.
11. Gootenberg JE, Pizzo PA. Optimal management of acute toxicities of therapy. Pediatr Clin North Am 1991; 38:269–288.
12. See reference 7a.
13. Hazinski MF. Cardiovascular disorders. In Hazinski MF (ed): Nursing Care of the Critically Ill Child, 2nd ed. St. Louis: Mosby–Year Book, 1992, pp 172–181.
14. Hughes WT. *Pneumocystis carinii* pneumonia: New approaches to diagnosis, treatment and prevention. Pediatr Infect Dis J 1991; 10:391–399.
15. Kendig EL, Inselman LS. Tuberculosis in children. In Barness LA (ed): Advances in Pediatrics. St. Louis: Mosby–Year Book, 1991, pp 233–254.
16. Mason C. Septic shock. J Assoc Pediatr Oncol Nurses 1987; 4:25–31.
17. McGaw WT, Belch A. Oral complications of acute leukemia: Prophylactic impact of chlorhexidine mouth rinse regimen. Oral Surg Oral Med Oral Pathol 1985; 60:275–280.
18. Pizzo PA, Rubin M, Freifeld A, et al. The child with cancer and infection. II. J Pediatrics 1991; 119:845–857.
19. Pizzo PA, Walsch TJ. Fungal infections in the pediatric cancer patient. Semin Oncol 1990; 17(suppl 6): 6–9.
20. Pizzo PA, Rubin M, Freifeld A, et al. The child with cancer and infection. I. Empiric therapy for fever and neutropenia and preventive strategies. J Pediatr 1991; 119:679–694.
21. Rutledge DN, Holtzclaw BJ. Use of Amphotericin B in immunosuppressed patients with cancer. I. Pharmocology and toxicities. Oncol Nurs Forum 1990; 17:731–736.
22. Rutledge DN, Holtzclaw BJ. Use of Amphotericin B in immunosuppressed patients with cancer. II. Pharmacodynamics and nursing implications. Oncol Nurs Forum 1990; 17:737–742.
23. Saag MS, Dismukes WE. Azole antifungal agents: Emphasis on new triazoles. Antimicrob Agents Chemother 1988; 32:1–8.
24. Saral R. Varicella zoster virus: Clinical manifestations. Nurs Acumen 1991; 3:1, 6.
25. Sauer SN, Atwood P, Sohner D. The challenges of physical care. In Fochtman D, Foley GV (eds): Nursing Care of the Child with Cancer. Boston: Little, Brown & Co, 1982, pp 233–315.
26. United States Department of Health and Human Services. Surveillance of congenital cytomegalovirus disease, 1990–1991. MMWR 1992; 41:35–44.
27. Zackrison LH, Tsou E. *Pneumocystis carinii*: A deadly opportunist. Am Fam Physician 1991; 44:528–541.
28. Ziegler EJ, Fischer CJ Jr, Spring CL, et al. Treatment of gram-negative bacteremia and septic shock with HA-1A human monoclonal antibody against endotoxin. N Engl J Med 1991; 324:429–436.

NURSING MANAGEMENT OF THE CHILD OR ADOLESCENT WITH BLOOD COMPONENT DEFICIENCIES

Mary Kay Foley

Causes for blood component deficiencies in children with cancer include marrow involvement by tumor, marrow suppression as a result of aggressive multidrug chemotherapy or radiation therapy, and/or increased peripheral destruction of blood cells. Before a blood component is administered to a child, a thorough evaluation to determine the cause of the deficiency should be completed. Table 13–1 describes blood components used to correct deficiencies in children with cancer. The use of growth factors may influence the prevalence and severity of blood component deficiencies in the future.

RED BLOOD CELL DEFICIENCY: ANEMIA

Normal hemoglobin levels in children vary with age; however, anemia is defined by a hemoglobin level below 11 g/dl. Approximately 90% of children with cancer develop anemia at some point in the course of their illness.[43] Patients with leukemia or a solid tumor with metastatic involvement of marrow are often anemic at diagnosis. The child with cancer and a low hemoglobin level may also have preexisting iron deficiency anemia.

Children have multiple sites of red blood cell (RBC) production through most of childhood. The bone marrow of most bones produces RBCs until a child is 5 years old, but the marrow of the long bones becomes fatty and produces no more RBCs after approximately the age of 20 years.[22] This has clinical importance for the child receiving radiation to the femur or tibia because RBC production will be reduced significantly by radiation therapy to these sites.

RBC formation is affected in varying degrees, depending on the disease and the intensity of chemotherapy. Production of RBCs is decreased in patients with disease metastatic to bone marrow. Intensive high-dose chemotherapy causes suppression of the bone marrow (myelosuppression) and also decreases RBC formation.

Gradual reduction in hemoglobin level (<7 g/dl) and hematocrit value ($<22\%$) to exceedingly low levels can occur without apparent symptoms as the body adjusts. When the decrease in tissue oxygenation is gradual, compensatory mechanisms such as hyperventilation and increased cardiac output can satisfactorily counterbalance the decreased number of circulating RBCs.[35] Weakness, fa-

TABLE 13—1. *Table of Blood Components*

COMPONENT	APPROXIMATE VOLUME	INDICATIONS
Albumin or plasma protein fraction	5%–25%	Volume expansion, replacement therapy
Cryoprecipitate	15 ml	Hypofibrinogenemia (disseminated intravascular coagulation treatment) Correct certain coagulation deficiencies
Factor concentrate	25 ml	Correct coagulation factor deficiency
Fresh frozen plasma	220 ml	
Frozen and thawed deglycerolized red blood cells (RBCs)	250 ml	Increased RBC mass in patient with antibody problem; frozen RBCs usually from rare donors negative for unusual antigens
Granulocyte-platelet concentrate	220 ml	Provide granulocytes for neutropenic patient with fever and sepsis; usually granulocytes and platelets given together to increase both white blood cells and platelets
Immune serum globulin	Varies	Treatment of hypogammaglobulinemia or agammaglobulinemia; disease prevention; autoimmune thrombocytopenia
Leukocyte-poor RBCs by filtration	200 ml	Increase RBC mass; prevent febrile reactions from leukocyte antibodies; decrease alloimmunization
Platelet apheresis	300 ml (8-unit pheresis pack)	Bleeding due to thrombocytopenia; preferred in multiply transfused pediatric patient
Platelet concentrate (random donor)	50 ml	Bleeding due to thrombocytopenia
Red blood cells	250 ml	Increase RBC mass in patient with symptomatic anemia; usual volume transfused to pediatric patient, 10 ml/kg; 1 U RBCs should increase hematocrit level 3%
Saline solution–washed RBCs	180 ml	Increase RBC mass in patient with allergic reactions to plasma proteins or child with high serum K level
Varicella-zoster immune globulin	1 ml per vial	Provide temporary immunity to varicella; give 1 vial/10 kg within 96 hr of exposure; maximum of five vials
Whole blood	500 ml	Increase RBC mass and plasma volume; rarely used in pediatrics; causes hypervolemia

tique, headaches, shortness of breath, pallor, and weight loss may occur in association with a malignancy with or without anemia. Whether these symptoms are due to anemia or to the malignancy can be difficult to determine. Patients with chronic anemia can be asymptomatic with a hemoglobin level as low as 8 g/dl or less, especially if activity is limited.[15]

Children receiving chemotherapy and regular RBC transfusions have a decreased capacity to compensate for anemia because of depressed erythropoiesis and the inability of older circulating RBCs to increase RBC enzyme production that assists in delivery of oxygen to tissues. In the majority of cancer patients the RBC survival time is 60 to 90 days as compared to 120 days in healthy individuals. Other causes of anemia are splenic sequestration (intrasplenic pooling of large amounts of blood), hemodilution (increased volume of blood plasma), hemolysis (often due to bacterial toxins), inflammation, infection, liver and renal disease, and folate deficiency.

Indications for Transfusion

The most common cause of anemia in children with cancer is lack of new RBC production.[43] Children with a hemoglobin level of 5 to 7 g/dl who are expected to have continuing interference with RBC production from disease or therapy are often electively transfused to maintain a hemoglobin value above that level. Transfusion of RBCs may improve the child's ability to tolerate chemotherapy by relieving the bone marrow of RBC production, thus permitting formation of new granulocytes and platelets. With elective transfusions, the child generally feels better and stronger and has a more adequate reserve of blood should sudden hemorrhage develop. Also in the patient receiving radiotherapy, adequate hemoglobin levels (>10 g/dl) provide better oxygenation of the tissues being irradiated, thus theoretically increasing the effectiveness of treatment.

The following is a helpful guideline in estimating the rise in hemoglobin or hematocrit level after transfusion:

1. 3 ml/kg of packed red blood cells (PRBCs) will increase hemoglobin level by 1 g/dl.

2. 20 ml/kg of PRBCs will increase hematocrit count by 10 points.

Pediatric infusion rates are calculated on the basis of weight, size, and condition of the patient. Patients are usually given 10 to 15 ml/kg of PRBCs. A unit of PRBC contains approximately 250 ml. Understanding all the guidelines and implications involved in the administration of blood products is a nursing responsibility.

Basic knowledge of ABO and Rh typing is required. ABO and Rh typing and an antibody screening test are done on the patient's cross-match specimen. In most cases patients should receive blood products matched for the patient's blood type. Table 13–2 outlines ABO compatibility and is applicable only when blood products containing RBCs will be administered.

The rate of blood loss is an indication of how rapidly the RBCs should be replaced. A whole blood transfusion is rarely indicated. With more gradual reduction in hemoglobin levels, transfusions of packed RBCs are carried out slowly. The standard rate for pediatric RBC transfusions is 2 to 5 ml/kg/hour; hence 1 U of PRBC is generally ordered for administration over 2 to 3 hours. The biggest risk to the patient with chronic anemia is the development of congestive heart failure resulting from a rapid infusion of fluid volume. Children with hemoglobin levels near 5 g/dl may already have mild heart failure as evidenced by fatigue, effort intolerance, anorexia, abdominal pain, and cough.[3] A partial exchange transfusion may be necessary to prevent cardiac failure. Partial exchange transfusion is the repeated administration and withdrawal of small amounts of blood until the RBC component has been increased without administration of excess fluid volume. The nurse's role in the administration of the blood product is very important: regulating the rate; continually observing the patient for any signs of fluid overload; and monitoring vital signs because pulse rate, respiratory rate, and blood pressure are important indicators of fluid status. Vital signs are taken before administration of the PRBC, then every 15 minutes for 1 hour, and then every hour until completion of the transfusion.

Risks of Blood Product Administration

Blood component transfusions pose risks for the patient. Incompatibility, alloimmunization, graft-versus-host disease (GVHD), and potential exposure to infectious diseases are four major hazards associated with blood

TABLE 13–2. *Red Blood Cell Compatibility*

PATIENT RBC TYPE	FREQUENCY OF OCCURRENCE IN GENERAL POPULATION (%)	ANTIBODY PRESENT IN PATIENT	COMPATIBLE RBC TYPE
O	44	Anti-A, Anti-B	O
A	45	Anti-B	A, O
B	8	Anti-A	B, O
AB	3		O, A, B, AB

component transfusion.[29] Improvements in identification of major and minor blood groups have reduced the chances of the child's receiving an incompatible blood transfusion. However, 30 fatal transfusion reactions are reported yearly in the United States.[35] Approximately 1 in 100 transfusions is accompanied by fever, chills, or urticaria, and 1 in 6000 RBC transfusions results in an acute or delayed hemolytic reaction.[22] Transfusion reactions are more common in children who have received multiple transfusions.[43]

Alloimmunization is a frequent problem for children who receive multiple blood transfusions. Despite accurate cross-matching for ABO, Rh, and other major blood group antigens, contaminating leukocytes may have human leukocyte antigens (HLAs) on their surface that are not present in the host. These disparate HLAs can stimulate the production of HLA alloantibodies in the transfusion recipient. These alloantibodies can cause nonhemolytic febrile transfusion reactions and bone marrow transplant rejection.[39] A single transfusion from a future donor to a potential recipient can endanger the marrow graft from that donor.

In a chronically transfused patient it becomes difficult to obtain donor cells to which the patient is not sensitized. This is the major limitation to effective transfusion therapy, especially platelet and granulocyte transfusion, in the child with cancer.[33] Leukocyte filtration is an effective and economic method for reducing alloimmunization.[40] Leukocyte filters used during RBC transfusions remove 90% to 99% of leukocytes simply and effectively.[39] Other methods to decrease alloimmunization include the following[33]:

1. Avoidance of transfusion from family members if a histocompatible family donor is available for marrow transplantation

2. Use of single-donor pheresis products

3. Use of HLA-matched donors if the child is refractory to unrelated single- or random-donor platelets

GVHD may result after administration of blood components containing viable lymphocytes to immunologically compromised patients. In an effort to prevent transfusion-induced GVHD, pediatric oncology patients receiving intensive chemotherapy and/or who are severely immunocompromised should receive only irradiated blood products. A dosage of 1500 to 5000 rads of irradiation to the blood product is recommended.[43] Irradiation eliminates the ability of the T lymphocytes to proliferate without impairment of RBC, platelet, or granulocyte function.[26]

Transmission of infectious disease is another risk of transfusions. Hepatitis, human immunodeficiency virus (HIV), and cytomegalovirus (CMV) are reported as the most significant transmissible diseases.[6,17]

The most prevalent disease causing serious clinical problems is hepatitis.[5] All donor blood currently is tested for hepatitis B surface antigen. However, 90% of posttransfusion hepatitis is due to non-A, non-B (NANB) hepatitis.[36] A screening test for NANB hepatitis, now called *hepatitis C*, is currently performed on all donor blood and may reduce the risk of NANB hepatitis to 1% per unit transfused.[34]

HIV has been transmitted to children by blood component transfusion.[20,29] The risk of HIV transmission has been highest in patients receiving factor VIII concentrates for treatment of hemophilia before 1985[18] (since 1985 all blood donors are tested for antibody to HIV[17]). These patients were exposed to factor concentrates from large pools of donors. Approximately 2% of children with HIV were infected by other blood products such as platelets, RBCs, cryoprecipitate, and plasma.[29] The proportion of acquired immunodeficiency syndrome (AIDS) cases related to transfusion as a mode of exposure in children has declined from 11% to 5.6% during the past decade.[7] Identification of HIV transmission by blood transfusion has led to stricter standards for screening donors and preparing blood products.

Blood donors are carefully screened and excluded from donation if identified as high risk.[36] Technology has developed to inactivate viruses in blood products by using heat, detergent and monoclonal treatment of factor concentrates, and ultraviolet irradiation of cellular blood products.[29] Blood banks have developed directed donor, autologous donor, and designated donor programs. Such programs, when appropriate, allow patients and families an opportunity to participate in obtaining potentially eligible donors. Directed donors complete the same screening and infectious workup as random donors.

Despite screening for antibodies against HIV, transmission of the virus from a seronegative donor is still possible because of the "window" period occurring from the time of exposure to development of antibody.[17] Screening tests may also fail to detect HIV antigens in the window period if mutations occur during replication of the virus.[11] The risk of HIV transmission by blood transfusion is approximately 1:40,000 to 1:1,000,000 per blood component exposure.[36]

CMV infection is a risk to immunosuppressed bone marrow transplant recipients. In allogeneic bone marrow transplantation platelet recovery is delayed when CMV infection is present.[41] Blood products are screened for CMV status in these patients, and CMV-seronegative products are given when appropriate. Leukocyte filtration also decreases the risk of CMV transmission because CMV infects white blood cells (WBCs).[13]

Blood product contamination by bacteria may occur during and after collection of blood. All blood products should be visually checked before transfusion for clots and unusually dark color (indicating hemolysis). Patients are observed for signs and symptoms of septic shock during and after transfusion.[17]

Hyperkalemia may be a complication for the child with renal failure who receives massive transfusions and has an increase in potassium level from the plasma. Using washed RBCs or units less than 7 days old alleviates this risk.[17]

Allergic reactions to blood transfusions are caused by recipient antibodies against plasma proteins in the transfused blood.[36] The symptoms of allergic reaction vary from hives, rash, and urticaria to anaphylaxis. Allergic reactions occur in 1% to 2% of recipients.[36] Most allergic reactions respond to oral or parenteral antihistamines. If symptoms subside after administration of antihistamines, the transfusion is continued. If anaphylaxis occurs, epinephrine and/or steroids are given. The child who experiences an anaphylactic reaction to a blood transfusion should receive washed RBCs.[36] RBCs are washed in normal saline

solution to remove plasma proteins and WBCs.

Volume overload is another risk of blood transfusion. Administration of a large volume of blood or smaller amounts given too rapidly can cause congestive heart failure because of circulatory overload.[29] Children should receive 10 to 15 ml/kg of packed RBCs per transfusion.[38] If the child's hemoglobin level is less than 7 g/dl, the transfusion should be given over 3 to 4 hours.

Nursing Implications

Transfusion reactions can occur from giving incompatible cells in error or because of improper patient identification. The first 15 minutes of blood product administration is the most critical time for RBC hemolytic transfusion reactions to occur. Acute hemolytic transfusion reactions are usually the result of ABO incompatibility.[36] An ABO incompatibility reaction is the most dangerous type for the child and can result in death. Intravascular hemolysis occurs when incompatible donor RBCs are destroyed by antibodies in the recipient's circulation.[17] When infusing PRBCs, whole blood cells, leukocyte-poor RBCs, frozen deglycerolized RBCs, or granulocyte concentrates, begin administration very slowly. Observe the child closely for transfusion reactions, not only in the initial 15 minutes, but periodically throughout the administration of the blood product. If the patient has no untoward reactions after 15 to 20 minutes, begin the ordered rate of infusion.

It is the nurse's responsibility to know the symptoms of transfusion reactions:

1. Hemolytic reaction—restlessness, anxiety, chills, rapid temperature increase, headache, chest pain, dyspnea, lumbar or thigh pain, red urine, nausea, vomiting, pulse increase, blood pressure decrease, oliguria

2. Febrile reaction—chill with increase in temperature, nausea, muscle aching (if child is already febrile, note baseline temperature at start of transfusion; suspect transfusion reaction if temperature increases at least 1° C above baseline)

3. Allergic reaction—rash, hives, facial swelling, respiratory distress

If a transfusion reaction does occur, do the following:

1. Stop the administration of the blood product; change the tubing but keep the intravenous line open with isotonic saline solution or maintenance intravenous fluids.

2. Notify the doctor immediately.

3. Notify the blood bank of the transfusion reaction immediately; obtain the blood specimens necessary for confirmation of the reaction.

4. Send the patient's first urine voided after the transfusion reaction to the blood bank for detection of hemoglobinuria.

5. If symtoms are acute, remain with the patient; monitor blood pressure, pulse, and respiration every 10 minutes; monitor temperature and urinary output each hour.

6. Record in the chart the volume of blood product infused.

7. Save the transfusion tubing and the blood product container and return them to the blood bank.

8. Check identification of the patient and blood bank identification tags to ensure there has been no mistake in identifying the patient or product.

9. Monitor the patient's output for 4 hours after a transfusion reaction to ensure adequate urinary output.

10. Document the transfusion reaction.

PLATELET DEFICIENCY: THROMBOCYTOPENIA

Thrombocytopenia, a decrease in the number of circulating platelets in the peripheral blood, is the principal cause of bleeding in children with cancer. Thrombocytopenia is defined as a platelet count less than 100,000/mm.[3] The three major causes of thrombocytopenia in the child with cancer are (1) decreased production of platelets in association with marrow infiltration by malignant cells; (2) intensive chemotherapy or wide-field radiation, producing transient suppression of megakaryocyte function; and (3) platelet sequestration in various organs (primarily spleen) or destruction in association with widespread activation of the clotting cascade.[19]

The mechanisms responsible for hemorrhage in children with cancer include the following[10]:

1. Quantitative platelet abnormalities
2. Qualitative platelet abnormalities
3. Plasma coagulation factor deficiencies due to decreased synthesis or increased consumption
4. Sepsis and antibiotic-induced platelet dysfunction
5. Neoplastic replacement of marrow

In addition to selected chemotherapy agents, platelet dysfunction is associated with use of several drugs. Aspirin inhibits platelet aggregation. Several antibiotics, including penicillin G, ampicillin, carbenicillin, and ticarcillin, can cause transient platelet dysfunction. Amphotericin B has also been implicated as a cause of transient platelet dysfunction.[43] Antidepressants such as amitriptyline inhibit platelet function.[19] Drugs alter platelet function by prevention of platelet activation and platelet adherence to endothelium.[8]

Nursing Implications

The occurrence of bleeding does not always correlate with the platelet count. There is no specific platelet count level at which bleeding occurs for every child. In general, however, the likelihood of hemorrhage is inversely related to the platelet count. The lower the platelet count, the more severe is the hemorrhage.

It is uncommon for bleeding to occur with platelet counts greater than 50,000/mm[3], and serious bleeding is unusual when the platelet count is greater than 20,000/mm[3].[10] The risk of bleeding is higher in patients with infection, rapid tumor lysis, disseminated intravascular coagulation (DIC), uremia, protracted vomiting, and/or mucositis.[25] Other risk factors associated with bleeding in the child with cancer include the specific disease (e.g., acute promyelocytic leukemia), the degree of marrow replacement by tumor, and the intensity of induction chemotherapy. Minor bleeding episodes evidenced by petechiae, ecchymosis, or microscopic hematuria occur more frequently when the platelet count is less than 20,000/mm[3].[10] Life-threatening hemorrhage, particularly intracranial, is a concern when the platelet count is less than 10,000/mm[3].[38]

Teaching the patient and family measures to reduce the risk of bleeding is important.

The following information will help the patient and family manage during periods of thrombocytopenia[12]:

1. Avoid contact sports and rough activities (e.g., bicycle riding).

2. Adolescents should use an electric shaver rather than a razor.

3. Use a file instead of clipping nails.

4. Use a soft toothbrush and/or swabstick for oral care.

5. Prevent constipation (add stool softeners and increased fiber and fluid in diet if patient can tolerate).

6. Provide a safe environment to prevent falls and bumps (e.g., siderails up, no clutter).

7. Inform dentist of platelet count before dental work.

8. Sexually active adolescents should avoid trauma during sexual relations.

9. Report signs and symptoms of bleeding promptly—bruising; bloody stools, urine, or secretions; nosebleeds or gingival bleeding.

The nurse must frequently assess the child's skin, stools, urine, gums, vomitus, sputum, and nasal secretions for bleeding.[30] Prophylactic antiemetics are useful to minimize nausea and vomiting. Rectal manipulations (i.e., enema, suppository, thermometer) are avoided. Invasive procedures such as intramuscular injections, venipuncture, and bone marrow aspirations are kept to a minimum, and puncture sites are monitored closely afterward for bleeding. Adolescent females may experience increased bleeding during menses.[23] This can be monitored by history and a pad count during menstrual periods. Hormone therapy to inhibit menses may be needed to minimize profound blood loss.[23]

Epistaxis occurs frequently in children, usually in the anterior nasal septum.[30] These nosebleeds stop after pressure is applied. However, nosebleeds from the posterior nasal septum are not stopped by pressure and may require packing. When a nosebleed occurs, the child should be placed in a sitting position and instructed to breathe through the mouth. Firm, constant pressure is applied on the lateral aspects of the nose against the septum.[30]

Platelet transfusion is used to terminate an episode of bleeding or to prevent the development of hemorrhage. The use of prophylactic versus emergent platelet transfusion is an area of controversy.[19] Children with severe thrombocytopenia due to myelosuppressive therapy may benefit from prophylactic platelet transfusion aimed at maintaining the platelet count greater than 20,000 to 50,000/mm³. Thrombocytopenic patients with bleeding need platelet transfusions to maintain a platelet count above 50,000/mm³ and produce hemostasis. However, unless the child is bleeding or is at high risk for hemorrhage (e.g., an allogeneic or autologous bone marrow transplant patient), platelet transfusion should be avoided. Repeated exposure to donor platelet antigens increases the likelihood of alloimmunization.

A platelet unit is defined as the number of platelets normally available in 1 unit of blood. The transfusion of 1 platelet unit usually results in an average increase in the circulating platelet count of approximately 12,000/mm³ in a child with a body surface area of 1 m². The usual platelet dose for pediatric patients is 1 U/10 kg body weight.[36] The life span of the transfused platelets is shortened by the presence of infection, fever, gross bleeding, significant splenomegaly, or platelet antibodies.[29] The nurse must monitor the child's clinical condition and response to the platelet transfusion and observe for signs of bleeding or infection. Vital signs are taken before administration of the platelets, after 15 minutes, and every 30 minutes until the transfusion is completed. A posttransfusion platelet count can document posttransfusion increment.

There are two methods of platelet collection: (1) preparing platelet concentrates from individual units of whole blood by centrifugation and (2) collecting apheresis platelets from a single donor, yielding 6 to 8 units of platelet concentrate. Apheresis platelets obtained from a single donor are recommended for patients receiving multiple transfusions to limit exposure to multiple donors and decrease the risk of infectious disease transmission. Platelet transfusions may also be ordered as *leukocyte poor, irradiated, CMV negative, washed,* or *HLA matched,* depending on the special needs of the child. Table 13–3 provides a guide for understanding the uses for specific platelet products.

A platelet transfusion should be ABO specific if the correct one is available. When ABO-

TABLE 13—3. *Indications for Specific Platelet Products*

PLATELET PRODUCT	INDICATION
Leukocyte poor	Repeated febrile nonhemolytic transfusion reactions
Washed	Repeated minor allergic transfusion reactions or respiratory compromise
CMV negative	CMV seronegative allogeneic bone marrow transplant patients
Irradiated	Severely immunocompromised oncology patients
HLA matched	Alloimmunization

From Fuller AK: Semin Oncol Nurs 1990; 6:123–128.

specific platelets are not available, the plasma suspending the platelets should be ABO specific, or most of the incompatible plasma should be removed.[4] The Rh type of the platelets should be compatible with the patient's Rh type.[4] Rh sensitivity is especially important in an Rh-negative female because Rh-antigen sensitization could affect an Rh-positive fetus in a future pregnancy.

Platelets are always administered through a specific platelet filter administration set. Often this administration set contains a leukocyte depletion filter. Platelets are fragile, and the container should be handled carefully to prevent their destruction. Many mechanical infusion devices have been tested and have not been found to alter platelet function or viability; therefore they are considered safe for platelet transfusion.[42] Platelets should be administered as rapidly as the patient can tolerate (usually over 20 to 30 minutes). Chills, fever, and allergic reactions may occur. These symptoms must be noted and reported promptly. Antihistamines (e.g., diphenhydramine) usually provide symptomatic relief. For a mild reaction the drug may be given orally. If the reaction is severe, the antihistamine should be given intravenously, and discontinuation of the transfusion may be necessary. Prophylactic antihistamines can reduce the number and severity of platelet transfusion reactions. Epinephrine should be available in the event of anaphylaxis.

COAGULATION FACTORS

In the body's defense against bleeding, there are two phases of coagulation. The first phase is referred to as *primary hemostasis*. In this phase blood vessels and platelets interact to form a temporary platelet plug.[28] Coagulation factors are responsible for the second phase of coagulation, referred to as *secondary hemostasis*.

During the second phase of coagulation, plasma proteins (coagulation factors) interact in a sequence of reactions to produce fibrin. Fibrin forms a clot around the primary hemostatic platelet plug. Both primary and secondary hemostasis are necessary for clot formation.[32]

There are 13 coagulation factors, and all but factor VIII are synthesized in the liver. The coagulation factors are divided into three specific groups, which interact to form the coagulation cascade. The coagulation cascade consists of three interacting pathways: the intrinsic, extrinsic, and common.[32]

A child with a dysfunction in secondary hemostasis will develop the following symptoms: ecchymoses, often with an associated hematoma; hematomas; and spontaneous or traumatic hemorrhage into deep tissues, especially muscles and joints.[9] Bleeding may occur simultaneously in any body cavity or from any body orifice.

The partial thromboplastin time (PTT; normal, 25 to 35 seconds) and prothrombin time (PT; normal, 11 to 15 seconds) are initially used to evaluate coagulation function. Coagulation abnormalities in the child with cancer are associated with multiple underlying problems.

Malignancy, liver disease, and/or infection can cause coagulation abnormalities. Drugs are known to affect the hemostatic mechanism. L-asparaginase interferes with fibrinogen synthesis. Aspirin significantly prolongs the bleeding time of healthy persons by altering platelet function.[29]

Vitamin K deficiency may occur after prolonged broad-spectrum antibiotic therapy. Without vitamin K the liver is unable to synthesize coagulation factors correctly. Thrombosis may occur with the use of indwelling catheters such as central lines and venous access ports.

Dilution of clotting factors and platelets during massive transfusion (>6 U PRBCs) can cause dilutional coagulopathy and bleeding.[27] However, it is no longer common practice to transfuse fresh frozen plasma and platelets routinely in this situation. Current practice is to monitor coagulation levels for deficiencies and to replace them as needed.[24]

Nursing Implications

Once the cause of a coagulation disorder is identified, treatment of the disorder and the underlying cause should begin. Treatment of the malignancy, administration of broad-spectrum antibiotics, and correction of the coagulation factors should occur simultaneously.

Fresh frozen plasma is used to correct abnormalities rapidly.[21] Albumin is given as a volume expander if hemorrhage has occurred. If a vitamin K deficiency exists, parenteral vitamin K should be given.

Nursing assessment and documentation of symptoms, treatment, and response are critical in planning care to correct the coagulation abnormality.

Disseminated Intravascular Coagulation

DIC is the most common serious coagulopathy that occurs in cancer patients.[21] DIC is an intricate process resulting from several chemical conditions in which clotting occurs throughout the vascular system.[8] While multiple clots form in the microvasculature of many organs, fibrinolysis causes consumption of clots and clotting factors, resulting in bleeding. DIC is usually associated with shock, sepsis, hemolytic reactions secondary to incompatible transfusion, or malignancy (e.g., acute promyelocytic leukemia).[8]

DIC begins when tissue thromboplastin is released as a result of tissue breakdown, thereby activating the extrinsic pathway of coagulation, or when endothelial damage activates the intrinsic pathway.[8] Excessive coagulation consumes clotting factors and platelets, activating the fibrinolytic system and causing diffuse fibrinolysis. The body becomes unable to respond to vascular or tissue injury by stable clot formation, and bleeding begins. Because coagulation factors and platelets are consumed or prevented from functioning, a cycle of bleeding, clotting, and fibrinolysis continues.

The onset of DIC in a patient with malignancy is usually gradual. The most common presentation is overt bleeding from at least three sites simultaneously. The child may experience epistaxis, gastrointestinal bleeding, ecchymoses, oozing from needle puncture sites, hematuria, and petechiae. Dysfunction of the pulmonary, renal, hepatic, and central nervous system as a result of DIC occurs when microthrombi occlude small vessels.

The laboratory profile associated with DIC includes prolonged PT, low platelet count, and decreased fibrinogen levels (<200 to 400 mg/dl). The measurement of a specific fibrin degradation product (implying both coagulation and fibrinolysis) such as D-dimer is a sensitive indicator of the presence of DIC.[9]

Nursing Implications

In general, the best treatment for pediatric DIC involves aggressive treatment of the triggering disease process. Depleted clotting factors, confirmed by laboratory findings, are replaced by administration of fresh frozen plasma and cryoprecipitate (factor VIII). Platelets are given if the platelet count drops below 20,000/mm³. RBCs are replaced if the child is anemic and symptomatic. Heparin therapy is usually reserved for situations in which thrombosis produces clinical symptomatology or the underlying disease process is not amenable to rapid reversal (e.g., release of tissue thromboplastin in a child with acute promyelocytic leukemia).

The nurse plays a vital role in the assessment of the child's condition. The nurse monitors vital signs, sensorium, intake, output, hydration; administers fluids, electrolytes, blood products; and notes trends in laboratory values. In addition to treating DIC, the nurse continues treatment to eliminate the underlying cause of DIC.

GRANULOCYTE DEFICIENCY: GRANULOCYTOPENIA

Three general types of WBCs, or leukocytes, are found in blood: (1) granulocytes (cells with numerous granules) and the nongranular cells, (2) lymphocytes and (3) monocytes. Neutrophils, the most numerous of the granulocytes, are phagocytic, functioning in the destruction of pathogenic microorganisms and other foreign material.[22] Granulocytopenia is defined as an abnormally low level of granulocytes in the blood (usually <1000 cells/mm³).[38]

Granulocytopenia occurs when bone marrow function is altered by malignancy, its treatment, or both. Deficiency of circulating granulocytes is the most important predisposing factor to infection in the child with cancer.[18]

Granulocyte Transfusion

The use of granulocyte transfusions has declined because of the risk of transfusion-associated complications, development of more effective antibiotics, and lack of effectiveness.[25]

The following are indications for giving a course of granulocyte transfusions in children with chemotherapy- or malignancy-induced severe granulocytopenia (absolute neutrophil count less than 500/mm³) that may last another week but who are expected to recover[29]:

1. Gram-negative septicemia
2. Significant bacterial or fungal infection unresponsive after 48 to 72 hours of appropriate antibiotic or antifungal therapy
3. Infection in a life-threatening parenchymal site
4. Antibiotic-resistant organisms
5. Additional medical abnormalities complicating documented infection
6. Multiple sites of infection

Granulocyte transfusions are given daily for 4 days in a volume of 15 ml/kg collected by leukapheresis. The granulocyte transfusion should be CMV negative, hepatitis B surface antigen negative, erythrocyte compatible, and irradiated.[29] A high incidence of complications is associated with granulocyte transfusions.[1] Fever and chills frequently occur, and other risks include possible pulmonary complications, fluid overload, and alloimmunization.

With the development of colony-stimulating factors such as granulocyte colony-stim-

ulating factor (G-CSF), the need for considering granulocyte transfusion will diminish. Use of G-CSF increases production of neutrophilic granulocytes,[14] stimulates the functional activity of the granulocytes already present,[31] and shortens the duration of severe neutropenia after chemotherapy.

Nursing Implications

Granulocyte transfusions are obtained through the process of leukapheresis in which the WBCs are separated from other blood constituents and collected for transfusion and the remaining blood is returned to the donor. In general, granulocytes should be irradiated before transfusion to kill any immunocompetent lymphocytes and reduce the possibility of transfusion-related GVHD.

The following guidelines should be used when administering granulocyte transfusion[43]:

1. Granulocyte concentrates should be ABO and Rh compatible because of the large number of RBC contaminants.
2. Granulocyte concentrates should be given as soon as possible after collection to minimize cell damage with storage. They should never be refrigerated.
3. A routine 170 µm blood filter should be used, followed by flushing with normal saline solution. Microaggregate filters should *not* be used.
4. Slow transfusion rate (2 to 4 hours) minimizes the incidence and severity of transfusion reactions.
5. Premedication with an antihistamine, acetaminophen, a glucocorticoid, and meperedine helps control chills and temperature elevations.
6. The granulocyte transfusion must be stopped immediately if a severe reaction occurs.

The transfused granulocytes generally go immediately to areas of infection. Administration of both amphotericin B and granulocytes has been associated with fatal pulmonary reactions.[25] If the patient must receive both treatments, they should be administered several hours apart and the granulocytes given slowly and carefully.[25]

Patients may complain of pain in a particular area during the infusion. This may be the result of migration of granulocytes to the infected area, and patient complaints should be noted. Vital signs should be monitored carefully and the patient observed for chills, high fever, urticaria, and variations in pulse and respiration. If symptoms develop during the transfusion, additional diphenhydramine is given intravenously. If the symptoms persist and are especially severe, the transfusion is stopped temporarily, the intravenous line is kept open, and hydrocortisone is given intravenously. The transfusion may be restarted and further reaction evaluated. If the recipient has unusual antibodies directed against the donor cells, a severe transfusion reaction could occur. This is a medical emergency and requires immediate therapy with epinephrine, antihistamines, corticosteroids, and oxygen.

Occasionally a blood component transfusion is refused by the patient or parents because of religious beliefs. A religious doctrine of Jehovah's Witnesses prohibits blood transfusions.[16] Although the courts have permitted adults to refuse transfusions, in all past cases in which a child's life is clearly in danger they have intervened to allow blood transfusion over the religious objection of the parents.[2]

In these cases a petition is made to the appropriate court for judicial declaration that the minor is a "neglected child" and for appointment of a guardian.[2] The petition is filed by a hospital representative, and the medical evidence is presented by the pediatric hematologist documenting the necessity for blood transfusion. This may be done by telephone if necessary. A hospital representative is usually appointed as guardian for the child and has authority to consent to transfusion.

If an adolescent refuses blood transfusion, it is critical to assess his or her understanding of the disease and the risks and benefits of blood transfusion. Recent court cases have affirmed a mature minor's (age 15 to 18 years) right to refuse blood transfusions on religious grounds.[37]

If possible, the use of blood transfusion should be avoided in dissenting adolescents and children whose parents object to blood transfusion because of religious beliefs. The nurse's role in this ethical dilemma is to advocate for the child, assess parental understanding, and coordinate the multidisciplinary team in sensitive management of the dilemma.

REFERENCES

1. Anderson KC, Braine HG. Specialized cell component therapy. Semin Oncol Nurs 1990; 6:140–149.
2. Baush LC. Blood transfusions and the Jehovah's Witness—Neonatal perspectives. Nebr Med J 1991; 76:283–284.
3. Behrman RE. Nelson Textbook of Pediatrics. Philadelphia: WB Saunders, 1992.
4. Butch SH, Coltre MA. Techniques of transfusion. In Kasprisin DO, Luban N (eds): Pediatric Transfusion Medicine, vol 1. Boca Raton, Fla.: CRC Press, 1987, pp 91–137.
5. Centers for Disease Control. Successful strategies in adult immunization. MMWR 1991; 40:700–709.
6. Centers for Disease Control. Surveillance of congenital cytomegalovirus disease, 1990–1991. MMWR 1992; 41:35–39.
7. Centers for Disease Control. Second 100,000 cases of acquired immunodeficiency syndrome—United States, June 1981–December 1991. MMWR 1992; 41:28–29.
8. Cipriano PS, McCance KL. Alterations of leukocyte, lymphoid and hemostatic function. In McCance KL, Huether SE (eds): Pathophysiology: The Biologic Basis for Disease in Adults and Children. St. Louis: CV Mosby, 1990, pp 800–824.
9. Corrigan JJ. Coagulation disorders. In Miller DR (ed): Blood Diseases of Infancy and Childhood. St. Louis: CV Mosby, 1990, pp 837–899.
10. Corrigan JJ. Platelet and vascular disorders. In Miller DR (ed): Blood Diseases of Infancy and Childhood. St. Louis: CV Mosby, 1990, pp 777–836.
11. Crowe S, Mills J. Infections of the immune system. In Stites DP, Terr AI (eds): Basic and Clinical Immunology. Norwalk, Conn.: Appleton & Lange, 1991, pp 697–712.
12. Daeffler RJ. Potential for bleeding. In Daeffler RJ, Petrosino BM (eds): Manual of Oncology Nursing Practice: Nursing Diagnoses and Care. Rockville, Md.: Aspen Publishers, 1990, pp 93–97.
13. De Graan-Hentzen YCE, Gratana JW, Mudde GC, et al. Prevention of primary cytomegalovirus infection in patients with hematologic malignancies by intensive white cell depletion of blood products. Transfusion 1989; 29:757–760.
14. Demetri GD, Griffin JD. Granulocyte-colony stimulating factor and its receptor. Blood 1991; 78:2791–2808.
15. Eiseman B. Perioperative transfusion: An overview. Bethesda, Md.: NIH Perioperative Red Cell Transfusion Consensus Development Conference, 1988, pp 17–18. (Abstract.)
16. Fox V. Caught between religion and medicine. AORN J 1990; 52:131–139.
17. Freedman S, Haisfield ME, Mcguire DB, et al. Nursing considerations in the administration of blood component therapy. Semin Oncol Nurs 1990; 6:155–162.
18. Frenck R, Kohl S, Pickering LK. Principles of total

care: Infections in children with cancer. In Fernbach DJ, Vietti TJ (eds): Clinical Pediatric Oncology, 4th ed. St. Louis: Mosby–Year Book, 1991, pp 249–271.

19. Fuller AK. Platelet transfusion therapy for thrombocytopenia. Semin Oncol Nurs 1990; 6:123–128.
20. Gjerset GF, Clements MJ, Counts RB, et al. Treatment type and amount influenced human immunodeficiency virus seroprevalence of patients with congenital bleeding disorders. Blood 1991; 78:1623–1627.
21. Gobel BH. Plasma and plasma derivative therapy for coagulation disorders. Semin Oncol Nurs 1990; 6:129–135.
22. Guyton AC. Textbook of Medical Physiology. Philadelphia: WB Saunders, 1991.
23. Haeuber D, Spross JA. Alterations in protective mechanisms: Hematopoiesis and bone marrow depression. In Baird SB, McCorkle R, Grant M (eds): Cancer Nursing: A Comprehensive Textbook. Philadelphia: WB Saunders, 1991, pp 759–781.
24. Hazinski MF. Cardiovascular disease. In Hazinski MF (ed): Nursing Care of the Critically Ill Child, 2nd ed. St. Louis: Mosby–Year Book, 1992, pp 117–394.
25. Hutter JJ. Principles of total care: Physiologic support. In Fernbach DJ, Vietti JJ (eds): Clinical Pediatric Oncology, 4th ed. St. Louis: Mosby–Year Book, 1991, pp 231–248.
26. Jassak PF, Godwin J. Blood component therapy. In Baird SB, McCorkle R, Grant M (eds): Cancer Nursing: A Comprehensive Textbook. Philadelphia: WB Saunders, 1991, pp 370–384.
27. Kreis DJ, Baue AE. Clinical Management of Shock. Baltimore: University Park Press, 1984.
28. Larson L. Primary hemostasis. In McKenzie SB (ed): Textbook of Hematology. Philadelphia: Lea & Febiger, 1988, pp 363–379.
29. Luban NLC. Blood groups and blood component transfusion. In Miller DR (ed): Blood Diseases of Infancy and Childhood. St. Louis: CV Mosby, 1990, pp 52–101.
30. Maul-Mellott SK, Adams JN. Childhood Cancer: A Nursing Overview. Boston: Jones & Bartlett Publishers, 1987.
31. McGuire P, Moore K. Recent advances in childhood cancer. Nurs Clin North Am 1990; 25:447-460.
32. McKenzie SB. Secondary hemostasis. In McKenzie SB (ed): Textbook of Hematology. Philadelphia: Lea & Febiger, 1988, pp 381–416.
33. Miller DR, O'Reilly RJ. Aplastic anemia. In Miller DR (ed): Blood Diseases of Infancy and Childhood. St. Louis: CV Mosby, 1990, pp 464–497.
34. National Institutes of Health Consensus Development Conference. Perioperative red blood cell transfusion. JAMA 1988; 260:2700–2703.
35. Pavel JN. Red blood cell transfusion for anemia. Semin Oncol Nurs 1990; 6:117–122.
36. Pisciotto PT (ed). Blood Transfusion Therapy, A Physician's Handbook, 3rd ed. Arlington, Va.: American Association of Blood Banks, 1989, pp 1–105.
37. Rhodes AM. A minor's refusal of treatment. MCN 1990; 15:261.
38. Rostad ME. Current strategies for managing myelosuppression in patients with cancer. Oncol Nurs Forum 1991; 18(suppl):7–15.
39. Sirchia G, Wenz B, Rebulla P, et al. Removal of white cells from red cells by transfusion through a new filter. Transfusion 1990; 30:30–33.
40. Sniecinski I, O'Donnell MR, Nowicki B, et al. Prevention of refractoriness and HLA-alloimmunization using filtered blood products. Blood 1988; 71:1402–1407.
41. Verdonck LF, deGast GC, van Heugten HG, et al. Cytomegalovirus infection causes delayed platelet recovery after bone marrow transplantation. Blood 1991; 78:844–848.
42. Walker RH (ed). Blood transfusion practice. In Walker RH (ed): Technical Manual, 10th ed. Arlington, Va.: American Association of Blood Banks, 1989, pp 287–288.
43. Warkenten PI. Transfusion therapy for the pediatric oncology patient. In Kasprisin DO, Luban N (eds): Pediatric Transfusion Medicine, vol 2. Boca Raton, Fla.: CRC Press, 1987, pp 19–43.

NURSING MANAGEMENT OF PSYCHOSOCIAL CARE NEEDS

Carolyn L. Walker
Linda Wells
Sue P. Heiney
Debra P. Hymovich
DeLois P. Weekes

Just as the physical care needs for each child vary, so the psychosocial needs vary. Each child is at a different developmental stage, and each child, along with his or her family, is confronting different psychosocial concerns. To provide comprehensive nursing care, the oncology nurse must be knowledgeable in assessing, planning, implementing, and evaluating all aspects of patient and family care.

The goal of pediatric oncology nursing is not just to rid the child of cancer but to have both the child and family either maintain or gain a higher level of psychologic functioning. The strengths and weaknesses of each family member must be assessed to individualize psychosocial interventions effectively. Nurses must encourage the child's and the family's expression of thoughts and feelings concerning the diagnosis and treatment, both as a means of establishing a baseline assessment and as a therapeutic intervention.

Interventions that meet psychosocial care needs are developed with respect to the cultural background of the individual family.[177] Identifying each specific cultural variation is beyond the scope of this chapter. In general,

nurses must be sensitive to cultural diversity within the American-born population and to cultural variation within peoples from other lands; furthermore nurses must not stereotype families from a given region, religion, or culture. An assessment is needed to determine the degree to which the family adheres to the values and beliefs of a given culture. Important elements of assessment include the family's education, socioeconomic status, and length of time and degree of enculturation into the resident country's culture.

THEORETIC FRAMEWORK
Stress, Appraisal, and Coping

The term *stress* has been widely used for several centuries with definitions pertinent to both the physical and psychologic sciences. Until the 1960s the major stress theorists investigated what constituted a stressful situation (the stressor) and the physiologic and psychologic reactions of the individual to stress (the stress response).[89,169,170] The work of Lazarus[123] began to shift the emphasis of study from a stimulus-response perspective to a process orientation of psychologically *coping* with stress.

Lazarus and Folkman[125] define psychologic stress as "a particular relationship between the person and the environment that is appraised by the person as taxing or exceeding his or her resources and endangering his or her well being." A *stressor* may be social, cultural, psychologic, physiologic, or a combination of stimuli impinging on the individual. For the stressor to cause stress, the individual must perceive the stressor as a source of threat, harm, loss, or challenge. The mental judgment about a stressor is referred to as *cognitive appraisal*, which is "an evaluative process that determines why and to what extent a particular transaction or series of transactions between the person and environment is stressful."[125] Cognitive appraisal refers to the mental processes that intervene between the encounter with the stressor and the resulting reaction. *Coping* is not a static event but is the "process through which the individual manages the demands of the person-environment relationship that are appraised as stressful and the emotions they generate."[125] The process of coping does not imply success, but effort.

Once the stimulus is judged stressful, the individual performs a secondary appraisal to determine what can or might be done. Once the stressful situation is appraised, the individual uses some form of cognitive and/or behavioral coping effort. Affecting the choice of coping efforts are the individual's personal resources and constraints. Young developmental age or limited life experiences are often constraints on the child's coping efforts. Coping efforts may be problem focused (e.g., learning more about cancer and management of the side effects of treatment), emotion focused (e.g., expressing fears about dying), or a combination of both (e.g., wearing a wig to cover the effects of alopecia and to look the same as one's peers). The results or outcome of the coping efforts are either adaptive or maladaptive.

According to Kitchener's model of cognitive processing,[107] psychosocial responses to the acute and chronic natures of cancer stem from four cognitive appraisal processes: (1) information about self, (2) information about the problem, (3) memory, and (4) information about the goal. Information about the self refers to what the child believes about his or her ability to carry out the necessary strategies to deal successfully with a problem. It also refers to awareness of his or her own feelings, actions, and appearance. Information about the problem refers to information about the nature and structure of the problem (whether it is an acute episode or a chronic remission). Using this information, the child defines the problem, evaluates its level of difficulty, and decides whether he or she has predeveloped strategies for coping with it. Once the problem has been defined, the memory process enables the child to recall strategies used to deal with similar problems in the past. He or she may also remember reading about or seeing others who have dealt with such problems. Information about the goal refers to information about possible approaches or solutions. This information helps the child make decisions about the usefulness of a particular strategy and the likelihood of its bringing about the desired results. Cognitive appraisal focuses on the meaning or significance of the stressor, and it takes place continuously.[125] However, the cognitive processes involved in appraisal are difficult to study in children because of their limited abilities to articulate precisely what they are thinking.

Coping is an interactive process between the person and environment that requires repeated cognitive appraisals leading to an action (cognitive, behavioral, or both) for the purpose of dealing with strong, upsetting emotions and problem resolution. Although the majority of research on coping has been done with adults, several studies with children raise the possibility that the stress, appraisal, and coping process is similar for children and adults[166,174,191]; however, further research, including replication studies, is needed on all age groups.

Lazarus[124] cautions about determining whether a given coping effort is adaptive or maladaptive. Nurses must be acutely aware of their own value system and culture, which can impinge on the determination of what is an adaptive or maladaptive coping effort. For example, one nurse may believe that directly confronting strong emotions is adaptive and therefore will determine that psychologic denial is maladaptive. Lazarus[124] states that the use of denial as a coping effort may indeed be adaptive for one individual (or in one situation) and maladaptive for another. Furthermore, the use of a coping effort is also related to time; that is, denial may be adaptive from a short-term perspective but maladaptive over the long term. When interpreting the benefits or limitations of a coping effort, the perspective of the individual and the function the effort serves (short- or long-term) must be considered. Cultural factors may also affect the choice of coping strategies.

Developmental Theory

In addition to understanding how people cope with stress, an essential framework for working with children and families involves knowledge of normal growth and development throughout the life span. Developmental theory provides the basis for all nurse-child interpersonal communication. Since developmental theory is taught in all nursing schools, only a brief summary is provided here. Piaget's theory of cognitive development[152] and Erikson's theory of psychosocial development[50] are outlined in Tables 14–1 and 14–2, respectively.

Knowing cognitive development theory is instrumental for nurses in understanding how children conceptualize events and how best to explain the disease and treatment. For example, when the nurse tells the child that only a "little bit" of blood is needed and then draws 10 ml of blood in several test tubes, how does a five-year-old child conceptualize the amount of the specimen? Young children perceive the amount in the test tubes as "a lot" of blood and may fear that it is "too much." Children need an explanation grounded in their own experiences. Using Piagetian theory, the nurse could explain that the child has approximately a "half gallon milk carton" worth of blood in his or her body and that the blood specimen is only 2 teaspoons. Since young children do not understand volume well, the nurse needs to demonstrate removing 2 teaspoons of water from an appropriate-sized container. Additionally,

TABLE 14–1. *Jean Piaget's Theory of Cognitive Development*

STAGE	AGE (YR)	CHARACTERISTICS
Sensorimotor	0–2	Immediate perceptual and motor events dominate Interacts actively with environment Develops reflex activity into purposeful actions Develops hand-mouth, eye-hand coordination Learns objects exist when out of sight (object permanence) Learns limits of own body Separates self as person apart from others
Preoperational Preconceptual Intuitive	2–7	Uses language to express thinking Begins to use symbols mentally Thinks egocentrically (e.g., "The sun follows me wherever I go") Uses self as a standard for others Subjective judgments still dominate perceptions
Concrete operational	7–11 or 12	Begins various forms of conservation (holds one-dimension invariant when changes in other dimensions of an object occur) Grasps reversibility of objects (water → steam → water) Can solve concrete problems Organizes objects and events into classes (classification) or along a continuum of increasing values (seriation)
Formal operational	12–15	Can deal with hypothetical-deductive situations Can plan and implement scientific approach to problem solving Systematically handles combinations

Data from references 68a and 168a.

TABLE 14–2. *Erikson's Theory of Psychosocial Development*

STAGE	AGE	CONFLICT
Trust versus mistrust	Infancy	Learns basic trust (feeling of security with self, others, and world in general) or mistrust from person who meets needs for food, comfort, shelter
Autonomy versus shame and doubt	Toddler	Learns independent actions acceptable (autonomy) or unacceptable (shame and doubt)
Initiative versus guilt	Preschool	Explores skills, even to the point of being intrusive (initiative) Believes tasks, questions, actions are inappropriate (guilt)
Industry versus inferiority	School-age	Seeks to master and refine physical, social, and intellectual skills learned in preschool years (industry) or if unable to excel or meet expectations, may want to quit (inferiority)
Identity versus role confusion	Adolescent	Perception of self is internally consistent (identity) or internally inconsistent (role confusion)
		Perception of self is in harmony with perception of others (identity) or is in disagreement with perception of others (role confusion)
		Tries out roles in all areas of life (e.g., moral, intellectual, sexual)
		Uses peer group for reality testing
		Condemns or ridicules those unlike self
Intimacy versus isolation	Young adult	Shares self with others in friendships and love relationships (intimacy) or keeps self uninvolved with others (isolation)

Data from references 68a and 168a.

children should be reassured that their body will make more blood.

Before the age of formal operations, children are not capable of abstract thought. Since most of the concepts relevant to cancer and its treatment are abstract and foreign to children, explanations must be related to their world of experience and in simple concrete terms. Blood running through a vein can be likened to water going through a garden hose. Cancer cells could be understood as an enemy army being tracked down by a good army of chemotherapeutic medicines.

Erikson's psychosocial developmental

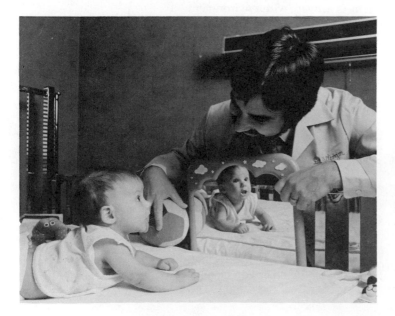

FIGURE 14–1. Encouraging normal development promotes long-term coping. *(Courtesy Sandi Ettinger and others, Center for Cancer and Blood Disorders, Children's Hospital at Richland Memorial, Columbia, South Carolina.)*

theory helps nurses identify age-related developmental tasks. The resolution of some developmental tasks are influenced by nurses in planning and implementing nursing care that fosters the child's successful progression through each stage. For example, an infant's development of trust can be enhanced by encouraging parental presence or performing procedures in a treatment room rather than in the infant's bed. A toddler's or preschooler's autonomy can be encouraged by giving the child choices. A school-age child's sense of industry can be enhanced by his or her mastering the skills needed to perform a central venous line flush. The adolescent's sense of independence can be encouraged by recognizing his or her responsibility for an action or by including the adolescent in decision making.

Cognitive appraisal is also associated with the child's level of cognitive development. According to Piaget and Inhelder,[153] children ages 2 to 7 years engage in preoperational thought in which the world is represented through images and words. Thus it is through imaginative play, questions and talking, listening, and experimentation that the preschool child collects and processes information about self and the world. Preschool children need opportunities to explore and gain experience with pretend objects and situations before they actually experience them. This can be achieved by allowing them time for imaginative play (e.g., with dolls and syringes without needles) and by providing simple answers to their questions. The preschool child typically attributes life qualities to the doll (animistic thought) and through the doll acts out his or her appraisal of procedures such as peripheral chemotherapy and lumbar punctures.

School-age children are capable of conceptual thinking in combination with concrete images.[153] Through the memory process, they integrate information about self, the problem, and the goal to arrive at an appraisal that is associated with a concrete object (e.g., needles used for procedures) or a recurrent aspect of the situation (e.g., being stuck repeatedly for a procedure). Through the same cognitive appraisal processes, adolescents who are capable of hypothetical-deductive thought typically arrive at appraisals that focus on "if, then" scenarios related to desired goals (e.g., if the treatments don't work, I won't be able to spend time with peers, to graduate high school, to drive a car).

IMPACT OF CANCER ON THE CHILD

Despite recent advances in the treatment of pediatric cancers, children with malignancies remain at risk for psychologic dysfunction. Although very few patients develop a major depression or thought disorder,[112] adjustment disorders have been reported.[155] The focus of psychosocial nursing care is to identify stressors or periods of distress and develop ways to mediate such stressors. The long-term goal is to promote the child's mental health and development. The psychologic impact on the child with cancer begins with the shock and disbelief at diagnosis and continues with the discomfort and inconvenience of treatment.[12] These are overlaid with the constant stressor of living with a life-threatening illness.[25] Peak times that are stressful for the child occur at diagnosis, during induction, at completion of therapy, and during relapse. Although some stressors occur or recur throughout treatment, the various stages of treatment often present different areas of concern for the patient.

Phases of Treatment

Diagnosis and Beginning Treatment. The child may begin to feel the impact of cancer on his or her life before diagnosis. The child may have pain and undergo multiple physical examinations, blood tests, and courses of antibiotic therapy before a diagnosis of cancer is suspected. The child may arrive at the pediatric hematology-oncology clinic with preconceived fears and mistrust of hospital staff and treatments. During the diagnostic period, the necessary workup does not alleviate these fears. Instead, the child may develop procedural needle and pain distress that makes further testing and treatment more difficult.

Before the 1970s most children were not told the diagnosis and prognosis in an effort to protect the child from additional anxiety. Waechter's landmark study[190] in 1971 showed that despite not being told, children were usually aware of their diagnosis and prognosis. Furthermore, instead of being protected, these children showed heightened anxiety and isolation. Based on these and other findings, currently once the diagnosis is confirmed, the parents and the child are told the diagnosis. The child's reaction may be disbelief, anger, fear, or frustration, which is exhibited through tears, outbursts of temper, inappropriate laughter or remarks, or even silence. Denial may be so great that the child physically and emotionally turns away from the discussion. Additionally, the child may have greater emotional stress if feelings of fear and apprehension must be masked to protect the parents and other family members. The child's response may change or become more intense as the physician and nurse discuss treatment issues. These emotions are even more heightened as induction, the first phase of treatment, begins.

During induction, the child is faced with a multitude of stressors that arise from the aggressive schedule of treatment and the resultant psychologic distress.[111,162] Stressors related to the actual diagnosis and treatment include pain and invasive procedures.[188]

PAIN AND INVASIVE PROCEDURES. Physical pain caused by the cancer itself may be present before the diagnosis of cancer. That pain is compounded by the diagnostic workup, particularly the pain of invasive procedures such as bone marrow aspirations, lumbar punctures, venipunctures, and surgery.[162,189] Although recent studies have demonstrated the safety and efficacy of intravenous medications for providing conscious sedation for painful procedures,[41,171] psychosocial interventions remain an important component of the nursing care plan. The pain is compounded by an overlay of psychologic stressors, including restraint, fear of the unknown, loss of control, and behavioral reactions. Often the child cannot see what is happening, and the anxiety the child is already experiencing about the procedure may be increased by the fear of the unknown. Not knowing when the procedure will end or how much pain must be endured may increase the child's stress level. Young children have a poor concept of time, and anxiety influences

the child's perception of time. Nursing research has identified strategies for patient teaching that include telling the child what will be seen, heard, felt, and/or smelled.[92] Additionally, other strategies such as distraction, relaxation, or allowing the child some control over the situation may be used to reduce stress.

Anxiety is often the hallmark response to pain associated with diagnosis and treatment of cancer. Behavioral distress is a combination of pain and anxiety and is inversely related to age.[101] Younger children demonstrate more diffuse verbal and physical expressions of distress such as crying, kicking, and biting than do older children and adolescents. In fact, the distress levels of children under 7 years of age are at least five times that of older children and adolescents.[91] The sharp decrease in anxiety and distress between the ages of 6 and 7 years suggests that increased reasoning ability (concrete thought) mediates selected anxiety responses.

Research findings are mixed regarding whether children become less distressed and anxious as a result of experience with procedures,[91] remain the same,[101] or become more anxious.[180] Emotion-focused efforts used by preschool and young school-age children include self-comforting behaviors such as thumb sucking, cuddling a favored object, and engaging in ritualistic behaviors.[32] Problem-focused efforts include withdrawing or attempting to avoid the situation, engaging in imaginative play, and asking questions.[32] Older school-age children and adolescents use efforts such as tense compliance, sleeping, crying, cursing, rigidity, hope and prayer, verbal and cognitive distraction, questioning, attempts to control, and denial.[195,196]

Children and adolescents with cancer report that procedure-related pain and anxiety are the worst problems they face.[205] Adolescents reported that treatment procedures were the most painful, difficult, and anxiety-producing aspects of their cancer experience.[147] Adolescents ages 11 to 19 years perceive and appraise cancer treatments as physically, psychologically, and mentally painful.[195] Physical pain is directly related to needle sticks, especially lumbar punctures and bone marrow aspirations. Mental dis-

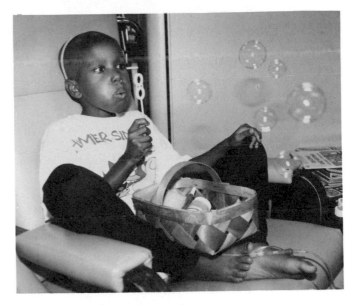

FIGURE 14–2. Practicing blowing bubbles helps the child relax. *(Courtesy Sandi Ettinger and others, Center for Cancer and Blood Disorders, Children's Hospital at Richland Memorial, Columbia, South Carolina.)*

comfort includes thoughts about the pain, which are believed worse than the actual pain.

SURGERY. Some children will have a surgical procedure, either to complete the diagnostic workup, establish staging of the tumor, complete resection of a tumor, or place a central venous catheter. Regardless of the severity of surgery, the patient will experience fears and some degree of pain.[42] Certain types of surgery such as amputation or creation of an ostomy can result in long-term stressors, including loss of function and changes in body image. Occasionally an adolescent's fears appear out of context to an adult; displaying more of a reaction to the cosmetic effect of the incision (how she or he will look in a bathing suit) may indicate that the adolescent is more concerned with the developmental issue of body image than with the meaning of the surgery or cancer.

RADIATION THERAPY. Although noninvasive and painless, radiation treatment may cause the child considerable emotional and physical stress. During simulation and treatment, the child must remain very still on the treatment table. This is a difficult process because concentration is required to prevent movement. The stress is compounded if the child worries about remaining motionless. Another emotional stressor is the stigma of the radiation marks and the misconceptions

about radiation (e.g., becoming "radioactive"). The side effects of radiation therapy may also be stressful and include nausea and vomiting, mucositis, skin reactions, and extreme fatigue.

CHEMOTHERAPY-INDUCED SIDE EFFECTS. Chemotherapy-induced side effects may result in high levels of stress and anxiety throughout treatment. For example, chemotherapy-related nausea and vomiting are aversive experiences,[46,111,189] and painful mucositis is a significant stressor.

Conditioned anxiety in anticipation of the actual treatment is concomitant with recurrent diagnostic and treatment procedures.[99,111] It can manifest as nausea, vomiting, anorexia, withdrawal, or insomnia. For example, some children become nauseated and begin vomiting as soon as the nurse enters the treatment room to set up for the procedure. The best intervention to deal with conditioned anxiety is prevention. Thus appropriate premedications to deal with treatment side effects are given before the side effect occurs.

Hair loss is a common side effect of chemotherapy that creates anxiety for the patient, especially the adolescent. The child may develop a negative self-image and avoid contact with friends, which further increases the sense of isolation and loneliness. Even if the patient is old enough to understand intellectually that the hair will grow back, baldness is a visible reminder that the child is different from the peer group and is still a major stressor.

Depending on treatment center protocol and if colony-stimulating factors are used, chemotherapy-induced neutropenia may require the child to stay away from friends and classmates. Also the child may need to avoid crowds, which means no trips to the movies, shopping, or even a favorite fast food restaurant. These restrictions add to the child's loneliness and sense of separation.

PERCEIVED VULNERABILITY. Perceived vulnerability is associated with acute and chronic aspects of cancer. During periods of exacerbation, the child feels vulnerable because of hospitalization, which evokes dormant fears of death and ultimate separation from parents, friends, and familiar environment.[25] Acute episodes herald frustration and boredom born of waiting for test results, for information, and for people. This precipitates feelings of helplessness, which increase perceived vulnerability. The experience of repeated painful medical treatments also contributes to feelings of vulnerability.

Perceived vulnerability is inextricably bound to the child's appraisal of cancer treatments as taxing or exceeding his or her resources, thus endangering physical well-being (threat related to being stuck with needles) and personal control (competence, autonomy).[25,53,205] Consequently, vulnerability constitutes a major source of stress for the child.

Maintenance. In the maintenance phase of therapy as treatment proceeds, the child faces a different set of challenges related to emergency hospital admissions and restrictions in normal routines. An emergent medical situation requiring hospitalization such as fever and neutropenia may reawaken fears faced at diagnosis. For the toddler or preschooler hospitalization may increase the normal developmental fear of separation or abandonment, whereas in older children the main concern is the disruption of their routine, especially isolation from peers. School-age children miss normal activities such as birthday parties, sporting events, and special school programs. Also older children may not be allowed to

have overnight visits, go on weekend trips, or participate in other peer-involved social events.

Most children are able to return to school or day-care centers on a fairly regular basis once maintenance therapy is begun. Although young school-age children may have some concerns about reactions of peers, both the school-age child and the adolescent worry about their friends' and schoolmates' reactions to the diagnosis, particularly to the loss of hair or other body disfigurement. Children may also be concerned about their grades and ability to compete academically with peers.[161]

UNCERTAINTY. Uncertainty is a lack of information about an event, resulting in an inability to predict an outcome. It is perhaps the most unsettling feature of cancer. Previous uncertainty centered around whether the child would live or die[188]; now it centers more on whether the cancer treatment will or will not bring about remission and cure.[132] Consequently, the children can never be entirely certain when to relax their worries about the appearance of additional problems.[110,126,183,195]

DEVELOPMENTAL ISSUES. Uncertainty extends beyond the question of physical survival; it permeates the entire fabric of the child's life. The unpredictability of onset of acute episodes induces considerable uncertainty about attainment of developmental tasks such as achievement of autonomy.

The struggle between dependence and independence is often exacerbated by the need for reliance on the skills and support of parents, medical and nursing staff, and the health care system.[25] Lability of illness and fluctuation between acute and chronic periods create imbalance in the child's life and require constant redefinition of self-identity (whether to view self as an ill or not ill person). They also necessitate constant change in expected performance ability on the part of both the child and parents. For example, adolescents may perceive their parents as overprotective, as trying to help too much, and as being unwilling to include them in treatment decisions, and this parental overprotectiveness may continue even during periods of chronicity when adolescents can be more autonomous.[147]

Incongruence between the child's actual

performance ability and the parent's perception of his or her ability represents a source of tension and potential conflict within the family that may be attenuated through counseling.[156,183] Parents are counseled to provide opportunities for children to participate in decision making about tasks within the family and to allow graded independence and flexibility.[156] Almost every aspect of cancer treatment has potentially negative implications related to separation-loss and control-compliance.[25] Separation from important people (e.g., peers, family members) and school activities may result in loss of self-identity, self-esteem, academic achievement, and attainment of developmentally appropriate interpersonal relationships. Family relations are altered during times of acute illness by increased dependence on parents and decreased personal control, whereas during remission there is a resurgence of striving for autonomy and independence, often in relation to control of activities of daily living, privacy, relationships with peers and to management of the illness and its treatment.[21,103,165]

Cancer treatments are described as intruding into school activities and peer relationships and causing body changes.[195] Studies indicate that uncertainty about the reaction of peers to changes in physical appearance, the loss of friends, difficulty keeping up with school work, and extreme separation anxiety contributes to disruption in return to school and participation in school-related activities.[45,90,94,103] Side effects of treatment serve as constant reminders that the child is different.[94,101] Body changes may precipitate withdrawal from peers and precipitate anxiety about performance.[94]

Challenging aspects of cancer treatment related to disruption of peer, social, and school activities may in part be explained by Erikson's theory[49] of identity development. Erikson indicates that a sense of identity ensues from interaction with significant others and peers. Significant others aid in the search for personal identity by providing information and feedback about specific behavior and by serving as role models. Adolescents experiencing the effects of cancer treatment may have problems in the area of identity devel-

opment and as a result feel unsure of themselves and others.

Children and adolescents cope with uncertainty by (1) preoccupation with the risk of recurrence, (2) belief that prior treatment provides immunity, thus precluding the possibility of recurrence, or (3) adoption of a "not worrying" stance.[113] Although all three coping postures may be assumed, the attitude of not worrying (which allows escape from distress engendered by matters over which no immediate preventive action may be taken) is perhaps a useful indicator of the child who is coping well with uncertainty. These children also tend to function by attending to day-to-day tasks (e.g., schoolwork, school activities, social activities with peers or sports) and not continuously thinking about their illness.[113,195] Adaptive denial is a coping strategy that calls for a positive, optimistic outlook and filling one's thoughts with daily tasks and concerns rather than with worries about the disease.

End of Therapy and Long-Term Follow-Up. Once the patient has completed the prescribed course of therapy, active treatment is stopped. The younger child is usually delighted. The older child or adolescent may experience ambivalence about completing therapy and may vacillate between happiness over stopping therapy and fear of recurrence. Once the therapy has been completed, the child may be frightened each time he or she feels ill. Routine tests such as computed tomography (CT) scans, bone marrow aspirations, and lumbar punctures may induce apprehension about results. Long-term follow-up may also produce anxiety because children are aware of possible late effects.

POSITIVE ASPECTS OF CANCER AND CANCER TREATMENT. The effects of repeated stressful events may alter sensitivities to stress or modify ways of coping that then protect from harmful effects later on in life.[165] Exposure to and mastery of stressful encounters enhances beliefs about the ability to enact behaviors necessary to produce desired outcomes.[7,48]

The chronically ill adolescent learns (over time) to live with varying degrees of ongoing life disruption and thus develops increased tolerance for stress and change.[105,147,205]

Other positive outcomes of cancer or cancer treatment include (1) the benefits of mastery such as becoming more confident and outgoing after completion of cancer treatment, (2) developing a sense of "I made it, I was tough, I succeeded," (3) a sense of having emerged as a better person who can handle almost anything and who has increased sensitivity to the needs of others, and (4) becoming more religious.[147]

Relapse. A recurrence or relapse of disease causes an intense period of anxiety. The child's focus is on the required treatments, which may be very aggressive and require inpatient treatment. The child may also react to parental distress and have behavioral changes, nightmares, or increased separation anxiety.[54] The same stresses experienced at diagnosis may recur and be even more intense because of negative memories of treatment. If remission is not attained, the child faces additional stressors related to death (see Chapter 16).

Stressors Throughout the Cancer Trajectory

Some common stressors—separation fear, loss of control, and loss of self-image and confidence in one's body—are present throughout the continuum of cancer treatment, from before the time of diagnosis through the off-treatment phase. The life-threatening nature of cancer creates fears of separation and even death, leading to a sense of loss.[12,25] The younger child particularly suffers separation anxiety when parents must leave the hospital for periods of time. The school-age child experiences loss and separation when isolated from friends and school events. Issues of control and competence are present in almost every aspect of the disease and its treatment.

The child with cancer experiences numerous assaults to the sense of control and competence. Basic doubts about competence and self-worth often develop because of major changes in daily routines, body weakness, need for protection from others by isolation, and the inability to keep up with schoolwork. Problems may develop so that the child regresses, abandoning competence achieved at an earlier stage.[25]

Another major area of stress for the child relates to low self-esteem and negative body image. These effects may emerge from a sense of loss over self-image and having a healthy body. The side effects of cancer therapy such as hair loss, acne, weight gain or loss, and body disfigurement affect the child's perceptions of self-worth. These perceptions may be compounded by negative reactions of peers and the previously discussed loss of control. These overall stressors may contribute to the development of major psychologic problems in some children.[25,63,151,155,189,201]

Psychologic Problems

Most children cope with the emotional upheaval related to having cancer and demonstrate not only adaptation but positive psychosocial growth and development. However, a minority of the children develop psychologic problems, including depression, anxiety, sleep disturbances, behavioral problems (including acting out), difficulties in interpersonal relationships, and nonadherence with treatment.[4,47,108,155,173] These issues require intensive interventions by a mental health specialist.[63,151,155,189,201] The nurse's priority concern should be the initiation of strategies to promote adaptive coping efforts.

Assessment

Before initiating any particular strategy, the nurse completes an assessment to assist in choosing appropriate support techniques. The overall assessment determines the child's level of emotional maturity and his or her ability to cope with illness and treatment, which depend on the family situation, the child's age and stage of development, previous experience with illness, hospitalization, and treatment, and personal ego strength.

Assessment Factors. The child's cultural background, family situation, and the general anxiety and distress experienced by the parents influence the child's coping abilities.[139] Extremely stressed parents are less able to meet the child's needs and to encourage coping strategies that result in an adaptive outcome. They may have such a need for support that they have difficulty giving support to the child. The child may feel insecure and act out as an expression of distress.[70] External events may affect the family, or the child's diagnosis may reawaken a previously unresolved crisis. One or both parents may decompensate because of these circumstances.[206] For example, a death in the family may have occurred, or the parents may be getting a divorce; therefore the nurse must carefully explore the family situation. Whatever the cause of the parents' anxiety and distress, the child's adjustment partially depends on the support from parents.[70,111]

Assessment of psychosocial and cognitive development will suggest to the nurse particular conflicts that a child may have at a given age and the limits of the child's cognitive understanding of situations. For example, the toddler focuses on learning control, possesses very basic reasoning skills, and is beginning to play make-believe. The nurse observes the child, listens to verbal expression, and talks with the parents to obtain an accurate assessment. Integrating the assessment into normal care routines is an efficient method. For example, while checking vital signs, the nurse asks the child to explain what is being done and why. Another approach is to ask the child to tell a story. These approaches give valuable clues to the child's stage of development and level of cognitive maturity.

A third factor to assess is the child's previous experiences with illness, hospitalization, and treatment. Asking the child and parent about them helps the nurse understand the child's expectations and determine if misconceptions exist. Particularly, the nurse should ask if the child knows someone who had cancer. The child may have known an elderly person who died from cancer or who experienced severe side effects and may expect the same to happen to him or her. Also, if the child has had positive experiences with doctors and nurses during well-child visits or trips to the dentist, the level of fear may be decreased. The nurse might also ask if the child has seen any television programs about being sick or being in the hospital. The child's perceptions of events are important to understand as the nurse begins to select supportive strategies.

Finally the nurse must attain an understanding of the child's personality and general ego strength. The parents are asked how the child coped in the past to new or different situations such as changing schools or moving. The nurse observes the child in unfamiliar situations. Does the child cringe and avoid the situation or does the child ask questions, look around, and try to understand? In general, the child who has weathered previously stressful situations is better able to cope with the diagnosis and treatment. The child who demonstrates problematic behavior at diagnosis such as difficulty in school, poor peer relations, or poor impulse control may have minimal ego strength from which to draw while coping with this crisis.[128] Such a child may need extra support during treatment.

Differentiating Stress Reactions From Psychopathology. Although the diagnosis and treatment of cancer are very stressful, most children adapt to the situation and exhibit minimal psychologic difficulties, usually having only mild adjustment reactions.[113,155] However, some children, because of preexisting psychosocial situations or particular reactions to drugs, exhibit psychopathology.[4,69,120,201] The nurse has a particular advantage in the early detection of difficulty because of the intimate nature of the contact with the patient and family. Therefore the nurse must be aware of signs of psychopathology and must differentiate them from simple adjustment reactions or stress responses. Stress responses are usually seen as simple regressive behaviors, such as thumb sucking, that improve over time, especially as supportive measures are instituted for the child and parents.

Psychopathologic difficulties include depression, severe anxiety, intractable nausea and vomiting, or psychosis.[25,151,155,189] Problems that warrant follow-up care include severe regressive behaviors such as bed-wetting, declining grades or poor attitude in school, increased fighting with siblings or friends, and school phobia.

If the child's behavior exceeds that expected for a normal stressful experience, further assessment of the child's *a*ffect, *b*ehavior, and *c*ognition (ABC) is warranted.[136] Using this simple ABC formula easily and quickly identifies the child who needs referral to a mental health specialist. To assess affect, determine if the child seems excessively sad or scared. Ask the child if he or she feels "blue" or "down." Asking the child to draw a picture of how he or she feels also yields good results. To assess behavior, observe if the child seems very withdrawn, is having excessive outbursts of temper, is not sleeping or eating well, does not engage in usual play, or is not interacting with others. Observe for signs of hallucinative behaviors such as talking to self, saying strange or unusual things, reaching into the air, or putting hands over his or her ears. Other behaviors might be those not usually seen as normal for the particular age or a disproportionate reaction to a situation.[120] To assess cognition, ask questions to determine mental status, including assessment of the child's orientation and judgment and the presence of psychotic thinking. Ask the child if he or she is having scary thoughts.

The following questions may help determine if referral is needed. Has the problem persisted longer than several weeks? Is the symptom or problem intense? Does the problem increase in the presence of anxiety-producing situations? Has the child's behavior changed significantly from the prediagnosis personality? Is the behavior at great variance to normal development? Does the ABC assessment reveal excessive sadness or the presence of abnormal thoughts? Four or five positive responses to the previous questions warrant further investigation.

A picture of dysfunction is not always easy to identify. To validate the accuracy of the assessment, consult with other team members such as the pediatric social worker or child-life specialist. Their observations may add insight that will aid in assessment. After consultation, the child may be referred to the mental health clinical nurse specialist, child psychologist, child psychiatrist, or behavioral pediatrician.

Mediating the Stress of Diagnosis and Treatment

Especially during the initial period of diagnosis and treatment, patients may be over-whelmed by the myriad of stressors they are facing. The goals of psychosocial support are to encourage ventilation of fears and concerns, increase cognitive understanding of the situation, provide a sense of mastery over the stressors, promote the use of adaptive coping strategies, maintain open communication, promote the child's self-esteem, and develop a supportive network.[12,149,178] To attain these goals, the nurse uses a variety of supportive techniques directed to the individual patient and to groups of patients. Since any single approach may not be appropriate for a specific child, the nurse should be prepared to try several until one is selected that seems to "fit" that particular child. Parents must be involved in any strategy selected for the child, using a collaborative, cooperative approach. Parents also help the child by reinforcing strategies and supporting the child in using a strategy. Serendipitously, parents may benefit from using the strategies, especially relaxation training, themselves.

Individual Approaches. Selecting the appropriate strategy for a particular child depends on the assessment, the stage of treatment, and the identified problem. Approaches effective in decreasing stress and increasing adaptation include communication techniques, education, anticipatory guidance and debriefing, behavioral techniques, expressive therapies such as bibliotherapy, play therapy, and art therapy, and imaginative strategies.[25,96,108] These strategies may be used alone or in various combinations, depending on the nature of the stressor and the individual child.[101]

COMMUNICATION TECHNIQUES. Supportive communication techniques assist the child in labeling feelings and clarifying concerns. Guidelines to keep in mind when talking to the child include to (1) recognize the individuality of the child; (2) match communications to the child's age, level of development, and experience; (3) attend to process over content; (4) be honest; (5) allow the child to express emotions; and (6) permit the child to sort out what is bothering him or her.[178] Communication skills of attending, reflecting, rephrasing, paraphrasing, and naming feelings work well for children. The goals of communication are to develop a trusting relationship so that the child feels comfortable to continue to ask questions and bring up concerns.

EDUCATION, ANTICIPATORY GUIDANCE, AND DEBRIEFING. An important element in coping is cognitive understanding of events. Therefore the nurse must create opportunities to help the child understand what is happening. Explain medical terms, tests, and treatments in simple terms. Use of books and videotapes improves the child's understanding, especially when undergoing unfamiliar procedures. Using puppets or dolls to explain complicated medical procedures such as central venous catheter insertion furthers the child's understanding. Rehearsing procedures or at least verbally "walking the child through" a procedure enhances coping. Telling the child what to expect, clearly indicating the things the child will see, hear, smell, and feel, also provides cues for coping.[92] For example, the nurse might say, "You will lie on a hard table and hear strange sounds." The nurse might add, "When you hear the sounds, think about something you enjoy doing." After the procedure is over, ask the child to describe what happened. This debriefing allows the child to ventilate negative and positive feelings and to identify the effective coping strategies. Also, the nurse is able to clarify areas of concern and reduce possible misconceptions resulting from the child's anxiety.

BEHAVIORAL TECHNIQUES. Behavioral strategies to reduce anxiety and increase coping are derived from behavioral psychotherapy, which posits that problematic behaviors occur as a response to stimuli and that the resulting distress is learned. Simply stated, learned behaviors may be unlearned. The use of positive reinforcement to improve coping is one example of this theory's implementation. A child who has "learned" to be anxious, to cry, and to resist is given a reward for cooperating or helping with a procedure. The reward—a coupon, sticker, toy or trophy—is given to increase the likelihood of future cooperation.[60,197] The tangible reward also is reinforced by praise and positive comments from the nurse and the parents.

EXPRESSIVE THERAPIES. Children engage in a variety of expressive therapies to help them cope more effectively. The benefits of these therapies, regardless of the specific modality, are that the child has an outlet for the expression of feelings and release of tension, may act out psychic problems associated with diagnosis and treatment, may attain a sense of mastery and competence from facing the stressor even symbolically, and may develop insight into the stressor.[60,61,93,158,168] The child may problem solve as he or she plays; thus problems are reworked and fears are allayed.[68] Additionally, expressive therapies are used as a way of assessing the child's understanding and perceptions and gaining access to the child's inner world.[11] These techniques include play therapy, art therapy, story telling, and bibliotherapy.

PLAY THERAPY. Play therapy has been used in child psychotherapy for many years and, with the advent of Petrillo and Sanger's landmark work,[150] has been adapted as a major modality for helping children cope with diagnosis, hospitalization, treatment, and chronic illness. Play therapy may be directive or nondirective. Typically, the child with cancer engages in play therapy to understand treatments and procedures and to work through fears and anxieties associated with the illness.[52] A variety of materials can be used in the play experience, including a play hospital with equipment and supplies, hand puppets, teaching dolls, and medically related flannel boards.[52,56]

ART THERAPY. Art therapy involves using the child's drawings as a means of communicating with the child and helping the child to express inner feelings nonverbally.[163] Through art, the child brings emotional conflicts to resolution, gains self-understanding, and experiences personality change and growth.[193] Encourage the child to draw a picture about being in the hospital, getting treatments, and other situations that can foster self-awareness and personal growth; or simply provide art materials, paper, markers, and crayons and permit the child to draw whatever he or she wishes. This allows the child to project into the drawing fears and concerns without having to face them directly. After the drawing is complete, ask the child to tell about the picture. Thus the child attains some emotional distance from stressful situations and in telling about the picture, may experience mastery. For children who are more in-

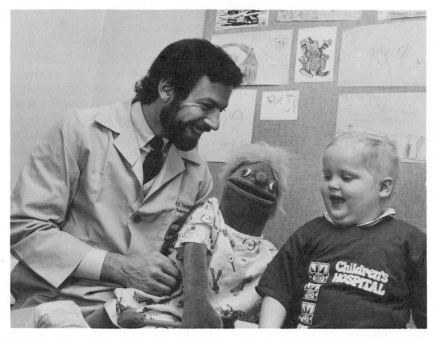

FIGURE 14–3.   Puppets may be used to help prepare patients for procedures. *(Courtesy Sandi Ettinger and others, Center for Cancer and Blood Disorders, Children's Hospital at Richland Memorial, Columbia, South Carolina.)*

hibited, using partially completed pictures that act as incomplete sentences may facilitate expression. For example, draw a key ring and tell the child to draw a picture of what the key fits. These are called *un-coloring books*.

STORYTELLING AND BIBLIOTHERAPY. A variation of expressive therapy that capitalizes on both normal development and the child's imagination is the use of storytelling and bibliotherapy. The child projects his or her own fears and concerns into fictional stories or characters in a book. Additionally, the child attains mastery through symbolic acting out of his or her own fears or identification with the characters in the book or story.[127] More importantly, the child can learn new coping methods for dealing with a particular experience.

Bibliotherapy involves reading the child a story that reflects some of the issues and problems confronting the child. Through the story a process of identification, catharsis, and insight occurs.[39] The theme of the story should be one similar to the difficulties the child is having and should contain positive resolution of fears or problems. The child may project his or her own concerns into the story without

losing any self-esteem by admitting to the fears. Parents may be given books to read and discuss with the child at home. An extensive list of books is included in Fosson and Husban's article,[55] "Bibliotherapy for Hospitalized Children." Often books for younger children can be used with older children by explaining that the child is too old for the book but you need his or her opinion about its usefulness for the younger child.

Storytelling involves encouraging the child to make up his or her own story or telling the child stories made up by the nurse that are similar to the child's situation. Variations to telling a story include writing a television script, acting in a play, putting on a puppet show, or making a videotape.

IMAGINATIVE STRATEGIES. Children have an active fantasy life and easily are engaged in techniques using their imagination. Children are less inhibited than adults and readily play "let's pretend." For this reason children as young as 3 years old are excellent candidates for using imaginative strategies to control anxiety and pain. Relaxation, imagery, and hypnosis capitalize on the natural abilities of children to focus their concentration so strongly that they do not attend to anxiety-producing situations or even pain.[78,145] Although hypnosis requires specialized training, no extensive training is needed to teach children relaxation and imagery.[100] Children naturally move from the imaginative to the real with great ease. The idea is introduced by explaining that the nurse needs the child to do a special part of the procedure or test. Explain that the child will be in control and can take care of himself or herself by using the special "magic" or energy that is inside each person. This magic can help the child control scared or bad feelings. The important focus is to help the child be less fearful. Once the child knows what to do to control fear, the child will be more amenable to helping. The goal is to help the child relax and feel good about his or her ability to help.

Relaxation is accomplished by encouraging the child to begin to breathe very slowly (i.e., breathe in to a count of 3 and breathe out to a count of 6). Children are encouraged to breathe by using blow bubbles, pinwheels, or party blowers. Most children do not like to close their eyes, viewing this as a loss of control or associating it with going to sleep. Instead, encourage the child to watch the stars float down a magic wand or look at a picture in the room. The child is directed to relax specific parts of the body in succession, using elements from progressive relaxation.[15]

Even toddlers can begin to use this strategy. As the child focuses on the breathing, the attention is directed away from the anxiety-producing event.

Once the attention is engaged, the child is encouraged to relax further by playing let's pretend or thinking of a pleasant time such as going to the beach. The child's imagination is used even more by telling a story, taking a special trip on a magic carpet, or seeing a favorite cartoon or television hero on a magic movie screen. The child is asked about favorite times or fun activities, and they can be integrated into the story. Elements of the story should incorporate strength, control, and good feelings.[61,93,168] Similarly, the child is engaged in distracting activities to such an extent that the anxiety-producing event (e.g., venipuncture) is ignored. The nurse or parent might read a pop-up book to the child, do finger plays, sing songs, or say nursery rhymes.[182]

Group Approaches. Participation in a support group has many benefits for the child with cancer. The therapeutic factors of being in a group include catharsis, universality, reality testing, interpersonal learning, and instilling of hope.[202,203] The group provides the child with a forum for ventilation of feelings, for learning coping methods from others, for decreasing loneliness and fear, and for learn-

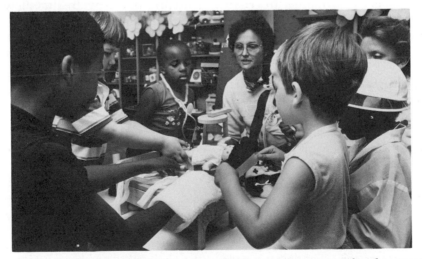

Figure 14–4.   Play group helps younger patients master stresses related to treatment. *(Courtesy Sandi Ettinger and others, Center for Cancer and Blood Disorders, Children's Hospital at Richland Memorial, Columbia, South Carolina.)*

ing realistic aspects about treatment. Through group participation, the child develops insight into concerns, learns new coping strategies, and acquires a sense of responsibility for behavior.[40,198]

Children may be involved in groups as inpatients or as outpatients.[13,67,82,200] Typical goals for the group are to increase a sense of support through peer interaction, decrease the feeling of isolation, promote self-esteem, and increase ventilation of feelings.[74] Children who especially benefit from group participation are those who are newly diagnosed, have relapsed, have a major change in treatment protocol, have undergone extensive hospitalization or surgery, have recently had a bone marrow transplant, or have problems with peer relations. The traumatic nature of these events is shared and discussed so that they become less anxiety producing. The child may learn that other children in the group have had similar feelings and experiences. Through discussion and expressive play, the child gains some mastery over the stressful nature of the events and feels more confident in his or her ability to cope.

Promoting Mental Health and Normal Development

A second overall purpose of psychosocial support is to promote the child's return to normalcy through mental health promotion strategies and fostering of normal development.[121] The nurse assists the child to attain these goals through individual or group approaches.

Individual Approaches. The majority of pediatric cancer therapy is given in an outpatient setting, including the home; therefore the child has more opportunities to participate in age-appropriate activities. However, parents may be so focused on coping with the disease that they fail to initiate these activities or ignore the child's need to master developmental tasks. Encourage parents to engage the child in play that stimulates development. Assess if the child is becoming independent and is learning to function separate from parents. Age-appropriate activities may be included in playroom programs. Exercise pro-

grams, music, and arts and crafts are ways to promote growth and development, even while the child is receiving treatment.

Program Approaches. Recognizing the need to address the child's return to normalcy, programs have been developed that specifically promote the child's independence, mental health, and return to normal functioning. The two most prevalent programs are school reentry and summer camps.

SCHOOL REENTRY. Since school is a major part of a normal child's life, the child with cancer needs to become a productive learner in school.[44] School reentry for the child with cancer presents unique challenges for both the child and family. These challenges include dealing with teachers who may have minimal experience with cancer and with classmates who do not understand the child's problems and the cancer patient's own problems of dealing with a life-threatening illness and the side effects of treatment.[102,160,161] Research studies have focused on ways to help the child reenter the school system and return to his or her prediagnosis level of attendance and achievement.[108,160] Review of these studies identifies the importance of a three-pronged approach to school reentry: communicating directly with school personnel, educating the child's classmates, and determining the child's attitude toward school.

First, direct communication between the pediatric oncology treatment team and the school personnel is critical as the child returns to school. If a school nurse or health educator is available, his or her partnership with the pediatric oncology nurse is critical to assure a positive school reentry. This communication should include medical information about cancer and its effects on the child and the psychosocial impact of cancer on the child and family. Workshops incorporating this information have been successful in enhancing teachers' knowledge about cancer and decreasing their anxieties about working with students with cancer.[5,10,186]

The second important aspect of school reentry is educating the child's classmates. If the classmates understand the disease and side effects of treatment, social acceptance is more likely to occur. Classmate education can

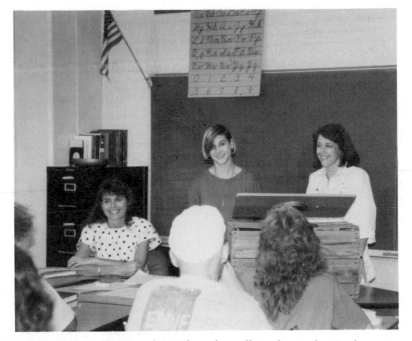

FIGURE 14–5.   Having a nurse and social worker talk to the student's classmates makes school reentry less stressful. *(Courtesy Sandi Ettinger and others, Center for Cancer and Blood Disorders, Children's Hospital at Richland Memorial, Columbia, South Carolina.)*

be accomplished by a member of the pediatric oncology team who talks to the class, by the cancer patient talking to his or her class about the disease, or by the use of puppet shows or videotapes to explain the process.[64,144]

Last, the child's attitude toward school attendance can contribute to the problem of reentry. Changes in appearance, stamina, coordination, and sense of well-being require physical and emotional adjustment and threaten the child's developing self-image and ability to compete successfully with classmates. The child may develop a fear of rejection and/or a fear of an inability to compete and refuse to attend school.[117,122,161] Recent studies of school attendance suggest that even 2 or 3 years after diagnosis, children with cancer miss a critical amount of time from school.[29,160] Attendance problems can be present even if the child and family are enthusiastic about the return to school.[77] Incorporate discussions about school attendance into routine clinic visits. Detailed questions about attendance, grades, peer relationships, and participation in school events can help uncover school problems that the child may

be experiencing.[117] Early recognition of problems may lead to early interventions, making school reentry an easier process for the child with cancer.

CAMPS. Returning to school is one method of normalizing the life of the child with cancer. However, the child needs other opportunities for independence and interaction with people outside the family unit. Summer camps for children with cancer provide the children with a normal childhood experience and a time to enhance their independence.[57] Goals of these camps include providing a normal camping experience for the child with cancer, a week of respite for the parents, a chance to develop a different relationship between patient and medical and nursing staff, and an informal support network for the patient.[57,66] Attainment of these goals often leads to increased self-esteem, increased self-worth, and improved self-image during and after camp.[83,172]

The structure used to accomplish the goals varies from camp to camp, but all of the camps are designed to provide a week of fun and excitement. Regardless of the camp's structure, the majority of the campers return from

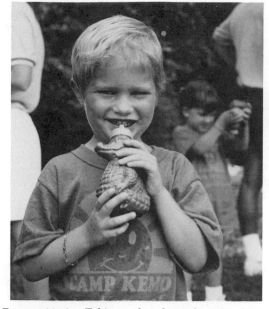

FIGURE 14–6. Taking a break at the zoo during CAMP KEMO. *(Courtesy Sandi Ettinger and others, Center for Cancer and Blood Disorders, Children's Hospital at Richland Memorial, Columbia, South Carolina.)*

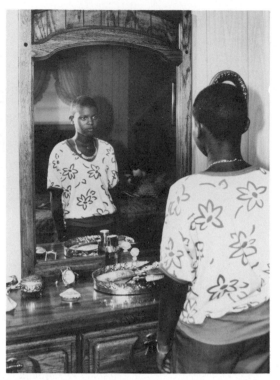

FIGURE 14–7. Hair loss in the adolescent is a major stressor. *(Courtesy Sandi Ettinger and others, Center for Cancer and Blood Disorders, Children's Hospital at Richland Memorial, Columbia, South Carolina.)*

camp with feelings of accomplishment and a host of new friends.

Special Needs of Adolescents

Adolescence is a tumultuous time characterized by conflicts with parents and concerns over peer relations, career, and sexuality.[143,157] The overall tasks of adolescence include the consolidation of identity, psychosexual differentiation, the development of life skills, and emotional separation from parents.[24] During adolescence, peer relations and peer acceptance are of major importance, along with forming close relationships with members of the opposite sex. Even under normal circumstances, the mastery of these tasks is fraught with difficulty. When the diagnosis of cancer is superimposed on these developmental issues, difficulties in coping may arise at any point on the treatment continuum (i.e., from diagnosis through long-term follow-up).

Stressors and Psychological Problems. The adolescent with cancer experiences many of the same stressors as the child diagnosed at an earlier age[146]; yet they may be more difficult to manage because of the adolescent's need to appear normal and to be coping well.[22] Although adolescents may experience situational anxiety, depression, and/or psychogenic reactions, particularly anticipatory nausea and vomiting,[81,104,105,184] overall their adjustment and reactions are within a normal range. As with younger children, the adolescent's challenge is to cope with the many stressors while continuing to deal with normal developmental demands. Major stressors include hair loss and other body changes that may lead to negative feelings about self-image.[205] Intrusive procedures, restrictions in activities, isolation from peers, hospitalizations, and fear of death are ongoing stressors that may cause the adolescent to feel a loss of control. These circumstances cause the adolescent, more than the younger child, to act out by being noncompliant with treatment (e.g., not taking prescribed medications),[12,185,206] taking unnecessary risks (e.g., ignoring precautions when white blood count is low), or having conflictual interpersonal relationships

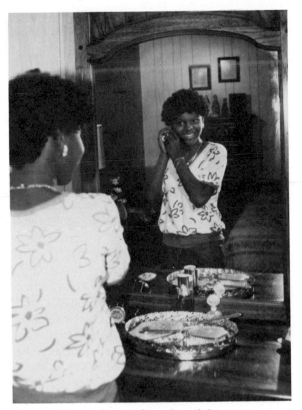

FIGURE 14–8. Persuading the adolescent to wear a wig may improve self-esteem. *(Courtesy Sundi Ettinger and others, Center for Cancer and Blood Disorders, Children's Hospital at Richland Memorial, Columbia, South Carolina.)*

with family, peers, and staff.[105,140] Some adolescents seem to have decreased social adjustment and lowered academic competence and may be unable to look to the future and make plans.[62] Because of the potential for these problems in the adolescent patient, the nurse should identify problems early and initiate interventions that seek to promote the attainment of developmental tasks and adaptation to the illness.[95] These approaches are implemented with the individual patient or in a group setting.

Individual Approaches. A variety of interventions directed to an individual patient may be implemented by nurses. They include working with the family, developing a relationship with the adolescent, and promoting adaptation.

COLLABORATION WITH THE FAMILY. Although adolescents are in the process of emancipation, they should still be viewed as part of a family system. The adolescent's needs for independence must be balanced with an understanding of the influence of the family system and culture on the adolescent's behavior. Collaboration with the parents, while respecting the adolescent's emerging independence, may work best. The parent's concerns must be addressed and fears allayed while allowing the adolescent to have input into care issues. Through a collaborative approach, the nurse is modeling for the parents ways to support the adolescent and get their own parental needs met. The nurse needs to establish clear boundaries between the nurse and parent and the nurse and adolescent. For example, the nurse may indicate that the physical examination will be private. If these boundaries are identified, the adolescent will feel comfortable to ask questions and will not need to feel adversarial toward the parents or the nursing staff. Clear messages about the adolescent's role in decision making should be given. The goal is to achieve a balance between the adolescent's and the parent's needs. This approach is particularly critical in matters involving the adolescent's sexuality.[71]

SUPPORTIVE RELATIONSHIP. To be effective in working with the adolescent, a supportive relationship must be established early. Techniques that may enhance the relationship include showing respect for the adolescent as an individual, listening attentively, using appropriate humor, and being genuine.[130] When the adolescent perceives the nurse is personally involved and committed in the care, the patient is able to use more coping mechanisms and become more hopeful. Therefore the nurse's relationship plays an important role in the adolescent's adaptation to the illness.[79]

ASSESSMENT OF PSYCHOSOCIAL STATUS. As the relationship with the adolescent begins, psychosocial status should be assessed. The nurse must determine the individual concerns of the adolescent. Assessment should include the adolescent's understanding of the illness, perception of his or her body and self, relationship with peers and family, school performance and extracurricular activities, and concerns over life and death.[19,189]

ANTICIPATORY GUIDANCE AND EDUCATION. Although seeming self-contained, the adolescent needs information and guidance about procedures, treatment, and side effects. Additionally, the adolescent needs assistance in mentally rehearsing potentially stressful social situations and how best to handle them. For example, the adolescent may need coaching on going back to school and answering classmates queries. The paradoxical problem is that the adolescent's need to appear competent may prevent asking about the issues. Therefore the nurse may intervene by saying, "By the way, some other teens wonder about . . ." Adolescents may benefit from watching videotapes or reading pamphlets about their illness because doing so may be done in privacy. Increasing the adolescent's cognitive understanding of the illness and treatment increases adaptation.

FACILITATING COPING WITH DIAGNOSIS AND TREATMENT. Assist the adolescent in overall adaptation by encouraging the ventilation of feelings and the use of adaptive coping skills. The adolescent may be hesitant to try relaxation and imagery because of concern over loss of control, misconceptions about the techniques, or a fear of appearing weak. Therefore offer the skills as a way to add to the many coping skills the patient already has. Another adolescent patient might be able to introduce the idea positively and increase acceptance.

An important area to address in helping the adolescent cope is the issue of compliance with treatment protocols. As a preventive measure when teaching is initiated at diagnosis, help the family clarify who is responsible for administering the medication, the parent or the adolescent. Once agreement is reached, teaching should include ways to help the patient take the medicine on time (e.g., use of calendar, pillbox). Also, seek feedback about the adolescent's and parent's satisfaction with the information given. All of these strategies appear to improve compliance with adolescents.[185]

PROMOTION OF COMMUNITY REENTRY AND MAINSTREAMING. The importance of school and community reentry should be discussed at diagnosis so that the goal of normalcy is introduced early. The actual timing of this preparation is based on treatment protocols. Involving the adolescent in discussions and plans for return to school increases the success of this effort and decreases the stress felt by the patient and family.

Group Approaches. The adolescent's ability to cope with the diagnosis and treatment and the reentry into school may be enhanced through group participation.[73] However, not all adolescents are comfortable in a group setting. Although groups largely replace the need for individual counseling, individual approaches such as relaxation training may still be beneficial. The adolescent support group may accomplish the following goals: (1) provide emotional support and understanding about common stresses; (2) promote the sharing of feelings and experiences among the members; (3) build self-esteem by promoting a sense of responsibility and pride in accomplishments; (4) enhance relationships with peers and family; (5) build socialization skills; (6) provide normalizing experiences; and (7) support career development and adult functioning.[3,20,26,75,134]

Activities within a support group may range from having a pizza party to making a videotape. By involving the adolescent in structured activities, anxiety is lessened. Additionally, interpersonal learning and support may emerge from activities and projects. Adolescents may write a newsletter, perform community service projects, visit newly diagnosed patients in the hospital, or attend weekend retreats. Usually, engaging the adolescents in a variety of projects assists in maintaining their interest in the group while helping them learn concrete ways to share and reach out to each other.

PSYCHOSOCIAL IMPACT OF CANCER ON PARENTS

Since children are part of a family system, all family members are affected by the cancer diagnosis. Parents are faced with the burden of coping with their own needs and feelings and with those of their child with cancer and the child's siblings. Like the child, parents experience many simultaneous stressors throughout the different phases of treatment.

There is some evidence that parents cope less well than children with cancer or their siblings.[12] The term *parents* denotes either a mother or a father and is not meant to imply only a married couple.

To help parents cope with their many stressors, nurses are called on to understand the commonalities and differences in coping styles and abilities and to provide support as necessary. Nurses are involved in helping parents meet their needs for trust, information, guidance, support, skills, and resources throughout the course of the illness.[85] At any given time, each parent may be at different stages of grieving and may use different coping strategies.

Parent Stressors and Challenges

Treatment Phases

DIAGNOSIS. The time of diagnosis is a very stressful period for parents. They are unprepared for the diagnosis of cancer, even though they may have suspected something was wrong with their child. Even if parents suspected the nature of the illness, they feel stunned. Parents typically react with profound shock, grief, disbelief, anger, guilt, and numbness.[2]

It is usually best for the physician and nurse together to tell parents the diagnosis in private and give them an opportunity to compose themselves before they return to tell their child. Seeing the parent distraught only adds to the child's fears. The parents may need to leave the hospital to share their concerns and emotions with one another before they are able to see their child. For single parents, finding someone with whom to share their initial feelings may be difficult. If there is not another involved relative, it may be useful for the nurse to help them mobilize an outside support person. The parents' previous means of coping with stress generally will be their initial manner of coping with the knowledge of their child's diagnosis. If usual strategies are perceived as inadequate, new coping strategies will be tried.[38]

Although given information about the probability of long-term survival and even the possibility of cure, parents still cognitively equate cancer with death. Regardless of actual risks quoted to them, parents appraise and interpret the information for themselves as either threatening or reassuring.[133] They may leave the initial conference with the certainty that their child has cancer and will die. Although they may accept the diagnosis intellectually, they are not likely to accept it emotionally.[112,116] Some parents cope by denying the reality of the diagnosis and even seek other opinions in an attempt to reverse it.

In addition to the diagnosis itself, parents are faced with numerous other stressors. While dealing with their own emotions, they must establish a relationship with the unknown oncologist or surgeon to whom they have been referred; settle into a strange hospital; learn about hospital bureaucracy; gain familiarity with medical language while making decisions about treatment options; support their child; and manage their family's life outside the hospital.[33] They must make a series of rapid decisions such as consenting to chemotherapy, surgery, and/or radiation therapy. They fear for their child's life and fear making the wrong decision. If the child is not treated, the child will die; if they agree to treatment, there are no guarantees of survival, and most likely the child will experience uncomfortable side effects.

A major parental task is to learn about their child's illness and treatment. This task creates many stressors for parents because they are given a tremendous amount of verbal and written information about the diagnosis, treatment, and prognosis. Helping them process this information is a major nursing intervention. Although parents need some information immediately, it is unlikely they will retain much of it, and frequent repetitions will be needed. It is essential that parents be told they are not expected to retain all of the information given to them. The nurse's availability when the parents are given the diagnosis can facilitate reinforcement in the following days. Parents should know that nurses, physicians, and social workers are there to repeat and clarify the information given. An offer to help explain the diagnosis and prognosis to other family members usually is appreciated.

The consent for all cancer treatment protocols is lengthy and extensive and involves words and concepts foreign to parents. Parents may not understand the technical information they are given about the treatment regimens and the role of informed consent.[164] Helping parents through the maze of terminology is often difficult because of their limited ability to comprehend so much while still in a state of shock. Reviewing the consent forms at a later date may help parents feel more in control of the situation. Because parents are often asked to consent to procedures and treatments throughout the course of their child's illness, consent is an ongoing process rather than a single event. Help parents understand the terminology as each new consent is required.

Regardless of the degree of knowledge or acceptance, parents are still able to fulfill their parental roles, mobilize themselves fairly rapidly, and act on their child's behalf. They are usually able to continue their parental role by providing their child with comfort, food, and social experiences.[133] As they are appraising the meaning of the diagnosis, they are also appraising their abilities to cope with the illness and care for their child (secondary appraisal). Although the parents are unable to control all events during this period, they do want to be informed and consulted and to participate to the greatest extent possible. Support the parents' strengths in caring for their child. Pointing out how they are helping the child through this period can foster parental self-esteem and confidence.

Parents are faced with multiple stressors and demands: the sick child needs special attention and care, frequent visits to (or remaining in) the hospital or clinic are necessary, and siblings require attention. The family system becomes disorganized as family plans and routines are disrupted. The frequent hospitalizations, cost of medical care, frequent changes in the child's physical condition, and extended parental absences associated with the child's care require alterations in the couple's role definition. For single parents, carrying the burden alone can be stressful, especially if they have no one with whom to share their concerns. Intense emotional focus on the ill child alters the frequency and energy with which family members express caring and support for one another.

A major stressor faced by parents at this time is telling their child about the illness, treatment, and prognosis. Although health care providers encourage openness, it is difficult for some parents to communicate openly with their children, and there is a wide range in the information parents disclose to their children.[34,35] Assess parent-child communication through observation and by asking in nonthreatening ways what parents have told the child and siblings. An important nursing task in helping parents maintain open communication with their children is to provide them with information about how young children think and respond to illness[179,187] and to changes (e.g., short temper, crying, or increased concern about the child's health) in their parents. In addition, point out to parents that children are aware of these changes in their parents and the children need help in understanding that this happens to parents when they worry about their child's health.

During their periods of anxiety and confusion, parents need to trust that their child is receiving the best possible care. Patience, consideration, and acceptance of the parents and their feelings are important. Open, courteous, and honest communication between parents and the health care team is important for parental adjustment and fosters trust in the health team. Cultural differences among families and health care providers may create communication barriers that must be bridged.[86] Unless parents believe they can trust the staff, they will not feel free to communicate openly about their feelings, fears, and hopes.[112] Being accessible, listening, providing individualized information, and providing telephone numbers and ways parents can contact you or other health team members engender trust. All health care team members must instill hope without giving false reassurances. Even when the diagnosis is associated with a poor prognosis, the nurse can reassure the parents that all that can be done will be done. Families need to know that they will not be abandoned.

Rapport established during this period lays the groundwork for support necessary to meet future challenges. Helping parents understand the feelings they are likely to experience is useful regardless of their ability to express those feelings. Helping parents realize that, in time, they will understand the illness and be able to work with the health care system may alleviate some of their initial feelings of fear and insecurity.

Assessment of social support and social networks available to the family should be done as soon as possible.[206] Encourage family members to maintain contact with those who have been helpful in the past, but remember that not all attempts at social support or all social networks are positive.[199] Inform the family of existing cancer support programs within the treatment center or in the community and facilitate contact if requested. These groups provide parents with an opportunity to discuss concerns and decrease their sense of isolation.[76] Insufficient data are available to indicate which parents respond best in a group setting or what group content or structure enhances parent coping and adjustment.[6]

Ongoing assessment of parents' problem-solving abilities is an important nursing role. Parents with effective problem-solving skills need to have them reinforced, whereas those with ineffective skills need additional help to enhance their abilities. Characteristics of effective problem solvers include an understanding of the nature of their child's illness from the outset; ability to communicate their knowledge to all family members, including the ill child; expressions of appropriate concern and sadness; and tolerance of expression of feelings by other family members. In addition, they are able to prepare themselves for the "long haul" and to support one another throughout the course of the illness.[97]

Beginning the necessary teaching early allows parents time to absorb what is being taught and to give return demonstrations of skills learned. It also enhances the parents' sense of control and usefulness while decreasing their sense of helplessness. While performing medical or nursing procedures, reinforce what was previously told and begin teaching the parents skills they will need to care for their child. Having written information and supplementing it with additional notes that parents can take home and study as they are ready facilitates comprehension. To assure that adequate support and information are provided for two-parent or blended families, include all parents. To do this may require juggling schedules of both the parents and the nurses. Because children are discharged as quickly as possible, teaching plans should be set up in both the ambulatory and the inpatient areas. Using checklists of information to impart and planning ways to facilitate communication among inpatient and ambulatory care nurses about their teaching should facilitate continuity between these areas. Having a clinical nurse specialist who can bridge these two areas is another way to facilitate adequate teaching.

Enlisting the assistance of the community health nurse is a nursing responsibility. Community-based nurses can assess family adjustment and the parents' ability to care for their child in the home setting. They can reinforce teaching, clarify questions, and explore concerns within the less-threatening environment of the family's home.

TREATMENT AND REMISSION. Initial treatment is typically begun in the hospital. The time from diagnosis to the start of treatment is brief, usually less than 24 hours. If surgery is required, there are additional stressors for the family.

Parents "search for meaning" as they deal with existential questions such as why this happened to them and their child. They search for an explanation of cause and may blame themselves. They may question their values and come to live one day at a time. They may become less materialistic and more child centered.

Many parents express concern about their ability to meet the challenge of caring for their child at home; however, their ability to manage their child's care gradually increases. Depending on the type of cancer, the child may return home with medications, instructions about side effects of medications or radiation, a central venous catheter or port, dressings from surgery, or any number of physical limitations resulting from the cancer and its treatment.

Parents benefit from discussion of child rearing throughout the treatment phase. Their natural tendency is to ease expectations and requirements of the child. Because the prognosis is good for many children, a discussion of the importance of continuing discipline and limit setting with their child is important. In addition, providing guidance about the child's normal developmental tasks keeps the child's normal developmental needs in focus.

As a result of initial treatments, the majority of children regain the external appearance of health. This is a time of hope for the parents.[112] There is evidence that the treatment modalities, regardless of how intense, are working. Yet parents fear a relapse each time their child suffers from any minor symptom, particularly those first noted at diagnosis. Medical checkups and treatment, even when not physically uncomfortable, are psychologically stressful. Anxiety increases as the family awaits test results because they could invalidate hope that the cancer is still under control.

As treatment progresses, parents begin the task of coping with the demands of a chronic illness. Frequent trips to the treatment center continue to disrupt the family's daily routine. Since many children with cancer are treated at regional cancer centers, many families must commute great distances for treatment, thus significantly increasing the disruption to their lives. During these visits, parents should receive further information about their child's treatment plan and illness. They are more able to assimilate information once the immediate threat to their child's life has been reduced. This is also a time to solidify a strong, trusting relationship between parents and the health care team. Nurses can do this by actively listening to parents, asking how parents are managing on a daily basis, expressing understanding of their difficulties, and providing support and guidance when indicated.

Perceived social support is significantly correlated with parental and child psychosocial adjustment during treatment.[141] Well-meaning relatives and friends, however, may deny the existence of cancer and question the parents for believing it, thus creating a burden of doubt for the parents to endure. Some parents cope by seeking a second opinion, and many isolate themselves from the people who raise their doubts. Asking parents about their contacts with family and friends will facilitate discussion of these issues. Since the relatives and friends who raise these issues

are also the people who could be sources of support, it may be helpful to talk with them.

During cancer treatment, parents come to realize that they are a vital part of the health care team. They are more knowledgeable about the illness and its treatment. Having information allows them to develop skills for interpreting their child's behavioral responses. However, parents vary in their ability to adapt to the changes brought on by the treatment. Although most parents become increasingly aware of their capabilities and become strong advocates for their child, some parents are unable to comprehend fully the needs of their children.[2] These parents need more time to adjust to the illness and benefit from assistance in finding a person (e.g., another family member, close friend) who can assume responsibility for the child's care.[80]

Treatment for the child involves major emotional challenges and stressors for parents. The emotional pain involved, the threat of loss of the child, and substantial practical stresses in day-to-day living affect the whole family as it mobilizes to cope with the crisis.[112] Parents express feelings of sadness, anger, and sometimes guilt during the first few months after the diagnosis.

Parental coping strategies during this period include continued seeking and using of information; managing their child's care at home; managing their emotional responses to the illness; modifying roles, routines, and plans; planning for potential stressors; educating others (extended family, friends, school personnel); and, for some, helping and supporting others such as other parents.[85] A certain level of temporary denial enables families to make necessary adaptations and maintain some sense of equilibrium.[53]

Anger is another common coping response of parents during this period. Their anger may be directed inward or toward their spouse, affected child, other children, and/or health care providers. Nurses can listen to parents without taking sides. When anger appears justified, encourage parents to confront the person directly and perhaps provide suggestions for handling the encounter. Much of the anger parents feel about the diagnosis itself may be displaced on the health team. Evidence that parents are coping successfully during the treatment period includes the ability to maintain a feeling of confidence (sense of self-worth, mastery, and control), maintain emotional and interpersonal equilibrium, and reorganize their lives.[112]

Parents grieve for the loss of their healthy child. In addition, anticipatory grief generally begins after diagnosis and continues throughout much of this period. Anticipatory grieving for the potential loss of their child is a common reaction of most parents. When the prognosis is uncertain, nurses can help parents by facilitating discussion of their concerns and supporting and encouraging their continued involvement in the child's care.

Although most parents of children undergoing invasive procedures are able to provide emotional support and coping guidance to their children during this period, other parents become so "procedure focused" that they are unable to help their children emotionally during the procedure.[30] Help these parents by listening to their concerns, explaining the procedures, correcting misinformation, and providing them with techniques such as relaxation and guided imagery to facilitate their dealing with the procedures. When the parents are ready, they can be given guidance in helping their child during the procedure.

END OF THERAPY AND CURE. The child's coming off therapy can be a particularly stressful time for the parents. They are faced with extreme ambivalence—glad the long phase of treatment is over but fearful that the medication is being discontinued too soon. Medication side effects were evidence that something was being done for their child. Now they must once again wait to see if the child will remain free of the illness or will develop late effects of the treatments or another cancer.

Parents need anticipatory guidance before termination of therapy and continued support during this period. Prepare parents for the feelings they are likely to experience. At this time there is a renewed need to protect and isolate their child, along with continued concern over each new minor symptom. They need frequent reassurance that their child is doing well. Although it is important to understand and support parents in their coping at this time, encourage them to move on with

their lives and to treat the child as normally as possible. Introducing them to parents who have been through this phase is another useful intervention.

LONG TERM SURVIVORS. Parents of children who survive childhood cancer may be at increased risk for psychosocial problems. Studies of parents of children off treatment indicate that they continue to fear their child will die, they do not believe their child is cured,[84] and they do not consider their child normal. They continue to worry about their child's future ability to marry, have children, and be healthy.[87] Parents continue to have financial and professional concerns and express anxiety when their child becomes ill or is scheduled for an annual checkup.[65] Provide parents with information and an opportunity to discuss their concerns. This is also the time to help parents understand their child's continuing need for increasing independence and information as development progresses.

RELAPSE. Relapse is an extremely difficult time for the parents since it resurrects initial fears and threatens hopes for a cure. Relapse shatters illusions, especially regarding the healing powers of the medical team.[181] Parents fear that eventually medical science will run out of treatments to use. They also fear successive treatments because of their increased toxicity and experimental status. Anticipatory grieving may return. Parents generally acknowledge the prognosis intellectually, even though hope persists. The nature of hope often evolves and changes focus throughout the course of the illness.[112] As hope diminishes, parental depression is likely to occur.

Continuing the open communication with and support of parents is essential during this time. Informing parents about available alternative therapy and helping them deal with the implications of the relapse for the child's prognosis must be done with support, compassion, and empathy. Parents need to trust that the medical and nursing staffs are doing all they can for their child.

TERMINAL PHASE AND DEATH. When chemotherapy, surgery, or radiation therapy is no longer beneficial, parents need continuing comfort and support from all members of the team. Care of the child continues, even though it is no longer cure oriented.

Parents are faced with acknowledging their child's impending death while maintaining hope; meeting their daily responsibilities while dealing with their disturbing feelings; and actually caring for, and emotionally providing for, the child while facing death and perhaps becoming emotionally detached. Parents attempt to meet their own needs and those of the other children while focusing their care on the sick child. In addition, they are faced with caring for the child while delegating responsiblity to medical personnel and with trusting the physician while accepting the limitations of medical technology.[59] After death, family relationships and life-style once more undergo alterations with which the parents and other family members must cope.

Providing comfort and support to the child is particularly supportive to the parents. Parents should be informed of alternatives regarding hospital or home death. Although home care is desirable for some families, it may not be the choice of others. Resources such as hospice and bereavement support groups should be identified. Greater discussion of the care of families during the terminal phase is covered in Chapter 16.

Economic Stressors. Although some families have resources to meet the financial obligations imposed by the child's cancer, a substantial number have limited resources. Some evidence suggests that families with lower socioeconomic status have poorer psychologic adjustment than those of higher status.[1] For some families, medical debts continue after the child's treatment ends. In addition, the nonmedical costs incurred are high, sometimes higher than the medical costs. Nonmedical costs include transportation, parking, meals and lodging away from home, telephone calls, gifts for the sick child and siblings, and baby-sitting costs.[18,118] Family savings may dwindle, and parents may have intangible losses such as missing work, having less time and energy to devote to career or salary advancement, or being tied to their current position because they fear losing insur-

ance coverage. They may have to take out loans or second mortgages on their homes to pay their debts.

Assess the adequacy of the family's third-party coverage, availability of community resources, cultural factors, and job-related issues. Nursing intervention includes referral for financial assistance and provision of resources. Parents may need financial aid in the form of assistance for medical and related services or social and counseling services.[154] Parents should be encouraged to keep track of their out-of-pocket expenses because some such as transportation may be deductible on their income taxes.[51]

Maintaining a Normal Family. During remission, the family begins to reestablish equilibrium. Parents need to normalize family life to the extent possible within the limitations imposed by the illness. Such normalization can assure well-being for the child who survives and give parents a sense the child lived as normally as possible if death occurs. Intellectually, parents may be able to accept the philosophy that raising a child normally is important; they may be unable to do so in actual practice. They usually are more lenient and indulgent and generally treat the child somewhat differently from other children in the family. Keeping a consistent approach is difficult because of the guilt they often feel about their child's illness. They are often faced with the dilemma of knowing the difference between drug-induced behavioral changes and behaviors consistent with normal growth and development. Overindulgence and overgenerosity may lead to fear and behavior problems in the sick child and aggravate sibling jealousy.[112]

Discuss the importance of promoting normal development and limit setting and discipline. Helping parents deal with these issues includes reassuring them that guilt feelings are a normal reaction but they are not to blame. Discussing child-rearing issues frequently throughout the course of the child's illness will reinforce their importance and perhaps encourage parents to change at some later date if they were not able to do so right away. Facilitating introduction to other parents may also be helpful.

Husband-Wife Relationship. The presence of cancer in their child brings individual parent coping styles into sharp focus. Both parents are likely to experience different stages of emotional response at different times and become "out of sync" with one another,[112] which can cause difficulty for spouses. Whereas one parent may cope by seeking information and freely expressing emotions, the other may be more reserved. One spouse, often the father, appears contained and controlled, concentrates on work, pays bills, and seems unsympathetic to the other, although he may cry privately. This difference in coping style, or "dis-synchrony," may be experienced as lack of empathy by a spouse.[1] Generally, more effective marital functioning is present when parents have similar problem-solving approaches.[9]

Marital quality and support from one's spouse are directly related to parents' psychologic well-being and ability to care for their child.[9] A history of marital difficulties and lack of support places the family at greater risk for psychosocial distress when coping with cancer. The sick child intrudes in the parents' relationship, and finding time for each other may be very difficult.[58] Assess family relationships and refer families for counseling if they have a history of marital difficulties or are currently having difficulty.

The passage of time and the child's health status may be critical determinants in how favorably parents evaluate their marital relationship.[135] Early in the illness parents work together on the child's behalf. As the child's condition becomes stable and favorable prognosis is likely, the "piled-up" issues of marital conflict rise to the surface and contribute to a sense of marital distress, dissatisfaction, and discord.[9] Approximately 4 to 6 months after diagnosis, the reality of the diagnosis makes its greatest impact, fatigue is present as a result of an intensive treatment regimen, and the flurry of activity abates.[53] Contrary to earlier beliefs, marriages generally survive, and although there may be heightened marital stress, the divorce rate is generally low.[119]

Failure to communicate makes adjustment very difficult and places greater strain on the marriage.[112] Although parents may talk to each other, they also are faced with the dilemma of how open they should be with one another.[131] One parent may wish to protect the other from painful feelings and thus projects an image of strength for the other's benefit. Although many parents report sharing feelings with one another, another relative, friend, or coworker, some parents report keeping their feelings to themselves. Communicating with parents individually and together can facilitate exploration and understanding of each spouse's coping strategies and feelings.

Although there is evidence the effects of childhood cancer on marriage and quality of life are not necessarily debilitating, a minority of parents report negative changes and lack of support from their spouse. Other parents report little change, and some report becoming closer as a consequence of the illness and treatment.[9,112] The sharpest decline in marital satisfaction and increased depression are likely to occur toward the end of the first year for both mothers and fathers.[53] Because relationships are likely to change at various times throughout the course of the child's illness, nurses must continually reassess how parents are doing and provide them with anticipatory guidance about possible fluctuations in marital relationships.

Early psychosocial intervention with parents can greatly promote adaptive coping strategies, for adequate support is needed to facilitate parental adjustment. When nurses develop supportive relationships with families, they also help family members support one another.[112] It is important to help parents take care of themselves because it is in the best interest of the child.[25] Parent support meetings are useful in helping parents to talk out some of their feelings and establish more open communication.[76] Many parents form strong bonds with parents of other children with cancer, thus providing emotional support to each other. Religion is also a source of support for some families.

Single-Parent Concerns. Single parents experience many of the same stressors as married parents and more. Their shock and grief at diagnosis are often borne alone. They may have friends and other family members with whom to talk and from whom to seek emotional support, but those people do not share the same parental bonds with the child as a spouse would. Single parents often state that their friends are simply not available at the times they most need them. The need to assist them in mobilizing a positive social support system and a supportive social network may be profound.

Single parents experience even more disruption in their family life. Whereas a married couple can share the workload of child care, transporting family members to clinic or other activities, and household chores, a single parent must juggle his or her time in doing all these activities while continuing as the family's breadwinner. Additionally, most single parents have less financial flexibility to absorb the out-of-pocket expenses involved in cancer treatment.

Single parents also feel the burden of making treatment decisions either alone or by reestablishing communication with their former mate. Either option creates additional stress. Furthermore, throughout treatment the single parent may have to share precious time with the child with a former spouse and possibly a stepparent. If the former spouse is supportive during the illness, the support usually is appreciated; however, if the former spouse withdraws from the situation, this withdrawal may be experienced as further abandonment. This may compound or reexpose original difficulties encountered in the marriage.

Some single parents are reluctant to join support groups or join in special oncology department activities (e.g., picnics, parties, or family camps) because they feel out of place if the group is composed primarily of married couples. Be sensitive to the single parents' concerns and find appropriate resources to meet their needs.

Extended Family and Friends. Maintaining relationships with extended family members may be problematic. Although some families become closer and offer considerable support, others may be unable to face the child's illness and pull away, and still others want additional support for themselves and create additional stressors for the child's parents.[58] Some grandparents are sources of additional

stress to the parents if they find it difficult to believe the diagnosis. Parents may find themselves forced to support the mourning grandparents rather than receiving comfort and help in their own grief.[112] Other grandparents provide needed resources and emotional support or share their experiences in dealing with similar crises that can enhance the parents' adaptation to the child's illness.

Grandparents may adjust even less well than parents because they lack sufficient information, have limited participation in decision making, and have less responsibility for the child's care.[12] They often feel helpless to provide assistance,[138] and communication problems with the parents may occur. Grandparents suffer two types of grief: for the child who is ill and for their children who are suffering. Behavioral disturbances such as disorganization, disorientation, and poor decision making, already problems in some elderly, may be exaggerated during grief.

For some parents friendships may be difficult to maintain because they have little time and energy for social engagements. Friends may withdraw for a variety of reasons such as fearing contagion, being uncomfortable with discomfort and pain, and feeling unable to help. This withdrawal leads to progressive social isolation among parents.[112]

Neighbors and other community members may display varied responses to the child's diagnosis. Some pry, some turn away, and some make tactless comments or ask inappropriate questions. Others will not let their children play with the child or siblings for fear of contagion or becoming attached to a child who might die. Parents may seek other parents of children with cancer for companionship. Their shared problems and mutual understanding provide a type of support they cannot find from friends, neighbors, or relatives.

Help parents understand the fears and concern of others and provide them with suggestions for communicating with their friends and relatives. In addition, talk directly with the people involved. For example, a meeting can be arranged with the grandparents to explain the child's disease and the impact the child's illness is having on the child's parent and to discuss the grandparents' concerns.

Relationship to the Community. Childhood cancer also creates potential stressors on parental participation in the larger community. Parents may become so involved in their child's care that participation in community activities suffers.[58] However, they should make every effort to continue participation in their prior community activities. Sometimes neighbors ask what they can do to help. Parents need to give specific suggestions (e.g., go grocery shopping, drive a child somewhere, do laundry) to make the help most beneficial. Many people expect parents to remain with their sick child and refrain from engaging in social engagements. Just when they need an opportunity to get out, parents find themselves excluded from invitations.

Many parents find their religious affiliation is a great source of support and solace. They rely on religion through praying, attending church, and seeking religious explanations for the illness. In addition, church members provide tangible resources such as meals, babysitting, and other needed services.

IMPACT OF CANCER ON SIBLINGS

Multiple studies indicate that siblings are a population at risk for anxiety and emotional suffering.[98,129] Studies comparing siblings to the child with cancer found that the siblings showed even more distress than did the patient on several important measures.[28,31,176] The literature clearly indicates that the siblings' needs are not being met adequately and that health care professionals need to identify ways to facilitate coping with the cancer experience.

Family Relationships

Like the patient and parents, the healthy siblings must adjust to multiple changes brought about by the diagnosis of cancer.[31] The first adjustment is often a temporary separation from the patient and parents while the ill child is in the hospital. The mother may stay in the hospital while the father tries to manage work and home responsibilities. Sometimes the father also is at the hospital, necessitating the delegation of care for the healthy siblings to relatives and friends. Understandably, siblings feel varying degrees of abandonment. Even after the patient and parents return home from the hospital, the siblings' needs for parental attention receive low priority. Research and clinical experience consistently identify loss of attention from parents as one of the major stressors for siblings.[31,88,109,114,191]

Major changes in parental roles often alter the roles of the children. If the parent is not available to prepare meals or clean the house, one or more of the healthy children may be asked to assume responsibility for these functions. In addition to functional role changes, interpersonal roles may be altered. For example, a child whose family role was the "socializer" may need to change and become the "supporter." Any change in the child's roles, functions, or expectations within the family system imposes additional stressors for the child.

Although siblings may not be thoroughly informed about financial changes that result from the direct and indirect costs of cancer treatment, they are aware of the impact of finances on their life-style. As parents' financial and emotional resources become more limited, family outings and vacations may be eliminated or severely curtailed.[14] The vacations that do occur are planned around the treatment needs of the ill child. In many families extra money that previously was available for children's activities is now spent on the ill child.

In most families there are coalitions between different members that vary in intensity and flexibility. Two siblings may be inseparable, or one parent may be exceptionally close to one child. When the treatment of cancer in one child leads to a separation between two coalesced members, additional emotional stress may result.

SIBLING BONDS. Siblings share the same cultural background and family value system. They share and compete for their parents' time, interest, and love. Sibling relationships are rarely static and display "varying degrees of loyalty, companionship, rivalry, love, hate, jealousy, and envy."[194] Sibling bonds are a connection at both the public and intimate levels.[8] To a large extent, the emotional bond depends on the degree of access. Similarity in age and sex, common friends, attendance in the same school, and sharing a bedroom and clothing are factors that contribute to "high access" between siblings. "Low-access" siblings have a greater difference in age, friends, and schools, sharing little time, space, and personal history.[8]

Stressors Affecting Siblings

Although stressors arising from the diagnosis and treatment of cancer may be social, cultural, or physiologic in origin, the vast majority that affect the siblings are psychologic.[37]

The overwhelming majority of siblings express feelings of *loss* and of being *deprived* of attention from their parents.[14,36,88,192] The loss of normal parental attention apparently is common among all age groups and may lead to feelings of abandonment. Developmentally, school-age and younger siblings lack the cognitive and emotional maturity to understand that the parents' focus on the ill child is based on medical need rather than a lack of love for them. Siblings experience a sense of loss of their own importance within the family. The ill child receives not only significantly more attention but also receives so many gifts from parents, relatives, and friends that the siblings feel left out and less valued. Many children feel *displaced* if they are forced to live with relatives or friends when the patient is in the hospital.[175] Feelings of displacement may also result from changes in family structure and roles that accompany changes to an illness-centered family system.

Loneliness may result from multiple sources. The patient and one or both parents may be absent from the home, or when they return home, they are often tired or preoccupied, thus leaving the siblings alone to cope with their own thoughts and feelings. Loneliness is heightened by a decreased participation in after school programs when the parents lack the time either to chauffeur or attend the siblings' activities. Siblings typically feel alone with their feelings about the cancer experience. They seldom know another child who has a brother or sister with cancer, so they often state that their friends do not appreciate what they are going through.[14]

Anger toward the patient or parents is a troublesome emotion with which the young child may cope. Children are frightened by their own anger and have limited ways to express it. They are angry with the patient for taking so much of the parents' time and for causing such parental anguish. At the same time they are angry with the parents for their own perceived lack of parental attention. Siblings may not share their anger with the parents; "this reluctance to express anger probably reflects insecurity about their precarious position in the family, a fear that anything they say or do may make things even worse."[28] The expression of anger is also hampered by an appreciation of their parents' burdens and worries. By understanding the patient's and parents' situation, the siblings are unable to assign blame for the family disruption; thus they are left anxious and confused.

Conflicting feelings are distressing to siblings. Young children have difficulty reconciling feeling two opposing emotions simultaneously. They feel empathy and anger toward the parents and patient. At times they have altruistic feelings of wanting to help, yet they are burdened by a sense of responsibility for caring for the ill child. They want to get out and enjoy their own lives but appreciate the limitations that cancer treatment is making on their brother's or sister's life. Confusion, ambivalence, anxiety, and guilt all too often result from the sibling's inability to resolve conflicting emotions.

Guilt is a troublesome emotion for siblings,[16,27] and they often feel guilt that somehow they have caused the cancer. When the patient is immunosuppressed and a sibling gets a cold, the sibling experiences extreme guilt if the patient then becomes ill. Even if the patient escapes an illness, the siblings are afraid that they may cause the patient's death.

It is not uncommon in any family for siblings occasionally to argue or fight. Sometimes in the heat of anger, one sibling may wish another dead. If that sibling later becomes ill with a life-threatening illness, memories of wishing for the sibling's death may cause tremendous guilt feelings.

Many of the thoughts and feelings the siblings experience create a sense of *vulnerability*. Most siblings quickly realize the ill child's frailty and vulnerability to death. Siblings' fear of the patient's death may begin and recur at any point from diagnosis to after therapy is completed.

Coupled with the patient's vulnerability for death, siblings come to appreciate that their own lives are just as vulnerable. There is a fear that if this could happen to someone they know and love, it could happen to them. Until the diagnosis, they thought their parents could protect them from harm. The reality that their parents cannot protect them is unsettling. They are left with a fear of getting sick and a fear of dying. The fear of the patient's death and their own death may be extended to a fear of a parent's death.

A nebulous *sense of danger* surrounds cancer treatment. Adolescent siblings worry about the danger for long-term sequelae from the toxic effects of radiation and chemotherapy. They know that radiation and powerful drugs are harmful. They may have witnessed serious treatment complications such as sepsis or hemorrhage. As medical science moves toward more aggressive and toxic treatment protocols, the siblings' fears of treatment effects and complications likely will increase.

Siblings may feel caught in a *double-bind* situation with their peers. Some siblings do not like it when their friends do not ask how the patient is doing but also resent it when everyone is overly solicitous of the patient and ignores them.

A sense of *isolation* is pervasive for many siblings. They may be highly selective about how, when, and to whom they share information about their sick sibling. They are afraid that friends or teachers will either pity them or engage in gossip. Faced with these equally undesirable alternatives, they may choose to isolate themselves by not sharing information. When the siblings choose to share the experience, they receive varied reactions from responsive empathy to disinterest. Supportive friends are appreciated, and siblings are angry with those who are unresponsive.

Many siblings relate that their parents have *increased expectations* for them. The parents become overprotective of the patient and demonstrate an increased tolerance for bad behavior in the patient while demonstrating the opposite expectations for the healthy sib-lings. Siblings often state that the patient "gets away with anything" while they must be good. The patient is seen as avoiding punishment while they experience an increase in punishment.

Sibling Coping Strategies

Children with cancer and their siblings are children first. One might suppose that all children use the same coping strategies. Indeed there may be core strategies common to all children such as receiving and processing information when confronting a new and stressful situation. However, the experience of personally having cancer or having a sibling with cancer subjects the child to stressors significantly different from those encountered by other children. Until research specifically verifies commonalities, caution must be used in applying findings from one group to another.

Relatively few studies have investigated the coping strategies used by well children,[142,148,166,174,204] and fewer still have specifically examined coping strategies of siblings of children with cancer.[109,192] Two studies identified coping strategies as secondary findings from exploring the illness experience for siblings.[88,114]

The most dominant cognitive coping strategies are related to *receiving and processing information.* Children need information and assistance in processing or understanding that information. Being apprised of the type of cancer and how it will be treated helps foster the siblings' coping and adaptation to all the changes that the diagnosis brings about within their family. Siblings have identified sources of information as videotapes, books, pamphlets, and talking to parents and health care professionals. Assess the siblings' understanding of the ill child's disease and do not wait for the siblings to initiate conversation or ask questions.

Deliberate and conscious attempts to think about a stressor in a different way have been reported by siblings as a means of coping. The technique of *thought stopping* is used by many children when stressful thoughts about the patient and illness are distressing them. Another strategy of *cognitive reframing* is used to think about the stressor in a different, less threatening, way.

Many children report a strategy of *"pep" talk*. With this strategy, children engage in a persuasive argument with themselves regarding why or how things will improve. They attempt to find real or imagined hope for the future. At times there may be elements of empathy in their argument: "When I get all upset that I don't get any attention, I think of what it's like for him."

Not all strategies are conscious attempts to cope with stress. *Denial* and *avoidance* are the child's subconscious attempt to refuse to acknowledge painful reality. Denial may serve to provide distance from the overwhelming impact of the situation. For this reason it is prudent not to strip children of this defense mechanism before they are willing to abandon it.

Regression is another subconscious coping strategy. The child copes with an overpowering stressor by reverting to a previous, more secure, developmental stage. The toddler who was previously quite autonomous may regress to clinging to the parent and have trouble with separation. The school-age child who seemed so sure of himself or herself now seeks parental approval or supervision. Regression is typically a short-term coping strategy used until the child regains a measure of security and confidence.

Solitary or group *play* is a common coping strategy that provides distraction or even a temporary escape from stressors. The child uses play as a means of gaining distance from troublesome emotions.

Many children admit to acting out behaviors as a means of *seeking attention* from their parents. They get in trouble at school, fight with other siblings, or even report getting sick so that their parents will have to pay attention to them. Other children seek attention by doing well in school or doing kind or generous acts to gain parental recognition. Siblings are empathetic to the patient's and parents' situations. To express their empathy, siblings want to be involved in the care of the patient. Performing needed services such as caring for a pet, getting homework assignments from the patient's teacher, or running errands provides the siblings with tangible evidence that they are needed and important and can be helpful.

Emotional expression provides an outlet for coping with a wide range of feelings. Crying when sad or venting anger is therapeutic and assists the child to cope with those emotions. Many children report that they are hesitant to express their emotions in front of the rest of the family, preferring solitude for catharsis.

A major contributor to the siblings' ability to cope with the illness experience is derived from *open communication*. Having someone with whom to talk or to whom to turn is a strategy that often reduces feelings of isolation and despair. In some families siblings do not believe they can talk to their parents, but they find someone else with whom they can communicate.

Another strategy relates to the process of *enduring* or *submitting* to the stressor. The child no longer fights the thoughts or feelings but rather reaches some level of acceptance that "this is just how it is right now." Apparently there is cognitive submission as well as behavioral endurance.

Interventions to Facilitate Coping and Adaptation

To facilitate coping, it is mandatory to develop a supportive relationship with the siblings. Although parents respond well to questions about how the healthy siblings are doing, evaluation of sibling concerns or problems should be based on direct assessment of the child. The parents are understandably preoccupied with the needs of the ill child and may not be observant of the siblings' needs. Meeting the siblings in person and documenting their names and ages clearly reinforces the siblings' importance and allows early preventive or therapeutic measures.[14] Meeting with the siblings soon after diagnosis provides the necessary baseline information for monitoring the physical, psychologic, and social status throughout treatment.[31]

The siblings of a child with cancer need opportunities to express their feelings about the diagnosis and treatment.[14,109] Since many siblings intuitively believe they should not express their emotions in front of the parents because to do so could increase the parents' distress, provide or suggest alternative opportunities for emotional expression or catharsis. Children can express emotions verbally by talking to an empathetic person, writing poetry, composing a song, or writing in a personal journal. Nonverbal expression through physical activity or a wide variety of art forms may help. Sibling drawings coupled with follow-up discussions have been shown to facilitate coping with disease-related and nondisease-related concerns.[159]

Siblings need accurate information about the disease (including causation), treatment, and prognosis from some reliable and sensitive source.[14,31,115,137] When health professionals inform and support the parents, many parents are then capable of relaying the information to the siblings and other family members. Recognize that because of individual emotional responses and varying intellectual capabilities, not all parents can meet the siblings' needs for information in a developmentally appropriate and supportive manner. Nurses and other health care providers must be prepared to assist siblings attain and process information either through individual or group interventions or by offering to be present or to assist parents when they speak to the siblings.

Establishing a sibling support group is one intervention that can address siblings' desire for disease-related information; a place for emotional expression; a place to receive attention and feel that their concerns are important too; support and identification with other children who are facing similar issues; developing their own identity; and decreasing the sense of isolation. Although several reports attest to the value of support groups for siblings,[43,72,106] only one study investigated the effects of group participation on sibling social adjustment.[72] Research into the short- and long-term effects of sibling support groups is needed.

Provide pivotal support for liberal sibling visitation policies, both while the patient is hospitalized and during outpatient care, and encourage contact between siblings, even when regular hospital visits are not possible. The siblings at home can maintain bonds with the patient by telephone calls, letters, exchanging audiotape recorded messages, and if resources are available, videotaped messages.

Open communication within the family has been cited as desirable and necessary for long-term adaptation for the child with cancer and the parents, but the findings for siblings have been mixed. Some siblings demonstrate an improved sense of well-being, whereas others appear more distressed.[17] The communication pattern in each family must be assessed to determine the degree of "openness" allowed. It may be that the change from a closed communication pattern to an open one is as or more distressing to the sibling than the actual communicated message. It may be helpful to maintain a more typical pattern of communication with siblings while assisting the parents to develop a more open communication pattern.

Teach parents to redirect some parental attention to the siblings. Sharing information with all family members can be encouraged by teaching parents how to interpret coping strategies, initiate discussions, and legitimize and acknowledge reasonable negative effects.[31] Parents must be taught what is known about stressors affecting siblings and ways children cope with stress so they can respond appropriately to their children.[23] Because few young children will ask spontaneous questions about emotionally sensitive issues, parents must be taught how to initiate such discussions.

Because so many siblings are fearful about how best to respond to questions posed by people outside of the family, either provide anticipatory guidance for the siblings or teach the parents to do so.[137] Siblings and parents should be forewarned that some people will ask only vague general questions and others will ask tactless, blunt, or probing questions. Family members need to know that seemingly insensitive remarks are usually a reflection of the person's distress over the diagnosis rather than a lack of caring.

Some treatment centers are exploring ways either to incorporate the siblings into the patients' summer camp, have a separate camp just for siblings, or have family camp weekends for all family members. It is very beneficial for the siblings to have a chance to relate to other children who also have a sibling living with cancer.

The sibling facing or experiencing the death of a brother or sister will benefit from emotional support provided by more than just the parents. The parents are struggling to deal with their own personal emotions and may have little emotional energy left to assist or be supportive of the siblings.

The goal of sibling care is to have siblings emotionally grow and develop while living through and beyond the cancer experience. Perhaps in the future professionals will talk not about the "truly cured child" but about the "truly cured family," for to cure the child who is ill and leave in the wake emotionally scarred siblings is equivalent to winning the battle but losing the war.

REFERENCES

1. Adams-Greenly M. Psychological staging of pediatric cancer patients and their families. Cancer 1986; 58:449–453.
2. Ahmed P. Living and Dying With Cancer. St. Louis: CV Mosby, 1981.
3. Altshuler A, Seidl A. Teen meetings: A way to help adolescents cope with hospitalization. MCN 1977; 2:348–353.
4. Armstrong G, Wirt R, Nesbit M, et al. Multidimensional assessment of psychological problems in children with cancer. Res Nurs Health 1982; 5:205–211.
5. Axelrod P. Cancer in the school-age child: The teacher's role in the return to the classroom. NC Med J 1986; 47:475–478.
6. Bakke K, Pomietto M. Family care when a child has late stage cancer: A research review. Oncol Nurs Forum 1986; 13:71–76.
7. Bandura A. Self-efficacy: Toward a unifying theory of behavioral change. Psychol Rev 1977; 84:191–215.
8. Bank SP, Kahn MD. The Sibling Bonds. New York: Basic Books, 1980.
9. Barbarin OA, Hughs D, Chesler MA. Stress coping and marital functioning among parents of children with cancer. J Marriage Fam 1985; 47:473–480.
10. Baskin C, Saylor C, Furey W, et al. Helping teachers help children with cancer: A workshop for school personnel. Child Health Care 1983; 12:78–83.
11. Bassin D, Wolle K, Their A. Children's reactions to psychiatric hospitalization: Drawings and storytelling as a data base. Art Psychother 1983; 10:33–44.
12. Baum BJ, Baum ES. Psychological challenges of childhood cancer. J Psychosoc Oncol 1989; 7:119–129.
13. Beck L, Lattimer J, Braun E. Group psychotherapy on a children's oncology service. Soc Work Health Care 1979; 4:275–285.
14. Bendor SJ. Anxiety and isolation in siblings of pediatric cancer patients: The need for prevention. Soc Work Health Care 1990; 14:17–35.
15. Benson H, Klipper M. The Relaxation Response. New York: William Morrow, 1976.
16. Binger C, Albin A, Feuerstein R, et al. Childhood leukemia: Emotional impact on patient and family. N Engl J Med 1969; 280:414–418.
17. Birenbaum LK. The relationship between parent-sibling communication and coping of siblings with death experience. J Pediatr Oncol Nurs 1989; 6:86–91.
18. Bloom BS, Knoor RS, Evans AE. The epidemiology of disease expenses: The costs of caring for a child with cancer. 1980; JAMA 253:1032–1035.
19. Blotcky A, Cohen D. Psychological assessment of the adolescent with cancer. J Assoc Pediatr Oncol Nurses 1985; 2:8–14.
20. Blum R, Chang P. A group for adolescents facing chronic and terminal illness. J Curr Adolesc Med 1981; 6:7–12.
21. Blum RW. Illness and Disabilities in Childhood and Adolescence. San Francisco: Grune & Stratton, 1984.
22. Bosworth T. Leukemia through a teenager's eyes. MCN 1989; 14:93–94.
23. Brett KM, Davies EM. What does it mean? Sibling and parental appraisals of childhood leukemia. Cancer Nurs 1988; 11:329–338.
24. Bru G. Adolescent and young adulthood. Cancer Nurs 1985; 8(suppl 1):21–24.
25. Brunnquell D, Hall MD. Issues in the psychological care of pediatric oncology patients. Am J Orthopsychiatry 1982; 52:32–44.
26. Byrne C, Stockwell M, Gudelis S. Adolescent support groups in oncology. Oncol Nurs Forum 1984; 11:26–40.
27. Cain A, Fast I, Erickson M. Children's disturbed reactions to the death of a sibling. Am J Orthopsychiatry 1964; 34:741–752.
28. Cairns N, Clark G, Smith S, et al. Adaptation of a sibling to childhood malignancy. J Pediatr 1979; 95:484–487.
29. Cairns N, Klopovich P, Hearne E, et al. School attendance of children with cancer. J School Health 1982; 52:152–155.
30. Carpenter PJ. Scientific inquiry in childhood cancer psychosocial research. Cancer 1991; 67(suppl 3):833–838.
31. Carr-Gregg M, White L. Siblings of paediatric cancer patients: A population at risk. Med Pediatr Oncol 1987; 15:62–68.
32. Caty S, Ellerton ML, Ritchie JA. Coping in hospitalized children: An analysis of published case studies. Nurs Res 1984; 33:277–282.
33. Chesler MA, Barbarin OA. Relating to the medical staff: How parents of children with cancer see the issue. Health Soc Work 1984; 9:49–65.
34. Chesler MA, Paris J, Barbarin OA. "Telling" the child with cancer: Parental choices to share information with ill children. J Pediatr Psychol 1986; 11:497–516.
35. Claflin CJ, Barbarin OA. Does "Telling" less protect more? Relationships among age, information disclosure, and what children with cancer see and feel. J Pediatr Psychol 1991; 16:169–191.
36. Cobb B. Psychological impact of long illness and death of a child on the family circle. J Pediatr 1956; 49:746–751.
37. Coddington RD. The significance of life events as etiologic factors in diseases in children. J Psychosom Res 1972; 16:205–213.
38. Cohen J, Cullen JW, Martin LR. Psychosocial aspects of cancer. New York: Raven Press, 1982.

39. Cohen L. Bibliotherapy using literature to help children deal with difficult problems. J Psychosoc Nurs Ment Health Serv 1987; 25:20–24.
40. Collison C, Miller S. The role of family re-enactment in group psychotherapy. Perspect Psychiatr Care 1985; 23:74–78.
41. Conner K, Sandler E, Weyman C, et al. Intravenous midazolam versus fentanyl as premedication for painful procedures in pediatric oncology patients. J Pediatr Oncol Nurs 1991; 8:86–87.
42. Cox N. Psychological effects of surgery on children. AORN J 1976; 24:425–432.
43. Cunningham C, Betsa N, Gross S. Sibling groups: Interactions with siblings of oncology patients. Am J Pediatr Hematol Oncol 1981; 3:135–138.
44. Cyphert FR. Back to school for the child with cancer. J Sch Health 1975; 43:215–217.
45. Deasy-Spinetta P. The school and the child with cancer. In Spinetta JJ, Deasy-Spinetta P (eds): Living With Childhood Cancer. St. Louis: CV Mosby, 1981, pp 153–168.
46. Dolgin M. Behavioral effects of chemotherapy in children with cancer. J Psychosoc Oncol 1988; 5:99–106.
47. Ducore J, Waller D, Emslie G, et al. Acute psychosis complicating induction therapy for acute lymphoblastic leukemia. J Pediatr 1983; 103:477–480.
48. Elder GH. Historical change in life patterns and personality. In Baltes PB, Brim OG (eds): Life-Span Development and Behavior, vol 2. New York: Academic Press, 1979, pp 1–57.
49. Erikson E. Identity and the life cycle: Selected Papers. Psychological Issues Monographic Series I, no 1. New York: International Universities Press, 1959.
50. Erikson EH. Identity, Youth and Crisis. New York: Norton, 1968.
51. Evans AE, Bloom BS. Out of pocket and medical costs of pediatric cancer. Proc Soc Clin Oncol 3:72, 1984. (Abstract C-279.)
52. Fernald C, Curry J. Empathic versus directive preparation of children for needles. Child Health Care 1981; 10:44–47.
53. Fife B, Norton J, Groom G. The family's adaptation to childhood leukemia. Soc Sci Med 1987; 24:159–168.
54. Fochtman D, Foley G (eds). Nursing Care of the Child With Cancer. Boston: Little, Brown & Co, 1982.
55. Fosson A, Husban E. Bibliotherapy for hospitalized children. South Med J 1984; 77:342–346.
56. Frick S, DelPo E. Play behaviors of children undergoing bone marrow aspiration. J Psychosoc Oncol 1986; 4:69–77.
57. Friedman F. Kids with cancer go to camp. Cancer News 1982; 6–9, 22.
58. Friedman MM. Intervening with families of school-aged children with cancer. In Leahey M, Wright LM (eds): Family and Life-Threatening Illness. Springhouse, Penn.: Springhouse, 1987, pp 219–234.
59. Futterman EH, Hoffman I. Crisis and adaptation in the families of fatally ill children. In Anthony EJ, Koupernik C (eds): The Child in His Family: The Impact of Disease and Death. New York: John Wiley & Sons, 1973, pp 127–143.
60. Gardner R. The mutual storytelling technique in the treatment of anger inhibition problems. Int J Child Psychother 1972; 1:34–64.
61. Gardner R. The mutual storytelling technique in the treatment of psychogenic problems secondary to minimal brain dysfunction. J Learning Disabilities 1974; 7:135–143.
62. Gavaghan M, Roach J. Ego identity development of adolescents with cancer. J Pediatr Psychol 1987; 12:203–213.
63. Goggin E, Lansky S, Hassanein K. Psychological reactions of children with malignancies. J Am Acad Child Psychiatry 1976; 15:314–325.
64. Goodell A. Peer education in schools for children with cancer. Compr Pediatr Nurs 1984; 7:101–106.
65. Greenberg HS, Kazak AE, Meadows AT. Psychological functioning in 8- to 16-year-old cancer survivors and their parents. J Pediatr 1989; 114:488–493.
66. Greenwood R, Day J. A very special camp. Am J Nurs 1982; 82:1218–1219.
67. Hagberg K. Social casework and group work methods in a children's hospital. Children 1969; 16:192–197.
68. Hahn K. Therapeutic storytelling: Helping children learn and cope. Pediatr Nurs 1987; 13:175–178.
68a. Hall M, Hardin K, Conaster C. The challenges of psychosocial care. In Fochtman D, Foley G (eds): Nursing Care of the Child With Cancer. Boston: Little, Brown & Co, 1982.
69. Harris J, Carrol C, Rosenberg L, et al. Intermittent high dose corticosteroid treatment in childhood cancer: Behavioral and emotional consequences. J Am Acad Child Psychiatry 1986; 25:120–124.
70. Heiney SP. Assessing and intervening with dysfunctional families. Oncol Nurs Forum 1988; 15:580–585.
71. Heiney SP. Adolescents with cancer: Sexual and reproductive issues. Cancer Nurs 1989; 12:95–101.
72. Heiney SP, Goon-Johnson K, Ettinger RS, et al. The effects of group therapy on siblings of pediatric oncology patients. J Pediatric Oncol Nurs 1990; 7:95–100.
73. Heiney SP, Ruffin J, Ettinger R, et al. The effects of group therapy on adolescents with cancer. J Assoc Pediatr Oncol Nurses 1988; 5:20–24.
74. Heiney SP, Wells LM. Strategies for organizing and maintaining successful support groups. Oncol Nurs Forum 1989; 16:803–809.
75. Heiney SP, Wells LM, Coleman B, et al. Lasting impressions: A psychosocial support program for adolescents with cancer and their parents. Cancer Nurs 1990; 13:13–20.
76. Heiney SP, Wells LM, Ettinger RS, et al. Effects of group therapy on parents of children with cancer. J Pediatr Oncol Nurs 1989; 6:63–69.
77. Henning J, Fritz G. School reentry in childhood cancer. Psychosomatics 1983; 24:261–269.
78. Hilgard R, LeBaron S. Hypnotherapy of Pain in Children with Cancer. Los Altos, Calif.: William Kaufmann, 1984.
79. Hinds P, Martin J, Vogel R. Nursing strategies to influence adolescent hopefulness during oncologic illness. J Assoc Pediatr Oncol Nurses 1987; 4:14–22.
80. Hockenberry MJ. Crisis points in cancer. In Hockenberry MJ, Coody DC (eds): Pediatric Oncology and Hematology. St. Louis: CV Mosby, 1986, pp 432–449.
81. Holt C. Psychosocial problems encountered in the management of the adolescent with cancer. J Curr Adolesc Med 1980; 9:44–48.
82. Hughes M. Chronically ill children in groups: Recurrent issues and adaptations. Am J Orthopsychiatry 1982; 52:704–711.

83. Hvizdala E, Miale T, Barnard P. A summer camp for children with cancer. Med Pediatr Oncol 1978; 4:71–75.

84. Hymovich DP. Unpublished data. 1989.

85. Hymovich DP. A theory for pediatric oncology nursing practice and research. J Pediatr Oncol Nurs 1990; 7:131–138.

86. Hymovich DP, Hagopian G. Chronic Illness in Children and Adults: A Psychosocial Approach. Philadelphia: WB Saunders, 1992.

87. Hymovich DP, Roehnert J. Psychosocial late effects of childhood cancer. Semin Oncol Nurs 1989; 5:56–62.

88. Iles P. Children with cancer: Healthy siblings' perceptions during the illness experience. Cancer Nurs 1979; 2:371–377.

89. Janis IL. Psychological Stress: Psychoanalytic and Behavioral Studies of Surgical Patients. New York: John Wiley & Sons, 1958.

90. Jannoun L. Are cognitive and educational development affected by age at which prophylactic therapy is given in acute lymphoblastic leukemia? Arch Dis Child 1983; 58:953–958.

91. Jay S, Ozolins M, Elliott C, et al. Assessment of children's distress during painful medical procedures. Health Psychol 1983; 2:133–147.

92. Johnson J, Kirchhoff K, Endress MP. Altering children's distress behavior during orthopedic cast removal. Nurs Res 1975; 24:404–410.

93. Johnson M, Whitt J, Barclay M. The effect of fantasy facilitation on anxiety in chronically ill and healthy children. J Pediatr Psychol 1987; 12:273–284.

94. Kagen-Goodheart L. Reentry: Living with childhood cancer. Am J Orthopsychiatry 1977; 47:651–658.

95. Kane N. The young adult with cancer: A developmental approach. Oncol Nurs Forum 1981; 8:16–19.

96. Kaplan DM. Interventions for acute stress experiences. In Spinetta JJ, Deasy-Spinetta P (eds): Living With Childhood Cancer. St. Louis: CV Mosby, 1981, pp 41–49.

97. Kaplan DM. Intervention strategies for families. In Cohen J (ed): Psychosocial Aspects of Cancer. New York: Raven Press, 1982, pp 221–233.

98. Kaplan DM, Grobstein R, Smith A. Predicting the impact of severe stress on families. Health Soc Work 1976; 1:71–82.

99. Katz ER. Illness impact and social reintegration. In Kellerman J (ed): Psychological Aspects of Childhood Cancer. Springfield, Ill.: Charles C Thomas, 1980, pp 14–46.

100. Katz E, Kellerman J, Ellenberg L. Hypnosis in the reduction of acute pain and distress in children with cancer. J Pediatr Psychol 1987; 12:379–394.

101. Katz ER, Kellerman J, Siegel SE. Behavioral distress in children with cancer undergoing medical procedures: Developmental considerations. J Consult Clin Psychol 1980; 48:356–365.

102. Katz E, Rubenstein C, Hubert N, et al. School and social reintegration of children with cancer. J Psychosoc Oncol 1988; 6:123–140.

103. Kellerman J. Psychological Aspects of Childhood Cancer. Springfield, Ill.: Charles C Thomas, 1980.

104. Kellerman J, Katz E. The adolescent with cancer: Theoretical, clinical, research issues. J Pediatr Psychol 1977; 2:127–131.

105. Kellerman J, Zeltzer L, Ellenberg L, et al. Psychological effects of illness in adolescence. I. Anxiety, self-esteem, and perception of control. J Pediatr 1980; 97:126–131.

106. Kinrade LC. Preventive group interventions with siblings of oncology patients. Child Health Care 1985; 14:110–113.

107. Kitchener KS. Cognition, metacognition, and epistemic cognition: A three-level model of cognitive processing. Hum Dev 1983; 26:222–232.

108. Klopovich P. Research on problems of chronicity in childhood cancer. Oncol Nurs Forum 1983; 10:72–75.

109. Koch-Hattem A. Siblings' experience of pediatric cancer: Interviews with children. Health Soc Work 1986; 11:107–117.

110. Koocher GP. Psychosocial care of the child cured of cancer. Pediatr Nurs 1985; 11:91–93.

111. Koocher GP. Psychosocial issues during the acute treatment of pediatric cancer. Cancer 1986; 58(suppl 2):468–472.

112. Koocher GP, O'Malley JE. The Damocles Syndrome: Psychosocial Consequences of Surviving Childhood Cancer. New York: McGraw-Hill, 1981.

113. Koocher GP, O'Malley JE, Gogan JL, et al. Psychological adjustment among pediatric cancer survivors. J Child Psychol 1980; 21:157–174.

114. Kramer RF. Living with childhood cancer: Impact on healthy siblings. Oncol Nurs Forum 1984; 11:44–51.

115. Kramer RF, Moore IM. Childhood cancer: Meeting the special needs of healthy siblings. Cancer Nurs 1983; 6:213–217.

116. Kupst MJ, Schulman JL, Maurer H, et al. Psychosocial aspects of pediatric leukemia: From diagnosis through the first six months of treatment. Med Pediatr Oncol 1983; 11:269–278.

117. Lansky S. Impediments to treatment and rehabilitation of the childhood cancer patient. CA 1985; 35:302–307.

118. Lansky SB. The high cost of cancer. Am J Pediatr Hemotol Oncol 1987; 9:89–91.

119. Lansky SB, Cairns NU, Hassanein JW, et al. Childhood cancer: Parental discord and divorce. Pediatrics 1978; 62:184–188.

120. Lansky S, Gendel M. Symbiotic regressive behavior patterns in childhood malignancy. Clin Pediatr 1978; 17:133–138.

121. Lansky S, List M, Lansky L, et al. The measurement of performance in childhood cancer patients. Cancer 1987; 60:1651–1656.

122. Lansky S, Lowman J, Vats T, et al. School phobia in children with malignant neoplasms. Am J Dis Child 1975; 129:42–46.

123. Lazarus R. Psychological Stress and the Coping Process. New York: McGraw-Hill, 1966.

124. Lazarus R. The costs and benefits of denial. In Spinetta JJ, Deasy-Spinetta P (eds): Living With Childhood Cancer. St. Louis: CV Mosby, 1981, pp 50–67.

125. Lazarus R, Folkman S. Stress, Appraisal, and Coping. New York: Springer-Publishing, 1984.

126. Levine AS, Hersh SP. The psychosocial concomitants of cancer in young patients. In Levine AS (ed): Cancer in the Young. New York: Masson & Cie, 1982, pp 367–387.

127. Levine E. Indirect suggestions through personalized fairy tales for treatment of childhood insomnia. Am J Clin Hypn 1980; 23:57–63.

128. Levine M, Carey W, Crocker A, et al. Developmental-Behavioral Pediatrics. Philadelphia: WB Saunders, 1983.

129. Lindsay M, MacCarthy D. Caring for the brothers and sisters of a dying child. In Burton L (ed): Care

of the Child Facing Death. London: Routledge & Kegan-Paul, 1974, pp 189–206.

130. Long K. Pitfalls to avoid and positive approaches in the nurse adolescent relationship. Perspect Psychiatr Care 1983; 23:22–26.

131. Maguire P. Can the parental psychological morbidity associated with childhood leukemia be reduced? Cancer Surv 1984; 3:617–631.

132. Marten GW. Psychological effects of cancer in the adolescent: Clinical management and challenge for research. In Shulman JR, Kupst MJ (eds): The Child With Cancer. Springfield, Ill.: Charles C Thomas, 1980, pp 156–165.

133. Martinson IM, Cohen MH. Themes from a longitudinal study of family reaction to childhood cancer. J Psychosoc Oncol 1988; 6:81–97.

134. McCallum L, Carr-Gregg M. Adolescents with cancer. Aust Nurs J 1987; 16:39–42.

135. McCubbin HI, Cauble AE, Patterson JM. Family Stress Coping and Social Support. Springfield, Ill.: Charles C Thomas, 1982.

136. McCubbin HI, Patterson JM. The family stress model: The double ABCX model of adjustment and adaptation. In McCubbin HI, Sussman M, Patterson J (eds): Social Stress and the Family: Advances and Developments in Family Stress Theory and Research. New York: Haworth Press, 1983.

137. McKeever P. Siblings of chronically ill children: A literature review with implications for research and practice. Am J Orthopsychiatry 1983; 53:209–218.

138. Miles MS. Helping adults mourn the death of a child. In Wass H, Corr CA (eds): Childhood and Death. Washington: Hemisphere, 1984, pp 219–241.

139. Moore A. Crisis intervention: A care plan for families of hospitalized children. Pediatr Nurs 1989:15:234–236.

140. Moore D, Holton C, Marten G. Psychological problems in the management of adolescents with malignancy. Clin Pediatr 1969; 8:464–469.

141. Morrow GR, Hoagland A, Carnrike LM. Social support and parental adjustment to pediatric cancer. J Consult Clin Psychol 1981; 49:763–765.

142. Murphy LB, Moriarty AE. Vulnerability, Coping and Growth: From Infancy to Adolescence. New Haven, Conn.: Yale University Press, 1976.

143. Nelms R. What is a normal adolescent? MCN 1981; 6:402–406.

144. Noll RB, Bukowski WM, Rogosch FA, et al. Social interactions between children with cancer and their peers: Teacher ratings. J Pediatr Psychol 1990; 15:43–56.

145. Olness K, Gardner G. Some guidelines for uses of hypnotherapy in pediatrics. Pediatrics 1978; 82:228–233.

146. Orr DP, Hoffmans MA, Bennetts G. Adolescents with cancer report their psychosocial needs. J Psychosoc Oncol 1984; 2:47–59.

147. Orr DP, Weller SC, Satterwhite MA, et al. Psychosocial implications of chronic illness in adolescence. J Pediatr 1984; 104:152–157.

148. Parkes KR. Locus of control, cognitive appraisal, and coping in stressful episodes. J Pers Soc Psychol 1984; 46:655–668.

149. Pearse M. The child with cancer: Impact on the family. J Sch Health 1977; 47:174–179.

150. Petrillo M, Sanger S. Emotional Care of Hospitalized Children, 2nd ed. Philadelphia: JB Lippincott, 1980.

151. Pfefferbaum B, Lucas R. Management of acute psychological problems in pediatric oncology. Gen Hosp Psychiatry 1979; 3:214–219.

152. Piaget J. The Origins of Intelligence in Children. New York: International Universities Press, 1952.

153. Piaget J, Inhelder B. The Growth of Logical Thinking from Childhood to Adolescence. New York: Basic Books, 1958.

154. Pless IB, Perrin JM. Issues common to a variety of illnesses. In Hobbs N, Perrin JM (eds): Issues in the Care of Children with Chronic Illness. San Francisco: Jossey-Bass, 1985, pp 41–60.

155. Rait D, Jacobsen P, Lederberg M, et al. Characteristics of psychiatric consultations in a pediatric cancer center. Am J Psychiatry 1988; 145:363–364.

156. Rankin SH, Weekes DP. Life-span development: A review of theory and practice for families with chronically ill members. Scholar Inq Nurs Pract 1989; 3:3–27.

157. Reres M. Stresses in adolescence. Fam Community Health 1980; 2:31–41.

158. Robertson M, Barford F. Story-making in psychotherapy with a chronically ill child. Psychother Theory Res Pract 1970; 7:104–107.

159. Rollins JA. Childhood cancer: Siblings draw and tell. Pediatr Nurs 1990; 16:21–27.

160. Ross J, Diserens D, Turney M. Evaluation of a symposium for educators of children with cancer. J Psychosoc Oncol 1989; 7:159–178.

161. Ross JW, Scarvalone SA. Facilitating the pediatric cancer patient's return to school. Soc Work 1982; 27:256–261.

162. Ross S. Childhood leukemia: The child's view. J Psychosoc Oncol 1989; 7:75–90.

163. Rubin J. Child Art Therapy. New York: Van Nostrand Reinhold, 1984.

164. Ruccione K. Informed consent with parents of children with cancer. Paper Presented at Annual Conference for the Association of Pediatric Oncology Nurses, Atlanta, 1989.

165. Rutter M. Stress, coping and development: Some issues and some questions. J Child Psychol Psychiatry 1981; 22:323–356.

166. Ryan NM. Stress-coping strategies identified from school age children's perspective. Res Nurs Health 1989; 12:111–122.

167. Sach MB. Helping the child with cancer go back to school. J Sch Health 1980; 50:328–331.

168. Schooley C. Communicating with hospitalized children: The mutual storytelling technique. J Pastoral Care 1974; 28:102–111.

168a. Schuster CS, Ashburn SS. The Process of Human Development: A Holistic Life-Span Approach, 3rd ed. Philadelphia: JB Lippincott, 1992.

169. Selye H. Stress Without Distress. Philadelphia: JB Lippincott, 1974.

170. Selye H. The Physiology and Pathology of Exposure to Stress. Montreal: Acta, 1950.

171. Sievers TD. Conscious sedation with midazolam for painful procedures. J Pediatr Oncol Nurs 1992; 9:53–54.

172. Smith K, Gottlieb S, Gurwitch R, et al. Impact of a summer camp experience on daily activity and family interactions among children with cancer. J Pediatr Psychiatry 1987; 12:533–542.

173. Smith S, Rosen D, Trueworthy R. A reliable method for evaluating drug compliance in children with cancer. Cancer 1979; 43:169–173.

174. Sorenson ES. Children's coping responses. J Pediatr Nurs 1990; 5:259–267.

175. Sourkes B. Siblings of the pediatric cancer patients. In Kellerman J (ed): Psychological Aspects of Child-

hood Cancer. Springfield, Ill.: Charles C Thomas, 1980, pp 47–69.

176. Spinetta JJ. The siblings of the child with cancer. In Spinetta JJ, Deasy-Spinetta P (eds): Living With Childhood Cancer. St. Louis: CV Mosby, 1981, pp 133–142.

177. Spinetta JJ. Measurement of family function, communication, and cultural effects. Cancer 1984; 53:2330–2338.

178. Spinetta JJ, Deasy-Spinetta P. Living With Childhood Cancer. St. Louis: CV Mosby, 1981.

179. Spinetta JJ, Deasy-Spinetta P, Kung FH, et al. Emotional Aspects of Childhood Leukemia: A Handbook for Parents. New York: Leukemia Society of America, 1986.

180. Spinetta JJ, Maloney LJ. Death anxiety in the outpatient leukemic child. Pediatrics 1975; 56:1034–1037.

181. Stolberg AL, Cunningham JG. Support groups for parents of leukemic children: Evaluation of current programs and enumeration of participants' emotional needs. In Shulman JR, Kupst MJ (eds): The Child with Cancer. Springfield, Ill.: Charles C Thomas, 1980, pp 26–36.

182. Suderman J. Pain relief during routine procedures for children with leukemia. MCN 1990; 15:163–166.

183. Susman EJ, Hollenbeck AR, Strope BE, et al. Separation-deprivation and childhood cancer: A conceptual re-evaluation. In Kellerman J (ed): Psychological Aspects of Cancer. Springfield, Ill.: Charles C Thomas, 1980, pp 155–170.

184. Tebbi C, Bromber C, Mallon J. Self-reported depression in adolescent cancer patients. Am J Pediatr Hematol Oncol 1988; 10:185–190.

185. Tebbi C, Cummings K, Zevon M, et al. Compliance of pediatric and adolescent cancer patients. Cancer 1986; 58:1179–1184.

186. Treiber F, Schramm L, Mabe P. Children's knowledge and concerns towards a peer with cancer: A workshop intervention approach. Child Psychiatry Hum Dev 1986; 16:249–269.

187. U.S. Department of Health and Human Services. Talking with Your Child about Cancer. NIH Publication 87-2761. Bethesda, Md.: National Cancer Institute, 1987.

188. Van Dongen-Melman JEWM, Sanders-Woudstra JAR. Psychosocial aspects of childhood cancer: A review of the literature. J Child Psychol Psychiatry 1986; 27:145–180.

189. Varni J, Katz E. Psychological aspects of childhood cancer: A review of research. J Psychosoc Oncol 1987; 5:93–119.

190. Waechter EH. Children's awareness of fatal illness. Am J Nurs 1971; 71:1168–1172.

191. Walker CL. Stress and coping in the siblings of children with cancer. University of Utah, Salt Lake City, 1986.

192. Walker CL. Stress and coping in siblings of childhood cancer patients. Nurs Res 1988; 37:208–212.

193. Walker CL. Use of art and play therapy in pediatric oncology. J Assoc Pediatr Oncol Nurses 1989; 6:121–126.

194. Walker CL. Siblings of children with cancer. Oncol Nurs Forum 1990; 17:355–360.

195. Weekes DP. Adolescents with cancer: Correlates of intraindividual change in type of coping strategy. Unpublished manuscript. University of California, San Francisco, 1989.

196. Weekes DP, Savedra M. Adolescents with cancer: Coping with treatment-related pain. J Pediatr Nurs 1988; 3:318–328.

197. Wells L. Clinical problems: Reward system for patients. J Assoc Pediatr Oncol Nurses 1986; 3:27.

198. Whitaker D, Lieberman M. Psychotherapy Through the Group Process. New York: Atherton Press, 1964.

199. Williams HA. Social support and social networks: A review of the literature. J Assoc Pediatr Oncol Nurses 1988; 5:6–10.

200. Williams K, Baeker M. Use of small group with chronically ill children. J Sch Health 1983; 53:205–207.

201. Worchel F, Nolan B, Willson V, et al. Assessment of depression in children with cancer. J Pediatr Psychol 1988; 13:101–112.

202. Yalom I. The Theory and Practice of Group Psychotherapy, 2nd ed. New York: Basic Books, 1975.

203. Yalom I. Inpatient Group Psychotherapy. New York: Basic Books, 1983.

204. Yamamoto K, Soliman A, Parsons J, et al. Voices in unison: Stressful events in the lives of children in six countries. J Child Psychol Psychiatry 1987; 28:855–864.

205. Zeltzer L, Kellerman J, Ellenberg L, et al. Psychologic effects of illness in adolescence: Impact on illness in adolescence—Crucial issues and coping styles. J Pediatr 1980; 97:132–138.

206. Zurlinder J. Minimizing the impact of hospitalization for children and their families. MCN 1985; 10:178–182.

HOME AND HOSPICE CARE FOR THE CHILD OR ADOLESCENT WITH CANCER

Patricia Benson
Edith D. Burkey
Belinda Martin Mitchell
Jane C. Clark

HOME CARE SERVICES

The early literature on home care for the child with cancer focused on caring for the child dying of disease or related complications.[7,14,17] Although home care for the child with end-stage illness is important, pediatric home care now is seen as a care option throughout the cancer experience.[18]

Provision of medical and nursing care in the home has been and continues to be an integral aspect of the health care delivery system. In recent decades proliferation of aggressive lifesaving and life-sustaining technologies has resulted in an increase in the number of long-term survivors of childhood cancer.[26] Advances in pharmaceuticals and durable and disposable medical equipment technology have been instrumental in allowing health care professionals to redefine the scope of home care services. The scope of pediatric oncology home care ranges from a single intervention such as teaching central line catheter care to a complex plan of care requiring intravenous therapy, physical and occupational therapy, nutritional support resources, or hospice services.

Clinical, psychosocial, and financial incentives also have contributed to the expansion of home care. With home care, exposure to nosocomial infections is decreased. Scheduling of routine treatment protocols is more predictable in the home than in the hospital where bed availability may be uncertain.[13] Home care services make it possible to provide care in a less restrictive and more familiar environment. The child and family are better able to maintain valued relationships and home and community activities. The child may be able to return to school. Involvement of family caregivers and normalization of the life of the child are valuable strategies in optimizing the quality of life for the child with chronic disease. Financially, the overall cost of care may be decreased by eliminating some of the expense associated with institutional care. Insurance payers currently are evaluating the cost-effectiveness of home-based care.[20]

Providing care to the child with cancer at home includes providing care to the entire family.[2] Thus attention to the structure of the family, cultural factors, roles and responsibilities shared by nuclear and extended family, communication patterns among family members, and the perceived impact of the illness of the child on the individual family members and on the family unit is essential in providing comprehensive home care.[3] As the primary caregiver, the family is an integral member of the home health care team.

To provide restorative, rehabilitative, and palliative care services in the home, professionals must collaborate with the family and community resources to

- Determine those services that can be offered safely in the home setting
- Identify children whose care demands can be met in the home setting
- Assess family strengths and resources needed to meet the care demands
- Develop and implement the care plan
- Select an appropriate provider(s) to meet the care demands
- Evaluate the effectiveness, quality, and costs of services

Determine Services to Offer in the Home Setting

Across the course of the cancer experience, the child with cancer receives intensive therapy that requires close monitoring for clinical effectiveness and for adverse physical and psychosocial effects. Yet because the treatment protocols for childhood cancers have a protracted time frame, evaluation of each child and family to determine those services that can be offered in an alternate care setting is warranted.

Once progress toward the clinical outcome is evident, the incidence and severity of adverse effects are determined, and effective treatment to minimize the incidence and severity of adverse effects implemented, the health care team begins to discuss the possibility of outpatient or home care. The primary factor the team considers in determining therapies to offer in the home setting is safety. Is the procedure well defined for safe delivery of the therapy? Is the risk of acute, life-threatening, adverse effects of the therapy high?

The second factor to consider is the availability of resources and support in the community. What supplies are needed to deliver the therapy in the home setting? Do agencies that provide such therapies exist in the community?

The appropriateness of home-based therapy is also determined by the scope of care needed, the level of responsibility required, and the availability of a health professional willing to assume such responsibility. Conditions requiring laboratory monitoring several times each day, children receiving antineoplastic therapy who require frequent monitoring, or treatments that have potential adverse reactions that require immediate emergency care may not be suitable for delivery in the home setting. If the responsibilities require the decision-making skills of a physician or frequent or complex assessment skills of a nurse, the child's condition is not stable enough to allow transfer of care to the home.

Identify Appropriate Children for Home Care

Children with cancer may have a variety of home care needs such as central line care, long-term antimicrobial therapy, nutritional support, ventilatory support, blood products administration, physical therapy, or occupational therapy. Likewise a variety of home care services and products are offered. The ideal child for home care is one whose demands of care match the available services and products (Table 15–1).

However, other factors contribute to whether an individual child is a candidate for successful home care. One factor is the desires of the child. Most children prefer being at home, in familiar surroundings, and in proximity to family and friends; yet for some children the hospital or outpatient care setting offers a sense of security with health care providers they know and trust. Treatment in these settings also offers children separation of the illness from their "normal" life at home. For an increasing number of children, the hospital setting is their only home.

Other factors include the commitment of the family to home care and the motivation of the family to learn the necessary knowledge and skills to maintain the child at home.

TABLE 15—1. *Home Care Services and Products*

CAREGIVERS	THERAPIES	EQUIPMENT
Nurse	Infusion	Wheelchair
Physician	Antimicrobials	Hospital bed
Social worker	Antineoplastic agents	Oxygen
Pharmacist	Total parenteral nutrition	Durable medical equipment
Laboratory staff	Pain management	Supplies
Physical therapist	Intravenous fluids	
Occupational therapist	Blood products	
Arts therapist	Restorative, rehabilitative, or palliative	
Teacher	Physical therapy	
Respiratory therapist	Respiratory therapy	
Speech therapist	Occupational therapy	
	Nutritional therapy	
	Art therapy	
	Speech therapy	

The family—parents, siblings, and significant others—must share a clear understanding of the anticipated demands of home care. In addition, they must be willing to accept resources and support from outside the family, if needed, to meet the home care demands.[19]

Assess Family Strengths and Resources

Care for children with cancer is provided successfully and safely in a variety of family systems with diverse structures, traditions, educational levels, incomes, and resources. However, the home care team can increase the likelihood of success of a home care plan by careful assessment of the unique characteristics of the family and the home environment.

Family Strengths. All families have strengths. Assessing four key areas of family functioning is critical in evaluating the family's strengths and potential to care for the child with cancer in the home: structure, roles and responsibilities, communication patterns, and decision-making processes.

STRUCTURE. The structure of families today is different from structures even two decades ago: the family may consist of one or two parents who may be heterosexual or homosexual; families may be blended; the extended family may be geographically close and contribute to the daily family life; and families may include people bound by factors other than blood lines (e.g., people who share a homeless shelter or a neighborhood). The home care provider assesses how the family is defined in each situation and determines the stability of the family structure. The more stable the family structure, the greater is the likelihood that the home care experience will succeed.[11]

ROLES AND RESPONSIBILITIES. The home care professional assesses the roles that each family member plays in the life of the family. In addition, the responsibilities associated with each role are identified. Do any members work outside the home? Who provides primary financial support for the family? Who usually cares for the child? What roles do each family member value? Can any of the responsibilities be assigned to other family members or friends? Through the assessment of roles and responsibilities, the home care provider gets a glimpse of how the family organizes to achieve common goals and thus is able to draw on the strengths and values of each family member in organizing home care responsibilities for the child with cancer.

COMMUNICATION PATTERNS. Communication patterns within the family are important in the assessment of the potential for home care. With the assumption of home care responsibilities, a family that already is stressed by the chronic illness of the child will be challenged even more. How do members of the family communicate with each other? When does the communication take place (e.g., at mealtime, during preparation for bed, at planned family conferences)? Is information shared among all members of the family? Is communication one way, or are all members encouraged to participate? Analysis of communication patterns allows the home care provider to identify channels of communication within the family unit. Plans for teaching and information sharing with the family about aspects of the home care experience can be developed.[11]

DECISION-MAKING PROCESSES. The family providing care to the child with cancer in the home must make many decisions. The home care provider must understand how the family makes decisions. Who makes the decisions? Are decisions made after evaluation of critical information or "on a hunch"? Is input from others outside of the family sought and welcomed? Are decisions flexible or final? How does each member of the family feel about the decision-making process used?

Home care professionals are confronted with recognizing their own definitions of the "ideal" family structure, role of family members, communication patterns, and decision-making processes. Most families have some degree of structural, psychologic, social, spiritual, or ethical turmoil.[12] "Normal" pathology occurs in family life. A prescription for a "correct" life, "perfect" behavior, or a "right" feeling is nonexistent. The challenge for professionals is to recognize the unique characteristics of each family and to develop a system of supports and services to assure the success of the family in providing needed care to the child with cancer in the home setting.

Family Resources. Three primary areas of family resources—the home environment, finances, and support systems—are evaluated in determining appropriateness of home care.

HOME ENVIRONMENT. Assessment of the home environment is critical to the provision of safe and effective care of the child with cancer. Basic elements of a safe home environment include the availability of electricity, plumbing, and access to a telephone. Other factors to assess include availability and accessibility of space for needed equipment and

supplies, electric outlets and adequate wiring to support both the usual household appliances and medical equipment, and adaptations that must be made to meet the care demands.[19] A sample of a home safety assessment form is shown in Figure 15–1.

In addition to the immediate home environment, the team member assesses the community environment. Access to transportation, emergency services, and medical care is evaluated.

FINANCES. Assessment of financial resources of the family can be divided into two parts: identifying the resources and negotiating payment. The resources most commonly include income, bank accounts, property holdings, and third-party insurance. Although financial information is considered a private matter by most individuals, accurate information about the finances of the family often dictates the availability of home care services. A social worker or discharge planner is instrumental in helping the family understand the need for others to know financial information to determine the feasibility of developing a home care plan for the child with cancer.

Three major categories of third-party insurance exist: (1) private, commercial, or indemnity insurance; (2) health maintenance organizations; and (3) publicly supported plans such as Medicare and Medicaid. Marked variability of benefits occurs across the plans; therefore the benefits for the individual plans must be verified. The parents can verify benefits for private, commercial, or indemnity plans through either the employer, the insurance benefits office, or insurance case manager. Medicare and Medicaid benefits can be verified through the local county Medicare or public assistance office.[19]

Once the treatment plan is developed, the second phase of financial assessment occurs. Payment for covered and noncovered services is negotiated. Usually a representative of the home care team discusses with a case manager the medical necessity of planned care and any limitations on frequency or length of care or on monetary payment. If noncovered services are critical to the safe and effective care of the child at home, the representative works with the family to seek assistance from

BASIC HOME SAFETY ASSESSMENT

Client Name: _____

Client ID#: _____

Signature/Date: _____

Complete the following checklist during the initial assessment to determine the safety of the client's home.

Safety Areas	Yes	No	N/A
1. Lighting is adequate in client care area(s).	❏	❏	❏
2. Furniture is arranged to allow free movement.	❏	❏	❏
3. Pathways are clear in heavy traffic areas.	❏	❏	❏
4. Stairways, hallways and exits are clear of clutter and loose objects.	❏	❏	❏
5. Throw rugs are eliminated or fastened down.	❏	❏	❏
6. Steps or stairs have accompanying sturdy hand rails or banisters.	❏	❏	❏
7. A flashlight, light switch or lamp is located within easy reach of the client.	❏	❏	❏
8. Electrical cords are placed close to walls and out of the pathway.	❏	❏	❏
9. There is a non-skid surface or mat on the bathtub or shower floor.	❏	❏	❏
10. Hand grippers are installed in the bathroom, when appropriate.	❏	❏	❏
11. Refrigeration is available for proper storage of solutions/medications.	❏	❏	❏
12. All medications are clearly labeled.	❏	❏	❏

Safety Areas	Yes	No	N/A
13. The following items are in secured areas and out of the reach of children and confused individuals:			
a. medications	❏	❏	❏
b. sharp objects	❏	❏	❏
c. cleaning substances	❏	❏	❏
d. poisons (*bug killer, weed killer, etc.*)	❏	❏	❏
14. Oxygen is placed in a non-smoking area and away from an open flame.	❏	❏	❏
15. Proper lifting aids are present for immobile clients or those clients requiring assistance with transfers.	❏	❏	❏
16. There is close access to a working telephone. If outside home, where: _____	❏	❏	❏
17. A list of emergency telephone numbers is present in the home.	❏	❏	❏
18. Client/caregiver verbalizes an understanding of the fire escape plan and route from the home.	❏	❏	❏
19. Smoke alarms are present on each floor of house.	❏	❏	❏
20. Home environment is suitable for care.	❏	❏	❏

INSTRUCTIONS GIVEN/MODIFICATIONS REQUIRED

_____

_____

_____

_____

_____

_____

_____

NHC9626   Original: Client   Yellow: Clinical Record   4/92

FIGURE 15–1. Sample home safety assessment form. (*Courtesy Norrell Health Care, Inc., Atlanta, Georgia.*)

other community resources to meet the identified needs.

Obtaining funding for home care for the child with cancer can be a time-consuming and tedious process. Families often feel overwhelmed by the demands made by the need for financial information while concerns about the ill child, other family members, and work responsibilities seem more urgent. The professionals on the home care team can simplify the complexities of the financing process [24]

SUPPORT SYSTEMS. Providing support for the family embarking on a home care experience for the child with cancer is essential. Assessment includes asking the following: Who or what has been a source of support in the past? What type of support was provided? Was the support offered or requested? Was the support provided effective in meeting the identified need? Once types of previous support and patterns of use are identified, the home care team must evaluate the perceptions of the family about anticipated support. Support must be perceived as needed and effective by the family.

Develop and Implement the Treatment Plan

Care is planned in collaboration with members of a multidisciplinary team that includes the child, as appropriate, the family, health care professionals, and representatives from a variety of community agencies or vendors (see Table 15–1). Generally the planning phase occurs within acute or long-term care settings. In general, the earlier home care planning is initiated, the smoother the transition for the child and family will be.

Coordination and communication are crucial to the success of the plan of care. If more than one agency or vendor is required to meet care demands, a coordinator, case manager, or primary nurse is identified as the liaison among all care providers and the family.

Parent-professional collaboration allows both providers to organize care responsibilities around valued roles in pursuit of common treatment goals.[4,25] As caregiving responsibilities are delineated, the ability to renegotiate roles of the parents and professionals at any time is stressed with all involved.

Select Appropriate Provider(s). Systematic evaluation of potential providers includes review of structure, process, and outcomes of services provided (Table 15–2). A variety of agencies provide home care services and products. The selection of home care vendors has become an arduous process in many institutions. Hospital joint ventures with home care agencies, physician joint ventures, preferred provider arrangements, and case man-

TABLE 15–2. *Considerations in Selecting Home Care Agency for Child With Cancer*

1. What type experience does the agency have in caring for children with cancer?
2. How does the agency recruit qualified pediatric oncology care providers?
3. Will the agency sign a contract or written agreement for care provision?
4. Will the agency accept the insurance plan and do the paperwork required?
5. What is the agency's policy for covering sick calls, vacations, and holidays?
6. Is the agency willing to send nurses to the hospital for training before discharge without additional costs?
7. Does the agency have written standards of care for the pediatric population in general and the pediatric oncology population specifically?
8. Is a nursing supervisor available?
9. Does the agency have a comprehensive, integrated program of services?
10. Who is responsible for providing updates and training for home care personnel?
11. What is the fee structure for services provided?
12. Is 24-hour coverage provided?
13. What rights do the parents have if they encounter problems with home care providers or the services provided?
14. Does the parent stay in the home while services are being provided?
15. Can the parents interview the care providers and other users of the services?

agers for third-party payers may influence the selection of home care providers.

Costs often are the determining factor in whether or not home care is a feasible alternative for some children with cancer. For instance, the cost for a comparable home infusion therapy varies by up to 700% nationwide. For example, the cost of 1 month of total parenteral nutrition ranges from $2,200 to $15,014.[8] Evaluation of the fee structures for services provided and comparison with other agencies providing the same services are recommended.

Referrals for home care may be made by a physician, nurse, social worker, family, or friend. Regardless of who makes the referral, evaluation of a range of options, recommendations based on safety and costs, and concensus with the desires of the family are essential. The majority of referrals to home care agencies are made when a child is discharged from an acute care setting; however, providers in ambulatory settings also make referrals.

Delineate Roles and Responsibilities. Ideally a member of the home care team, usually the nurse, visits the child and family before discharge. The case manager discusses aspects of the home care experience with the family. The plan of care is outlined in detail, with assignments for primary care responsibility negotiated among the family and other outside providers. Schedules of home visits and services are reviewed. The home care professional also discusses the assignment of benefits. Finally, the rights of the child and family are discussed (Fig. 15–2).

Home care demands and responsibilities change over time. The case manager discusses with the family the need to modify and update the plan of care continually. The family is also encouraged to keep the case manager aware of changes in family roles, responsibilities, and reactions to the home care experience that have implications for redistributing caregiver responsibility.

Teach Providers and Family Caregivers How to Implement Plan. As a teacher, the pediatric nurse, whether in the institutional or home care setting, is responsible for assessment of the learning needs of the child, family, and home care providers in anticipation of the transition to home care.[24]

- What information is critical for the child, family, and home care providers to know to provide safe and effective care at home?
- What psychomotor skills are needed to provide care to the child at home?
- What portion of the critical information or psychomotor skills has the child, family, and home care providers mastered?
- Do the child, family, and home care providers perceive a need for additional information or skills?

Assuming the responsibility for caring for a child with cancer in the home is stressful for the family and home care providers. The goal is to provide competent and safe care. The nurse plays a unique role in developing teaching-learning strategies that maximize the likelihood that the family and the home care providers will succeed in achieving the goal.

- What strategies are most effective in teaching the required information or skills to the variety of care providers?
- Is adequate time available for teaching to occur before transition to the home care setting?
- Are opportunities provided for demonstrating mastery of information and skills before transition?
- What methods are available to evaluate the effectiveness of the teaching-learning experiences?
- What written or audiovisual aids appropriate to the educational level, developmental stage, and sensory abilities of the variety of providers can be used to reinforce information given?[18,22]

The teaching-learning experience for the family and home care providers for the child with cancer is different for each situation. The challenge for the pediatric oncology nurse is to develop a teaching-learning plan that addresses the unique needs of the child, the family, and home care providers, that maximizes the likelihood of success in achieving

CLIENT RIGHTS AND RESPONSIBILITIES

As a client you have the _right_ to:

1. Competent, concerned, individualized health care without regard to race, color, creed, sex, age, national origin, handicap, ethical/political beliefs, ancestry, religion, sexual orientation or whether or not an advance directive has been executed.

2. Exercise your rights. In the event that you have been judged incompetent, your family or guardian has the right to exercise your rights.

3. Be free from verbal, physical and psychological abuse and to be treated with consideration, respect and full recognition of your dignity and individuality, including privacy in treatment and care for personal needs.

4. Your property being treated with respect.

5. Be admitted for service only if the agency has the ability to provide safe, professional care at the level of intensity needed.

6. Expect all personnel caring for you will be current in knowledge, duly licensed or certified as applicable, and have completed a training program or competency evaluation regarding his/her respective areas of employment.

7. Be informed that you may participate in the development of your plan of care or treatment, the periodic review and update, discharge plans, appropriate instruction and education in the plan of care, and be informed of all treatments the agency is to provide, the disciplines to provide care, and the frequency of visits/shifts to be furnished.

8. Know when and how each service will be provided and coordinated, the agency ownership, name and functions of any person and affiliated agency personnel providing care and services.

9. Choose care providers, to communicate with those providers, and to reasonable continuity of care.

10. Be fully informed, orally and in writing, at the time of admission, and in advance of care provided, a statement of services available by the agency, care and treatment provided by the agency, and related charges. This must include those items and services for which you may be responsible for reimbursement, eligibility for third party reimbursement, coverage available under Medicare, Medicaid, and any other federal program of which the home health agency is aware. Advance notification will be provided to you or your responsible guardian regarding any changes in the care, services, and items or as soon as possible no later than 30 calendar days in writing from the date Norrell Health Care was notified of any changes in any prior payment information.

11. Be taught and have your family members taught the treatment plan, so that you can, to the extent possible, assist yourself; and your family or other designated party can also understand and assist you.

12. Request information regarding the diagnosis, prognosis, and treatments including alternatives to care risk(s) involved. This information will be given in a language or format so that you and family members can readily interpret and understand so that informed consent may be given.

13. Refuse any/all treatment to the extent permitted by law after being fully informed of and understanding the possible consequences of such action, without relinquishing any other portions of the treatment plan, except where medical contraindication of partial treatment exists.

14. Be informed of the procedures for submitting client complaints with respect to client care, that is, or fails to be furnished, or regarding the lack of respect for property by anyone who is furnishing services on behalf of the agency with suggested changes in service or staff, without discrimination or reprisal for voicing such grievances.

15. Review all of your health records during normal business hours with prior approval of management, unless contraindicated in the clinical record by the physician.

16. Be referred elsewhere when denied services for any reason, and upon request, given a written explanation regarding the denial and availability of community resources; and upon transfer, informed of any financial benefits by Norrell Health Care.

FIGURE 15–2. Client's bill of rights and responsibilities. (*Courtesy Norrell Health Care, Inc., Atlanta, Georgia.*)

Client Name:_____ I.D.#:_____

17. Assistance in locating appropriate community resources before you run out of funds.
18. Privacy including confidentiality of all record communications, personal information, and to refuse release of records to any individual outside the agency; except in the case of your transfer to a health care facility, as required by law, or third party payment contracts. You shall be informed of the policy and procedure regarding disclosure of your clinical records.
19. Receive the care necessary to assist you in attaining optimal levels of health, and if necessary, cope with death.
20. Be informed of your state's home health agency hotline telephone number and the hours of its operation of service, in order to obtain information about home health agencies; or to report abuse, neglect or exploitation, as applicable:

    (Toll-Free Telephone Number)   **(Hours of Operation)**

21. Be informed of the procedure for submitting a written complaint/grievance to Norrell Health Care. You shall receive a prompt and reasonable response regarding the complaint/grievance within 15 days. All complaints/grievances are to be referred to NORRELL HEALTH CARE management at the following address and telephone number: _____

Telephone Number   _____

22. Be informed of the procedure for filing a complaint/grievance with the appropriate State Department of Health at the following address and telephone number: _____

Telephone Number   _____

As a client you have the responsibility to:

1. Remain under a physician's care while receiving agency services.
2. Provide the agency with a complete and accurate health history.
3. Provide the agency with all requested insurance and financial records.
4. Sign the required consents and releases for insurance billing.
5. Participate in your Plan of Care.
6. Accept the consequences for any refusal of treatment or choice of non-compliance.
7. Provide a safe home environment in which your care can be given.
8. Cooperate with your Physician, agency staff and other caregivers.
9. Treat agency personnel with respect and consideration.
10. Advise the agency of any problems or dissatisfaction with the care being provided, without being subject to discrimination or reprisal.
11. Notify the agency when unable to keep appointments.

All of the above rights and responsibilities shall be referred to the appointed committee authorized to act on behalf of the client if adjudicated incompetent.

This agency is an affirmative action/equal opportunity employer and does not discriminate on the basis of race, color, national origin, religion, sex, handicap, age, ethical or political beliefs, ancestry, sexual orientation, or whether or not an advance directive has been executed.

NHC0083   Original: Client   Yellow: Clinical Record

      1/92

FIGURE 15–2 *Continued*

safe and effective care, and that normalizes the life of the child and family to the greatest degree possible.

Health care services in the home should be instituted after a sufficient trial in the hospital or clinic setting has been conducted. Caregivers, both professional and family, should have had an opportunity to learn and should have successfully demonstrated knowledge and skills necessary for care of the child.

Evaluate Home Care Experience

Evaluation of home care services is essential for the well-being of the child with cancer and family and for third-party payers. The goal of home care for the child with cancer is the normalization of life for the child and the family. Home care provides the opportunity for the child and family to maintain valued relationships and activities within their own community.[18]

Clinical Effectiveness. Evaluation of the clinical effectiveness of the treatment plan is paramount in the plan for home care. With each home visit, members of the home care team are responsible for assessing the health status of the child and the compliance with the prescribed treatment plan. Clear evaluation criteria for clinical effectiveness of care are established in collaboration with the primary care provider before initiation of home care.

Impact of Responsibilities on Family. Home care responsibilities in caring for the child with cancer change the life of the family. Parents must juggle the demands of the ill child with needs of other family members, job responsibilities within and outside the home, and individual physiologic and psychosocial needs. Numerous home care providers may be in and out of the home during a 24-hour period. Scheduling of visits and coping with the interruptions to the daily routine may be perceived as challenges or burdens to the family. Research studies have indicated that the changes in family life resulting from home care are underestimated by most families.[5,18]

Many families can cope with the various changes in roles, responsibilities, time commitments, privacy, and finances associated with home care. The advantages of having the ill child in the home environment may overshadow the adaptations required. However, for some families, the demands of caring for the child at home are perceived as detrimental to the physical or psychosocial development or well-being of individual family members or the family unit. The pediatric nurse plays a vital role in discussing both the positive and negative outcomes of the home care experience with the family. As an advocate, the nurse troubleshoots problem areas, communicates problems to other members of the team, and works collaboratively with the team to enhance the support for the family or to recommend transfer to an alternate care setting.

Quality of Services Provided. The evaluation of the quality of service by the home care providers is accomplished through evaluation against both federal and professional standards of care and a quality improvement program within the agency. The focus of the evaluation of quality centers on the structural elements of the services, the process of service and product delivery, and the outcomes of the services delivered.

Quality of structural elements of home care agencies and services is determined by the presence and content of a written philosophy, purpose, goals, and objectives, organizational charts that describe the relationship among components of the agency and the responsibilities of each component, written standards of home care for the agency, and job descriptions of key personnel within the agency.

A plan to evaluate the process of service and product delivery may include the following:

1. Completeness of the assessment conducted before transition to home care
   - Was an assessment done before planning the transition to home care?
   - Did the child, if appropriate, the family, and participating health care professionals take part in the assessment?

■ Were unanticipated problems experienced as a result of lack of information about the clinical, psychosocial, and developmental status of the child, family strengths and needs, family resources, or services offered by coordinating agencies?

2. Appropriateness and timeliness of the services, equipment, and products provided in the home

■ Was the need for all services, equipment, and products documented and ordered by the appropriate care providers?

■ Were standards for storage, preparation, packaging, labeling, and dispensing of intravenous solutions followed?

■ Was equipment needed for home care delivered before transition to the home care setting?

3. Clear delineation of roles and responsibilities for family and agency care providers

■ Was the systematic preparation of the family to assume responsibility for selected aspects of care documented?

■ Was the family aware of steps to take in the event of a clinical emergency?

■ Were the decisions of the family respected by agency care providers?

Given that structure and process standards that reflect state-of-the-art home care are in place, the final component of a quality improvement program is the focus on the child- and family-focused outcomes of care.

■ Was the physical, psychosocial, and developmental status of the child with cancer maintained, improved, or restored?

■ Were significant adverse effects of therapies delivered in the home experienced by either the child or the family?

■ Did the family perceive that they had access to and knowledge of information about the status of the child?

■ Did the family possess the necessary skills to provide competent care?

■ Were significant changes in the condition of the child reported to the appropriate care professional in a timely manner?

■ Did the family perceive that life for the ill child and the family members was "normalized" by the delivery of home care services?

Cost of Services. Cost of provided services is the final area included in a quality improvement package. A continuous process of cost comparisons with agencies offering comparable services occurs. The issue of containing costs while providing quality services is of concern to care providers and receivers. Many agencies offer a program of incentives for home care providers to implement cost-saving, quality-enhancing strategies.

Conclusion. The evaluation of the home care experience is a process that involves the referral source, the home care agencies and providers, and the child with cancer and his or her family. Quality in-home care is measured not only by the quality of services provided but also by the impact of those services in allowing the child and family to maintain as normal a life as possible within the limits imposed by cancer.

HOSPICE SERVICES

Unfortunately, some children are not cured by current treatment, and their disease continues to progress. The terminal phase may last from several weeks to months. During this phase of illness, a transition from curative to palliative care occurs.[23]

Research studies have demonstrated that families are able to care for their terminally ill child at home and that the child, family, and community can experience many benefits from such an experience. Benefits include the child's remaining in the secure environment of home, the parents' maintaining a sense of control, the family members' reunifying among themselves and with the community, and siblings' participating in the care of the ill child and feeling a part of the family unit.[5,17,18]

Models of Hospice Care

Models of home care for children in the terminal phase of illness have been described in the literature.[14,15,17] In addition, the hospice philosophy of care has been recommended as one method of supporting terminally ill children and their families.

Four primary models of hospice services have been described: the freestanding hospice, the hospital-based hospice unit or team, the home health agency hospice, and the community-coordinated hospice. Regardless of the setting for the services, commonalities of services and philosophy exist.

Hospice Philosophy. The hospice philosophy is based on the provision of palliative and supportive services designed to control adverse physical and psychosocial symptoms and improve the quality of life for the patient and family. Care is provided through the involvement of an interdisciplinary team, which commonly consists of a physician, nurse, social worker, chaplain, home care aids, trained volunteers, and a bereavement counselor.[1,5,23] Health care professionals provide 24-hour consultation to primary care providers. Trained volunteers may be available to assist with routine home activities such as shopping, performing errands, and providing transportation or to serve as caring and supportive listeners for the patient and family.

Eligibility criteria for enrollment in hospice programs usually include a prognosis of less than 6 months and the decision to focus the goals of care on palliative support rather than aggressive curative treatment.[16] The use of hospice services by pediatric populations has been limited in the past. Many children and parents are unable to meet these eligibility criteria in that the child may be deteriorating and have a guarded prognosis but the family does not want to give up the option of trying any treatment they believe may extend or save the life of their child. The second factor influencing the use of hospice services is the availability of professional pediatric caregivers in many hospice systems. To provide the child and family with competent care, the professionals involved with that care must have specialized knowledge, skills, and attitudes about the care of children and families. Thus the decision to seek hospice care for the child with cancer involves careful considera-

tion by the child, family, primary care provider, and potential hospice care providers.

Clinical Issues in Hospice Care

Once the option of hospice care is introduced, a family conference is scheduled. The purposes of the conference are to review the health status of the child, discuss options for terminal care, and address any family questions or concerns.

Certain clinical issues may need clarification in the initial family conference so that appropriate care can be planned. One major issue is the type and amount of medical treatment to provide. Therapies often used in the acute phase of the illness such as radiation therapy or steroids may also be used for palliative care. Without clear explanation, parents may be confused about the goals of care with the use of such therapies in the terminal phase.

A second issue is to determine those interventions that will be continued or initiated to assure the comfort of the child. The child may require supportive care for problems such as pain, dehydration, seizures, nausea, or vomiting. The goal of symptom control is to allow the child to function at a maximal level that allows sharing of quality time with the family unit.

A third issue in hospice care is the status of resuscitation orders for the child. Since curative cancer therapy is not available, death is the anticipated outcome. If families are clear on the goals of hospice care, the decision not to resuscitate the child will be apparent. A letter or state-approved form from the primary physician that defines the medical prognosis and code status may be given to the family to use if they need to clarify the condition of the child to emergency personnel or care institutions. If the family is not ready to make a resuscitation decision, the team should develop a plan for emergency services to use in the case of a life-threatening event. In either case, the hospice team clarifies the procedures to follow when the child dies. Are there cultural or religious ceremonies that are important to the family? Who will be notified of the death—the hospice team, funeral home, and the primary physician? Will an autopsy be done? Who will receive the body and how will the body be transferred? Who will sign the death certificate? Dealing with these issues before the actual death can assist the family with anticipatory grieving.

The location where the child dies is a final concern expressed by parents. Parents may feel guilty if they desire to return to the hospital before the death of the child. Studies have shown that many families cared for their children at home the majority of the remaining time but less than 50% of the children actually died in the home.[9,10,15] Interviews with 103 primary caretaker parents after the death of their children revealed 55.7% of children returned to the hospital to die. All families expressed a high degree of satisfaction with the ultimate location of their child's death.[15]

Parental Concerns About Home-Hospice Care

For parents who decide to use home-based hospice care, the anxieties associated with taking the terminally ill child home may be great. Identified fears of families caring for the dying child include the unknown, abandonment by care providers, not being able to control symptoms, and those fears associated with the child's dying at home.

To address some of these fears, the nurse may suggest that the parents talk with other parents who have selected hospice care for their child. Incorporation of the hospice team in planning care with the primary care providers during the active treatment phase of the illness reinforces the commitment of the health care team to the well-being and continued care of the child and family. Home visits are scheduled at regular intervals according to the desires of the family. Also family members are reminded that the hospice team is available 24 hours a day. Anxiety levels often can be reduced by letting the parents know that if the condition of the child changes suddenly or they need additional help in care for the child, the hospice team is only as far away as the telephone. Some families are more comfortable if they approach the experience of home-hospice care 1 day at a time.

Care of the Dying Child and His or Her Family

A detailed description of the critical elements of care for the child with cancer who is dying and his or her family is presented in Chapter 16. However, three factors that affect the care of the dying child—communication, consistency, and compassion—deserve additional attention.

Communication is the key to hospice care. The hospice team is responsible for assuring that the family identifies ways to contact the team with any concerns. Accessible and open communication contributes to confidence in the care and empowerment of the family. Communication between the hospice team and the primary care providers is necessary also. Reports on the initial visit, weekly updates, and reports of any significant change in the condition of the child help the providers keep current on the status of the child and family and provide needed information should admission to the hospital become necessary.

Consistency helps establish trust and confidence in the hospice care. The hospice care provider schedules routine visits at a time convenient with the family. Appointments are kept. A 24-hour on-call service is offered, and response to calls from the family is timely. Needs for adjustment in symptom management are noted, and adjustments are made in a timely manner. The hospice care provider evaluates parental and sibling responses with each visit and discusses concerns with the family and the team.

By providing care, the hospice provider shares in the experience of the child's dying with the family. For most families the experience of losing a child is new. The hospice care provider is the guide through the experience. Counsel, empowerment, kindness, caring, and relief offer compassion to the child and family.

Grief and Bereavement Services

The loss of a child is one of the most significant losses anyone can experience. Parental grief appears exaggerated when compared to other types of bereavement.[10,21,22] Siblings also are affected significantly by the death of a brother or sister.[6] Hospice programs by definition offer bereavement support groups; however, the focus of such groups may be on support after the loss of an adult. Parents or siblings may not find them helpful. Self-help groups such as Candlelighters or Compassionate Friends may be more helpful as parents deal with the death of a child.

In the course of bereavement follow-up care for the family who has experienced the death of a child, the hospice professional continually assesses the progress of the individual family members and the family unit toward grief resolution. As members of the family begin establishing new relationships, planning for future experiences, recalling rich memories or past experiences with the child, and assuming previous roles, the professional will know that resolution has begun.

Symptoms of prolonged or unresolved grief reaction may occur. Withdrawal, social isolation, extreme emotional reactions, developmental regression, and a decline in physical or psychologic functioning are cues that additional professional assistance may be needed. The bereavement coordinator may recommend referral to mental health clinics or private counselors.

SUMMARY

Because the survival rate from childhood cancer has increased, cancer is being viewed as a chronic disease. As with other chronic diseases, the setting for care shifts during the course of illness from the acute, professionally controlled care settings to the restorative, rehabilitative, or palliative family-controlled setting of the home. Home care and hospice care are not for every child with cancer, nor are they for every family. Yet when the needs of the child, availability of services, and commitment and skill of the family and home care providers are compatible, home care can be a successful and valuable experience. The role of the pediatric oncology nurse remains indispensable in the assessment of factors that affect the ultimate success of the home care plan, the development of the interdisciplinary plan of care, the preparation of families, and the evaluation of the quality, effectiveness, costs, and satisfaction of children and families with home or hospice care.

REFERENCES

1. Amenta MO, Bohnet NL. Nursing Care of the Terminally Ill. Boston: Little Brown & Co, 1986.
2. APON. Scope of Practice and Outcome. Standards of Practice for Pediatric Oncology Nursing. Richmond, Va.: Author, 1988.
3. Bru G. Using the revised APON Standards of Practice. J Pediatr Oncol Nurs 1990; 7:17–21.
4. Bruder MB. Parent and professional partnerships under PL 99-457. Early Child Update 1989; 5:1–2.
5. Corr CA, Corr DM (eds). Hospice approaches to pediatric care. New York: Springer Publishing, 1985.
6. Davies B, Martinson IM. Care of the family: Special emphasis on siblings during and after the death of a child. In Martin BB (ed): Pediatric Hospice Care: What Helps. Los Angeles: Children's Hospital of Los Angeles, 1989, pp 186–197.
7. Edwardson SR. The choice between hospital and home care for terminally ill children. Nurs Res 1983; 32:29–34.
8. Fins A. AIDS home care may be due for some housecleaning. Bus Week June 1990; 20–21.
9. Foley GV, Whittam EH. Care of the child dying of cancer: Part I. CA 1990; 40:327–354.
10. Foley GV, Whittam EH. Care of the child dying of cancer. Part II. CA 1991; 41:52–60.
11. Friedman MM. Family Nursing: Theory and Practice, 3rd ed. Norwalk, Conn.: Appleton & Lange, 1992.
12. Kohrman A. Home-based services: Today's challenge for handicapped children and their families. Proceedings Second Annual Pediatric Research and Training Center Conference. University of Connecticut, 1986, pp 13–14.
13. Lange BJ, Burroughs B, Meadows AT, et al. Home care involving methotrexate infusions for children with acute lymphoblastic leukemia. J Pediatr 1988; 112:492–495.
14. Lauer ME, Camitta BM. Home care for dying children: A nursing model. J Pediatr 1980; 97:1032–1035.
15. Martin B, Landsverk J, Schweitzer S, et al. Home care for children with catastrophic diseases: Implementation of a hospital-based pediatric hospice care program. MCH Grant no. MCH-063703-03-0, 1989. (Monograph.)
16. Martin BB. Care of the terminally ill child. In McCoy PA, Votroubek WL, (eds): Pediatric home care: A comprehensive approach. Rockville, Md: Aspen Publishers, 1990, pp 255–267.
17. Martinson IM, Armstrong GD, Geis DP, et al. Home care for children dying of cancer. Pediatrics 1978; 62:106–113.
18. Martinson IM, Widmer A. Home Health Care Nursing. Philadelphia: WB Saunders, 1989.
19. McCoy PA, Votroubek WI. Pediatric Home Care: A Comprehensive Approach. Rockville, Md.: Aspen Publishers, 1990.
20. O'Keiff H. Pediatric diversification. Caring 1986; 5:50–55.
21. Rando TA. Grieving: How to go on living when someone you love dies. Lexington, Mass.: Lexington Books, 1988.

22. Rice R. Home Health Nursing Practice: Concepts and Application. St Louis: Mosby–Year Book, 1992.
23. Smith SN, Bohnet N. Organization and administration of hospice care. J Nurs Adm 1983; 13:10–16.
24. Stair J, McNally J. Home care. In Groenwald SL, Frogge MH, Goodman M, et al. (eds): Cancer Nursing: Principles and Practice, 2nd ed. Boston: Jones & Bartlett, 1990, pp 1106–1131.
25. Thomas RB. The struggle for control between families and health care providers when a child has complex health care needs. Zero to Three 1988; 8:15–18.
26. Wong DL. Transition from hospital to home for children with complex medical care. J Pediatr Oncol Nurs 1991; 8:3–9.

THE TERMINALLY ILL CHILD OR ADOLESCENT

Dianne Fochtman

Although the cure rate for childhood cancer has increased dramatically over the last two decades, the pediatric oncology nurse must approach each child newly diagnosed with cancer with optimistic honesty. No one knows at the time of diagnosis which child will live and which child eventually will succumb to the illness or to the side effects of therapy. Pediatric oncology nurses must be prepared to deal not only with issues of survivorship, but also with the care of the terminally ill child when death is inevitable. This includes learning to deal with personal feelings in order to help the child and family traverse the terminal phase with as much comfort, dignity, and strength as possible.

CHILDREN'S CONCEPTS OF DEATH

Helping children and their families in the terminal stages of the illness requires an understanding of how children's ideas and concepts about death develop.[31] Social, scientific, and technologic advances over the years have produced changes that have influenced a child's experience with death. Until recently children were common witnesses to death.[75] When the infant mortality rate was high and the average life expectancy was short, a child often witnessed the death of siblings and/or parents. The modern child is much less likely to lose a parent or sibling through death. In fact, recent generations are the first known in history

in which many middle-aged adults have not experienced the death of an immediate family member.[75]

On the other hand, technologic advances have brought the facts of death into the child's world through the media. Even if parents refuse to allow their child to watch "violent" television shows, they cannot completely remove the idea of death from the child's world. The mass media—television, radio, newspapers, even books designed especially for children—expose a child to death: the bad guy gets killed; the cartoon character dies, often violently, only to be resurrected immediately or in the next sequence; war and the death it brings are presented nightly in news broadcasts; notices of death, violent and otherwise, appear daily on television broadcasts and in newspapers; and even a common bedtime prayer contains a reference to death—"If I should die before I wake . . ." In addition, children are exposed to death in other ways: the dead animal along the highway; the death of a pet; or the death of a grandparent.

All of these factors have varying consequences for the intellectual and emotional development of the child. Sooner or later the terminally ill child will be faced with a situation that makes it necessary for his or her parents or other adults to talk with him or her about death. Unfortunately, the adult may not respond to the need. Ideally the subject should be introduced before a situation is encountered (e.g., when a dead animal is observed along the road).[35] How the subject is handled depends on many variables, one of which is the meaning of death to the child.

Early landmark studies in the development of the concept of death in children were done by Anthony[2] in prewar London (1937 to 1939) and Nagy[57] in Budapest in the 1940s. Anthony found that younger children in her study tended to interpret death as sleep or temporary departure. She believed that the idea of death develops in the child as intellect advances, rather than as age or personal experiences increase.[35,82] Magical thinking often pervaded, and almost all of the children had spontaneous death-related thoughts.

Nagy[57] identified three stages in the development of the death concept in children.

1. Death is seen as separation, departure, or disappearance, with no definitive death, only a state of being less alive. Death is seen as reversible, and there is no understanding of the finality of death (ages 3 to 5 years).

2. Death is personified and thought of as a contingency. Death is understood as final, and the dead do not return (5 to 9 years).

3. Death is perceived as a universal, inevitable, and final process and a cessation of body activities (9 years and older).

Since the 1960s further research has added to the knowledge of how children view death at different stages of development. (See references 3, 11, 18, 33, 34, 39, 46, 66, 71, 76, 77, and 85.) Children's concepts of death at various developmental stages are presented in Table 16–1.

TABLE 16–1. *Common Concepts of Death in Childhood*

COMMON CONCEPTS OF DEATH	REPRESENTATIVE BEHAVIORS AND RESPONSES	IMPLICATIONS FOR COMMUNICATION
Infancy		
No concept of death; death is experienced as separation.	Infant reacts strongly to separation from parents or caregivers and experiments with object permanence and separation with "throwaway" and "peekaboo" behaviors.	Understand strategies for dealing with separation anxiety. Help other family members cope with death so they can be available to the infant who is dying or who has experienced the death of a parent or caregiver.
Early Childhood		
Concepts about death are greatly influenced by attitudes of parents. Young child learns the words *dead* and *death* but understands little or nothing of their meaning. As the concept begins to form, death is viewed as temporary, gradual, reversible, and a continuation of life on a reduced level. Popular media and magical thinking may reinforce these beliefs. Egocentrism may lead the child	Child displays increased curiosity about things related to death and spontaneity about discussing the topic. Child retains a sense of the dead person's being and may be concerned that the corpse can sense cold or discomfort or may worry about how it goes to the bathroom. Child may look forward to the dead person's return or carry on imaginary conversations with the dead person.	Expect children to be open and honest in asking questions about death if given the freedom of expression. Children may discuss death by parroting what they have heard from adults without really understanding. They often have an incomplete or erroneous understanding about death. Assess the need to correct misconceptions, especially if they are causing fear and anxiety. Help children to understand death as a part of life and to comprehend the nature of death while allowing their

Modified from Miles MS, Burman SI. Nursing care of the dying child. In Mott SR, James SR, Sperhac AM (eds): Nursing Care of Children and Families, 2nd ed. Redwood City, Calif.: Addison-Wesley, 1990. Sources include references 7, 19, 71, 72, 80, 81, and 84.

Table continued on following page.

TABLE 16—1.   *Common Concepts of Death in Childhood* Continued

COMMON CONCEPTS OF DEATH	REPRESENTATIVE BEHAVIORS AND RESPONSES	IMPLICATIONS FOR COMMUNICATION
Early Childhood— cont'd		
to believe that wishes, misbehavior, or unrelated actions can cause death. Young children who have experiences related to death may have a relatively mature concept of death long before they are able to verbalize it.		own positive fantasies to linger. Bereaved siblings may fear that their thoughts or feelings caused the serious illness or death of a brother or sister. Dying children need the opportunity to share concerns and ask questions of their parents. However, some parents are not able to handle the anxiety this causes, and the child may share primarily with a special nurse. Children of this age often communicate best through play. Since separation remains an important issue, dying and grieving children need special considerations to remain close to their parents.
Middle Childhood		
The majority of children between the ages of 4½ and 8 years achieve at least some level of understanding of the universality (all living things die), irreversibility (the dead cannot be made alive again), and nonfunctionality (all life-defining functions cease) of death. Mutilation fears may be linked to death anxiety. Children may be superstitious and may view death as an unnatural event caused by random, violent external forces. Children begin facing the fact that family members, including parents, may die.	Child asks more specific questions about death, being dead, and death-related rituals such as burial. Burial and closure rituals for coping with the death of a pet are highly important. Child may want to touch the corpse to see how it feels. Child may use play to develop further understanding of death and to cope with feelings.	Expect children in this period of development to give concrete explanations about the physical causes of death. Play may be used to facilitate a child's understanding of death and related rituals. Children may need to discuss fears about the potential loss of a parent. Siblings need opportunities to ask questions about the illness and death of a brother or sister and may need more specific information about the cause of death. Be alert to feelings of guilt in bereaved siblings and dying children. Dying children continue to need to discuss their concerns with parents and may choose a special nurse as a confidant. They are still concerned about separation and often have concerns about pain, mutilation, and other suffering that may be involved. Dying children during this developmental stage begin to worry about the impact of their death on parents and may try to protect them by closing down communication.

TABLE 16–1. *Common Concepts of Death in Childhood* Continued

COMMON CONCEPTS OF DEATH	REPRESENTATIVE BEHAVIORS AND RESPONSES	IMPLICATIONS FOR COMMUNICATION
Late Childhood Universality, irreversibility, and nonfunctionality of death are understood. Children begin to face anxiously the reality of their own mortality; personal fear of death may surface. They begin to incorporate family and cultural beliefs and attitudes about death and show an interest in exploring views about afterlife.	Child may use rituals to decrease anxiety. Reckless behavior, tough demeanor, or humor may be used to cope with sense of vulnerability and fear.	Opportunities are needed for children to verbalize fears and understand that such fears are normal. They need more detailed explanations about why an individual has died, along with opportunities to share feelings and ask questions. Children may need to discuss realistic consequences of reckless activity. Dying children need to discuss concerns with family and staff but may have difficulty in doing so. Normal emotional responses of this age may become more complex as children deal with feelings about dying. It is important to help the dying child feel that life has been important and meaningful.
Adolescence Adolescents reach an "adult" perception of death, but strong focus on "here and now" and intense search for personal identity make death emotionally unacceptable. The thrill of reckless behaviors may outweigh safety factors. Adolescents derive comfort from the concept of having a long life yet to live. They may still hold concepts from previous developmental levels depending on actual experiences and family communication. They are working through religious and philosophic views about life, death, and afterlife.	Anxiety about death may be particularly acute because body image and the emerging self-concept are threatened. Denial and avoidance of death may be used to reduce personal death anxiety.	Use opportunities in daily life to open conversation about death. Avoid assumptions of an adult understanding by assessing the adolescent's specific perceptions. Be alert to feelings of guilt, hostility, confusion, and anxiety when communicating with the adolescent. Treat the feelings and concerns with utmost respect and confidence. Be open in sharing views and concerns about death. Correct misperceptions without being judgmental. The dying adolescent and bereaved sibling may have difficulty in sharing concerns with family. The dying adolescent often feels isolated from the usual channel of communication, the peer group, and may choose a nurse as a confidant regarding concerns and fears. He or she needs support in maintaining self-esteem, help in gaining positive closure about the meaning of a relatively short life, and assistance in completing things undone or wishes unfilled.

Like Piaget's theory of cognitive development,[59] the early studies of children's death concept development proposed a series of stages, with fixed corresponding ages, during which specific kinds of behaviors and conceptual development occurred.[2,57] "Current research, however, demonstrates that sequence is more reliable than correlating stages of understanding to ages in describing how children learn about death."[16] Although there is support for the cognitive-developmental approach to children's concepts of death, . . .

> Development involves more than maturation, it results from an interaction of biological readiness with environmental factors. Life experiences, intelligence levels, family attitudes and values, self-concepts, and many other as yet unexamined factors all seem to play a part in each child's individual attainment of meaning for death.[75]

The modern consensus is that "children attain a mature concept of death through a process more dependent on developmental level than chronological age."[20] Some children, for various reasons, come to an adult understanding of death at a very early age, whereas others, for other reasons, may not fully understand death until late childhood. Children with chronic illnesses may come face to face with death through relationships with other children in the hospital who die. Earlier researchers generally concluded that the cognitive resources necessary to conceive of death as final and inevitable were acquired near the age of 9 years.[57] However, the evidence now suggests that children between the ages of 5 and 7 years may attain a beginning understanding of these concepts.[16]

EXPLAINING DEATH TO CHILDREN

Eventually the child will ask questions about death. Answers to these questions depend on the child's age, the intensity and extent of interest, the reasons for the interest, the kind of questions asked, and the situation promoting the question. Questions should be answered clearly, directly, and as truthfully as possible without burdensome detail. Philosophic interpretations should be avoided, and

adults must remember that children easily mistake the meaning of words and phrases or take literally what is only an idiom.

The parent or other adult should not attempt to hide the meaning of death with fiction that someday must be repudiated. Some unhelpful explanations of death to avoid include (1) the dead person has gone on a long journey—the child may react with anxiety and resentment at apparent desertion; (2) God took the dead person away because He wants and loves the good in heaven—the child may develop fear, resentment, and hatred against a god who capriciously took a loved one because that person was loved by God; (3) the dead person is now living in heaven—introduction of the traditional concepts of "living" in heaven may create far more questions than it answers; (4) the person died because he or she was sick—this linking of sickness and death without any additional information (e.g., saying "The doctors could not fix it") only prolongs and intensifies the fear of death and may add new fears about illness; and (5) to die is to sleep—this explanation, besides being inaccurate, may cause a pathologic fear of sleep.

The specific answers of the adult depend very largely on personal resources, attitudes, social, cultural and religious traditions, and an understanding of the child. The adult must respond to the child's questions with genuine sincerity and conviction because what is said is important; but *how* it is said has even greater bearing on whether the child will develop anxiety and fears or will accept (within his or her capacity) the fact of death.[72] When communicating with a child, the adult should remember that words, although important, are never as important as the feelings imparted to the child.[20]

Art and play may help gain insight into the young child's feelings and may be used as a medium to share concerns and fears. Many children's books are very useful in helping children at various stages of development to understand death.[55] For example, several books deal with the death of a child's pet and help the child to understand and grieve (e.g., Fred Rogers' *When a Pet Dies*[64] for 3 to 8 year olds and Judith Viorst's *The Tenth Good Thing About Barney*[78] for 3 to 10 year olds).

As a child matures, parents may find other books useful in helping a child understand the concept of death (e.g., *Talking About Death: A Dialogue Between Parent and Child* or *Explaining Death to Children*, both by Rabbi Earl Grollman[24,25]).

The death of a loved one (e.g., a grandparent) is difficult for a child to understand and accept. Whether the death presents a barrier to appropriate psychologic development or an opportunity for development and maturation depends largely on how the adults in the child's environment handle the loved one's death. If a death is expected, the child should gradually be prepared for the inevitable outcome. Although the death may be due to illness, the differences between a terminal illness and the routine illnesses of life should be emphasized. Feelings commonly related to someone's dying, particularly anger and sadness, should be acknowledged, with emphasis on the fact that feelings do not cause death.

DEATH SITUATIONS IN PEDIATRIC ONCOLOGY

In pediatric oncology a child's dying trajectory, or his or her individual course of dying, may be long or short.[22] Death may occur while the child is in remission in a sudden and unexpected way (e.g., from septic shock or cranial hemorrhage), and death may occur unexpectedly, even when expected (e.g., the child with a poor prognosis at diagnosis may die from complications of therapy). Finally, there is the child in whom death is the expected outcome. The child who has relapsed or for whom therapy has proven to be ineffective falls into this category.

Although no situation is without hope, there is a time when discontinuing disease-oriented therapy is appropriate.[63] When cure of the disease is no longer possible, "hope is then centered on palliative care, moving toward hope that the child will die with dignity, without pain either to the child or the significant others surviving with subsequent grief."[26] Parents, and sometimes the child, are involved in the decision-making process, but the ultimate decision to terminate disease treatment should be made by the oncology team. If parents believe they made the medical decision to stop medical treatment, they later may feel guilt that such a decision was premature, inaccurate, or inappropriate.

Some families believe it is unacceptable to give up hope for a cure and that it is their obligation to fight death at all costs.[17] Such families are a challenge to the oncology team. Ethical dilemmas can develop when the desires of the parents are contrary to those of the older school-age child or adolescent or even the oncology team. Open and frequent communication between all participants is necessary to attempt to support both parents and child and determine the most appropriate plan of care. Patience and understanding, offered in a nonjudgmental way, are necessary since the conflicts are often not resolved quickly.

PHYSICAL NEEDS OF THE DYING CHILD

The terminally ill child may require treatment aimed at palliation of symptoms. For example, radiation therapy may be given to reduce the size of a tumor mass and thereby make the child more comfortable. Surgery and chemotherapy may be given for similar reasons. The parents and the staff must be clear that the purpose of these modalities is to make the child more comfortable, *not* to cure the child. Everyone must understand the purpose so that unrealistic expectations are discouraged.

A terminally ill child has many of the same physical needs as any seriously ill child. Sleep deprivation can occur, particularly if the child has been in the hospital for a long period of time. It is important to set a time schedule and provide an environment conducive to sleep at the appropriate times of day or night. Administering a mild sedative may be helpful at night, although this is usually not required.

The dying child may be restless and have nightmares or frequent waking.[27] It may be helpful to provide a nightlight, keep the door open, or reinforce that loved ones are near. At home a portable intercom may give reassurance to both the parents and the child. As the terminal phase progresses, the child may sleep for longer and longer periods, and waking moments may be minimal. Such moments are treasured, and at this point "family time may need to be geared around the child's waking and alert moments."[27]

Nutritional status is an important consideration in the terminally ill child. Oral nutritional intake should be maintained as long as it is physically possible and enjoyed by the child. Oral intake should never be allowed to become a point of contention between parent and child. If the child cannot or does not want to take adequate oral intake, the family can choose to provide no further intake or nutrition can be supplemented with tube feedings or hyperalimentation as needed.[6] Antiemetics may be helpful if nausea and vomiting are a problem.

Problems with elimination present another important consideration in the care of the terminally ill child. Methods to deal with these problems must take into account the child's desires and comfort. For example, if the child has diarrhea, the health care professional may recommend dietary restrictions to control the diarrhea. The child, on the other hand, may have few pleasures left in life except for dietary intake. Thus the parent and child may decide how to live with the diarrhea, maintaining cleanliness and comfort, so the child can continue eating what he or she wants. For a variety of reasons, including the use of narcotics, constipation may be a problem. Dietary manipulations (aimed first at preventing this complication), the early use of laxatives, and the use of enemas may be necessary, as may intermittent or continuous urinary catheterization if urinary retention occurs.

Some children require oxygen therapy to maintain respiratory status and provide comfort. Oxygen therapy can be provided by a mask or cannula, in the hospital or at home. It may be required only intermittently at first, but the need for supplemental oxygen may increase as the child approaches death.

Bleeding may be a problem for the terminally ill child. A low platelet count can occur because of marrow infiltration of disease or because of the intensive therapy previously received. Treatment of bleeding relates directly to the child's comfort. Increased bruising or petechiae may not produce discomfort in the child and may not interfere with activities of daily living; in that case a platelet transfusion is not given because it is not necessary for the child's comfort. However, in some cases a low platelet count results in severely bleeding gums or uncontrolled epistaxis. Both of these situations, and the vomiting of blood that they can produce, can increase the child's discomfort and fears. Platelet transfusions may be given in these cases to increase the comfort and decrease the fears of the child and family. Red blood cell transfusions may be given if the child is excessively fatigued and wants to remain active. However, parents must be reminded that anemia is not painful and transfusions may not improve a child's activity level. There may come a time when red blood cell transfusions prolong the dying process and not the living.

Although many children traverse the terminal phase of illness without significant discomfort, pain control is often the biggest challenge in the nursing care of the terminally ill patient. Pain control can be achieved using a variety of methods, including positioning and providing emotional support, massage, and cuddling. Imagery,[45] storytelling, diversion, socialization, talking through fears, and play therapy often provide comfort.[27] Medication should be used as needed in adequate doses on an appropriate schedule to relieve the pain. Multiple agents are available, varying from acetaminophen to opiates, which can be given through several routes.

The fear of pain is perhaps the greatest concern of both the parents and the child. A major nursing challenge is to give sufficient medication to relieve the child's pain while maintaining as much alertness as possible. Concerns about addiction and the amount of pain medicine sometimes required to eliminate the pain must be addressed.[51] The amount of pain medication required is whatever it takes to eliminate the pain. There is no "ceiling" on the amount that eventually may be given. The family needs to know that, although the suffering related to a child's dying may not be totally eliminated, there is no reason the child should be in pain.

PSYCHOSOCIAL NEEDS OF THE DYING CHILD

The terminally ill child has the same rights as any other human being approaching the last stages of life—the right to be treated with respect and to die with dignity. Independence should be fostered and stressed as long as possible, and the child should be given some degree of control over how, where, and with whom he or she spends the last days of life.

Some children choose to attend school, even if only for a few hours a day, up until shortly before their death. "The terminally ill child needs to learn, to have the opportunity to socialize and spend time with other children, to develop increased independence and control over the environment, and to experience success."[15] Attending school can help counter boredom and depression, increase peer contacts, enhance dignity, and normalize life-style.[10]

The terminally ill child may be emotionally labile for a variety of reasons (e.g., anxiety, central nervous system disease, discomfort, anger, or medication side effects).[27] He or she may be irritable and act out in negative ways (e.g., being nasty or obstinate, swearing, or throwing temper tantrums). Some children choose to touch as many lives as possible in their few remaining days or weeks, whereas others narrow their focus of relationships and interactions as death approaches. Staff and extended family may need help in understanding the child's narrowed focus of relationships as his or her energy decreases.

The child's spiritual needs must be respected. They may intensify as death approaches, or they may diminish as the child finds peace. Discussions of God, Heaven, or an afterlife will depend on the family's beliefs, the child's beliefs, and the family and child's openness to discussing them. Such discussions should take place only when the child indicates a willingness to participate. "Toward the end of the terminal phase, the work of the dying child (depending upon his age, maturation and experience) is to center on himself, his beliefs, his concepts. He, in essence, puts his life together."[27]

The issue of fulfilling a dying child's last or final "wish" often arises. The parents and many lay people are often willing to go to great lengths to fulfill these wishes. The desire for wish fulfillment must be tempered with a realistic expectation of the child's energy level and what he or she can actually enjoy.

C. was a 3-year-old girl diagnosed with ALL at age 2 years. Six months into therapy she relapsed and successfully underwent a bone marrow transplant. However, the leukemia recurred, and remission was not induced. The parents elected to take her home to die. C. had little energy at home, but she did enjoy watching children's movies. Her wish fulfillment was a new couch and lounge chair. C. greatly enjoyed alternating between her couch and lounge chair, playing with her younger brother and watching videos of children's movies over and over.

Although C. might have expressed a desire to visit a theme park in another state, fulfillment of a such a wish was really beyond the scope of her energy and ability at that time in her life. Fulfillment of a simpler wish, although somewhat unusual, did much more to enhance the remaining weeks of her life.

In 1970 Eugenia Waechter,[79] a pediatric nurse, conducted a hallmark study that demonstrated fatally ill children's awareness of death. Further studies by Spinetta, Rigler, and Karon[74] and Spinnetta and Maloney[73] supported Waechter's findings and indicated that despite efforts to keep the child with a fatal illness from becoming aware of his or her prognosis, the child still somehow senses that his or her illness is not ordinary and is in fact very threatening.

Often the adults in the child's world, both the staff and sometimes the parents, are very uncomfortable if they are anticipating conversations with the child about dying, but . . .

The dying child, depending on his age, maturation, and condition should be an active participant in his dying process. Often families (and sometimes staff) overprotect, cover-up, hedge, evade, stifle, or even lie to a terminally ill child, to make his life, short as it is, "easier." This closed approach not only makes his death more difficult, and increases the tension between family members and staff, but it disallows appropriate communication, grieving, honesty and completion of unfinished business.[27]

The most important thing to remember is that it is not so much *what* you say, as *how* you say it. However, an open approach does not mean that a child is blatantly and uncaringly told he or she is dying.[27] Be alert to cues, both verbal and nonverbal, from the child. Check what the child needs. "Although all patients have the right to know, not all patients have the need to know."[41] There are no clear-cut guidelines on what to say and what not to say. Every child and every situation are different. "Children need the opportunity to complete their own unfinished business. . . .The requests are as varied as each unique child who makes them. They are usually painful for staff and family to hear, for by acknowledgement of the request we acknowledge reality."[41]

Perhaps the child's question most feared by adults is "Am I going to die?" The response to this question depends on many factors—the adult's relationship with the child and/or the family, what the adult believes the child really is asking, the child's degree of pain, discomfort, or suffering, and knowledge of the child's fears and concerns. Reflecting the question back to the child, "What do you think?" will check the accuracy of the adult's understanding and perception of the child's meaning. A response such as "not right now" may suffice for the child who is not imminently dying but is afraid of going to sleep for fear of dying that night. In some cases a "no" answer is appropriate if in fact the child feels very sick but is not dying. In some situations a simple "yes" is appropriate, but be prepared for a possible floodgate of feelings that may then be communicated. Be thoughtful with your answer and do not use platitudes or cliches to hide your discomfort.

Older children and adolescents may question directly or indirectly if they are dying.[80] A child who has the stamina to pose this question usually wants and can handle the answer.[58] Some may discuss death openly with family and staff; others may want to protect their parents and choose instead to share their feelings with staff. "For the nurse who can tolerate listening to the adolescent's feelings about dying, the moments are privileged ones. They are a time to listen openly and let the patient know he will not be abandoned. They are a time to share silently, and in the silence, compassion, empathy, and humanness will be communicated."[58]

Often children need someone to listen to them and someone who is comfortable with silences with them rather than someone to talk to them. Some children work out in their own mind what their feelings are about dying, and they do not necessarily need to discuss dying with anyone. Others need help to express their feelings. Reflecting their comments or describing the feelings of other children may help them to express their concerns.

Some children have last wishes or want to "will" their possessions to a loved one. "It is during the terminal phase that the dying child completes his unfinished business. That can include delegating who gets his belongings, writing/recording letters, poems, his story, or making amends to others; essentially leaving his mark in life as he is losing his."[27] Other children have specific ideas about their funeral or burial. Some children may not realize they can express their desires, or they may be concerned about the effect such statements would have on parents or other loved ones. They need reassurance that such desires are appropriate and can be expressed, or they need to "test out" the expression of such desires on staff.

> L. was a 14-year-old girl dying of leukemia. During one hospitalization she indicated a need to talk with one of the staff members at 4 o'clock in the morning. During this conversation she expressed her desire to plan her funeral. At her funeral she wanted everyone to receive a daisy because daisies to her were a sign of hope and life. Once she found that the expression of such desires was accepted by the staff person, she felt ready to explain her wishes to her mother.

Staff members who work with terminally ill children must remember to make each moment count. Even silences are moments shared. Do not make unreasonable promises, but keep promises that are made. If you promise to play a game or stop by for a short visit, do so. There may not be a tomorrow to make up for times missed. Staff members need to come to a closure in some way. Closure may be indirectly confronted (e.g., withholding the usual "see you next week" after a clinic visit) or may involve the direct situation of saying good-bye.

L. came to clinic on what was to be her last visit. Although not in pain, she was very weak and lay quietly on the cart. While her parents discussed her terminal care with her physician, she expressed a desire to talk with the staff on the inpatient unit where she had spent so much time. With great difficulty I wheeled her around the unit and listened to her as she said her good-byes with simplicity and honesty to some very special friends. It was only as I approached the front door of the hospital with her that I realized that I, who had been so supportive to both her and the other nurses, had not said my own good-byes. With a mixture of tears and laughter and hugs, we expressed our love and caring for each other in our last conversation.

The above situations can occur only when the child's death is an expected event. When the child dies unexpectedly or in an unresponsive state such as when a child is on a ventilator, both the parents and the staff may need to work out their feelings about not being able to share certain things with the dying child. Such feelings include guilt, anger, and disappointment. The staff must be willing to listen to the hurt and the anger in a nonjudgmental, caring way. Parents and staff should be encouraged to communicate with the child, both through touch and words, even though the child appears unresponsive. Parents must be reminded of their past everyday expressions and actions that made the child feel loved. Staff members need to remember the "good" days or moments they had with the child. Both parents and staff should be encouraged to say their good-byes.

When Death Occurs

In pediatric oncology nursing a child's death most often is an anticipated event. In many cases the parents, and sometimes the child, choose to have the child die at home. Home care for dying children is both a feasible and desirable alternative to hospitalization during the final days.[4,27,41,46,47,65] Ambulatory care may continue during this period to provide reassurance to the family and supportive care. Home visits often are made by the nursing staff, or a hospice agency may be involved.

Preparing the family to take the child home to die requires patient and family education.

> The physical environment, as well as the physical and emotional support for the child and family should be assessed . . . .Teaching the family what to expect throughout the terminal and dying process can provide more support and cooperation, as well as make the death of a child an experience in living . . . . The appropriate preparation is not only for the dying process, but in essence, is a preparation for a lifetime of grief, healing and recovery the family faces.[27]

The family must be taught how to manage pain and other side effects. Most parents wish to be prepared for any eventuality, including seizures, bleeding, or respiratory problems. Parents who are prepared for these possibilities are less likely to panic if they should occur at home.

Parents must be aware of potential changes in respiration (e.g., irregular breathing, Cheyne-Stokes respirations, and sounds of pulmonary congestion) as death approaches. If the family is not prepared for the unusual sounds of the respirations, they may become frightened.[27] For example, the child may moan loudly with each breath. However, close observation will demonstrate that the moaning occurs with exhalation and has nothing to do with pain or fear.

As death approaches, the child's physical appearance may change dramatically. Physical disfigurement from tumor growth may progress rapidly. The child's color may change as he or she becomes more pale, bluish, mottled, and/or blotchy.

If the parents are alone with the dying child, they may have some concerns that they will not be able to know when the child has died. They must be prepared for this event, including information on things such as the final agonal breathing, described as "puffing" or "fish-out-of-water" breathing,[27] or the late "gasps" that commonly occur after a child dies.

If the child will die at home, it helps the parents if they make funeral arrangements ahead of time.[41] This is often very difficult for the parents but will make things much easier at the actual time of the child's death. Although state laws differ, in many instances the funeral home personnel will come to the home to pick up the child's body if the pediatric oncologist agrees ahead of time to sign the death certificate.

Parents need to know that when a child dies, it is not an emergency. Paramedics, if called, must attempt to resuscitate the child unless they have a do not resuscitate (DNR) order from a physician. On the other hand, the parents do not need to call the funeral home immediately. They may spend as much time as they wish with their child. This time may include bathing, dressing, or holding their child or other family or cultural rituals. "After the last breath (gasp), there needs to be no rush for the stethoscope, but a calm period in which the family holds, prays and/or cuddles their precious child without medical intervention disrupting or validating the obvious."[27]

If the child dies at the cancer center, the family often is asked to consent to an autopsy. They need to know that it is their right to refuse one or to request certain restrictions. However, the autopsy may be helpful if they have some unanswered questions about their child's course, or it may provide information useful to the care of other children with cancer. If the child dies at home, it may be more difficult to obtain an autopsy because of cost and transportation issues. Nevertheless, it is possible in many situations to make the necessary arrangements, and the family should be assisted so that their wish for a home death does not preclude autopsy.

Whether the child dies at home or in the hospital, the family should be given as much time as they need with the child to say goodbye and absorb the reality of the child's death. A supportive nurse, clergy member, or appropriate family friend should stay with them throughout this time to provide support, answer questions as needed, and facilitate the various procedures that must be followed. Even when death is anticipated, the family will be in shock and will be grieving and will need compassionate support and direction.

Siblings. Several studies have described the effects of childhood cancer on healthy siblings. In some families the siblings were described by parents as having problems with enuresis, depression, separation anxiety, somatic complaints, and feelings of guilt.[29,40,44] In a study by Lauer et al.[43] children who participated in the home care of their dying brother or sister described a significantly different experience than those whose sibling died in the hospital. Data from Lauer et al. revealed multiple factors that appeared to favor more positive adjustment for the children who participated in home care. The children's reports indicated that a major advantage of home care was the opportunity for increased family communication and intimacy. Martinson, Davies, and McClowery[50] found that the self-concept ratings of bereaved siblings who had been involved in the Home Care Project[49] were significantly higher than would be expected for "normal" children. Children clearly demonstrated their desire for involvement in the ill child's care.[29,43]

Siblings of the dying child should not become the "forgotten people." In one way or another they have been a part of the child's entire illness and should be allowed to participate in the final processes of the child's life, if they wish, in a way that is comfortable for them. Siblings must be asked. It should not be assumed that they do or do not want inclusion. Parents may believe they should protect the siblings from the reality of death; however, the sibling's fears and fantasies about the dying process may be more detrimental than the reality. If possible and if the siblings wish, they should be present when the death occurs, although their presence should not be forced. Since the parents may be overwhelmed with their own grief, the presence of a supportive adult other than the parent can help the siblings during this process.

"The well siblings of terminally ill children live in houses of chronic sorrow. The signs of sorrow, illness and death are everywhere, whether or not they are spoken of."[8] When a brother or sister is terminally ill, many changes can produce role confusion and conflict and disruption of usual relationships. If siblings are not fully informed, they may feel deceived and rejected by parents. The care of the ill child may occupy so much of the parent's time and attention that the siblings are forced to take on increased responsibilities at home. The relationship between the ill child and sibling may change as death approaches and the terminally ill child withdraws.

The siblings' feelings must also be addressed, particularly those of anger, guilt, and ambivalence.[23] Young children particularly may have wished that their sibling would die during the child's illness. They may need help to understand that their death wish did not cause the actual death. All children have feelings of anger about the special attention and concern given to the child who is ill. They may be frustrated because they cannot express their feelings and fears to preoccupied parents.[35] Such feelings of anger and resentment may lead to feelings of guilt, particularly when the child dies. These children need a caring, nonjudgmental adult who can help them deal with these feelings. All siblings need help from their parents and other caring adults as they deal with their feelings of grief and loss.

Classmates. If the child has attended school, his or her classmates will need help to deal with their own feelings of grief and loss at the death of their classmate. Many of these children will have had no experience with death, and the death of a classmate, no matter how remote from them, will be a profound life experience for them. The child's death should be confronted in an open and forthright manner, dispelling any myths or misconceptions. The classroom teacher, school nurse, school psychologist, and/or school social worker may all become involved in helping the children deal with their feelings. Voluntary attendance at the child's wake or funeral may help some children terminate the relationship and work through their feelings, but no child should be forced to attend.

Staff. The needs of staff members working with dying patients vary according to their level of maturity and past experiences. Contrary to popular belief, one does not "get used to" working with dying children. Staff members who work effectively with dying children throughout the years develop appropriate styles of coping. They are alert to situations

having potential for overidentification. Some staff members, for example, have difficulty caring for a patient similar in age or with characteristics reminiscent of members of their own family. They recognize their own feelings, allow time and space for their own grieving, and gain personal satisfaction from helping the child and family throughout the child's illness and death. Each individual develops an awareness of how best to help the child and family through the illness and dying process. Skill in dealing with death is an experienced-based personal growth process developed over many years.[12]

Other staff members do not cope as effectively with the dying child. They become overly involved or detach themselves as the child's death approaches. The overly involved staff member may make the dying child and family the entire focus of his or her life to the exclusion of personal needs. Although this happens occasionally to almost every pediatric oncology nurse, if it occurs frequently, it is often a danger signal. Frequent overinvolvement can only lead to burnout. On the other hand, the nurse who continuously backs away from the situation when death is inevitable may require as much assistance to deal with his or her feelings as the overly involved nurse.

For the staff "emotional adaptation involves dealing with the reality of the child's death."[10] The inevitability of death may engender feelings of anger, frustration, and depression. Efforts to support the family members in their grief and to relate to the dying child may produce feelings of helplessness and inadequacy that lead to guilt and anger. At the same time, the nurse must deal with personal feelings of sadness and grief over the loss of the child he or she has come to know and love and the changed relationship with parents and family members with whom the nurse has established emotional bonds.

The individual nurse may choose to express these feelings in a destructive or constructive manner.[12] Destructive expressions can include counterproductive or inappropriate behavior such as distancing oneself, becoming defensive, and becoming easily upset or frustrated[5]; overindulgence in food, alcohol, or drugs; or preoccupation with death and dying.[12] Constructive expression includes sharing and working through feelings on a regular basis; personal sensitivity to emotional exhaustion and stress; and coming to terms with his or her own concept of death.[12]

Recognizing the dying child as an independent human being "enables the nurse to work in a partnership rather than a protectorship."[12] Dealing openly and honestly with the dying child means having a willingness to be available as a confidante with whom the child can share his or her fears and feelings. "Availability is a physical, emotional, and spiritual presence; a willingness to respond honestly and compassionately to the child's needs at all times. Such a commitment often leads to extremely high self-expectations."[12] After the child's death, the nurse has the responsibility to replenish himself or herself. Some staff members take a physical and mental break from intense patient involvement to reevaluate, gather strength, and rekindle efforts.[1,28] Others use institutional resources such as psychiatric nurse clinicians or staff support groups. Still others find nonhospital friends and family the best sources for renewal. Strengthening the intellectual, emotional, and philosophic base enables a nurse to remain available day after day to children who might die.[12]

With experience comes the professional maturity to deal effectively with the dying child, the child's family, and oneself.[21] Working with dying patients can help nurses face their own immortality. Each dying child and every family can teach something about life and about dying. In pediatric oncology when death is inevitable, the natural course of the events cannot be changed. However, nurses can make things easier, can help alleviate some of the pain and suffering, can facilitate coping, and can provide physical and emotional support that will make a difference.

Bereavement. The process of grieving is long and painful. Parents and siblings will need support as they go through the grieving process, which will take months or even years.[52,53]

Staff members, however, cannot provide grief support until they do their own grieving. How they support others depends on how they manage their own grieving. Unresolved grief accumulates and interferes with the ability to help others. The staff's feelings must be permitted, acknowledged, felt, and expressed to others. Staff support groups are useful in helping nurses and others deal with their grief. Some guidelines for staff on being helpful and supportive can be found in Table 16–2.

For parents and siblings the grieving process takes much longer than most realize,[56,60] typically 1½ to 2½ years or longer.[69] "The loss of a child is the most painful of human experiences."[69] The grief of losing a child is indescribably painful, both emotionally and, at times, physically.[5,26,30,37,38,62,67–69] Physical manifestations include sleeping problems, lethargy, eating difficulties, weight fluctuations, crying, chest pain, headaches, menstrual irregularities, or muscle spasms.[26] Emotional responses include numbness, denial, anger, sadness, depression, apathy, jealousy, insecurity, guilt, or fear.[26] Although the probability of emotional swings is predictable, the nature and timing of these feelings are not.[69] The grieving persons may actually feel they are going crazy because of the intensity, duration, and unpredictability of their emotions. They need reassurance that they are not going crazy and that their feelings and behavior are normal.[69]

Some may try to avoid grieving by keeping too busy to feel or by using drugs or alcohol to numb their feelings. The hard reality is that grief hurts, the painful energy of grief needs release, and "the only way beyond grief is through it."[26] Some parents and siblings have sufficient inner resources to deal with this grief on their own. Others need help from a caring, supportive staff.[61,72,83] One of the most important things that a staff member can provide is being a good listener as family members express their grief because healing can occur only in a safe, trusting, accepting, compassionate, and nonjudgmental environment.[26] Feelings can be released through talking or writing about the experience, crying, or even screaming. Support groups may be helpful,[9,13,14,36,70] and many families draw strength from their spiritual resources. Referral can be made to community agencies for group or individual counseling.

No words can take the pain away, and

TABLE 16—2. *Do's and Don'ts for Helping Bereaved Parents*

DO'S	DON'TS
Do let your genuine concern and caring show.	Don't let your own sense of helplessness keep you from reaching out to a bereaved parent.
Do be available . . . to listen, to run errands, to help with the other children, or to do whatever else seems needed at the time.	Don't avoid the parents because you are uncomfortable (being avoided by friends adds pain to an already intolerably painful experience).
Do say you are sorry about what happened to their child and about their pain.	Don't say you know how they feel (unless you have lost a child yourself, you probably do not know how they feel).
Do allow them to express as much grief as they are feeling at the moment and are willing to share.	Don't say "you ought to be feeling better by now" or anything else that implies a judgment about their feelings.
Do encourage them to be patient with themselves and not to impose any "shoulds" on themselves.	Don't tell them what they *should* feel or do.
Do allow them to talk about the child they have lost as much and as often as they want.	
Do talk about the special, endearing qualities of the child they have lost.	Don't change the subject when they mention their dead child.
	Don't avoid mentioning the child's name out of fear of reminding them of their pain (they have not forgotten it).
Do give special attention to the child's brothers and sisters—at the funeral and in the months to come (they too are hurt and confused and in need of attention that their parents may not be able to give at this time).	Don't point out that at least they have their other children (children are not interchangeable; they cannot replace each other).
	Don't say that they can always have another child (even if they wanted to and could, another child would not replace the child they have lost).
	Don't suggest that they should be grateful for their other children (grief over the loss of one child does not discount parents' love and appreciation of their living children).
Do reassure parents that they did everything they could and the medical care their child received was the best or whatever else you know to be *true* and *positive* about the care given their child.	Don't make any comments that in any way suggest that the care given their child at home, in the emergency room, in the hospital, or wherever was inadequate (parents are plagued by feelings of doubt and guilt without any help from their family and friends).

healing and recovery do not take place in any systematic sequence of stages. In fact, "one never gets over the loss of a loved one; one learns to live with the loss."[26] Over time the painful episodes become less intense, less frequent, and of shorter duration. Life takes on meaning again as parents and siblings learn to live in a world without the loved child. The hurt becomes "a muted sadness rather than a wrenching agony"[69] as the bereaved learn that, although life will never be the same, it can be good.

CONCLUSION

One of the most painful aspects of pediatric oncology nursing is learning to accept and cope with the death of a terminally ill child. It can also be one of the most personally satisfying and professionally rewarding. Nurses often begin their relationship with the child and family on a hopeful note, stressing the curability of many childhood cancers. When death becomes a probability, nurses must change course to maintain quality of life and facilitate death with dignity. They cannot change the inevitable outcome for the terminally ill child, but they can help make his or her remaining time comfortable and peaceful and help his or her parents and siblings cope with their grief.

REFERENCES

1. Adams JP, Hershatter MJ, Moritz DA. Accumulated loss phenomenon among hospice caregivers. Am J Hospice Palliative Care 1991; 8:29–37.
2. Anthony S. The Child's Discovery of Death. New York: Harcourt, Brace & World, 1940.
3. Anthony Z, Bhana K. An exploratory study of Muslim girls' understanding of death. Omega 1988–1989; 19:215–228.
4. Armstrong GD, Martinson IM. Death, dying, and terminal care: Dying at home. In Kellerman J (ed): Psychosocial Aspects of Childhood Cancer. Springfield, Ill.: Charles C Thomas, 1980.
5. Arnold J, Gemma P. A Child Dies: A Portrait of Family Grief. London: Aspen, 1983.
6. Bendorf K, Meehan J. Home parenteral nutrition for the child with cancer. Issues Compr Pediatr Nurs 1989; 12:187–197.
7. Betz CL. Death, dying and bereavement: A review of the literature, 1970–1985. In Krulik T, Holaday B, Martinson IM (eds): The Child and Family Facing Life-Threatening Illness. Philadelphia: JB Lippincott, 1987.
8. Bluebond-Langner M. Worlds of dying children and their well siblings. Death Studies 1988; 13:1–16.
9. Burnell GM, Burnell AL. The Compassionate Friends: A support group for bereaved parents. J Fam Pract 1986; 22:295–296.
10. Cairns N, Klopovich P, Moore R, et al. The dying child in the classroom. Essence 1980; 4:25–32.
11. Childers P, Wimmer M. The concept of death in early childhood. Child Dev 1971; 42:705–715.
12. Coody D. High expectations: Nurses who work with children who might die. Nurs Clin North Am 1985; 20:131–142.
13. Corr CA. Support for grieving children: The Dougy Center and the hospice philosophy. Am J Hospice Palliative Care 1991; 8:23–27.
14. Davis CB. The use of art therapy and group process with grieving children. Issues Compr Pediatr Nurs 1989; 12:269–280.
15. Davis KG. Educational needs of the terminally ill student. Issues Compr Pediatr Nurs 1989; 12:235–245.
16. DeSpelder LA, Strickland AL. The Last Dance. Mountain View, Calif.: Mayfield, 1987.
17. Dufour DF. Home or hospital care for the child with end-stage cancer: Effects on the family. Issues Compr Pediatr Nurs 1989; 12:171–186.
18. Fetsch SH. The 7- to 10-year-old child's conceptualization of death. Oncol Nurs Forum 1984; 11:52–56.
19. Fetsch SH, Miles MS. Children and death. In Amenta MO, Bohnet NL (eds): Nursing Care of the Terminally Ill. Boston: Little Brown & Co, 1986.
20. Foley GV, Whittam EH. Care of the child dying of cancer, Part I, CA 1990; 40:327–354.
21. Foley GV, Whittam EH. Care of the child dying of cancer, Part II. CA 1991; 41:52–60.
22. Glaser BG, Strauss AL. Time for Dying. Chicago: Aldine, 1968.
23. Grogan LB. Grief of an adolescent when a sibling dies. MCN 1990; 15:21–24.
24. Grollman EA (ed). Explaining Death to Children. Boston: Beacon Press, 1967.
25. Grollman EA. Talking About Death: A Dialogue Between Parent and Child. Boston: Beacon Press, 1970.
26. Gyulay J. Grief responses. Issues Compr Pediatr Nurs 1989; 12:1–31.
27. Gyulay JB. Home care for the dying child. Issues Compr Pediatr Nurs 1989; 12:33–69.
28. Herrle SM, Robinson B. Helping staff cope with grief. Nurs Manage, 1987; 18:33–34.
29. Iles P. Children with cancer: Healthy siblings' perceptions during the illness experience. Cancer Nurs 1979; 2:371–377.
30. Johnson SE. After a Child Dies: Counseling Bereaved Families. New York: Springer, 1987.
31. Johnson-Soderberg S. The development of a child's concept of death. Oncol Nurs Forum 1981; 8:23–26.
32. Kalkofen RW. After a child dies: A funeral director's perspective. Issues Compr Pediatr Nurs 1989; 12:285–297.
33. Kane B. Children's concepts of death. J Genet Psychol 1979; 134:141–153.
34. Kastenbaum RJ. The child's understanding of death: How does it develop? In Grollman EA (ed): Explaining Death to Children. Boston: Beacon Press, 1967.
35. Kastenbaum RJ. Death, Society and Human Experience, 4th ed. New York: Macmillan, 1991.
36. Klass D. Bereaved parents and the Compassionate Friends: Affiliation and healing. In Kalish RA (ed): The Final Transition. Farmingdale, N.Y.: Baywood, 1985.
37. Klass D. Parental Grief. Solace and Resolution. New York: Springer, 1988.
38. Knapp RJ. Beyond Endurance: When a Child Dies. New York: Schocken, 1986.
39. Koocher G. Childhood, death and cognitive development. Dev Psychol 1973; 9:369–375.
40. Kramer RF. Living with childhood cancer: Impact on healthy siblings. Oncol Nurs Forum 1984; 11:44–51.
41. Kuykendall J. Death of a child: The worst kept secret around. In Sherr L: Death, Dying and Bereavement: An Insight for Carers. Boston: Blackwell Scientific, 1989.
42. Lauer ME, Camitta BM. Home care for dying children: A nursing model. J Pediatr 1980; 97:1032–1035.
43. Lauer M, Mulhern R, Bohne J, et al. Children's perceptions of their siblings death at home or hospital: The precursors of differential adjustment. Cancer Nurs 1985; 8:21–27.
44. Lauer M, Mulhern R, Wallskog J, et al. A comparison study of parental adaptation following a child's death at home or in the hospital. Pediatrics 1983; 71:107–112.
45. LeBaron S, Zeltner LK. The role of imagery in the treatment of dying children and adolescents. J Dev Behav Pediatr 1985; 5:252–258.
46. Lonetto R. Children's Conceptions of Death. New York: Springer, 1980.
47. Martin BB. Predictors of length of home and hospital stay, types of services received, cost and family response in an established pediatric hospice program. J Assoc Pediatr Oncol Nurses 1988; 5:27.
48. Martinson I. Home Care for the Dying Child: Professional and Family Perspectives. New York: Appleton-Century-Crofts, 1976.

49. Martinson I, Armstrong G, Geis D, et al. Home care for children dying of cancer. Pediatrics 1978; 62:106–113.
50. Martinson I, Davies E, McClowery S. The long term effects of sibling death on self-concept. J Pediatr Nurs 1987; 2:277–335.
51. Meehan J. Pain control in the terminally ill child at home. Issues Compr Pediatr Nurs 1989; 12:235–245.
52. Miles M. Helping adults mourn the death of a child. In Wass H, Corr C (eds): Children and Death. New York: Hemisphere, 1984.
53. Miles MS. Emotional symptoms and physical health in bereaved parents. Nurs Res 1985; 34:76–81.
54. Miles MS, Burman SL. Nursing care of the dying child. In Mott SR, James SR, Sperhac AM (eds): Nursing Care of Children and Families, 2nd ed. Redwood City, Calif.: Addison-Wesley, 1990.
55. Mills GC. Books to help children understand death. Am J Nurs 1979; 79:291–296.
56. Moore IM, Gilliss CL, Martinson I. Psychosomatic symptoms in parents 2 years after the death of a child with cancer. Nurs Res 1988; 37:104–107.
57. Nagy MH. The child's theories concerning death. J Genet Psychol 1948; 73:2–27.
58. Pazola KJ, Gerberg AK. Privileged communication—Talking with a dying adolescent. MCN 1990; 15:16–20.
59. Piaget J. The Origin of Intelligence in Children. New York: Harcourt, Brace & World, 1932.
60. Rando TA. An investigation of grief and adaptation in parents whose children have died from cancer. J Pediatr Psychol 1983; 8:13–20.
61. Rando TA. Bereaved parents: Particular difficulties, unique factors and treatment issues. Social Work 1985; 30:19–23.
62. Rando TA (ed). Parental Loss of a Child. Champaign, Ill.: Research Press, 1986.
63. Reimer JC, Davies B, Martens N. Palliative care: The nurse's role in helping families through the transition of "fading away." Cancer Nurs 1991; 14:321–327.
64. Rogers F. When a Pet Dies. New York: GP Putnam, 1988.
65. Ross-Alaolmolki K. Supportive care for families of dying children. Nurs Clin North Am 1985; 20:457–466.
66. Safier G. A study in relationships between the life and death concepts in children. J Genet Psychol 1964; 105:283–294.
67. Schiff HS. The Bereaved Parent. New York: Penguin Press, 1978.
68. Schiff HS. Living Through Mourning: Finding Comfort and Hope When a Loved One Has Died. New York: Penguin Press, 1986.
69. Schmidt L. Working with bereaved parents. In Krulik T, Holaday B, Martinson IM (eds): The Child and Family Facing Life Threatening Illness. Philadelphia: JB Lippincott, 1987.
70. Soricelli BA, Utech CL. Mourning the death of a child: The family and group process. Social Work 1985; 30:429–434.
71. Speece MW, Brent SW. Children's understanding of death: A review of three components of a death concept. Child Dev 1984; 55:1671–1686.
72. Spinetta JJ, Deasy-Spinetta P. Talking with children who have a life-threatening illness. In Spinetta JJ, Deasy-Spinetta P (eds): Living With Childhood Cancer. St. Louis: CV Mosby, 1981.
73. Spinetta JJ, Maloney LJ. Death anxiety in the outpatient leukemic child. Pediatrics 1975; 56:1034–1037.
74. Spinetta JJ, Rigler D, Karon M. Anxiety in the dying child. Pediatrics 1973; 52:841–849.
75. Stillion J, Wass H. Children and death. In Wass H (ed): Dying: Facing the Facts. New York: Hemisphere, 1979.
76. Tallmer M, Formanek R, Tallmer J. Factors influencing children's concepts of death. J Clin Child Psychol 1974; 3:17–19.
77. Vianello R, Lucamante M. Children's understanding of death according to parents and pediatricians. J Genet Psychol 1988; 149:305–316.
78. Viorst J. The Tenth Good Thing About Barney. New York: Atheneum, 1984.
79. Waechter E. Children's awareness of fatal illness. Am J Nurs 1971; 71:1168–1172.
80. Waechter EH. The adolescent with life-threatening chronic illness. In Mercer RP (ed): Perspectives on Adolescent Health Care. Philadelphia: JB Lippincott, 1979.
81. Waechter EH. Dying children: Patterns of coping. In Wass H, Corr CA (eds): Childhood and Death. New York: Hemisphere, 1984.
82. Waechter EH. Death, dying and bereavement: A review of the literature. In Krulik T, Holaday B, Martinson IM (eds): The Child and Family Facing Life Threatening Illness. Philadelphia: JB Lippincott, 1987.
83. Waechter EH. How families cope: Assessing and intervening. In Krulik T, Holaday B, Martinson IM (eds): The Child and Family Facing Life Threatening Illness. Philadelphia: JB Lippincott, 1987.
84. Wass H, Corr CA (eds). Childhood and Death. New York: Hemisphere, 1984.
85. Wenestam C-G, Wass H. Swedish and U.S. children's thinking about death: A qualitative study and cross-cultural comparison. Death Studies 1987; 11:99–122.

LATE EFFECTS IN LONG-TERM SURVIVORS

Wendy Hobbie

Kathleen Ruccione

Ida (Ki) Moore

Susie Truesdell

At least 60% of children diagnosed with cancer will become long-term survivors, defined by the absence of disease for 5 years and being off therapy for at least 2 years.[119,131] Most are considered cured of their disease. As of 1990, it was estimated there are 125,000 to 150,000 long-term survivors of childhood cancer.[18] Projecting from the number of children diagnosed with cancer each year and the current survival rate, 5000 additional survivors of childhood cancer can be expected annually.

Survival rates have increased over the past 30 years in response to advances in surgery, radiation, chemotherapy, and supportive care. Components of modern multimodality treatment regimens also affect normal cells and organs adversely, as does the disease itself. Persistent injuries to normal tissues that may become apparent months to years after completion of therapy are commonly called *late effects*. This terminology is used in this text, although *long-term effects* is probably a more accurate term. Lack of nourishment to healthy cells, chronic cell injury, death of cells with subsequent loss of normal functioning tissue, and scar tissue formation result in these late effects. They may manifest themselves as (1) clinically obvious effects that interfere with activities of daily living (e.g., pulmonary fibrosis resulting in respiratory distress); (2) clinically subtle effects noticeable to the trained observer (e.g., learning impairment after treatment of the central nervous system); and (3) subclinical effects detectable only by laboratory screening or x-ray studies (e.g., elevated liver enzyme levels).[61]

Survivors of childhood cancer must be evaluated in a systematic manner. Early identification and intervention may attenuate late effects of treatment. Knowledge gained from survivors assists in modifying current protocols to decrease the late effects for future generations. Although some late effects can have a profound effect on a child's life, the cost for cure must be balanced with the "richness of surviving."[136]

The nurse plays a pivotal role in the systematic evaluation and follow-up care of long-term survivors. Sound knowledge of potential long-term consequences of therapy and clinical expertise in detecting abnormalities based on history and physical examination are essential. A broad background in growth and development is necessary to change the focus from "sick child" to the promotion of normalcy.[79]

The nurse coordinates services among multiple disciplines. Organizing referrals and transferring information to other services and then back to patients facilitate comprehensive care and identification of the nurse as a key resource person and case manager. Providing education to change the stigma of cancer is an important role of the nurse. Patients, parents, and the general, medical, and nursing communities need education about survival rates, life expectancies, and quality of life issues. Educating insurance companies and the military has also become important as the survivors become young adults. The clinical nurse also can collaborate with nurse researchers to address the many unanswered questions of the survivorship experience.

ASSESSING ENDOCRINE SYSTEM FOR LATE EFFECTS

The endocrine system often is affected by cancer treatment. The dysfunction of this system can result from either direct damage to the end organ (ovaries, testes, thyroid gland) or the controlling hypothalamic-pituitary axis.

Hypothalamic-Pituitary Axis

The hypothalamus and pituitary gland work synergistically to maintain endocrine homeostasis and are connected by the pituitary stalk. Releasing and inhibiting hormones are produced in the hypothalamus and carried to the anterior pituitary gland via the portal vessels. The releasing and inhibitory hormones act on the anterior pituitary (hypophysis) to regulate production and storage of thyroid-stimulating hormone (TSH), luteinizing hormone (LH), follicle-stimulating hormone (FSH), growth hormone (GH), adrenocorticotropic hormone (ACTH), and melanocyte-stimulating hormone (MSH). Oxytocin and antidiuretic hormone are produced in the hypothalamus and released into the posterior pituitary gland (neurohypophysis).[88]

Effect of Radiation. Radiation delivered to the cranium or nasopharynx can cause hypothalamic-pituitary dysfunction. The hypothalamus is adversely affected by doses ≥2400 cGy, but the pituitary gland is more radioresistant, requiring doses ≥4000 cGy to cause dysfunction.[170]

GH production and release are usually affected first by radiation damage. Some children with acute lymphocytic leukemia (ALL) treated prophylactically with cranial irradiation equaling 2400 cGy have had growth disturbances.[157] However, it is generally with doses greater than 3000 cGy that growth is severely compromised. Studies have found that 50% of children treated for brain tumors with more than 3000 cGy have severe growth retardation.[139,145]

Radiation to the spine such as that used with some patients treated for brain tumors or central nervous system (CNS) disease with ALL and whole abdominal irradiation compromise spinal growth and result in a shortened trunk.[14,169] This alone or in combination with GH failure compromises linear growth.

Patients treated with total body irradiation have GH deficiency characterized by a decreased rate of growth (<5 cm/year), delayed bone age (documented by x-ray studies), short stature, and documented low GH and somatomedin-C levels.

Subnormal levels of GH have been found in as many as 87% of children who received cranial irradiation, followed by total body irradiation before bone marrow transplant.[36] However, 42% of patients have documented low secretion of GH after total body irradiation alone.[165] Several factors such as damage to the epiphyseal growth plate, poor nutrition, and thyroid dysfunction also play a role in bone marrow transplant patients' poor growth patterns.[165]

Other factors that may contribute to the radiation effects on the hypothalamic-pituitary axis are the age of the child (younger children are affected more than adults), the method of radiation, number of fractions, fraction size, and duration of treatment.[157,170]

Precocious puberty has been noted following radiation to the hypothalamus. Generally this is noted after doses >2500 cGy but occasionally has been seen in patients treated with 1800 cGy cranial irradiation. These patients begin to exhibit secondary sex characteristics at early ages (8 years for females, 10 years for males) and if untreated, will have early halted growth from premature fusion of epiphyses.[174] The patient exhibiting early secondary sex characteristics should be referred to an endocrinologist for evaluation and treatment.

Assessment Guidelines for Late Effects on Hypothalamic-Pituitary Axis. Standing height must be obtained every 6 months (in children who exhibit growth problems), preferably with a stadiometer (device to measure linear height), and plotted on a growth chart. Sitting height should also be taken at each visit. Diagnostic studies should be completed on any child who demonstrates deceleration in growth. Sitting height, thyroid function studies, and bone age are part of a growth evaluation. In addition, determination of sexual maturation is important to rule out precocious puberty since, as noted previously, an early growth spurt can mask a GH deficiency and prematurely close the epiphyses.[174] The Tanner staging system[183] gauges sexual maturation by penile and scrotal development, breast development, and pubic hair growth. A score of 1 on this scale indicates no secondary sex characteristics, and a 5 indicates an adult.

Provocative testing is necessary to document GH deficiency before treatment with GH. One way of testing for GH deficiency is by the administration of oral L-dopa and intravenous (IV) arginine to measure GH secretions.[204] Synthetic GH replacement is given to patients with documented GH deficiency. Treatment generally improves final heights, but patients have a wide range of growth response from this therapy.[80] Those treated with spinal radiation and bone marrow transplantation generally have poorer responses to therapy because of multiple factors affecting growth.[174]

There has been concern that the use of GH could promote recurrence and relapse of disease in long-term survivors. However, results of current studies suggest that survivors are not at increased risk for relapse or recurrence when GH is used.[6,34] Treatment centers are beginning to monitor children treated with anthracyclines and GH because of concern about GH increasing cardiac overload and placing the children at greater risk for cardiac problems.

Thyroid Gland

TSH is produced and secreted by the anterior pituitary gland in response to thyrotropin-releasing hormone (TRH), which is produced in the hypothalamus. TSH stimulates the thyroid gland to produce thyroxine (T_4) and triiodothyronine (T_3).[88] Function of the thyroid gland can be compromised by direct irradiation to the gland or by damage to the hypothalamic-pituitary axis.

Overt or Compensatory Hypothyroidism. Overt hypothyroidism is characterized by lethargy, weight gain, dry skin, anemia, hair loss, poor growth rate, and delay in intellectual development. Patients with hypothyroidism have elevated TSH levels and decreased T_3 and T_4 levels. Clinically, compensatory hypothyroidism is demonstrated by elevated TSH levels with normal serum levels of T_3 and T_4.

Radiation doses of >2600 cGy delivered to the thyroid gland result in hypothyroidism in 4% to 79% of the patients based on an elevated TSH level.[124,154] Studies have revealed that patients receiving <2600 cGy to the thyroid gland (mantle) have a 17% rate of hypothyroidism, whereas doses >2600 cGy cause hypothyroidism in 78% of the population.[37] Thyroid dysfunction usually appears 3 to 5 years after treatment.[37,124] Thirty-five percent of patients treated with a single total body irradiation dose of 750 cGy demonstrated an elevated TSH level.[173]

Occasionally, hyperthyroidism has been noted following radiation therapy to the thyroid gland.[132]

Secondary Hypothyroidism. Secondary hypothyroidism is found in patients who receive radiation doses >5500 cGy to the hypothalamic-pituitary axis. These patients are hypothyroid (clinically and chemically) with a low TSH level. TSH stimulation testing will confirm the diagnosis.[163] TSH response to TRH can be used to determine whether the anterior pituitary gland is damaged (TSH level remains low) or the hypothalamus is damaged (TSH level increases).

Assessment Guidelines for Late Effects on Thyroid Gland. Treatment of hypothyroidism with thyroid supplements is recommended for patients with either overt or compensatory hypothyroidism. Patients with compensatory hypothyroidism probably are overstimulating the thyroid gland, which may place them at an increased risk for second malignant neoplasms in the thyroid gland because of the stress placed on the gland.[37]

Patients at high risk for thyroid gland dysfunction should have an annual examination of the gland. In addition, to determine free T_4 and TSH levels, blood should be drawn annually for 15 to 20 years after treatment and only if symptoms arise thereafter. A referral to an endocrinologist is necessary if any abnormalities are noted.

Testes

Testicular function is controlled by the release of FSH and LH from the pituitary gland. Gonadotrophin-releasing hormone (Gn-RH) is released from the hypothalamus and controls LH and FSH secretions. The Leydig cells located in the testes produce testosterone, and the germinal epithelia produce spermatozoa. The testosterone-producing Leydig cells affect secretion of LH and FSH by a negative feedback mechanism.[88] Germinal cell epithelia are very sensitive to cancer therapy and are damaged more easily than the Leydig cells.

Primary Testicular Failure. The signs and symptoms of primary testicular failure are lack of secondary sex characteristics, lack of or change in libido (if Leydig cells are affected), and low sperm counts. Elevations in LH and FSH with possible decrease in testosterone are indicative of dysfunction. Alkylating agents primarily affect the germinal epithelia. Age at diagnosis, nutritional status at time of treatment, and combination therapy affect the degree of dysfunction.[114] Total doses of more than 11 g of cyclophosphamide can cause azoospermia; some patients who received fewer than 11 g seem to retain normal function.[153] Patients treated with combinations of mustard, vincristine, procarbazine, prednisone (MOPP) therapy experienced changes with as few as three to five cycles of treatment. In general, greater than six cycles of MOPP will cause permanent infertility.[47]

Radiation to the testicle is very damaging to the germinal epithelia. As little as 10 cGy can temporarily reduce the number of spermatozoa.[35] Doses of radiation between 400 and 600 cGy cause azoospermia that may be reversible within 3 to 5 years after completion of therapy. However, doses >600 cGy appear to cause permanent azoospermia.[7] Leydig cell function is rarely affected by radiation doses <2000 cGy. Some boys treated with 2400 cGy for testicular leukemia have been found to have Leydig cell damage.[16]

Secondary Testicular Failure. Secondary testicular dysfunction is caused by radiation to the hypothalamic-pituitary axis. Doses >5500 cGy cause hypothalamic damage, resulting in a decreased production of prolactin-inhibiting factor (PIF) that causes hyperprolactemia. In men this condition is characterized by decreased libido and impotence and decreased testosterone levels. Treatment with bromocriptine resolves these symptoms.[38]

Assessment Guidelines for Late Effects on Testes. The testes of every male at risk for testicular damage should be examined to determine if they are the appropriate size for their stage of sexual development. A recent study has correlated the size of the testicle with degree of function.[172] In addition, every patient should be graded on the Tanner scale to determine their stage of sexual development to identify patients with halted or delayed pubertal progression.

Serum LH, FSH, testosterone, and prolactin (if appropriate) levels should be determined at the age of 12 years on any patient at risk for dysfunction and annually until full sexual maturation is achieved. If symptoms of dysfunction arise, reevaluation is necessary. Semen samples can be obtained, starting at the age of full sexual maturation, to determine the number and condition of sperm.

This examination should be repeated every 3 to 5 years to evaluate sperm production and possible recovery.

Sperm banking before treatment should be an option offered to all males who are producing sperm. The only reliable means of ascertaining if a male has a sufficient sperm count is performing a semen analysis. Adult levels of testosterone are produced when a male is Tanner IV.[202] Therefore if a male is at least a stage IV, the option of testing should be offered. However, many young men are initially seen with low sperm counts as a result of their illness.[31]

The physiologic changes associated with gonadal failure can be treated with hormones. However, the psychologic impact of infertility may require counseling to help these patients deal with their feelings and explore alternate methods of becoming a parent (e.g., adoption). Genetic counseling may be indicated if their treatment (e.g., MOPP therapy) may have affected the viable sperm or if they had a genetic form of cancer (e.g., retinoblastoma). It is important to stress to these patients that infertility does not mean impotence; in most cases the adolescent or young adult will function as a normal male.

Ovaries

Ovarian function is controlled by the release of FSH and LH from the pituitary gland. The release of LH and FSH is controlled by Gn-RH from the hypothalamus. Estrogen production in the ovary regulates the LH and FSH secretion from the hypothalamus through a negative feedback mechanism.[88]

Primary Ovarian Failure. Ovarian failure is characterized by lack of or halted pubertal progression, amenorrhea, decreased libido, vaginal dryness, mood swings, and hot flashes. Elevated levels of serum LH and FSH with low levels of estradiol are noted with primary ovarian failure.[29] The severity of ovarian dysfunction is related to a number of factors: (1) the dose of chemotherapy and/or radiation; (2) stage of puberty at diagnosis; (3) patient's nutritional status at the time of diagnosis; (4) duration of therapy; and (5) surgical removal of ovaries.[138]

The prepubescent ovary was once believed protected against treatment effects. However, a decreased number of ova are found after cancer treatment in prepubescent females, particularly in those patients with poor nutritional status and those who have undergone a longer duration of treatment.[138]

MOPP chemotherapy, which is used for Hodgkin's disease, includes a number of alkylating agents. Women over the age of 30 are more likely to become amenorrheic than younger women or girls after receiving this combination chemotherapy.[3] Cyclophosphamide-induced ovarian dysfunction occurs after doses of 4 g in women >40 years, whereas doses of 20 g in prepubescent females usually do not interfere with the attainment of puberty after completion of treatment.[99,123] On the other hand, it is hypothesized that the latter population will be at risk for ovarian dysfunction or early onset of menopause because of treatment-induced reduction in the number of ova.[80]

Radiation to the ovary in doses up to 800 cGy does not cause ovarian failure.[7,196] Doses over 1200 cGy have been administered to children with preservation of ovarian function in some patients.[179] Fifty percent of girls treated with 1200 cGy of spinal radiation therapy for ALL experience ovarian failure.[74] Ovarian failure is common after pelvic radiation (3000 to 4000 cGy) for Hodgkin's disease unless the ovaries are surgically moved out of the radiation field (oophoropexy).[85] The use of oral contraceptives (suppression of ovulation is thought to protect the ova) and oophoropexy are two methods used in an attempt to preserve ovarian function.[30] However, conflicting data make it difficult to determine their efficacy. Oophoropexy does not protect the ovary if systemic chemotherapy is used, and actual manipulation of the ovary may also cause damage to the ovary because of possible disruption of blood flow.[63] Results from studies of the protective mechanism of oral contraceptive use while patients are receiving therapy are mixed. One study revealed five out of six women preserved normal gonadal function after treatment for Hodgkin's disease and concomitant use of oral contraceptives,[30] whereas other researchers have documented ovarian failure even with the use of oral contraceptives.[202]

Surgical removal of the ovaries is a rare event in pediatric oncology. However, it would cause primary ovarian failure, and the patient would require hormonal replacement to attain full sexual maturation and prevent long-term consequences of estrogen depletion (e.g., osteoporosis).

Secondary Ovarian Failure. Secondary ovarian failure is caused by radiation damage to the hypothalamic-pituitary axis. The type of radiation, fraction dose and number of fractions, and the duration of treatment are all factors affecting the degree of dysfunction. In patients with secondary ovarian failure serum studies reveal decreased LH, FSH, and estradiol levels.

Higher doses of radiation ($\geq$5500 cGy) to the hypothalamus decrease PIF. This decrease can cause irregular menstrual bleeding and anovulatory periods. Patients who demonstrate these symptoms and who have received high doses of cranial radiation should be evaluated for hyperprolactinemia. Bromocriptine is used to suppress the secretion of prolactin.[38]

Precocious puberty has also been documented after cranial irradiation as a result of hypothalamic damage.[20] Precocious puberty is defined as any secondary sex characteristics in a female before the age of 8 years. If early sexual development is noted, the child should be referred to an endocrinologist for treatment to halt the maturational process.

Assessment Guidelines for Late Effects on Ovaries. Careful monitoring of sexual development and menses is imperative for early identification of problems and for initiation of appropriate treatment. A baseline determination of LH, FSH, and estradiol levels should be made at 12 years and annually until puberty is completed. If symptoms of ovarian failure arise, LH, FSH, estradiol, and prolactin levels should be determined. A referral to an endocrinologist should follow the evaluation. Patients at risk for ovarian failure but currently with normal functioning ovaries (and who plan to have children) are encouraged to have children before 30 years of age because of the risk of early menopause. Furthermore, these patients should not wait the usual 1 year before obtaining an infertility referral, for their referral to a fertility clinic is imperative for complete evaluation and presentation of options. In addition, genetic counseling may be necessary if the survivor had a congenital tumor (e.g., retinoblastoma) or if treatment may have affected the ova (e.g., with Hodgkin's disease).

ASSESSING CENTRAL NERVOUS SYSTEM FOR LATE EFFECTS

Neuropsychologic deficits and neuroanatomic abnormalities can occur as a result of whole brain radiation therapy and intrathecal (IT) chemotherapy.[146,148,149] The combination of 2400 cGy or more of radiation therapy and IT methotrexate has been most closely associated with CNS late effects that usually become apparent 2 to 5 years after treatment.[121,181] However, children treated with lower radiation therapy doses (e.g., 1800 cGy) can also experience long-term neurologic toxicities.[156] Greater doses of chemotherapy can increase the severity of CNS late effects because of synergism between radiation therapy and drugs such as methotrexate.[160]

Neuropsychologic Effects of Treatment. Neuropsychologic, or cognitive, impairments are typically manifested as significant declines (10 to 20 points) in IQ and academic achievement scores and as specific deficits in visual motor integration, memory, attention and motor skills.[39,52,60,66,101,133,148,150] Nonverbal skills (e.g., abstract reasoning, visual spatial skills, arithmetic) are particularly vulnerable to the damaging effects of radiation therapy and IT chemotherapy. Deficits in these areas often appear first. Children who receive CNS therapy before the age of 5 years are at great risk for cognitive impairments. This "age-at-time-of-treatment" effect is believed due to the vulnerability of the developing brain to the delayed toxicity associated with radiation and IT therapy.[91,130]

Neuroanatomic Effects of Treatment. Atrophy and decreased subcortical white matter are the most common neuroanatomic abnormalities after CNS treatment. Calcifications and leukoencephalopathy (progressive white matter deterioration) occur less frequently. These structural changes can be detected by computerized tomography (CT) and magnetic resonance imaging (MRI) studies. Atrophy is typically seen as dilation of the ventricles and widening of the subarachnoid space. Periventricular hypodensity is a frequent CT finding and generally is thought to represent decreased white matter.[23,46,146,147,149] Children with leukoencephalopathy, the most severe form of persistent neurologic toxicity, may also have elevated levels of myelin basic protein in the cerebral spinal fluid.[64]

Although radiation is the type of treatment most closely associated with neuroanatomic pathology, less severe changes have also been observed in up to 20% of children who receive only IT methotrexate.[140] Risk factors for neuroanatomic abnormalities include whole brain radiation therapy, IT chemotherapy doses, and younger age at the time of treatment. The recent use of hyperfractionated radiation (e.g., in the treatment of medulloblastoma) may be less damaging to normal CNS tissues and therefore result in less severe neuroanatomic abnormalities and neuropsychologic deficits.

Assessment Guidelines for Late Effects on Central Nervous System. A comprehensive assessment for CNS late effects involve parental and teacher appraisal of school performance, neuropsychologic evaluation, and neuroimaging studies. The neuropsychologic evaluation should consist of measures of general intelligence (e.g., Wechsler Intelligence Scale for Children–Revised) and academic achievement (e.g., Wide Range Achievement Test of Reading, Spelling and Arithmetic) and tests of more specific areas of cognitive functioning, especially for those children whose CNS treatment places them at high risk for late effects. However, factors such as the physical and emotional stress associated with a very recent cancer diagnosis, physical fatigue after induction chemotherapy, and surgery in the brain tumor population make it difficult to obtain reliable neuropsychologic data before the child receives CNS therapy. Because acute toxicity usually resolves within

3 months and cognitive impairments do not become measurable for approximately 24 months after whole brain radiation therapy and IT chemotherapy, baseline evaluations can be completed 3 to 6 months after CNS treatment. Subsequent evaluations should be conducted on an annual basis, especially in high-risk patients. The importance of serial evaluations is based on the fact that learning deficits often progress over time.

Coordinating the multidisciplinary care required and interpreting the evaluation results to the family and the school are important roles for the pediatric oncology nurse. If educational needs can be identified and appropriate interventions initiated as soon as possible, it may be possible to minimize the child's academic problems. It is essential to seek the consultation of educational specialists when planning for the child's unique educational needs.

The teacher may be unaware of the child's previous cancer treatment or that CNS treatment can have long-term adverse effects on school performance. It is essential that the parents keep in close communication with the school about the child's progress. An Individual Educational Program (IEP) can be established for the child who has special needs as a result of previous cancer treatment. The pediatric oncology nurse has a central role in encouraging parents to be advocates for the child's educational needs (e.g., providing teachers with essential information about the long-term educational effects of cancer treatment).

ASSESSING CARDIOVASCULAR SYSTEM FOR LATE EFFECTS

Acute and/or chronic cardiovascular sequelae occur in children treated with anthracyclines, mediastinal radiation, and/or cyclophosphamide.[2,21,53,69] The presence or absence of acute complications does not correlate with the development of late complications. In most cases the total dose delivered correlates directly with the development of late complications and long-term sequelae.[21] However, there are isolated cases of cardiovascular complications in children receiving low-doses of these agents. Early recognition of the myocardial dysfunction may improve long-term survival.

Effects of Anthracyclines

Anthracycline-induced cardiovascular abnormalities are seen in approximately 25% of patients; the frequency of abnormal findings increases with total doses >350 mg/m². Anthracyclines affect cardiac myocytes, causing loss of muscle fibers and shifts in intracellular calcium. A decrease in the number of myocardial muscle fibers coupled with diminished available calcium may predispose these children to myocardial dysfunction and arrhythmias.

Although cardiomyopathic changes are more common, electrocardiographic (ECG) changes that may predispose these children to serious ventricular arrhythmias have also been reported.[2,178] In addition to diminishing QRS voltages seen in children with increasing anthracycline cardiotoxicity, other ECG changes are now being appreciated. QT_c (the heart rate corrected time in milliseconds from the onset of the Q wave to the termination of the T wave), which measures the repolarization phase, is prolonged in many of these children. The normal QT_c is less than 0.43 msec. Many of these children have QT_c measurements near 0.5 msec. Prolongation of the QT_c puts the heart at risk for ventricular arrhythmias, and 24-hour ECG recordings have shown short runs of ventricular tachycardia or multiple premature ventricular contractions (PVCs) in some of these patients.[11,168]

Cardiac failure can occur at times of increased cardiovascular stress such as during anesthesia, pregnancy, illness, illicit drug ingestion, or heavy weight lifting. There are isolated reports of patients previously treated with anthracyclines who experience cardiovascular collapse while undergoing anesthesia.[19] All patients who have received anthracyclines must be considered to have abnormal myocardium and therefore at risk during procedures that stress the cardiovascular system.

Assessment Guidelines for Late Effects of Anthracyclines on Cardiovascular System. Careful health history and examination of patients should include history of exercise in-tolerance, dizziness, palpitations or syncope, vital signs, the presence of S_3 or S_4 heart murmurs, an echocardiogram (to measure fractional shortening, velocity of circumferential fiber shortening or ejection fraction, and diastolic function indices), and electrocardiography with QT_c measurement. Multiple gated acquisition (MUGA) scans may be done to evaluate cardiac function further. Patients with exercise intolerance, dizziness, palpitations, syncope, or prolonged QT_c should be referred to a cardiologist. The cardiologist's evaluation may include an exercise test with serial measurements of QT_c and pulmonary function, use of a 24-hour Holter monitor for evaluation of ventricular arrhythmias, and/or cardiac catheterization for endomyocardial biopsy. Treatment of cardiomyopathy may include the following medications: digoxin, diuretics, and under certain circumstances afterload-reducing agents such as enalapril. For those patients who are not helped with this regimen, cardiac transplantation may be considered.

Effects of Mediastinal Radiation

Mediastinal radiation has at least three separate effects on the heart. First, thickening of the atrioventricular (AV) valves and pericardium may cause mitral or tricuspid insufficiency or restrictive pericardial changes. Second, histologic changes in the coronary arteries occur and predispose these children to early coronary atherosclerosis and early myocardial ischemia and infarction.[78] Third, there is often damage to the right ventricle (which is anterior to the chest and therefore receives the highest radiation dose) with areas of myocardial fibrosis.[53] The general incidence of these changes is 35% to 40%.[78] However, mild abnormalities may escape detection and thus are recognized only when the abnormality becomes clinically significant. Surgical approaches to restrictive pericarditis are difficult, with varying results. AV valve insufficiency, if severe, would warrant surgical valve replacement. Coronary artery disease would be managed with coronary artery bypass graft (CABG) surgery or balloon dilation angioplasty. Right ventricular (RV) dysfunction is not amenable to surgery but could be managed in the same manner as anthracycline-induced cardiomyopathy.

Assessment Guidelines for Late Effects of Radiation on Cardiovascular System. For all mantle radiation patients, a careful history should be taken to evaluate exercise tolerance, chest pain, and dizziness. Physical examination should include evaluation of vital signs, the presence of S_3 or S_4 heart murmurs, and cardiac rhythm. An echocardiogram can be performed to evaluate fractional shortening and diastolic function indices. Evaluation of the AV valves for valvular insufficiency and the pericardium for unusual thickening should be completed by a cardiologist.

Effects of Cyclophosphamide

High-dose cyclophosphamide such as is used in preparatory regimens for bone marrow transplantation can cause acute cardiotoxicity with decreased QRS voltages, diminished ventricular function, pericardial effusions, pericardial tamponade, and acute congestive heart failure.[69] In those who survive this treatment, these abnormalities usually return to baseline within a few months. Long-term effects of this agent remain unknown.

Assessment Guidelines for Late Effects of Cyclophosphamide on Cardiovascular System. Until more information is available about children who have been treated with cyclophosphamide for bone marrow transplantation, obtaining an ECG and echocardiogram in conjunction with history and physical examinations is recommended.

ASSESSING RESPIRATORY SYSTEM FOR LATE EFFECTS

Acute pneumonitis and chronic fibrosis result from radiation damage to type II pneumocytes and endothelial cells. Chronic changes result from impairment in the growth of new or established alveoli. Chronic changes are enhanced by decreased growth of the muscle, cartilage, and bone of the chest wall.[73]

Acute Pneumonitis. Acute pneumonitis usually appears 3 to 6 months after therapy.

Acute changes are seen in 5% to 15% of patients and generally do not develop until 3000 cGy are delivered to more than 50% of the lung volume.[198] Chronic changes may appear months to years after treatment; however, most changes are apparent within 1 to 2 years.[73] Symptoms of pulmonary fibrosis include dyspnea, dry cough, and low exercise tolerance. Symptoms may progress to cyanosis, progressive respiratory distress, and occasionally respiratory failure and death.[10,162]

The dose of lung radiation considered consistent with life is 2500 cGy without dactinomycin and 1500 cGy with dactinomycin.[73] Even with these dose limitations, chronic changes are noted on pulmonary function studies in patients treated for Ewing's sarcoma, Wilms' tumor, and Hodgkin's disease.[89,120] Lung capacity and vital capacity are 70% of predicted volumes after standard treatment for metastatic Wilms' tumor.[13] Patients treated with 3500 to 4000 cGy to the mantle for Hodgkin's disease generally exhibit a 5% incidence of pneumonitis.[92,124] Most of these patients are asymptomatic, but pulmonary function tests reveal decreases in maximal breathing capacity and tidal volumes. Chest x-ray studies may reveal linear streaking, regional contraction, pleural thickening, and tenting of the diaphragm.[36]

Total body irradiation is also associated with acute and chronic lung changes. The rate for pneumonitis is generally 5% after autologous transplant and 20% after allogeneic transplant.[165]

Chronic Fibrosis. Bleomycin, busulfan, and nitrosoureas (CCNU/BCNU) can cause pulmonary fibrosis. Doses >400 U of bleomycin and >800 of CCNU/BCNU apparently are correlated with a higher incidence of damage.[10,141,164] Concurrent lung irradiation increases the damaging effect.[162] The incidence of chronic fibrosis after doses >400 U of bleomycin is approximately 10%. At lower doses the incidence is approximately 5%.[10,163] BCNU toxicity is seen with as little as 800 mg/m², although with doses >1500 mg/m² the incidence of symptoms of chronic fibrosis is 50%.[5] Melphalan, cyclophosphamide, vinblastine, and methotrexate have all been implicated in causing pulmonary fibrosis but not at a significantly high incidence.

Assessment Guidelines for Late Effects on Respiratory System.   Careful follow-up is required, including assessment for signs and symptoms of pulmonary fibrosis. A chest x-ray study and baseline pulmonary function tests with perfusion studies to evaluate the condition of the lung tissue and to follow any changes should be done every 3 to 5 years if no or mild abnormalities are noted. If moderate to severe changes are present, referral to a pulmonologist is recommended in addition to more frequent pulmonary function tests. Treatment may include steroids or bronchodilators. Patients treated with bleomycin must be aware that they are at increased risk for pulmonary complications if high concentrations of oxygen are administered during surgery or postoperatively. Recommendations are to reduce the oxygen concentration intraoperatively and postoperatively to levels slightly above or at room air. In addition, careful monitoring of fluid replacement with administration of more colloid versus crystalloid fluids is important to decrease the risk of pulmonary interstitial edema.[68]

ASSESSING MUSCULOSKELETAL SYSTEM FOR LATE EFFECTS

Growth and development are often used as indicators of health in a child. Radiation therapy and surgery may greatly affect a child's growth and development.

Effects of Radiation on Bone Growth.   Aside from the endocrine effects of treatment, radiation therapy delivered directly to growing bones, epiphyses, and soft tissue most dramatically affects growth. Doses of 1000 to 2000 cGy cause partial growth arrest. Doses >2000 cGy completely arrest endochondral bone formation.[73,201] Bones, soft tissue, and blood vessels are most susceptible to damage during phases of rapid growth. Therefore the effects of radiation on growth are most pronounced in children less than 6 years of age and during the pubertal growth spurt.[152]

Decreased bone growth after irradiation is associated with a decrease in muscle and soft tissue mass in the area. This change in the soft tissue and muscle mass results in asymmetry of the body referred to as *hypoplasia.* The development of fat in the irradiated areas is also compromised, which will make the asymmetry even more pronounced, particularly in overweight patients.[73]

Irradiation to the vertebral bodies results in end-plate irregularities, loss of vertebral height, abnormal contour, lateral wedging, atrophy of the pedicle and/or lamina, and growth arrest lines.[73] These deformities and the development of scoliosis, kyphosis, and shortened sitting height (crown to rump) are prevalent following doses >2000 cGy to the spine. Studies have documented scoliosis in 67% to 80% of patients treated with 2000 to 6200 cGy to the spine.[36] Hypoplasia of the ilium often occurs after flank irradiation (for Wilms' tumor) and may affect the degree of scoliosis.[161,189] Marked progression of scoliosis occurs during the pubertal growth spurt regardless of when the child was treated. Careful monitoring is necessary at this time.[36]

Avascular necrosis of the femoral head is most frequently associated with combination radiation and chemotherapy for the treatment of Hodgkin's disease and non-Hodgkin's lymphoma. A combination of steroids and radiation is considered the cause of this late effect.[36] Slipped capital femoral epiphysis is noted after doses >2500 cGy of radiation therapy to the femoral head. In one study 50% (7 out of 15) children less than 4 years of age who were treated had slipped capital femoral epiphysis compared to 1 out of 21 patients treated between 5 and 15 years of age. Shielding the femoral head greatly decreases this effect.[50] Changes may also be seen after prolonged steroid administration.

Treatment Effects on Dentition and Maxillofacial Area.   Dental and maxillofacial changes are prevalent after radiation to the head and neck area. Dental abnormalities occur with 2000 to 4000 cGy to the head and neck region and include poor root development, incomplete calcification, delayed or arrested tooth development, and multiple caries.[90] Forty percent of children treated for leukemia with 1800 to 3000 cGy show root and crown abnormalities.[36] Patients treated for leukemia with chemotherapy alone have demonstrated shortening and thinning of premolar roots.[90] Thirty to 50% of bone marrow transplant patients receiving 1000 cGy total body irradiation demonstrated impaired root development, microdontia, enamel hypoplasia, and premature apical closure.[43]

Radiation directly to the salivary gland results in decreased secretions, causing mouth dryness. In one study 40% of patients treated for head and neck sarcomas had absent secretions.[36] Fifty-five percent of patients treated for Hodgkin's disease with 4000 cGy to the submandibular area showed a decreased flow rate of secretions.[24]

Maxillofacial abnormalities may include asymmetry, abnormal occlusion, and symmetric hypoplasia (e.g., with bilateral retinoblastoma).[90,111]

Patients who have undergone amputation, disarticulation, or limb salvage procedures must be followed for compensatory scoliosis, leg length discrepancies, and back pain, and to determine the condition of the internal prosthesis or the stump.

Assessment Guidelines for Late Effects on Musculoskeletal System. Follow-up focuses on the condition of the bones and soft tissues in the field of radiation therapy. X-ray films are used to evaluate changes. X-ray studies of the irradiated bones are recommended every 3 to 5 years. Patients with trunk irradiation are encouraged to maintain their ideal body weight to decrease the noticeable asymmetry of the muscle mass. The condition of the prosthesis must be updated at least annually by a prosthetist, especially during periods of rapid growth. Growing limbs require careful measurements and follow-up to evaluate for discrepancies. Referrals to an orthopedist should be made before a period of rapid growth for assessment. Adequate dental care and follow-up are imperative during treatment and long term to preserve the teeth and the tissues of the oral cavity.

ASSESSING URINARY TRACT FOR LATE EFFECTS

The kidney and bladder are both affected by chemotherapy and radiation. Chronic ne-

phritis and cystitis are the most commonly noted effects. Chemotherapy, including dactinomycin, cisplatin, methotrexate, anthracyclines, azacytidine, and nitrosoureas can cause renal failure or enhance the radiation effects on the urinary tract.[14,59] Cyclophosphamide causes hemorrhagic cystitis, bladder fibrosis, atypical bladder epithelium, and renal tubular necrosis. Ifosfamide may have similar effects. Concurrent radiation to the pelvis increases the risk of these effects.[12]

Effects of Treatment on Kidney. The severity of radiation damage to the urinary tract is dose dependent. The risk of significant renal damage increases with doses exceeding 2500 cGy to both kidneys.[14,65] These doses are reported to cause chronic nephritis, especially in patients treated for soft tissue sarcomas of the abdomen and pelvis and patients with Wilms' tumor and abdominal lymphomas. The signs and symptoms of chronic nephritis include fatigue, nocturia, proteinuria, anemia, hyposthenuria, edema, salt wasting, hyperuricemia with or without gout, and progressive renal failure. Acute renal toxicity resulting from cisplatin administration occurs in 50% to 75% of patients. The degree of toxicity is dependent on the duration of therapy and the dose of cisplatin. Dysfunction is rarely documented with doses below 50 mg/m² per course. Reversibility has been noted in this population, although several studies documented up to 40% decrease in creatinine clearance 2 to 4 years after treatment.[207]

Other factors that may increase the risk of renal failure include the use of antimicrobial agents such as vancomycin, inadequate alkalinization before methotrexate administration, ectopic kidneys, radiation fibrosis with subsequent hydronephrosis, and chronic urinary tract infections.[14]

Nephrectomy results in compensatory hypertrophy of the remaining kidney. Patients with this condition must protect their remaining kidney from damage as a result of trauma or infection. Early treatment of infection and wearing extra protection (kidney guard) during contact sports will decrease the risk of damage. There apparently is no significant increase in hypertension after nephrectomy and treatment of Wilms' tumor.[93]

Effects of Treatment on Bladder. There is a 5% incidence of hemorrhagic cystitis following doses <4000 cGy to the bladder.[14] Larger doses of radiation to the pelvis (e.g., with pelvic rhabdomyosarcoma) can result in decreased bladder wall elasticity, resulting in strictures of the urethra (which may require dilation and bladder training), small bladder capacity requiring frequent urination, and enuresis at a late age, especially in boys.[187] Radioenhancers such as dactinomycin can lower the threshold dose and cause earlier onset of dysfunction.[73]

The incidence of cystitis has been documented at approximately 10% and occasionally occurs years after therapy.[104] The incidence of hemorrhagic cystitis following ifosfamide therapy has been reported as high as 45%.[95] Adequate hydration in conjunction with administration of mesna at time of treatment appears to attenuate these long-term effects.[54,171,207]

Assessment Guidelines for Late Effects on Urinary Tract. Annual evaluation of blood pressure and routine urinalysis to screen for protein, blood, and bacteria and to determine serum urate and creatinine levels are necessary to evaluate the urinary and renal status of these patients. A health history should include questions to evaluate status of the urinary tract and any problems such as frequency of urination, blood in the urine, painful urination, and enuresis. The early detection and treatment of urinary tract infections are imperative to decrease the risk of pyelonephritis and to preserve the function of the remaining kidney.

ASSESSING GASTROINTESTINAL TRACT FOR LATE EFFECTS

Methotrexate alone or in combination with 6-mercaptopurine can cause hepatic dysfunction.[41,55] Occasionally children treated for ALL with this combination of therapy have developed hepatic fibrosis and cirrhosis with portal hypertension.[137] It is unclear whether these changes are due to chemotherapy or viral hepatitis from blood transfusions.

Hepatic Fibrosis. Radiation treatment alone or in combination with radio-enhancers results in hepatic fibrosis, which may result in portal hypertension. The incidence of hepatic fibrosis is small as documented by the Late Effects Study Group.[116] However, subclinical abnormalities are thought to go undetected, and the incidence is most likely higher.[41] Veno-occlusive disease is a rare but usually fatal effect after 750 cGy single-dose total body irradiation.[206] Children's livers apparently are more sensitive to damage than those of adults, especially when radiation is given in conjunction with dactinomycin. Doses of 1200 to 2500 cGy delivered to the liver caused abnormal liver function study and radionuclide scan results in 50% of patients, whereas doses of 2300 to 3500 cGy caused abnormalities in 63% of patients.[36] Severe hepatitis has been noted with as little as 2000 cGy when given in conjunction with dactinomycin.[36]

Fibrosis and Enteritis. Fibrosis and enteritis are the most common effects noted on the gastrointestinal GI tract.[49] These late effects can affect the tract from the esophagus to the rectum, resulting in adhesions, stricture formation obstructions, ulcers, and malabsorption syndromes. The stomach and small intestine apparently are more radiosensitive than the colon and rectum.[14,200] The incidence of fibrosis is 5% at 4000 to 5000 cGy and as high as 36% after 6000 cGy.[159]

GI stricture can arise 5 to 20 years after treatment and may be progressive and/or recurrent.[159] Abdominal surgery and radioenhancers increase the occurrence of late effects on the GI tract.[200] Abdominal surgery (e.g., laparotomies) has been associated with bowel obstruction weeks to years after treatment of diseases such as Hodgkin's disease.

Assessment Guidelines for Late Effects on Gastrointestinal Tract. Annual physical examination and health histories to assess for hepatomegaly, icterus, and malabsorption are necessary for early detection. Signs and symptoms such as severe, intermittent abdominal pain, diarrhea, and constipation should be evaluated thoroughly. Transaminase and bilirubin levels should be determined every 2 to 5 years to monitor liver function. Persistently abnormal laboratory study results should be evaluated in conjunction with a gastroenterologist and may require liver scans and biopsy.

Special diets may be required for malabsorption syndromes. Low-fat, low-residue, gluten-free, and lactose-free diets may be required to aid in controlling symptoms associated with GI dysfunctions.

ASSESSING HEMATOPOIETIC SYSTEM FOR LATE EFFECTS

Immunosuppression and myelosuppression are possible late effects after radiation, chemotherapy, and removal of the spleen. Bone marrow transplantation places the patient at highest risk for hematopoietic late effects.

Immunosuppression. After bone marrow transplantation, immune function is severely compromised for the first 6 months.[205] Patients who do not have graft-versus-host disease (GVHD) demonstrate normal immunologic function 1 year after the transplant. Patients with GVHD are further delayed in normal immune function. It has been documented that non-GVHD patients have normal levels of IgG and IgM 3 to 4 months after transplant.[8] T and B cells are restored to normal, and suppressor cells are within normal limits 1 year after transplant. Recovery of all of these parameters are delayed in patients with GVHD. Even when patients with chronic GVHD have normal numbers of T and B cells, they have nonspecific suppressor cells that affect their immunologic response and place them at risk for infection. Approximately one third of patients with chronic GVHD develop serious and potentially fatal infections.[165]

Patients whose spleens have been removed have impaired humoral immunity and decreases in serum levels of IgM and IgA.[75] Studies have found that 7.9% of them develop fulminant infections, usually from encapsulated organisms (e.g., pneumococci, *Haemophilus influenzae, Neisseria meningococcus*).[103] Splenic atrophy after radiation (4000 cGy) to the spleen results in similar infection patterns.[42]

Myelosuppression. Radiation to the bone marrow may affect lymphocytes and other bone marrow lineages. The degree of marrow damage depends on the dose and volume irradiated. After 4000 cGy of total nodal radiation therapy, peripheral granulocyte counts and bone marrow reserve can be decreased up to 7 years from treatment.[175,194]

The long-term chemotherapy effects on bone marrow function have not been well documented. However, it appears that chemotherapy given up to 3 years after radiation for Hodgkin's disease or methotrexate given up to 18 months after craniospinal radiation may result in long-term myelosuppression.[40,116]

Assessment Guidelines for Late Effects on Hematopoietic System. Annual examinations with a detailed history to elicit symptoms of recurring infection, anemia, or bleeding disorder are important for early detection.

Patients whose spleens were removed should receive pneumococcal vaccine, *Haemophilus* b conjugate vaccine, and meningovax, followed by daily prophylactic penicillin or erythromycin. Temperature at or above 101° F should be treated immediately with empiric antibiotics that affect encapsulated organisms.

ASSESSING VISION AND HEARING FOR LATE EFFECTS

The eye is composed of several layers of tissues that vary in radiosensitivity. Long-term effects include cataracts, retinopathy, optic neuropathy, corneal vascularization and scarring, glaucoma, and eyelid atrophy with ectropion and entropion.[36]

Radiation Effects on Eye. Low-dose radiation results in cataract formation due to damage to the germinal zone of the epithelium.[22,36] Researchers vary in the dose they believe is required to cause damage. Doses varying from 750 to 2000 cGy have been reported to cause cataracts. Studies have reported a 60% frequency of cataracts after 750 to 950 cGy doses and 100% frequency after 1150 cGy doses.[22,126] Cataracts after bone marrow transplantation have been documented in 80% of patients who received a 1000 cGy single dose compared to 19% in those who received fractionated doses.[48] All patients who receive total body irradiation should be evaluated for dry eye syndrome. This is most commonly noted with GVHD and can be prevented with the use of artificial tears.[165] Patients who undergo prolonged steroid use and/or high-dose therapy are at greatest risk for steroid-induced cataracts.[14]

Injury to the optic nerve is rarely noted with doses below 5000 cGy. Optic nerve damage is most commonly manifested by visual field deficits. Higher doses and prolonged therapy increase the incidence.[197]

Surgical removal of the eye is most commonly associated with treatment for retinoblastoma. These surgical patients require a prosthetic device to replace their globe for cosmetic purpose.

Effects of Treatment on Hearing. Hearing loss, most commonly in the high frequency ranges (6000 to 8000 Hz), may occur after the administration of cisplatin. As hearing loss progresses, the frequency range becomes lower. Patients receiving radiation to the auditory system in conjunction with cisplatin are at greater risk for hearing loss.[54] Hearing loss can greatly affect speech, language, and social development.[162] Recurrent ear infections, with subsequent damage to the tympanic membrane, may further compromise hearing, as can the use of antibiotics such as gentamicin and amikacin.

Assessment Guidelines for Late Effects on Vision and Hearing. A careful health assessment to ascertain diminished vision or hearing should occur annually. A Snellen chart eye evaluation should be done annually, and all high-risk patients should be examined by an ophthalmologist to evaluate for the development of cataracts or diminished vision. Vision problems may necessitate removal of cataracts and fitting with corrective lenses for cosmetic repair of the orbital area. After enucleation, a well-fitting ocular prosthesis enhances the cosmetic appearance of the patient and should be resized for an appropriate fit as the child grows.

A baseline hearing test should be completed for patients treated with cisplatin and, if the results are normal, repeated every 3 to 5 years or if symptoms arise. If abnormalties are noted, a referral to an otolaryngologist is necessary for thorough evaluation. A hearing aid may be required to accommodate hearing loss.

ASSESSMENT FOR SECOND MALIGNANT NEOPLASMS

The development of a second malignant neoplasm (SMN) is probably the most feared consequence of therapy. The general risk of SMNs is approximately 10 to 20 times greater than the risk of first neoplasms in the general population.[127] Other factors that determine potential risk include genetic predisposition (e.g., retinoblastoma), radiation therapy, certain chemotherapeutic agents,[96] and other genetic conditions such as neurofibromatosis, nevoid basal cell carcinoma, and xeroderma pigmentosa.[73,117] The lifetime risk of developing an SMN has not been defined; however, the risk of developing an SMN within the first 20 years after treatment for a tumor is estimated at 3% to 12%.[117,118,127]

Genetic Predisposition. Retinoblastoma comprises 3% of pediatric malignancies, but up to 17% of the SMNs occur in children with retinoblastoma.[117] Up to 70% of the SMNs occur in the field of radiation, although unirradiated children with bilateral disease also develop SMNs. Soft tissue sarcomas are the most frequently noted tumor, with osteogenic sarcoma being the most common. The chromosomal 13 and 14 homozygosity that has been noted in familial retinoblastoma patients is also found in patients with osteogenic sarcoma when it occurs as an SMN in this population.[77] A report of 2300 retinblastoma patients revealed SMN risks of 20% at 10 years, 50% at 20 years, and 90% at 30 years from the date of their original tumor.[1] Other reports document a risk of 8% at 20 years.[51]

Patients treated for Ewing's sarcoma have a risk of developing an SMN up to 35% at 10 years from diagnosis.[180] Tumors in the field of radiation and acute nonlymphocytic leukemia have been reported.[167,176]

Patients treated for Wilms' tumor have been reported as having a 6% cumulative risk for developing SMNs 20 years after treatment.

The SMNs seen in this population include tumors of the thyroid gland, bone, connective tissue, GI tract, and CNS and the leukemias.[192] Children with bilateral Wilms' tumor and certain congenital anomalies may be at higher risk. Breast cancer after chest wall irradiation has been documented.[106]

As much as a twentyfold risk of developing brain tumors following prophylactic treatment (i.e., cranial radiation and IT methotrexate) of the CNS for leukemia has been noted.[113,155] However, CNS tumors following the treatment of leukemia have been noted in the absence of radiation therapy. Families have also been identified with both malignancies (brain tumors and leukemias), and it is possible that this represents a cancer syndrome.[117] Other SMNs in this population include thyroid cancers,[182] and muscle, pancreas, and liver tumors.[117,127]

Treatment Causes of Second Malignant Neoplasms. The risk of SMNs after the treatment of Hodgkin's disease has been well documented. A report from Stanford University (Palo Alto, California) documented the mean 15-year risk of all SMNs after treatment of Hodgkin's disease as 17.6%.[190] Seventy-five percent of these tumors were solid and included lung cancer, non-Hodgkin's lymphomas, stomach cancer, bone tumors, connective tissue malignancies, breast cancer,[26] and thyroid tumors. The risk for these tumors increases with time. The risk of leukemia (usually nonlymphocytic) appears to plateau at 3.3% at 10 years after therapy.[4,17] SMNs were characterized further in this study by treatment. Leukemia was noted after chemotherapy and radiation therapy or chemotherapy alone at the same frequency (6% at 15 years). Solid tumor frequency was 7% at 15 years following radiotherapy alone, 11.7% when chemotherapy was used, or 16.5% when salvage chemotherapy was used. Alkylators were frequently used in those patients who developed SMNs.[190]

Radiation-Induced Sarcomas. A distinction between radiation-induced sarcomas and other SMNs has been made over the years: (1) the radiation-induced sarcoma must be in the field of radiation; (2) more than 4 years

must have lapsed since the primary diagnosis; (3) the radiation-induced sarcoma must be histologically proved; and (4) if the radiation-induced sarcoma is a bone tumor, the bone must have been normal (e.g., genetically) before treatment of the first tumor. A dose response for radiation-induced sarcoma has not been clearly defined. However, a fortyfold risk of developing a radiation-induced sarcoma is present after 6000 cGy. This risk decreases to a 22½-fold risk at 5000 cGy.[73] The reduced risk is believed related to destruction of potentially transforming cells or to a decrease in the doubling time of the surviving cells. If alkylating agents are used in conjunction with radiation therapy, there is a higher risk of radiation-induced sarcoma.[191]

Dactinomycin (although a radio-enhancer) decreases the risk of SMNs in the field of radiation. This protective effect was not noted when children were also given antifolates, the vinca alkaloids, or alkylating agents.[44,45] Breast tumors after chest radiation for the treatment of Hodgkin's disease or metastatic lung disease are now more prevalent.[26, 106]

Assessment Guidelines to Evaluate for Development of Second Malignant Neoplasms. A routine annual evaluation of asymptomatic survivors will not detect most SMNs. However, educating the patient and family to have persistent symptoms evaluated by a health care professional will achieve better overall surveillance. As a final note, all patients should be encouraged to follow the recommendations for risk reduction and early detection of cancer, including *no* smoking, moderate or no alcohol intake, a low-fat, high-fiber diet, the use of sunscreens, and simple screening methods such as testicular and breast self-examination. Some centers are recommending a baseline mammography at 25 years for female patients who received chest wall radiation in view of the increased risk of breast tumors.

ASSESSING PREGNANCY OUTCOMES AFTER TREATMENT

Cancer treatment may affect the patient's offspring in two ways. The children may inherit the genes that caused the parent's disease, or they may possess new genetic abnormalities induced in the parent's germ cells by cancer treatment.[123] An inherited defect may be seen in some patients with retinoblastoma, Wilms' tumor, and neuroblastoma.[96,105] These patients should be apprised of the potential risk and obtain genetic counseling.

It is now clear that chemotherapy is most hazardous to a developing fetus during the first trimester and less so when used later in pregnancy.[14] However, the effect that chemotherapy and radiation have on the long-term survivors' offspring is somewhat more confusing.

Treatment Effects on Pregnancy. A variety of studies have evaluated the risk of having abnormal offspring after cancer treatment.[3,83,115] One study found a 7.5% risk of significant fetal malformation following the treatment of Hodgkin's disease. This same study noted a 15% fetal wastage, and another 15% of pregnancies resulted in premature or low-birth-weight babies. These numbers exceed the risk noted in the general population.[115] Another report found a low son-to-daughter ratio following treatment for non-Hodgkin's lymphoma.[142] Yet another study revealed that women treated with chemotherapy and radiation therapy for Hodgkin's disease had a greater risk for having abnormal offspring when compared to women treated with chemotherapy alone.[83] It has also been documented that female patients treated for Wilms' tumor with abdominal radiation experience fetal perinatal death and premature offspring.[107]

However, several other studies have found cancer survivors who have undergone intensive chemotherapy regimens before pregnancy have had normal offsprings. In these studies major and minor birth defects were noted but not at a greater rate than in the general population.[15,108] One large study evaluated survivors' offspring at 0 to 12 years of age and did not detect any significant major or minor abnormalities.[15]

Teratogenic and Mutagenic Effects on Pregnancy. The teratogenic effect of chemotherapy and/or radiation in men has been poorly addressed. However, one study documented an increase in spontaneous abortions in offspring who were fathered by survivors of Hodgkin's disease.[83]

The mutagenic (versus teratogenic) effect of cancer treatment has been raised; however, there are no studies that have documented excess cancer in the offspring of survivors. Patients who possess a genetic predisposition (e.g., those with retinoblastoma, Wilms' tumor, neuroblastoma) have offspring with the same genetic predisposition for the same tumor.

Assessment Guidelines for Pregnancy Outcomes. Patients with suspected genetic tumors should be referred for genetic counseling. In addition, those survivors who have received treatment damaging to the gonads (e.g., those with Hodgkin's disease) should also be referred for genetic counseling. The general consensus is that survivors should wait at least 1 year after treatment before having children. However, the data regarding survivors' offspring are limited.

SUMMARY OF PHYSIOLOGIC EFFECTS

With increasing survival rates in pediatric oncology, the long-term physical impact of multimodality treatment is becoming an important area of focus and follow-up for pediatric cancer survivors. Table 17–1 provides a summary of the long-term physiologic effects of pediatric cancer treatment and recommended assessment and management strategies.

ASSESSING PSYCHOSOCIAL EFFECTS OF THERAPY

Cancer in childhood leaves an indelible imprint on all whose lives are touched by it. By the mid-1980s a sizable body of literature had begun to emerge that addressed the psychosocial adjustment of childhood cancer survivors. (See references 25, 27, 28, 58, 62, 67, 84, 97, 98, 100, 102, 112, 122, 129, 134, 143, 144, 166, 177, 185, 186, 188, and 199.) Although the findings of most studies suggested that the majority of the survivors are functioning well, nearly all were time-limited cross-sectional studies, and many had methodologic limitations.[166] This has made it difficult (1) to

Text continued on p. 486.

TABLE 17–1. *Evaluation of Long-Term Effects*

BODY SYSTEM	HEALTH PROBLEM	ASSOCIATED TREATMENT MODALITY	METHOD OF ASSESSMENT	MANAGEMENT AND NURSING CONSIDERATIONS
Endocrine				
Ovaries	Ovarian dysfunction	Procarbazine, cyclophosphamide, nitrogen mustard, busulfan	Careful health history and physical examination	Oophoropexy before treatment Refer to endocrinologist
	Primary Secondary	400–800 cGy High risk 　Older patients 　Poor nutrition 　Longer length of treatment 　Combination therapy	Tanner staging Serum determinations of LH, FSH, estradiol at age 12 yr if no secondary sex characteristics	Replacement hormones Refer for counseling Anticipatory teaching: 　Lack of secondary sex characteristics 　Loss of menses, irregularities 　Decreased libido, vaginal dryness
Testes	Testicular dysfunction	Procarbazine, cyclophosphamide, nitrogen mustard, busulfan	Careful health history and physical examination	Sperm banking at treatment
	Primary	400–600 cGy; azoospermia	Tanner staging	Refer to endocrinologist
	Secondary	≥2400 cGy; Leydig cell damage High risk 　Poor nutrition 　Combination therapy 　Longer length of treatment	Testicular volumes Semen analysis Serum determination of LH, FSH if no secondary sex characteristics after 14 yr of age	Replacement testosterone Refer for counseling Anticipatory teaching: 　Small testicles 　Possible impotence 　Decreased libido 　Lack of secondary sex characteristics
Thyroid	Hypothyroidism 　Overt and compensatory	No known chemotherapy >2000 cGy; overt or compensatory hypothyroidism; Graves' disease	Careful health history and physical examination Free T$_4$, TSH, T$_3$	Refer to endocrinologist Replacement hormones Anticipatory teaching: 　Hypothyroidism or hyperthyroidism—signs and symptoms
	Graves' disease	≥750 cGy total body irradiation; hypothyroidism High risk 　Younger patients		
Hypothalamic-pituitary axis	Hypothalamic dysfunction Panhypothalamic dysfunction Panhypopituitary dysfunction	No known chemotherapy ≥2400 cGy; hypothalamic dysfunction ≥4000 cGy; pituitary dysfunction	Careful health history and physical examination Growth charts Tanner staging GH: stimulation tests, pulsatile tests Somatomedin-C LH, FSH, estradiol, testosterone, prolactin, Free T$_4$, TSH, T$_3$	Refer to endocrinologist Replacement hormones Bromocriptine (for hyperprolactinemia) Anticipatory teaching: 　As above 　Poor growth 　Short stature

Data from references 80 and 162.

TABLE 17–1. *Evaluation of Long-Term Effects* Continued

BODY SYSTEM	HEALTH PROBLEM	ASSOCIATED TREATMENT MODALITY	METHOD OF ASSESSMENT	MANAGEMENT AND NURSING CONSIDERATIONS
Cardiovascular	Cardiomyopathy	Anthracycline chemotherapy Risk increased with Lifetime cumulative dose >550 mg/m² Mediastinal radiation	ECG, echocardiogram, or MUGA History of symptoms of congestive heart failure (CHF) Stress testing	Careful monitoring of anthracycline dosage to limit lifetime dose If CHF develops, supportive care with Referral to cardiologist Digoxin, diuretics Sodium restriction
	Pericardial damage	Mediastinal radiation	Physical examination, echocardiogram History of chest pain, dyspnea, fever, pulsus paradoxus, venous distension	May be subclinical If pericardial effusion develops, treatment may include Referral to cardiologist Anti-inflammatory drugs Pericardial tap If restrictive pericarditis occurs, treatment may include pericardiectomy
	Early coronary artery atherosclerosis	Mediastinal radiation	ECG, echocardiogram History of chest pain with exertion, decreased exercise tolerance	Referral to cardiologist Dietary restriction of fat and salt intake Program of moderate exercise If significant obstruction to coronary artery flow develops, treatment may include Thrombolytic drugs Calcium channel blocking agents Balloon dilation angioplasty Coronary artery bypass surgery
	Atrioventricular (AV) valve tissue damage	Mediastinal radiation	Physical examination, ECG, echocardiogram	Referral to cardiologist If significant AV valve insufficiency develops, treatment may include Diuretics Afterload reducing agents Surgical implication of replacement of valve
	Ventricular arrhythmias	Anthracycline chemotherapy	ECG, Holter monitor, exercise test	Referral to cardiologist If significant arrhythmias develop, treatment may include antiarrhythmic drugs

Table continued on following page.

TABLE 17–1. *Evaluation of Long-Term Effects* Continued

BODY SYSTEM	HEALTH PROBLEM	ASSOCIATED TREATMENT MODALITY	METHOD OF ASSESSMENT	MANAGEMENT AND NURSING CONSIDERATIONS
Musculoskeletal	Scoliosis, kyphosis	Radiation therapy for intraabdominal tumor in which vertebrae absorb radiation unevenly	Regular physical examination May not become apparent until adolescent growth spurt	Referral to orthopedist for rehabilitative measures Instruction about normal weight maintenance to make problem less noticeable
	Spinal shortening (sitting height)	Spinal irradiation (e.g., for medulloblastoma); direct effect of radiation on growth centers of vertebral bodies	Serial measurements of sitting height (crown to rump)	Referral to orthopedic surgeon Anticipatory teaching about disproportion between shorter-than-usual trunk and normal leg length as full growth is attained; reassurance that disproportion probably will not be obvious to others but may be a problem in fitting clothing
	Increased susceptibility to fracture, poor healing, deformities of shortening of extremities	Irradiation to lesions in long bones (e.g., with Ewing's sarcoma)	Regular physical examination	Referral to orthopedic surgeon Teaching about protective measures such as avoiding rough contact sports
	Facial asymmetry	Surgery plus irradiation to head and neck area (e.g., for rhabdomyosarcoma), causing altered growth of facial bones	Physical examination Early evaluation by reconstructive surgeon	Anticipatory guidance about possible adjustment problems with visible deformity Referral to family counseling to manage or prevent adjustment and behavioral problems
	Dental problems Gingival irritation and bleeding, tooth loosening, migration (can lead to peridontal disease) Delayed or arrested tooth development	Radiation therapy to maxilla and mandible Chemotherapy	Clinical observation with dental examination	Many dental problems can be minimized or prevented with Good oral hygiene with flossing and brushing, gingival massage, use of plaque-disclosing tablets or solutions Preradiation therapy fluoride prophylaxis Frequent dental evaluation Extraction of damaged, nonfunctional teeth

TABLE 17–1. *Evaluation of Long-Term Effects Continued*

BODY SYSTEM	HEALTH PROBLEM	ASSOCIATED TREATMENT MODALITY	METHOD OF ASSESSMENT	MANAGEMENT AND NURSING CONSIDERATIONS
Vision	Cataracts	Cranial radiation Corticosteroids (long term)	Eye examination Visual inspection Slit-lamp examination	Ophthalmology consult Surgical removal Corrective lense fitting
Hearing	Hearing loss (high-tone range)	Cisplatin Increased risk Recurrent ear infections Ototoxic antibiotic therapy Radiation to auditory area	Monitor with hearing tests	Hearing aid Speech therapist consult
Respiratory	Pulmonary fibrosis	Lung irradiation Some chemotherapeutic agents Risk increased with Larger lung volume in radiation field Dose, 4000 cGy Radiation-sensitizing chemotherapeutic agents	Clinical observation for dyspnea, rales, cough, decreased exercise tolerance, pulmonary insufficiency Monitor with Physical examination Chest x-ray studies Pulmonary function tests	Health education for smoking prevention or cessation Supportive care with provision of adequate rest periods Vigilance for development of pulmonary infection Pneumococcal vaccine Yearly influenza vaccination Careful oxygen administration (busulfan)
Gastrointestinal	Chronic enteritis	Radiation therapy Risk increased with Dose, 5000 cGy Previous abdominal surgery Radiation-sensitizing chemotherapeutic agents	Clinical observation for pain, dysphagia, recurrent vomiting, obstipation or constipation, blood or mucous-containing diarrhea, or malabsorption syndrome	Nutritional consultation for diet plan to diminish symptoms while providing adequate nutrition for growth and development and to fit family routine, ethnic, or cultural customs Dietary modifications may include low-fat, low-residue, gluten-free diet free of milk and milk products If enterostomy is performed, coordination with enterostomal therapist for patient and family teaching about stoma care
	Hepatic fibrosis, cirrhosis	Radiation therapy Some chemotherapeutic agents	Clinical observation for pain, hepatomegaly, jaundice Monitoring with liver function tests and liver scans may be inconclusive so periodic liver biopsy may be necessary	Supportive care with nutritional consultation

Table continued on following page.

TABLE 17–1. *Evaluation of Long-Term Effects* Continued

BODY SYSTEM	HEALTH PROBLEM	ASSOCIATED TREATMENT MODALITY	METHOD OF ASSESSMENT	MANAGEMENT AND NURSING CONSIDERATIONS
Kidney and Urinary Tract	Chronic nephritis (may lead to renal failure, cardiovascular damage)	Radiation to renal structures Risk increased with concomitant chemotherapy	Clinical observation and monitoring with Blood pressure readings Urinalysis Creatinine levels Complete blood count (CBC)	If progressive renal failure develops, supportive care (possibly dialysis and/or transplantation)
	Chronic hemorrhagic cystitis	Chemotherapy (cyclophosphamide) Risk increased with Pelvic irradiation Inadequate hydration before, during, and after chemotherapy	Clinical observation for dysuria, urinary frequency, hematuria Monitoring with urinalysis, blood pressure	Assure adequate hydration before, during, and after chemotherapy (3000 ml/m²/24hr) Bladder hemorrhage may be treated with formalin instillation and/or fulguration of bleeding sites
	Unilateral kidney	Nephrectomy for Wilms' tumor	Clinical observation for dysuria, urinary frequency, hematuria Monitoring with urinalysis, blood pressure	Health education to avoid injury to remaining kidney (e.g., avoid contact sports) Wear kidney guard during sports If urinary tract infection develops: Identification of causative organism Antibiotic treatment Urinalysis Medic-Alert identification bracelet
Hematopoietic	Prolonged immunosuppression	Chemotherapy (high dose, extended periods) Radiation to marrow-containing bones Splenectomy (e.g., for Hodgkin's disease)	Monitoring with: CBC, platelet count Tests of immune function Bone marrow examinations as indicated	Health education about infection Pneumococcal vaccine and prophylactic antibiotics for asplenic individuals Prompt treatment if infection occurs

predict who will function well after cancer treatment; (2) to understand the impact of cancer among different age groups; and (3) to develop appropriate preventive measures for high-risk individuals.[110] For the 1990s and beyond, prospective longitudinal studies are needed.

Meanwhile, there are clinical and intuitive reasons to believe that the lingering effects of a cancer experience are determined by many factors, including the type of cancer and the way it is treated, the age of the child at the time of diagnosis and treatment, the child's intrinsic characteristics, family functioning and resources, and the quality of care provided. Two recent surveys highlighted several global concerns of childhood cancer survivors and their parents, including the ability to marry and have healthy children, risks of other or recurrent disease, psychologic normality, schooling and relationships with family and friends, employment discrimination, getting insurance, and access to future good medical care.[32,195]

Personal-Emotional Issues

Living With Uncertainty. Living with uncertainty and living with compromise are two personal-emotional issues described by Fitzhugh Mullen,[135] a physician and cancer survivor. Prolonged uncertainty is the phenomenon Koocher and O'Malley[97] labeled the *Damocles syndrome*—a metaphor comparing the predicament faced by the families of children with cancer to the plight of the Greek mythologic figure, Damocles, as he sat at a sumptuous feast and contemplated the sword dangling by a thread over his head.

Anecdotal experience suggests that long-term survivors of childhood cancer may respond to uncertainty with a heightened sense of vulnerability. One effect may be a fear of recurrence expressed by hypervigilance and worry that every routine illness is a harbinger of the cancer's return or through denial expressed in behavior that says, "Not me—I really don't have any health problems." The parents of childhood cancer survivors may perceive their child as especially vulnerable. This is nothing new to cancer; the "vulnerable child syndrome" was first described in the general pediatric literature 25 years ago.[70]

On the other hand, living with uncertainty and a heightened sense of vulnerability can have positive effects. Survivors of cancer and other serious illnesses often are irrevocably changed by the experience. They may reorder their priorities in life and reconsider their values. Personal growth can and does come out of surviving a life-threatening illness.

Learning how to live with compromise is a major challenge in a society that fosters the myth that after diagnosis and treatment of cancer, survivors can pick up where they left off.[33] This myth ignores the high personal price paid by cancer patients for their biologic cure and the developmental disruptions cancer causes in young people.

Living With Compromise. Living with compromise can have repercussions in self-concept, self-esteem, body image, and other aspects of personal life.

One might predict that survivors with marked or residual physical disability would have a more difficult adjustment. Results of studies in this area are inconclusive, however, and the literature about children with physical handicaps and other chronic illnesses does not support a straightforward association between severity and adjustment.[62,71,94,134,145,203]

Marriage and family decisions, indicators of adult adjustment, have been studied but with contradictory findings.[25,67,109,184,186] Data from these studies cannot be compared accurately because of differences in the ways the studies were conducted. In the largest study so far, however, Byrne et al.[25] interviewed 2506 cancer survivors and 3266 matched sibling controls. Survivors were slightly less likely to marry than controls, with survivors of brain tumors least likely to marry. In addition, survivors who married and who were not known to be infertile were only 87% as likely to report a pregnancy as controls. These and other personal-emotional issues are currently undergoing further study.

Social-Political Issues

Coping with the reactions of friends and society in general is a major challenge for the survivor. Van Eys[193] contends that as long as survivors are viewed as persons rescued from the dead, strangers in a strange land, they may be perceived with open arms but, by virtue of their special status, excluded from society.

Stigmatization. The essence of stigmatization is blaming the victim—a way to regard people as different and to justify treating them differently. Stigma is one of the reasons that some people feel the term *survivor* should be discarded, and in some centers the newer term *graduate* is used instead.[128]

By whatever name, individuals cured of cancer carry the stigma of survival when they are discriminated against in *education, employment,* or *health, life, and disability insurance coverage.* Instances of all these types of discrimination have been documented,[58,72,76,82,97,125,184,188,199] although the actual scope of the problem is not clearly delineated.[81] In fact, some studies have found few documented problems with vocation or insurance.[76,125,184]

For some individuals, however, it is the fear—rather than the fact—of discrimination that is harmful, forcing them to stay in undesirable jobs ("job-lock") because they are afraid to risk losing employee benefits.[72] In addition, studies that demonstrate that cancer survivors have occupational status similar to matched population controls may not tell the entire story if these individuals are not reaching their own potential.[151]

Discrimination against cancer survivors grows out of three prevailing myths: (1) that cancer is a death sentence; (2) that cancer is contagious; and (3) that cancer survivors are not productive workers.[81] Public education, lobbying, and legal recourse are required to overcome these general misconceptions and specific instances of discrimination.

Laws protecting people with a history of cancer from discrimination in employment vary from state to state. On the federal level, the Vocational Rehabilitation Act of 1973 and the Americans With Disabilities Act enacted in July 1990 (effective 1992) offer certain protections, but they are an awkward fit for survivors with no physical or mental impairment who must argue that they are simultaneously cured but within the legal definition of "disabled." Opportunities in the armed forces were opened to childhood cancer survivors with a Department of Defense directive issued in 1986. Insurance coverage is a mine field of potential problems, with health insurance out of the reach of many Americans, including cancer survivors. Assistance is available from the American Cancer Society, the National Coalition for Cancer Survivorship, local cancer support groups, and state insurance commissions. The Candlelighters Childhood Cancer Foundation has published two informative resources: *Equal Employment Opportunity for People With a History of Cancer*[56] and *Insurance: Your Options and Your Child's*.[87] Additional print resources are listed in Table 17–2.

How Nurses Can Help Survivors Help Themselves

Assess Rehabilitation Needs. Assess rehabilitation needs well before the arbitrary 5-year survival point. This is the time when many of the challenges of survivorship occur, and it is the time when patient education and counseling can make a difference in the quality and nature of long-term survival.[135] For example, many families experience high anxiety during the period surrounding the completion of treatment, which is usually approximately 2 years after diagnosis. It is not unusual for families to relate that they were no more prepared for treatment to finish than they were for the diagnosis in the first place. It is surprising that this "season" in survival has received very little attention in the literature, but clearly families' needs for information and support must be anticipated at this critical point in survivorship.

When assessing patients and families, some of the general risk factors for personal-emotional problems include the following: temporal clustering of stressful medical and life events (the "pile up" of stresses); a cluster of poverty, ethnicity, and single adult family structure; poor prior coping resources; preexisting emotional problems or family discord; extent of disease, treatment modality, and degree of physical distress or residual disability; and a lack of social support.[9,86]

Psychologic cure requires two things: patient education and counseling. Through education, patients and families who understand and expect that fears of recurrence and feelings of loss and grief that accompany living with uncertainty and compromise are normal and are part of the recovery process may be less fearful about the future.

Through counseling, referrals can be made to peer support groups. Such groups or one-on-one linkage between newer patients and long-term survivors can provide the buffering effect of social support from others who have gone through similar experiences. Also, in comprehensive rehabilitation programs individuals and families with the highest levels of psychologic distress are referred to an individual therapist. Referring

TABLE 17—2. *Selected Print Materials About Cancer Survivorship*

TITLE/AUTHOR	SOURCE
After the Storm (Dasenbrock AI, Flynn BE, Kitson JK)	The Derald Ruttenberg Cancer Center Box 1129 1 Gustave Levy Place New York, NY 10029
An Almanac of Practical Resources for Cancer Survivors (Mullan F, Hoffman B, eds)	Consumer Reports Books 9180 LeSaint Drive Fairfield, OH 45014-5452
Cancer Survivorship: An Annotated Bibliography	National Cancer Institute NIH Publication No. 91-3173 1-800-4-CANCER
Facing Forward: A Guide for Cancer Survivors	National Cancer Institute NIH Publication No. 90-2424 1-800-4-CANCER
Networker (newsletter)	National Coalition for Cancer Survivorship (NCCS) 323 Eighth Street, S.W. Albuquerque, NM 87102 1-505-764-9956
Surviving (newsletter focusing on survivors of Hodgkin's disease)	Stanford University Medical Center Department of Radiology Division of Radiation Therapy, Room H013 300 Pasteur Drive Stanford, CA 94305
Taking Care of Yourself for Life: Your Personal Long-Term Follow-Up Guide and Treatment Record (Ruccione K, Hobbie W)	Kathy Ruccione, RN, MPH Children's Hospital of Los Angeles Division Hematology/Oncology Mail Stop 54 Los Angeles, CA 90027
Taking Charge of Your Health: A Guide to Cancer Prevention for Men (Women) Who Had Cancer in Childhood, Part 1 (Meadows AT, Gallagher J, Jarrett P, Blumberg B)	Children's Hospital of Philadelphia 34th and Civic Center Boulevard Philadelphia, PA 19104
Taking Charge of Your Health: A Guide to Medical Follow-Up for Adults Who Had Cancer in Childhood (Meadows AT, Gallagher J, Jarrett P, Blumberg B)	Children's Hospital of Philadelphia 34th and Civic Center Boulevard Philadelphia, PA 19104
Taking Control: 10 Steps to a Healthier Life and Reduced Cancer Risk	American Cancer Society Publication No. 2019.05 1599 Clifton Road, N.E. Atlanta, GA 30329 1-800-ACS-2345
Cancervive: The Challenge of Life After Cancer (Nessim S)	Houghton Mifflin Company Boston, Massachusetts

therapists are selected who are comfortable working with young people with cancer and their families and who are familiar with the medical situations these individuals face.

Provide Anticipatory Guidance. Provide anticipatory guidance about the disease, its treatment, and its likely aftereffects. Information must be clarified, reinforced, and reinterpreted over time. Children, in particular, must be taught and retaught in ways appropriate to their changing developmental stages.[57] A variety of print resources have been published recently for use by survivors. See Table 17–2 for a partial list of materials about survivorship that may be useful to families.

Convey Importance of Health Observation and Maintenance. Convey the importance to survivors of health observation and maintenance. This includes their participating in long-term follow-up care, including regular physical examinations with appropriate tests. Additional specific follow-up guidelines based on the disease and treatment have been discussed previously in this chapter.

Part of the health teaching for survivors should include health promotion and risk reduction.[158] A useful free publication is the American Cancer Society's booklet, *Taking Control*, which describes 10 steps to a healthier life and reduced cancer risk. Take advantage of "teachable moments" when cancer survivors may be particularly receptive to information about ways to help reduce the chances of the preventable cancers in the future.

In addition, teach survivors to stay in touch with the medical center where the original cancer treatment was given since that is where the detailed records are and because most centers are participating in long-range follow-up to learn more about disease and treatment sequelae.

Inform Survivors of Available Resources. Assist survivors to make use of available resources for information and support. These resources include the treatment center and organizations such as the Candlelighters Childhood Cancer Foundation, the American Cancer Society, the Leukemia Society, and the National Cancer Institute. Also, the National Coalition for Cancer Survivorship is a clearinghouse for information, publications, and programs about survivorship and serves as an advocate for survivorship concerns. Social cure requires effective political lobbying by well-informed groups. In sheer numbers, cancer survivors have the potential to be a strong political voice.

Social cure also requires public education. The public needs to adjust its view of the cancer survivor—the person who had cancer—to one more consistent with changing prognoses and technology. In addition, social cure requires true acceptance of the philosophy that underlies the Cancer Survivors' Bill of Rights, which was issued by the American Cancer Society in 1988. Its four major precepts are that (1) survivors have the right to assurance of lifelong medical care; (2) in their personal lives survivors, like other Americans, have the right to the pursuit of happiness; (3) in the workplace survivors have the right to equal job opportunities; and (4) since health insurance coverage is an overriding survivorship concern, every effort should be made to assure all survivors adequate health insurance, whether public or private.

Lobby for More Equitable Distribution of Resources to Care for Survivors. Lobby within the treatment centers for a more equitable distribution of resources to provide coordinated care for survivors. Individuals in the acute phase of illness and survivors have very different needs. Yet many institutions have no specific programs for survivors, despite strong reasons for them. Help persuade clinical administrators of the necessity for allocating limited resources to both groups.

Conduct Nursing Research Related to Survivorship. There is an urgent need for good survivorship research, and nurses should be doing it. In the psychosocial area in particular, previous research has been limited by a lack of sensitive instruments and appropriate control groups. Prospective collaborative studies are needed. One of the reasons nurses are the appropriate investigators is that they provide continuity of care over long periods and trust and communication are established. Also, patients may be reluctant to discuss late effects—especially if there are psychosocial concerns—with their physicians out of a feeling that they may seem ungrateful for their biologic cure.

SUMMARY

In summary, the problem of late effects must be seen in perspective. Late effects result from lifesaving treatment. Complications do come with cure. It is true that survivors will need lifelong monitoring and that taking care of a person with cancer is always a balancing act, weighing the need for cure against the risk of late effects. Someday it may be possible to prevent late effects completely. For now, it is fitting to keep in mind what Mullen[136] says: "There is a richness to surviving, a richness of having something that might never have been—whether it is 2 weeks of life or 50 years. We need to celebrate that richness. . . ."

REFERENCES

1. Abramson DH, Ellsworth RM, Kitchin FD, et al. Second nonocular tumors in retinoblastoma survivors. Ophthalmology 1984; 91:1351–1355.
2. Ali MK, Soto A, Maroongroge D, et al. Electrocardiographic changes after adriamycin chemotherapy. Cancer 1979; 2:465.
3. Andrieu J, Ochua-Molina ME. Menstrual cycle, pregnancies and offspring before and after MOPP therapy for Hodgkin's disease. Cancer 1983; 52:435–438.
4. Andrieu JM, Ifrah N, Payen C, et al. Increased risk of secondary acute non-lymphocytic leukemia after extended-field radiation therapy combined with MOPP chemotherapy for Hodgkin's disease. J Clin Oncol 1990; 8:1148–1154.
5. Aronin PA, Mahaley MS Jr, Rudnick SA, et al. Prediction of BCNU pulmonary toxicity in patients with malignant gliomas. An assessment of risk factors. N Engl J Med 1980; 303:183–188.
6. Arslanian S, Becker D, Lee P, et al. Growth hormone therapy and tumor recurrence. Am J Dis Child 1985; 139:347–350.
7. Ash P. The influence of radiation on fertility in man. Br J Radiol 1980; 53:271–278.
8. Atkinson K, Hansen JA, Storb R, et al. T-cell subpopulations identified by monoclonal antibodies after human bone marrow transplantation I. Helper-inducer cytotoxic-suppressor subsets. Blood 1982; 59:1292–1298.
9. Barbarin OA. Psychosocial risks and invulnerability: A review of the theoretical and empirical bases of preventive family-focused services for survivors of childhood cancer. J Psychosoc Oncol 1987; 5:25–41.
10. Bauer KA, Skarin AT, Balikian JP, et al. Pulmonary complications associated with combination chemotherapy programs containing bleomycin. Am J Med 1983; 74:557–563.
11. Bender KS, Shematek JP, Leventhal BG, et al. QT interval prolongation associated with anthracycline cardiotoxicity. J Pediatr 1984; 105:442.
12. Bennett AH. Cyclophosphamide and hemorrhagic cystitis. Urology 1974; 111:603–606.
13. Benoist MR, Lemerle J, Jean R, et al. Effects of pulmonary function of whole lung irradiation for Wilms' tumor in children. Thorax 1982; 37:175–180.
14. Blatt J, Copeland D, Bleyer A. Late effects of childhood cancer and its treatment. In Pizzo P, Poplack D: Principles and Practice of Pediatric Oncology, 2nd ed. Philadelphia: JB Lippincott, 1993, pp. 1091–1114.
15. Blatt J, Mulvihill JT, Ziegler JL, et al. Pregnancy outcome following cancer chemotherapy. Am J Med 1980; 69:828–832.
16. Blatt J, Sherin SR, Niebrugged, et al. Leydig cell function in boys following treatment for testicular relapse of acute lymphoblastic leukemia. J Clin Oncol 1985; 3:1227–1231.
17. Blayney D, Longo D, Young R, et al. Decreasing risk of leukemia with prolonged follow-up after chemotherapy and radiotherapy for Hodgkin's disease. N Engl J Med 1987; 316:710–714.
18. Bleyer WA. Impact of childhood cancer on the United States and the world. CA 1990; 40: 355–367.
19. Borgeat A, Chiolero R, Baylon P, et al. Perioperative cardiovascular collapse in a patient previously treated with doxorubicin. Anesth Analg 1988; 67:1189.
20. Brauner R, Czernichow P, Rappaport R. Precocious puberty after hypothalamic and pituitary irradiation in young children. N Engl J Med 1984; 311:920.
21. Bristow MR, Mason JW, Billingham ME, et al. Dose-effect and structure-function relationships in doxorubicin cardiomyopathy. Am Heart J 1981; 102:709.
22. Britten M, Halmon K, Meredith W. Radiation cataract—New evidence on radiation dosage to the lense. Br J Radiol 1966; 39:612–617.
23. Brouwers P, Riccardi R, Fedio P, et al. Long-term neuropsychological sequelae of childhood leukemia: Correlation with CT brain scan abnormalities. J Pediatr 1985; 106:723–728.
24. Bucker J, Fleming T, Fuller L, et al. Preliminary observations on the effect of mantle radiotherapy on salivary flow rates in patients with Hodgkin's disease. J Dent Res 1988; 6:518–521.
25. Byrne J, Mulvihill MH, Myers R, et al. Effects of treatment on fertility in long-term survivors of childhood and adolescent cancer. N Engl J Med 1987; 317:1315–1321.
26. Carey R, Linggood R, Wood W, et al. Breast cancer in four women cured of Hodgkin's disease. Cancer 1984; 54:2234–2236.
27. Carpenter PJ, Morrow GR, Schmale AH. The psychosocial status of cancer patients after cessation of treatment. J Psychosoc Oncol 1989; 7:95–103.
28. Chang PN, Nesbit ME, Youngren N, et al. Personality characteristics and psychosocial adjustment of long-term survivors of childhood cancer. J Psychosoc Oncol 1987; 5:43–58.
29. Chapman R, Sutcliffe S, Malpas J. Cytotoxic-induced ovarian failure in Hodgkin's disease. II. Effects on sexual function. JAMA 1979; 242:1882–1884.
30. Chapman RM, Sutcliffe SB. Protection of ovarian function by oral contraceptives in women receiving chemotherapy for Hodgkin's disease. Blood 1981; 58:848–851.
31. Chapman RM, Sutcliffe SB, Malpas JS. Male gonadal dysfunction in Hodgkin's disease. A prospective study. JAMA 1981; 245:1323–1328.

32. Chesler M, Lozowski S. Problems and needs of children off treatment: Candlelighters research and proposed programs. Candlelighters Child Cancer Found Q Newslett 1988; 12:1–3.

33. Christ GH. Social consequences of the cancer experience. Am J Pediatr Hematol Oncol 1987; 9:84–88.

34. Clayton P, Gattamaneni H, Shalet SM, et al. Does growth hormone cause relapse of brain tumors? Lancet 1987; 1:711–713.

35. Clifton DK, Bremmer WJ. The effect of testicular x-irradiation on spermatogenesis in man. J Androl 1983; 4:387–392.

36. Constine L. Late effects of radiation therapy. Pediatrician 1991; 18:37–48.

37. Constine L, Donaldson SS, McDougale IR. Thyroid dysfunction after radiotherapy in children with Hodgkin's disease. Cancer 1984; 53:878–883.

38. Constine L, Rubin P, Woolf P, et al. Hyperprolactinemia and hypothyroidism following cytotoxic therapy for CNS malignancies. J Clin Oncol 1987; 5:1841–1851.

39. Copeland DR, Fletcher JM, Pfefferbaum-Levine B, et al. Neuropsychological sequelae of childhood cancer in long-term survivors. Pediatr 1985; 75:745–753.

40. Curran RE, Johnson RB. Tolerance to chemotherapy after prior irradiation for Hodgkin's disease. Ann Intern Med 1970; 72:505–509.

41. Dahl MGG, Gregory MM, Scheuer PJ. Liver damage due to methotrexate in patients with psoriasis. Br Med J 1971; 1:625–630.

42. Dailey MD, Coleman CN, Kaplan HS. Radiation-induced splenic atrophy in patients with Hodgkin's disease and non-Hodgkin's lymphomas. N Engl J Med 1980; 302:215–217.

43. Dalhllof G, Barr M, Bolme P, et al. Disturbances in dental development after total body irradiation in bone marrow transplant recipients. Oral Surg Med Pathol 1988; 65:41–44.

44. D'Angio GJ, Meadows AT, Mike V, et al. Decreased risk of radiation-associated second malignant neoplasms in actinomycin D treated patients. Cancer 1976; 37:1177–1185.

45. D'Angio J, Farber S, Maddock CL. Potentiation of x-ray effects by actinomycin-D. Radiology 1959; 73:1975–1977.

46. Davis PC, Hoffman JC, Pearl GS, et al. CT evaluation of effects of cranial radiation therapy in children. Am J Neurolog Res 1986; 7:639–644.

47. DeCunha MF, Meistrich ML, Fuller LM, et al. Recovery of spermatogenesis after treatment for Hodgkin's disease: Limiting dose of MOPP chemotherapy. J Clin Oncol 1984; 2:571–577.

48. Deeg H, Flournoy N, Sullivan K, et al. Cataracts after total body irradiation and bone marrow transplantation: A sparing effect of dose fractionation. Int J Radiat Oncol Biol Phys 1984; 10:957–964.

49. Donaldson SS, Jundt S, Ricour C, et al. Radiation enteritis in children: A retrospective review, clinicopathologic correlation and dietary management. Cancer 1975; 35:1167–1178.

50. Donaldson SS, Kaplan HS. Complications of treatment of Hodgkin's disease in children. Cancer Treat Rep 1982; 66:977–989.

51. Draper G, Sanders B, Kingston J. Second primary neoplasms in patients with retinoblastoma. Cancer 1988; 62:1676–1679.

52. Duffner PK, Cohen ME, Parker MS. Prospective intellectual testing in children with brain tumors. Ann Neurol 1988; 23:575–579.

53. Dunsmore LD, LoPonte MA, Dunsmore RA. Radiation-induced coronary artery disease. J Am Coll Cardiol 1986; 81:239.

54. Einhorn LH, Williams SD. The role of cisplatinum in solid tumor therapy. N Engl J Med 1979; 300:289–291.

55. Einhorn M, Davidson I. Hepatotoxicity of mercaptopurine. JAMA 1964; 188:802–806.

56. Equal opportunity for people with a history of cancer. Washington, D.C.: Candlelighters Childhood Cancer Foundation, 1987.

57. Everhart C. Overcoming childhood cancer misconceptions among long term survivors. J Pediatr Oncol Nurs 1991; 8:46–48.

58. Feldman FL. Work and cancer health histories: Work expectations and experiences of youth with cancer histories (ages 13–23). Oakland, Calif.: American Cancer Society, California Division, 1980.

59. Fjelborg P, Sorenson J, Helkjaer PE. The long term effect of cisplatin on renal function. Cancer 1986; 58:2214–2217.

60. Fletcher JM. Neurobehavioral effects of central nervous system prophylactic treatment of cancer in children. J Clin Exp Neurol 1988;19:495–538.

61. Fochtman D, Fergusson J, Ford N, et al. The treatment of cancer in children. In Fochtman D, Foley G (eds): Nursing Care of the Child With Cancer. Boston: Little Brown & Co, 1982, pp 218–226.

62. Fritz GK, Williams JR, Amylon N. After treatment ends: Psychosocial sequelae in pediatric cancer survivors. Am J Orthopsychiatry 1988; 58:552–561.

63. Gabriel D, Bernard S, Lambert J, et al. Oophoropexy and the management of Hodgkin's disease: A reevaluation of risks and benefits. Arch Surg 1986; 121:1083–1085.

64. Gangji D, Reaman GH, Cohen SR, et al. Leukoencephalopathy and elevated levels of myelin basic protein in the cerebral spinal fluid of patients with acute lymphoblastic leukemia. Med Intell 1980; 303:19–21.

65. Garnick MB, Mayer RJ. Renal failure associated with neoplastic disease and its treatment. Semin Oncol 1978; 5:155–165.

66. Goff JR, Anderson HR, Cooper PF. Distractibility and memory deficits in long-term survivors of acute lymphoblastic leukemia. J Dev Behav Pediatr 1980; 1:158–163.

67. Gogan JL, Koocher GP, Fine WE, et al. Pediatric cancer survival and marriage: Issues affecting adult adjustment. Am J Orthopsychiatry 1979; 19:423–430.

68. Goldiner P, Schweizer O. The hazards of anesthesia and surgery with bleomycin treated patients. Semin Oncol 1979; 6:121–124.

69. Gottdiener JS, Appelbaum FR, Ferrans VJ, et al. Cardiotoxicity associated with high-dose cyclophosphamide therapy. Arch Intern Med 1981; 141:758.

70. Green M, Solnit A. Reactions to the threatened loss of a child: A vulnerable child syndrome. Pediatrics 1964; 34:58–66.

71. Greenberg HS, Kazak AE, Meadows AT. Psychologic functioning in 8- to 16-year-old cancer survivors and their parents. J Pediatr 1989; 114:488–493.

72. Greenleigh Associates. Report on the social, economic, and psychological needs of cancer patients

in California. In Proceedings of Western States Conference on Cancer Rehabilitation. Palo Alto, Calif.: Bull Publishing Co, March 1982.

73. Halperin E, Constine LS. Second tumors and late effects of cancer treatment. In Halperin EC, Kuhn LE, Constine LS, et al (eds): Pediatric Radiation Oncology. New York: Raven Press, 1989, pp 344–389.

74. Hamre M, Robinson L, Nesbit M, et al. Effects of radiation on ovarian function in long-term survivors of childhood acute lymphoblastic leukemia: A report from the Children's Cancer Study Group. J Clin Oncol 1987; 5:1759–1765.

75. Hancock BW, Bruce L, Ward AM, et al. Changes in immune status in patients undergoing splenectomy for the staging of Hodgkin's disease. Br Med J 1976; 1:313–315.

76. Hays DM. Personal communication, 1990.

77. Hensen M, Koufas A, Gallie B, et al. Osteosarcoma and retinoblastoma: A shared chromosomal mechanism revealing recessive predisposition. Proc Natl Acad Sci U S A 1985; 86:6216–6220.

78. Hicks GL. Coronary artery operations in radiation-associated atherosclerosis: Long term follow-up. Ann Thoracic Sur 1992; 53:670–674.

79. Hobbie WL. The role of the pediatric oncology nurse specialist in a follow-up clinic for long term survivors of childhood cancer. J Assoc Pediatr Oncol Nurs 1986; 3:9–12.

80. Hobbie WL, Schwartz C. Endocrine late effects among survivors of cancer. Semin Oncol Nurs 1989; 5:14–21.

81. Hoffman B. Cancer survivors at work: Job problems and illegal discrimination. Oncol Nurs Forum 1989; 16:39–43.

82. Holmes GE, Baker A, Hassanein RS, et al. The availability of insurance to long-term survivors of childhood cancer. Cancer 1986; 57:190–193.

83. Holmes GE, Holmes FF. Pregnancy outcome of patients treated for Hodgkin's disease: A controlled study. Cancer 1978; 41:1317–1322.

84. Holmes JA, Holmes FF. After ten years, what are the handicaps and life styles of children treated with cancer? Clin Pediatr 1975; 14:819–823.

85. Horning S, Hoppe R, Kaplan H, et al. Female reproductive potential after treatment of Hodgkin's disease. N Engl J Med 1981; 304:1377–1382.

86. Hymovich DP, Roehnert JE. Psychosocial consequences of childhood cancer. Semin Oncol Nurs 1989; 5:56–62.

87. Insurance: Your options and your child's. Washington, D.C.: Candlelighters Childhood Cancer Foundation, 1990.

88. Jacob S, Franconi C, Lossow W (eds): Structure and Function in Man. Philadelphia: WB Saunders, 1982.

89. Jaffe N. Late sequelae of cancer therapy. In Fernbach DJ, Vietti J (eds): Clinical Pediatric Oncology, 4th ed. St. Louis: CV Mosby, 1991, pp 647–674.

90. Jaffe N, Toth B, Hoer R, et al. Dental and maxillofacial abnormalities in long term survivors of childhood cancer: Effects of treatment with chemotherapy and radiation to the head and neck. Pediatrics 1984; 73:816–823.

91. Jannoun L. Are cognitive and educational development affected by age at which prophylactic therapy is given in acute lymphoblastic leukemia? Arch Dis Child 1983; 58:953–958.

92. Kadota RP, Burgert EO, Driscoll DJ, et al. Cardiopulmonary function in long-term survivors of childhood Hodgkin's lymphoma: A pilot study. Mayo Clin Proc 1988; 63:362.

93. Kantor A, Li F, Janov AJ, et al. Hypertension in long term survivors of childhood renal cancers. J Clin Oncol 1989; 7:912–915.

94. Kazak A, Clark MW. Stress in families of children with myelomeningocele. Dev Med Child Neurol 1986; 28:220–228.

95. Klein HO, Wickramanayake D, Coerper C, et al. High-dose ifosfamide and mesna as continuous infusion over 5 days, a phase I/II trial. Cancer Treat Rev 1983; 10A:167–173.

96. Knudson AG Jr. Genetics and the etiology of childhood cancer. Pediatr Res 1976; 10:513–517.

97. Koocher GP, O'Malley JE. The Damocles syndrome: Psychosocial consequences of surviving childhood cancer. New York: McGraw-Hill, 1981.

98. Koocher GP, O'Malley JE, Gogan JL, et al. Psychological adjustment among pediatric cancer survivors. J Child Psychol Psychiatry 1980; 21:163–175.

99. Koyama H, Wada T, Nishizawa Y, et al. Cyclophosphamide-induced ovarian failure: Therapeutic significance in patients with breast cancer. Cancer 1977; 39:1403–1407.

100. Kupst MJ, Schulman JL. Long-term coping with pediatric leukemia: A six year follow-up study. J Pediatr 1988; 13:7–22.

101. Lansky SB, Cairns NU, Lansky LL, et al. Central nervous system prophylaxis. Am J Pediatr Hematol Oncol 1984; 6:183–199.

102. Lansky SB, List MA, Ritter-Sterr C. Psychosocial consequences of cure. Cancer 1986; 58:529–533.

103. Lanzkowsky P, Shende A, Karayakin G, et al. Staging laparotomy and splenectomy: Treatment and complications of Hodgkin's disease in children. Am J Hematol 1976; 1:393–404.

104. Lawrence HJ, Simone J, Aur RJA. Cyclophosphamide-induced hemorrhagic cystitis in children with leukemia. Cancer 1975; 36:1572–1576.

105. Li F. Genetic studies of survivors of childhood cancer. Am J Pediatr Hematol Oncol 1987; 9:104–106.

106. Li FP, Corkery J, Vawter G, et al. Breast cancer after cancer therapy in childhood. Cancer 1983; 51:521–523.

107. Li FP, Gimbrere K, Gelber RD, et al. Adverse pregnancy outcome following radiation therapy. Proc Am Soc Clin Oncol 1986; 5:202.

108. Li FP, Jeffe N. Progeny of childhood cancer survivors. Lancet 1974; 2:704–714.

109. Li FP, Stone R. Survivors of cancer in childhood. Ann Intern Med 1976; 84:551–553.

110. Linuks PS, Stockwell ML. Obstacles in the prevention of psychological seqelae in survivors of childhood cancer. J Pediatr Hematol Oncol 1985; 7:132–140.

111. Maguire A, Craft AW, Evans RGB, et al. The long-term effects of treatment on the dental condition of children surviving malignant disease. Cancer 1987; 60:2570–2575.

112. Makipernaa A. Long-term quality of life and psychological coping after treatment of solid tumors in childhood. Acta Paediatr Scand 1989; 78:728–735.

113. Malone M, Lumley H, Erdohazi M. Astrocytoma as a second malignancy in patients with acute lymphoblastic leukemia. Cancer 1986; 57:1979–1985.

114. Matuse-Ridley M, Nicosia S, Meadows AT. Gonadal effects of cancer therapy in boys. Cancer 1985; 55:2353–2363.

115. McKeen EA, Mulvihill JJ, Rosner F, et al. Pregnancy outcome in Hodgkin's disease. Lancet 1979; 2:590.

116. McLennan IM, Ray HM, Festenstein M, et al. Analysis of treatments in childhood leukemia: Predisposition to methotrexate-induced neutropenia after craniospinal irradiation. Br Med J 1975; 1:563–566.

117. Meadows AT. Second malignant neoplasms. Clin Oncol 1985; 4:247–261.

118. Meadows AT, Baum E, Fossati-Bellani F, et al. Second malignant neoplasms in children. An update from the late effects study group. J Clin Oncol 1985; 3:532–538.

119. Meadows AT, Hobbie WL. The medical consequences of cure. Cancer 1986; 58(suppl):524–528.

120. Meadows AT, Krejmas NL, Belasco JB. The medical cost of cure: Sequelae in survivors of childhood cancer. In Van Eys J, Sullivan MP (eds): Status of the Curability of Childhood Cancer. New York: Raven Press, 1980, pp 263–276.

121. Meadows AT, Massari DJ, Fergusson J, et al. Declines in IQ scores and cognitive dysfunction in children with acute lymphoblastic leukemia treated with cranial irradiation. Lancet 1981; 2:1015–1018.

122. Meadows AT, McKee L, Kazak AE. Psychosocial status of young adult survivors of childhood cancer: A survey. Med Pediatr Oncol 1989; 17:466–470.

123. Meadows AT, Silber J. Delayed consequences of therapy for childhood cancer. CA 1985; 35:271–286.

124. Mefferd J, Donaldson S, Link M. Pediatric Hodgkin's disease: Pulmonary, cardiac and thyroid function following combined modality therapy. Int J Radiat Oncol Biol Phys 1989; 16:679–685.

125. Mellette SJ, Franco PC. Psychosocial barriers to employment of the cancer survivor. J Psychosoc Oncol 1987; 5:97–115.

126. Merriam G, Focht E. Radiation doses to the lens in the treatment of tumors of the eye and adjacent structures: Possibilities of cataract formation. Radiology 1958; 72:357–369.

127. Mike V, Meadows AT, D'Angio GJ. Incidence of second malignant neoplasms in children: Results of an international study. Lancet 1982; 2:1326–1331.

128. Monaco GA. Personal communication, 1990.

129. Moore IM, Glasser ME, Ablin AR. The late psychosocial consequences of childhood cancer. J Pediatr Nurs 1987; 3:150–158.

130. Moore IM, Kramer JH, Ablin AR. Late effects of central nervous system prophylactic leukemia therapy on cognitive functioning. Oncol Nurs Forum 1986; 13:45–51.

131. Morris-Jones PH, Craft AW. Childhood cancer: Cure at what cost? Arch Dis Child 1990; 65:638–640.

132. Mortimer RH, Hill GE, Gullingan JP, et al. Hypothyroidism and Graves disease after mantle irradiation: A follow-up study. Aust NZ J Med 1986; 16:347–351.

133. Mulhern RK, Crisco JJ, Kun LE. Neuropsychological sequelae of childhood brain tumors: A review. J Child Clin Psychol 1983; 12:66–73.

134. Mulhern RK, Wasserman AB, Friedman AG, et al. Social competence and behavioral adjustment of children who are long-term survivors of cancer. Pediatrics 1989; 83:18–25.

135. Mullen F. Re-entry: The educational needs of the cancer survivor. Health Educ Q 10(suppl) 1984; 88–94.

136. Mullen F. Needed: An agenda for survivors. Cope Magazine 1986; 66.

137. Nesbit M, Krivit W, Heyn R, et al. Acute and chronic effects of MTX on hepatic, pulmonary and skeletal system. Cancer 1976; 37:1048–1054.

138. Nicosia S, Matus-Ridley M, Meadows T. Gonadal effects of cancer therapy in girls. Cancer 1985; 55:2364–2372.

139. Oberfield SE, Allen JC, Pollack J, et al. Long term endocrine sequelae after treatment of medulloblastoma: A prospective study of growth and thyroid function. J Pediatr 1986; 108:219–223.

140. Ochs JJ, Berger P, Brecher ML, et al. Computed tomography brain scans in children with acute lymphoblastic leukemia receiving methotrexate alone as central nervous system prophylaxis. Cancer 1980; 45:2274–2278.

141. O'Dirscoll B, Hasleton P, Taylor P, et al. Active lung fibrosis up to 17 years after chemotherapy with carmustine (BCNU) in childhood. N Engl J Med 1990; 323:378–382.

142. Olsson H, Brandt L. Sex ratio in offspring of patients with non-Hodgkin's lymphoma. N Engl J Med 1982; 306:367–368.

143. O'Malley J, Foster D, Koocher G, et al. Visible physical impairment and psychological adjustment among pediatric cancer survivors. Am J Psychiatry 1980; 137:94–96.

144. O'Malley JE, Koocher G, Foster D, et al. Psychiatric sequelae of surviving childhood cancer. Am J Orthopsychiatry 1979; 49:608–616.

145. Onoyama Y, Mitsuyuki A, Takahashi M, et al. Radiation therapy of brain tumors in children. Radiology 1977; 115:687–697.

146. Packer R, Meadows AT, Rorke L, et al. Long-term sequelae of cancer treatments on the central nervous system in childhood. Med Pediatr Oncol 1987; 15:241–253.

147. Packer RJ, Zimmerman RA, Silaniuk LT. Magnetic resonance imaging in the evaluation of treatment-related central nervous system damage. Cancer 1986; 58:635–640.

148. Peckham VC, Meadows AT, Bartel N, et al. Educational late effects of long term survivors of childhood acute lymphoblastic leukemia. Pediatrics 1988; 81:127.

149. Peylan-Ramu N, Poplack D, Pizzo D, et al. Abnormal CT scans of the brain in asymptomatic children with acute lymphoblastic leukemia after prophylactic treatment of the central nervous system with radiation and intrathecal chemotherapy. N Engl J Med 1978; 298:815–819.

150. Pfefferbaum-Levine B, Copeland DR, Fletcher JM, et al. Neuropsychological assessment of long-term survivors of childhood leukemia. Am J Pediatr Hematol Oncol 1984; 6:123–128.

151. Phillips SL. Occupation and employment issues in pediatric oncology. In Pizzo PA, Poplack DG (eds). Principles and Practice of Pediatric Oncology. Philadelphia: JB Lippincott, 1989, pp 1037–1040.

152. Probert JC, Parker BR. The effects of radiation therapy on bone growth. Radiology 1975; 114:155–162.

153. Qureshi M, Pennington J, Goldsmith J, et al. Cyclophosphamide therapy and sterility. Lancet 1972; 2:1290–1291.

154. Ramsay N, Kim T, Coccia P, et al. Thyroid dysfunction in pediatric patients after mantle field radiation therapy for Hodgkin's disease. Proc Am Soc Clin Oncol 1978; 19:331. (Abstract.)

155. Rimm I, Li F, Tarbell N, et al. Brain tumors after cranial irradiation for childhood acute lymphoblastic leukemia. Cancer 1987; 59:1506–1508.

156. Robison LL, Nesbit ME, Sather HN, et al. Factors associated with IQ scores in long-term survivors of childhood acute lymphoblastic leukemia. Am J Pediatr Hematol Oncol 1984; 6:115–121.

157. Romske C, Zipf W, Miser A, et al. Evaluation of GH release and human growth hormone treatment in children with cranial irradiation associated short stature. J Pediatr 1984; 104:177–181.

158. Rose M. Health promotion and risk prevention: Applications for cancer survivors. Oncol Nurs Forum 1989; 16:335–340.

159. Roswit B. Complications of radiation therapy: The alimentary tract. Semin Roentgenol 1974; 9:115–131.

160. Rowland JH, Glidewell OJ, Sibley RF, et al. Effects of different forms of central nervous system prophylaxis on neuropsychological function in childhood leukemia. J Clin Oncol 1984; 2:1327–1335.

161. Rubin P, Puthie RB, Young LW. The significance of scoliosis in post irradiated Wilms' tumor and neuroblastoma. Radiology 1962; 79:539–559.

162. Ruccione K, Weinberg K. Late effects in multiple body systems. Semin Oncol Nur 1989; 5:4–13.

163. Samaan N, Schultz P, Yang KP. Endocrine complications after radiotherapy for tumors of the head and neck. J Lab Clin Med 1987; 109:364–372.

164. Samuels ML, Johnson PE, Holoye P, et al. Large-dose bleomycin therapy and pulmonary toxicity: A possible role of prior radiotherapy. JAMA 1976; 235:1117–1120.

165. Sanders J. Long-term effects of bone marrow transplantation. Pediatrician 1991; 18:76–81.

166. Sawyer M, Crettenden A, Toogood I. Psychological adjustment of families of children and adolescents treated for leukemia. Am J Pediatr Hematol Oncol 1986; 8:200–207.

167. Schmitt-Grat A, Jurgens H, Gobel U, et al. Acute monocytic leukemia complicating combined modality therapy for localized childhood Ewing's sarcoma. J Cancer Res Clin Oncol 1981; 102:93–97.

168. Schwartz CL, Hobbie WL, Truesdell SC, et al. QT$_c$ prolongation in anthracycline treated survivors of childhood cancer. Presentation at the American Society of Clinical Oncologists, May 1990.

169. Shalet SM. Growth and hormonal status of children treated for brain tumors. Childs Brain 1982; 9:284–293.

170. Shalet SM, Beardwell CG, Pearson, et al. The effect of varying doses of cerebral irradiation on growth hormone production in childhood. Clin Endocrinol 1976; 5:287–290.

171. Shaw IC, Graham MI. Mesna. A short review. Cancer Treat Res 1989; 14:67–86.

172. Siimes M, Rautonen J. Small testicles with impaired production of sperm in adult survivors of childhood malignancies. Cancer 1990; 65:1303–1305.

173. Sklar C, Kim T, Ramsey N. Thyroid dysfunction among long term survivors of bone marrow transplantation. Am J Med 1982; 73:688–694.

174. Sklar CA. Growth and pubertal development in survivors of childhood cancer. Pediatrician 1991; 18:53–60.

175. Slanina J, Mussoff K, Rhaner T, et al. Long term side effects of irradiated patients with Hodgkin's disease. Int J Radiat Oncol Biol Phys 1977; 2:1–19.

176. Smithson WA, Burgert EO, Childs DS, et al. Acute myelomonocytic leukemia after irradiation and chemotherapy for Ewing's sarcoma. Mayo Clin Proc 1978; 53:757–759.

177. Spinetta JJ, Murphy JL, Vik PJ, et al. Long-term adjustment in families of children with cancer. J Psychosoc Oncol 1989; 6:179–191.

178. Steinberg JS, Cohen AJ, Wasserman AG, et al. Acute arrhythmogenicity of doxorubicin administration. Cancer 1987; 60:1213.

179. Stillman RJ, Schinfeld JS, Schiff I. Ovarian failure in long-term survivors of childhood malignancy. Am J Obstet Gynecol 1981; 139:62–66.

180. Strong L, Herson J, Osborne B, et al. Risk of radiation-related subsequent malignant tumors in survivors of Ewing's sarcoma. J Natl Cancer Inst 1979; 62:1401–1406.

181. Tamaroff M, Salwen R, Miller D, et al. Neuropsychological sequelae in irradiated (1800 rads [r] and 2400 r) and non-irradiated children with acute lymphoblastic leukemia (ALL). Am Soc Clin Oncol 1985; C-644. (Abstract.)

182. Tang TT, Holcenberg JS, Duck SC, et al. Thyroid carcinoma following treatment for acute lymphoblastic leukemia. Cancer 1980; 46:1572–1576.

183. Tanner JM. Growth at Adolescence, 2nd ed. Oxford: Blackwell Scientific Publication, 1962.

184. Tebbi CK, Bromberg C, Piedmonte M. Long-term vocational adjustment of cancer patients diagnosed during adolescence. Cancer 1989; 63:213–218.

185. Tebbi CK, Mallon JC. Long-term psychosocial outcome among cancer amputees in adolescence and early adulthood. J Psychosoc Oncol 1987; 5:69–82.

186. Teeter MA, Holmes GE, Holmes FF, et al. Decisions about marriage and family among survivors of childhood cancer. J Psychosoc Oncol 1987; 5:59–68.

187. Tefft M, Lattin PB, Jerab B, et al. Acute and late effects of normal tissue following combined chemo- and radiotherapy of childhood rhabdomyosarcoma and Ewing's sarcoma. Cancer 1976; 37:1202–1213.

188. Teta MJ, Del Po MC, Kasl SV, et al. Psychosocial consequences of childhood and adolescent cancer survival. J Chronic Dis 1986; 39:751–759.

189. Thomas PRM, Griffith KD, Fineberg BB, et al. Late effects of treatment for Wilms' tumor. Int J Radiat Oncol Biol Phys 1983; 9:651–657.

190. Tucker M, Coleman C, Cox R, et al. Risk of second cancers after treatment of Hodgkin's disease. N Engl J Med 1988; 318:76–81.

191. Tucker M, D'Angio G, Boice J, et al. Bone sarcomas linked to radiotherapy and chemotherapy in children. N Engl J Med 1987; 317:588–593.

192. Tucker MA, Meadows AT, Boice J, et al. Cancer risk following treatment of childhood cancer. In Boice J, Fraumeni J (eds): Radiation Carcinogenesis: Epidemiology and Biological Significance. New York: Raven, 1984, pp 211–220.

193. van Eys J. Living beyond cure: Transcending survival. Am J Pediatr Hematol Oncol 1987; 9:114–118.

194. Vogel JM, Kimball HR, Foley HT, et al. Effects of extensive radiotherapy on marrow granulocyte reserves of patients with Hodgkin's disease. Cancer 1968; 21:798–804.

195. Wallace MH, Reiter PB, Pendergrass TW. Parents of long-term survivors of childhood cancer: A preliminary survey to characterize concerns and needs. Oncol Nurs Forum 1987; 14:39–43.

196. Wallace WHB, Shalet SM, Hendry JA, et al. Ovarian failure following abdominal irradiation in childhood: The radiosensitivity of the human oocyte. Br J Radiol 1989; 62:995–998.

197. Wara W, Irvine A, Neger R, et al. Radiation retinopathy. Int J Radiat Oncol Biol Phys 1979; 5:81–83.

198. Wara WM, Phillips TL, Margolis LW, et al. Radiation pneumonitis: A new approach to the derivation of time-dose factors. Cancer 1973; 32:547–552.

199. Wasserman AL, Thompson EEI, Wilimas JA, et al. The psychological status of survivors of childhood/adolescent Hodgkin's disease. Am J Dis Child 1987; 141:626–631.

200. Wellwood JM, Jackson BT. The intestinal complications of radiotherapy. Br J Surg 1973; 60:814–818.

201. Wharam MD. Radiation therapy. In Altman AJ, Schwartz AD (eds): Malignant Disease of Infancy, Childhood and Adolescence. Philadelphia: WB Saunders, 1983.

202. Whitehead E, Shalet S, Blockledge G, et al. The effects of combination chemotherapy on ovarian function in women treated for Hodgkin's disease. Cancer 1983; 52:988–993.

203. Whitt JK. Children's adaptation to chronic illness and handicapping conditions. In Eisenberg MG, Sutkin LC, Jansen MA (eds): Chronic Illness and Disability Through the Life Span: Effects on Self and Family. New York: Springer-Verlag, 1984, pp 69–102.

204. Wilson G, Foster D. Textbook of Endocrinology. New York: WB Saunders, 1985, pp 269–276.

205. Witherspoon RP, Storb R, Ochs H, et al. Recovery of antibody production in human allogeneic marrow graft recipients: Influence of time post-transplantation, the presence or absence of chronic graft-versus-host disease and antithymocyte globulin treatment. Blood 1981; 58:360–368.

206. Woods W, Dehner L, Nesbit M, et al. Fatal veno-occlusive disease of the liver following high dose chemotherapy, radiation and bone marrow transplant. Am J Med 1980; 60:285–290.

207. Womer RB, Pritchard J, Barratt M. Renal toxicity of cisplatin in children. J Pediatr 1985; 106:659–663.

Interdisciplinary Management of the Child or Adolescent With Cancer

Leslie Wagner McMahon

Advancing technology and the complexity of the health care system have resulted in increased specialization in oncology. Over the past 20 years significant improvements in survival rates for children with cancer have changed the focus from terminal care. Patients and families now must live with the disease and be prepared to minimize the stress of financial, marital, sibling, school, and community issues. The goal for a truly cured child is to be physically healthy and well-adjusted mentally and socially.[42]

Hammond[20] states that institutions expecting to provide state-of-the-art care for children with cancer should have interdisciplinary teams to provide the coordination that can produce good outcomes. He further recommends that if institutions do not establish such teams, they should refer patients to those that do. Interdisciplinary teams should include the patient and family and together should focus their efforts beyond the delivery of medical care objectives.[34]

Team members collaborate to determine necessary referrals and establish an ongoing treatment plan that includes the entire family. The treatment plan must continually be evaluated by the team and revised as needed. Administrative support for establishment of an interdisciplinary approach to patient care is necessary. Commitment to teamwork should be a part of a departmental or organizational philosophy. Cost effectiveness of a team is difficult to quantify and may become a factor in future prospective payment for health care.[37]

An interdisciplinary approach to patient care does not just happen by assigning people to work together. Teamwork depends on full use of the competency of individual members.[12] Many health care professionals are not experienced as part of an integrated team and often are not knowledgeable about specific competencies of other professions. Consequently, people who work together do not necessarily function as a team. Overlapping of roles on a health care team, along with status and viewpoint differences, may lead to conflict within the team.[12,34,38] Although some degree of difference is unavoidable, professional territoriality hampers coordination attempts.

Team structure is determined by the scope of care provided, the environment, and available resources. An interdisciplinary team may vary greatly in size but generally has a core, or primary, group of nurses, physicians, other health care providers, and psychosocial support members who routinely interact on behalf of the child and family. Other professionals within the treatment center or community may serve in a consultative capacity.

Two questions frequently asked concern where children with cancer should be treated, and by whom. Most health care providers insist that children and adolescents be referred for initial evaluation to university hospitals or cancer centers where totality of disciplines, resources, and current therapies is available. Referral of children and adolescents to centers participating in treatment protocols not only assures the best physical and psychosocial care for the patient and family but also contributes to future progress in pediatric oncology.[32] In the United States the majority of children with cancer are treated by pediatric hematologists and oncologists, many of whom are members of a cooperative study group (Pediatric Oncology Group and Children's Cancer Group).[8] Some treatment centers also offer institution-based research studies for some or all diseases. Some adolescents are treated within an adult practice. It is imperative that these adolescents receive age-appropriate physical and psychosocial care and that they participate in clinical trials.

After the diagnosis and treatment plan are determined, some families can return to their community for care. A partnership between the cancer center and community caregivers may be considered when the treatment protocol is not too complex, the distance to a major medical center is substantial, or there is an established trust relationship with the local medical staff. Successful collaboration between sponsoring protocol centers and community practitioners necessitates continuous exchange of medical and psychosocial information. Medical cost savings and decreased nonmedical expense and lost income may be realized for families who receive some care by community physicians. Such an arrangement decreases the family's financial burden caused by traveling and does not interfere as much with the child's normal activities. Although benefits to the family may be obvious, further research is needed to determine if community care has an adverse impact on survival data.

Often a child and family are overwhelmed by the number of individuals they encounter once a diagnosis of cancer is made. Staff members within the cancer center may participate in both inpatient and outpatient care, or their role may be based in only one area. If some of the child's treatment is provided through a local physician or nurse practitioner, additional community staff and resources are introduced to the family. Treatment at times may be provided in the home, and once again the child and family must interact with another group of professionals.

INTERDISCIPLINARY HEALTH CARE TEAM

Collaboration of team members is dependent on their ability to blend roles or blur boundaries.[37] Team members must strive to complement each other's roles and to avoid competitive behavior. A team should not concentrate on which discipline does what but should coordinate their work to meet the needs of the child or adolescent and family.

The health care team coordinates treatment and support services based on the premise that cancer affects not just the patient but the whole family (Fig. 18–1). Families need access to an unfragmented foundation of multidisciplinary support, which is achieved through the combined efforts of the primary health care team and the family's community.[27] Every effort is made to build a trusting relationship between the team and the family to minimize the effects of chronic illness. Children and families need to know that it is natural to develop different relationships with different team members. The team member who most effectively relates to the patient and the family needs to communicate

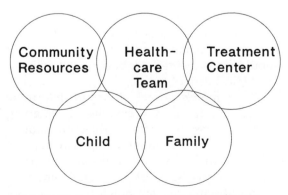

FIGURE 18–1. Health care team coordination.

frequently with other colleagues so they do not feel isolated. "It is important that the family know the role of each member, so they can better utilize their expertise."[5]

Physicians

The local pediatrician or family doctor often detects a suspected childhood cancer and initiates referral to a pediatric oncologist for diagnosis. Oncologists bring an understanding of the pathophysiology of the disease and are responsible for treatment decisions based on available protocols or randomized study results. Depending on the type of childhood malignancy, the oncologist may consult with various specialists who may not specialize in the treatment of young people (e.g., surgeon, pathologist, radiation oncologist, neurologist, ophthalmologist, endocrinologist, nephrologist). A psychiatrist may also be involved, depending on the psychosocial assessment.

Generally the pediatrician remains an important member of the treatment team even after the referral to a center better equipped for specialized pediatric oncologic care. The degree of continued involvement by the family physician is determined by a number of factors: the amount of therapy that can be done outside the hospital, the distance to the cancer center, and the past experience and interest of the pediatrician in treating childhood cancer. Whether cancer care will be delivered in a medical center or shared with the local community, the pediatrician usually continues to provide primary care for noncancer-related medical needs. Shared patient management makes it possible to provide the maximal benefits of current therapy and ensures that patients can be enrolled in research protocol studies.[15,40]

Van Eys[42] states that the medical care objective is to cure the child of cancer, and yet medical decision making must be in harmony with other elements of team care. Most team members agree that children and adolescents should be allowed to participate in decision making. They must be included in age-appropriate treatment discussions about potential benefits, risks, or side effect information related to the proposed treatment. Documentation of parental approval, in the case of minors, is required before initiation of any therapy.

Teaching hospitals may have fellows, residents, medical students, and physicians' assistants participating with the attending or primary physician. Families are often confused about the roles and inpatient and outpatient rotations of different physicians. Whenever feasible, care must be taken to consolidate questions and examinations so families do not feel they have been repeatedly asked for the same information. Attending pediatric oncologists usually are faculty members of a university and combine teaching responsibilities with patient care and research. The attending physician must be identified for the family so they know who is responsible for their care. Parents also have the right to obtain complete, current information from their child's physician in terms that can be reasonably understood. Some oncologists are in private practice and treat patients in community facilities. Fellows are physicians who are pursuing specialized training in childhood cancer and blood diseases. They function independently as practitioners who confer with attending physicians on treatment plans. Fellowship training includes clinical, teaching, and research responsibilities. Residents are physicians involved in a 3-year training program in general pediatrics. Patient care responsibilities are performed with the guidance of fellows or attending physicians. Oncology experience may be mixed with general pediatrics or may exist as a separate rotation if service size permits. Medical students generally rotate through the service in more of an observational role, performing limited functions. The physicians' assistant works under the overall medical direction of an attending physician. Institutional medical staff by-laws and state regulations vary regarding the physician assistant's appointment and practice privileges.

Nurses

Pediatric oncology nursing practice is a blend of theory with the findings of nursing research and those of related fields.[3] The specialty developed in response to the specific knowledge and skill required to care for children with cancer and their families.[6] The Association of Pediatric Oncology Nurses (APON) is dedicated to supporting quality care for children with cancer and their families. APON strives to promote high standards of nursing practice, education, and research. Bru[6] states that professional associations should assist in defining and evaluating specialty practice. In 1978 APON collaborated with the American Nurses' Association (ANA) to develop the standards for pediatric oncology nursing practice. APON revised the standards in 1988 and developed the first scope of practice statement.[3] There are seven APON outcome standards (Table 18–1). The first six refer to direct care of the child and family. The final standard refers to nurses'

professional practice responsibilities. The Joint Commission on Accreditation of Healthcare Organizations states that a registered nurse shall plan, supervise, and evaluate the nursing care for every patient.[23] Pediatric oncology nurses should use these documents to monitor practice, develop policies and procedures, and plan for the future.[6] Standards from the ANA and the Oncology Nursing Society (ONS) should be used together with the APON standards.

Pediatric oncology nursing includes various roles such as direct patient care provider, teacher, manager of resources, counselor, consultant, advocate, liaison, and researcher.[3] Nurses facilitate coordination among team members and representatives of the com-

TABLE 18–1. *APON Outcome Standards of Pediatric Oncology Nursing Practice*

Information Regarding Disease and Therapy

Standard: The child and family possess accurate current information about the disease, options for treatment, consequences or side effects of treatment, potential oncologic emergencies, alternative care settings and resources in order to be fully informed partners in the health care team. Information should be specific to the developmental level of the child and family.

Growth and Development

Standard: The child and family possess adequate information regarding the psychologic and physiologic effects of the diagnosis and treatment of cancer on the normal growth and developmental level of the child and family.

Physical Care

Standard: The child's physical care is provided by the nurse in collaboration with the child and family. The nurse is responsible for assessing and determining the child's and family's participation in the physical care of the child. The nurse selects interventions that facilitate an appropriate level of self-care.

Psychosocial Care

Standard: The child and family maintain psychologic, social and spiritual integrity while living with a diagnosis of cancer.

Prevention and Early Detection of Secondary Cancers and Malignancies in Adulthood

Standard: The child and family possess appropriate knowledge with regard to prevention and early detection of secondary cancer and adult malignancies.

Long-Term Survival

Standard: The child and family demonstrate optimal adaptation to long-term survival. This is demonstrated by the integration into the family's usual health care practice of current information about possible psychologic and/or physical late consequences from a diagnosis and treatment of cancer in childhood. The child and family also participate in long-term follow-up activities.

Professional Development

Standard: The nurse assumes responsibility for improving pediatric oncology nursing practice through evaluation of practice and an ongoing involvement in continuing education, professional development, and research.

From Association of Pediatric Oncology Nurses. Scope of Practice and Outcome Standards of Practice for Pediatric Oncology Nursing. McLean, Va.: The Association, 1988, pp 8–24.

munity to individualize care for the child and family. Family-centered care and rooming-in practices have changed the nurse's responsibility for total child care. Today the nurse's role is to facilitate the parents' desired level of participation to avoid family members' feeling neglected or usurped in their roles. In the hospital the parents' role often is poorly defined, and their rights and responsibilities are not clear.[4] A classic study examining parent participation on pediatric oncology units suggested that nurses who have had experience with parent participation find that method of care more desirable than do nurses without such experience.[19]

The child with cancer may receive care on a general medical-surgical unit, a unit limited to a particular age range, or a unit specific to diagnosis or specialty. The scope of practice on the unit in turn affects the nurses' care delivery focus. A separate oncology unit may not be feasible because of the relatively low incidence of childhood cancer. Nurses on a general medical-surgical unit are oriented to a generalist practice. They may feel inadequately prepared to administer protocol chemotherapy agents, or they may not have time to provide the intense symptom management care oncology patients require. Age-specific units are geared to the growth and development needs of those particular children; however, the nursing staff will be less familiar with oncology care, and the children will not benefit from socializing with other children of all ages who have cancer. Nurses should develop collaborative networks within organizations to identify experienced oncology nurses. Any nurse may then contact a resource nurse for consultation or for technical assistance (e.g., in administering chemotherapy or performing central line care). An oncology unit with dedicated personnel allows nurses to specialize in their practice, which should translate into high-quality patient care. The challenge for pediatric oncology nurses is to stay current with the rapidly expanding oncology literature and achieve skill in working with children of all ages.

Relationship building with the family is facilitated if the method of nursing care delivery provides for continuity, regardless of the unit's scope of practice. Some institutions use a case manager concept and assign families to a specific nursing staff member. This system provides a contact person from whom the family receives consistent communication throughout treatment. The case manager consults with and informs other team members as needed to meet the identified needs. Primary nursing generally limits the number of nurses caring for a child during hospitalizations. Orienting parents to hospital and patient care routines is important. Teamwork among the nursing staff is critical to promote a unified approach to all patient care needs and not just to those of assigned patients. Licensed practical nurses and nursing assistants, if included in the staffing plan, assist in providing direct patient care under the direction of a registered nurse.

Nurses within a cancer center may specialize further in nutrition, pain control, mental health, or other services. Clinical nurse specialists (CNS), nurse practitioners (NP), or clinicians have additional training, generally a master's degree, which has prepared them to assume advanced nursing roles. Although the origins of CNSs and NPs are different, recent studies found similarities in education curriculum and overlapping role functions, suggesting advantages for merging the two roles.[14,16]

Historically, the NP role evolved with a stronger medical model component, focused on more technical activities, and was based in the ambulatory care setting. Job descriptions for an NP include using comprehensive physical assessment and teaching skills, writing orders or prescriptions, and performing bone marrow aspirates or lumbar punctures. Teaching and counseling patients and their families are other major components of the NP's role. In recent years NPs have been seeking both legal coverage of their practice in state nursing practice acts and prescriptive practice. The question of supervision versus independent practice for NPs has led to issues with third-party reimbursement.

CNSs generally are oriented to advanced clinical specialization and work in direct and indirect patient care, often in the inpatient setting. They use their teaching, research, clinical, and consulting skills to assist in treating the child and family. The CNS also interacts with the nursing staff to facilitate patient care, support groups, and ongoing staff development.

Larger institutions may have doctorally prepared nurses in research roles. Nurse researchers contribute to nursing knowledge through scientific investigation of clinical and administrative problems. Nurse researchers are knowledgeable about design methodology and analysis. They often serve as consultants or coinvestigators with interested advanced practice nurses or staff nurses. Staff nurses should also be encouraged to implement research findings into clinical practice. A study aimed at establishing pediatric cancer nursing research priorities found professional issues dominated the cancer center sample, whereas psychosocial issues were more prominent in the APON sample.[22]

Systems should be developed to ensure continuity of nursing care, regardless of the setting. Consistency of care makes things easier for the family. The complexities of caring for a child with cancer have necessitated the role of the nurse as coordinator, for coordination is necessary among the treatment center staff, the patient, and the community to facilitate continuity of care. Collaborating with the physician to facilitate patient care is time consuming, and the responsibility must be shared by all the nursing staff. Some centers rotate staff members between inpatient and outpatient units to maximize continuity for the patient and family. Rotating the staff may also help mitigate the staff stress often associated with high-acuity inpatient nursing. Another benefit is that it allows all the nursing staff to see the increasing number of cancer patients who do well and who are seen only in the outpatient center. When staffing is separate, nurses in both areas want updates on the treatment progress of the child. Outpatient nurses often do not get the opportunity to visit patients while they are hospitalized. They may not realize when a child is very sick, or the nurses may feel uncomfortable seeing patients outside the ambulatory environment. Inpatient nurses, especially, verbalize the need for information as increasingly more therapy is done on an ambulatory basis. Inpatient medical rounds, outpatient clinic rounds, and psychosocial and discharge planning meetings provide opportunities for both inpatient and outpatient staff members to share communications. Information may also be obtained from other team members who routinely work in both inpatient and outpatient settings.

During treatment, nursing caregivers from community agencies may participate in meeting the child's health care needs. Availability of a school nurse is not consistent among schools. If available, a school nurse may assist in educating classmates as part of reintegrating the child into the school setting. On a long-term basis the school nurse may act as a liaison between the treatment center and the school, interpreting the ongoing health care needs while remaining cognizant of the school setting.[25] Academic personnel, including the school nurse, should collaborate in the development of individualized educational programs to meet the short- and long-term academic, social, and developmental needs of the student with cancer.[11]

Local community nurses may be an untapped resource for meeting the needs of the child and family. Treatment centers could provide educational programs and discharge conferences to prepare community nurses better to assist the team. Intervention by the community nurse enables patients to remain at home for longer periods, thus remaining close to family and friends while promoting the usual life-style of the family.

State funding agencies for children with chronic illness have been established in some states. Many are organized with case managers who work closely with the treatment center to keep current on the child's progress and to determine available funding and resources. As home care reimbursement continues to gain acceptance with federal, state, and third-party payers, an increasing number of services that historically required hospitalization or treatment in an outpatient center are provided in the home. Services with which home care nurses may assist include antibiotic therapy, blood product and chemotherapy administration, central line care, and enteral or total parenteral nutrition administration. Home care should not be recommended to a family simply because it costs less. Nurses must assess the family's desire to care for the child at home. A home care assessment should also include the family's cultural beliefs, support systems, and ability to provide care in the home.[13] If a decision is made for home health care, the agency nurses emphasize teaching the child and family to assume an active role in the care. Hospice care for the terminally ill child is also available in many communities to provide emotional support and increasingly to assist with physical care. This type of home care is also a cost-effective alternative to hospitalization and allows the family structure to remain intact.

Opportunities for nurses have grown to keep pace with changes in health care. Advanced technology, decreased hospitalization, and increased numbers of childhood cancer survivors will continue to present new challenges to nurses. Ongoing attention to professional development is necessary to keep pediatric oncology nursing practice current. Professional development can be enhanced through membership in a professional nursing organization such as APON. Pediatric oncology nurses may share ideas and become acquainted with each other during association conferences and through APON publications.

Clinical Social Workers

Central to the idea of social well-being is the role of the clinical social worker. Social work practice aims to make it possible for the family to use available health services more effectively. Social workers provide valuable input into treatment planning by contributing to the team's understanding of social factors that may influence the child's health care.

A professional social worker must have a master's degree plus supervised experience. Social workers have extensive training in human behavior and counseling skills. Clinical social workers are also trained to work with groups, and they often facilitate or cofacilitate support groups for parents, patients, and staff.

Clinical social work in health care assists people on a one-to-one basis to identify and use their own resources plus other available resources to solve the array of problems surrounding chronic illness. The trend in health care toward minimal hospitalization necessi-

tates social workers' assuming an active role in discharge planning from the time of admission. Planning may involve securing equipment or assessing potential for care in the home. Additionally, social workers support family members who are providing the home care.

Psychologists

The psychologist ideally works with the entire family as a designated member of the pediatric oncology interdisciplinary team but in some settings may be available only on a consultative basis. A doctoral degree is required to practice as a psychologist. He or she also has background in behavioral research methods.

The expertise of the psychologist may be limited to a particular specialty (e.g., clinical, developmental, school, physiologic, or educational). The field of psychology focuses on the understanding of behavior and on identification of the conditions that influence behavior.[44] Assistance from a psychologist is frequently sought to assess the emotional well-being of children with cancer in relation to their total environment.

The services generally provided by the psychologist include psychologic assessment, consultation, program evaluation, psychotherapy, and behavior modification. Psychologists have been leaders in the use of behavioral interventions such as hypnosis, relaxation therapy, and guided imagery. They have also played a central role in cognitive evaluation through skilled testing and interpretation of the impact of cancer treatment and the potential for long-term cognitive deficits.

Child Life Specialists

As integral members of the health care team in both the inpatient and outpatient settings, child life specialists strive to promote age-appropriate development and to minimize the adverse psychologic effects of chronic illness. Much has been written about the negative impact hospitalization has on children in terms of separation, regression, and emotional trauma. Child life programs seek to provide comprehensive care by decreasing stress and anxiety for the child, encouraging essential life experiences, and providing opportunities to retain self-esteem and appropriate independence.[2]

Academic preparation for the child life specialist as defined by the Association for the Care of Children's Health is a bachelor's degree, with supervised experience in the health care setting. Expertise of the child life specialist includes developmental observation, behavior management, medical play, and working with siblings. In the health care setting these specialists are involved with standardized developmental testing, establishment of behavior contracts with children, preoperative teaching, relaxation techniques for procedures, sibling support groups, or individual counseling.

Children often develop strong emotional relationships with child life personnel because they are viewed as nonthreatening and are generally removed from direct patient care. Child life staff members are responsible for planning recreational activities to foster normalcy and promote play. These activities are often supervised with the assistance of volunteers. Child life programs are generally small and may benefit by establishing ties with volunteer departments for assistance, particularly after hours and on weekends. Volunteers should receive some training before working with children with life-threatening illness. Initial training includes review of growth and development, explanation of childhood cancers and issues surrounding the child and family, and review of guidelines regarding follow-up communication to the health care team. Ongoing educational topics are identified by the volunteers and speakers obtained as needed.[30]

Observations and recommendations pertinent to the medical and psychosocial needs of children and families should be shared by child life personnel during interdisciplinary rounds and documented in the medical record. Patient care plans should also reflect nurses' and child life specialists' collaboration on individualizing interventions for identified psychosocial goals.

Teachers

Hospital-based teaching staff members provide educational services to inpatients and sometimes to outpatient children. Individualized education plans are developed based on the child's evaluated learning needs. The hospital teaching staff also facilitates early reentry of the child into the regular school classroom and continues to serve as a school liaison during the entire course of treatment. The school liaison can also facilitate informing the siblings' school personnel about the patient's cancer diagnosis and how it may affect the educational performance of the siblings.[11] School is the workplace for children to learn both academic and social skills. However, homebound teaching may be necessary for some children when classroom attendance is not possible.

Many health care teams offer community outreach programs for regular teachers and classmates, thus easing reentry for the child.[26] School personnel are instructed not to overprotect the child with cancer or lower academic standards for them. Successful reentry of the student with cancer into the classroom is an important aspect of reestablishing normalcy and enhancing quality of survival.[1] The child and parents must be included in planning the information to share about the diagnosis, treatment plan, and prognosis.

Staff members who visit the school may include the hospital teacher, a psychosocial team member, and a nurse to handle the variety of questions that may be asked. Children with cancer frequently decide to participate also in the classroom sessions. Their involvement provides them an opportunity to cope with their feelings and to help peers understand their situation. Educational materials for parents and teachers, including Charles Schultz' *Why, Charlie Brown, Why?*, a television videotape and corresponding teaching guide directed toward children with cancer, are available through the American Cancer Society. Research is needed to evaluate the effectiveness of different reentry programs.[36]

Since the goal of medical treatment for most children is cure, maintaining educational progress is vital. However, the majority of research shows that childhood cancer can have a negative impact on education.[7,17,24,31] Studies suggest that children experience difficulty in school because of numerous absences, lowered teacher expectation, and the side effects of treatment, especially cranial radiation, that may result in learning difficulties.

Hospital classroom attendance must be strongly encouraged unless prevented by extreme illness. Children should arrange in advance to bring schoolbooks and assignments when a scheduled hospitalization is planned. Bedside teaching assistance can be offered to children too ill to attend the unit classroom or for those in isolation.

Teachers are usually viewed as safe confidants for children since their relationship is removed from medical treatment concerns. The teachers' feedback to the interdisciplinary team is valuable because it includes both intellectual progress and socialization observations that indicate the coping ability of the child.

Clinical Pharmacists

Pharmacy services have traditionally been performed in a central location invisible to the patient. Continued progress in pharmacology has made it difficult for physicians and nurses to maintain current drug knowledge. Organizational changes in some pharmacy departments have resulted in attempts to use the pharmacist's knowledge and expertise more directly in patient care.

Clinical pharmacists dispense drugs and provide pharmacologic information to the health care team and families. Technicians are used for preparing and dispensing many of the drugs once accuracy has been verified by a pharmacist. These personnel changes may make a clinical pharmacy program economically feasible.

Some institutions have satellite or unit-based pharmacies. Medication orders may be given directly to the clinical pharmacist, who prepares the first dose immediately. Communication between team members is enhanced when a pharmacist works directly in the clinical area. The clinical pharmacist serves as the liaison to the central pharmacy for additional needs. Unfortunately, many clinical pharmacist programs do not function 24 hours a day, 7 days a week.

Physicians and nurses consult pharmacists on matters of drug compatibility, therapeutic serum drug levels, and methods of drug administration. Clinical pharmacists further advise on drug interactions and proper dosage and scheduling of drugs, sometimes suggesting drug therapy alternatives. Pharmacists coordinate investigational drug use and protocols with physicians. They provide new drug education to staff to ensure patient safety.

Another important aspect of the clinical pharmacist's role is to provide drug information to patients, their families, and the community. Cancer treatment often necessitates taking medications at home. Parents must understand proper drug administration, the importance of compliance, and the requirements for monitoring their child's clinical response and reaction to therapy.

Clinical Dietitians

Dramatic changes in the nutritional status of a child may occur in less than a week after oncologic treatment.[35] Nutrition services should begin at the time of diagnosis, and follow-up consultation should be continued in the outpatient center. The clinical dietitian serves as the nutrition resource for the team.

An initial patient assessment by the dietitian includes a diet history, estimation of basal energy expenditure, and baseline requirements. Anthropometric measurements of the size, weight, and proportions of the child may be obtained. Culture, age, and habits affect a child's food preferences. Parents can provide information on usual mealtimes, meal sizes, and the social dining habits of the family. A dietary care plan must be developed incorporating the data base.

A feeding-on-demand philosophy must be espoused for all cancer patients. Radiation therapy, drug therapy, and surgery all affect a child's dietary intake. Dietitians often advocate for unit-based kitchens, which stock beverages, soup, ice cream, and sandwich items to supplement between meals. They assist in interpreting the links between socialization and nutrition by encouraging taking meals in the cafeteria or in a unit communal dining room, if available. Parents and visitors are encouraged to visit during mealtimes to normalize the experience and may be asked to bring the child's favorite foods from home or from restaurants.

Dietitians help plan hospital menus designed to meet children's food preferences. Patient requests for non-menu items should be met whenever possible. The child's favorite food may not always be the most nutritious, but the dietitian can suggest ways to increase their nutritional quality.[29] Patient and family teaching is an important role of the dietitian.

Dietitians generally establish criteria with the physicians to identify children at high nutritional risk. Oral supplements may be offered to increase intake. However, if the patient falls below acceptable parameters, options for nutritional support must be explored. A nutrition support consultative team may be available. The combined disciplines of medicine, nursing, pharmacy, and dietary work together to offer comprehensive nutritional support. Enteral nutrition, usually by tube feeding, or parenteral nutrition are considered.

It may be necessary to continue nutritional support in the home. The complex issues of reimbursement and the need for family participation often surface and may affect the home treatment plan. Proper nutritional support in children with cancer has value in improving growth and organ system function and appears to improve treatment tolerance.[35]

Chaplain

The spiritual needs of the child and family vary greatly based on their culture and belief system. The chaplain should work with the staff to assess the degree of harmony between the religious beliefs of the parents and child or adolescent. Childhood cancer may affect previously held practices and beliefs of the family; thus periodic reassessment is suggested. Health care professionals must respect family beliefs and expressions of spirituality that are not part of organized religion. However, any spiritual or religious practice that interferes with the care of the child must be addressed with the family. One of the roles of the hospital-based chaplain is to educate the interdisciplinary team about different religious practices.

The family's specified spiritual needs should be included in the care plan. The diversity of organized religious beliefs necessitates that a hospital-based chaplain develop relationships with other community clergy. Clerical services may then be provided that are more closely aligned with the family's stated religious beliefs. A religious network also provides support to the community clergy members.

Rehabilitation Team

Several of the disciplines previously discussed may also be members of a rehabilitation team. In addition, physical therapists, speech therapists, and occupational therapists strive to enhance physical, social, and vocational functioning to improve the child's quality of life. Wells[45] defined *rehabilitation* as an active, ongoing process that begins at diagnosis and continues throughout the treatment process to minimize effects of treatment. Most rehabilitation programs require some form of referral or consultation before beginning services.[43,45]

Nurses must routinely assess the child's rehabilitation needs to ensure these services are not overlooked throughout the treatment course. Rehabilitation needs are often evident if amputation, limb salvage, or radiation is part of the treatment. All too frequently aggressive therapies such as bone marrow transplant produce lasting side effects such as graft-versus-host disease, which may require ongoing rehabilitative care. Long-term follow-up or survivor clinics have been developed in many large cancer centers as increasing numbers of children live and face adaption to the physical and psychosocial changes following cancer treatment.

Child and Family

In a team approach to patient management, parents provide the constant link between hospital, home, and family.[19] The child with cancer is also at the center of the interdisciplinary team. Health care members can better coordinate interventions if the child and family work directly with the team to identify their special needs. Patient and family participation is unique from that of other team members because their contribution to the planning and implementing of care is based on a personal perspective.

Years ago children with cancer often were "protected" from knowing anything about their disease. Child advocates now realize the importance of input from the child and stress the need to inform children of their disease from the time of diagnosis. Trust is a key developmental concept for children that the team can foster by providing honest, age-appropriate information to the child.

The family generally serves as the patient's main support system. In turn, the health care team should support the family caregivers. Active family participation in the child's care seems to enhance coping of the child and family members alike. Yet caregivers must be sensitive to those individuals who are not capable or who do not desire a high degree of involvement.

The environment must promote open, two-way communication between the family and the interdisciplinary team. The Association for the Care of Children's Health (ACCH) recognizes several components as key elements of a family-centered approach to care. It states the need to recognize the family as the constant in the child's life. However, each family has different strengths and methods of coping, and each child has unique developmental needs. Health care systems must be responsive to family needs. Comprehensive programs should be available that include emotional and financial support to families. Parents need to receive complete and ongoing information about their child to enable collaboration with health care professionals. Finally, ACCH encourages health care providers to facilitate parent-to-parent support.[41]

Team members are responsible for providing information and access to resources so families can make informed decisions, participate as team members, and ultimately function as primary caregivers. Health care systems must be designed to minimize barriers that separate the family unit. Open visitation, care by parent units, and evening or weekend clinics are attempts to keep the family intact as much as possible.[21,33]

Parent, patient, and professional collaboration can lead to more comprehensive and appropriate care plans. Health care members offer the expertise of their discipline, and parents and children individualize the experience.[44] Oncology treatment often extends over several years; thus staff acceptance and encouragement of family participation are vital for a positive long-term relationship.

TEAM EVALUATION AND EDUCATION

The value of varied and specialized professionals working together to coordinate patient care has been described in the literature; yet many wonder—does the team approach work?[12,28] Further research is needed to examine whether coordination of services does result in better patient care. Ducanis and Golin[12] recommend evaluation from the viewpoint of the patient, professional, and organization. Some variables to consider in evaluating effectiveness of the health care team include costs, consistency, and continuity (Table 18–2). Although many aspects of team-

---

TABLE 18–2. *Health Care Team Effectiveness: The Seven C's*

1. *Collaboration:* Does the team include the child and family in making treatment plan decisions? Does the team meet regularly to discuss and plan for the physical and psychosocial needs for each child and family?
2. *Continuity:* Are specific team members identified to interact regularly with the child and family?
3. *Consistency:* Does the entire team facilitate the agreed on plan of care?
4. *Communication:* Does the team provide information in a timely manner to the child and family?
5. *Coping:* Does the team continually reassess the child's and family's perceived level of stress and wellness and intervene as needed?
6. *Consultation:* Does the team routinely refer the child and family to available resources within the treatment center and community?
7. *Costs:* Do the team's interventions affect the child's length of hospital stay or treatment charges?

work are difficult to quantify, team evaluation can provide valuable data for the administrator who is faced with designing alternative delivery systems and allocating scarce resources.

Nason[28] notes there are not so many elements holding teams together as are potentially able to pull them apart. Many believe that internal conflict and professional struggles occur partly because of ignorance of the skills of other team members. One idea for optimizing health care professionals' ability to function as a group has been education for teamwork.[12] Team interaction education should include content on system or group and change theory, interpersonal communication skills, conflict resolution, and team building.

Although team skills can be integrated into an existing curriculum, the need for specific interdisciplinary education has also been voiced. Ducanis and Golin[12] surveyed 175 varying professional schools and reported that 90% of the respondents agreed with the need for health care team teaching. However, only 34% indicated they currently had such instruction.

Continuing education programs may be a better option for those who believe professionals should first be trained in their area of expertise or for individuals new to a health care team concept. Teamwork education strives to enhance understanding of the interrelatedness of roles and to promote effectiveness of the team delivery approach.

SUPPORT FOR THE CAREGIVERS

Health care professionals are frequently asked, "How can you work with children who have cancer?" The reality is caregivers can become overwhelmed as they attempt to assist families in coping with seemingly endless stressors plus deal with their own personal affairs. Maul-Mellott and Adams[25] state that few nursing specialties require more emotional reserve and technical expertise than pediatric oncology.

Changes in health care and working as part of an interdisciplinary team have left some nurses feeling unclear about their roles. Coker and Schreiber[10] described a workshop designed to clarify the roles of various disciplines and their perceptions and expectations of one another. Although the work nurses perform may be broader than that of other disciplines, the nurses who participated in the workshop were able to identify patient needs that would not be met by anyone else. The staff was successful in recognizing the centrality of their role and their unique contribution among health disciplines.

Brown[5] suggests caregivers learn to follow some of the advice they often give to patients and families. Specifically, be kind to yourself and to your coworkers. Caregivers often discover other team members are their greatest source of support and understanding. Professionals sharing work experiences with their own family members may obtain additional support, or it may prove too difficult a subject for others to discuss. Caregivers must be sensitive to the emotional burden disclosure may place on family members who are not trained health professionals.

Institutions should provide formal support groups that meet routinely or as a need is identified. Although psychologists, social workers, and mental health nurse specialists are trained in facilitating groups, team members from these disciplines may be too close to the situation. It may be necessary to seek psychosocial support from other professionals who are not members of the pediatric oncology team and thus remain more objective.

Sharing feelings and experiences, in a formal group or informally, provides opportunity to gain insight into management of stressful situations. Once sources of stress are identified, coping methods may be explored. Open communication among team members is comforting as individuals learn that others also experience feelings of confusion, anger, or grief. "Too often, lack of efforts to understand or manage work-related conflict contributes to professional burn-out."[18] Depression or apathy may be an early indication of coping difficulty, and professional help is advisable. Employee assistance counseling services may be available as a benefit from the hospital. Unfortunately, not everyone seeks help in time to prevent transfer from the unit, a decision to leave oncology nursing, or personal emotional harm.

Balancing professional, organizational, and personal lives is a daily challenge. Scharer[39] recommends that caregivers develop psychologic, social, and biophysical strategies for preventing burnout. The best way to cure burnout is to prevent its occurrence. Accept personal limitations, but also enjoy your successes, attend conferences to learn from and share with others, maintain interests outside of work, and deal with frustrations as they occur to avoid a buildup of problems later.[5,9]

Nursing administrators must strive to provide a supportive environment for the staff. Job satisfaction, retention, and turnover are critical concerns in today's health care climate. Most nurses believe the triumphs and rewards of caring for children with cancer outweigh the inherent emotional risks. There is no feeling quite as exhilarating as knowing you have made a difference in someone's life or have been a comfort at the time of someone's death.

REFERENCES

1. Adams-Greenly M. Psychosocial assessment and intervention at initial diagnosis. Pediatrician 1991; 18: 3–10.
2. Association for the Care of Children's Health. Child Life Position Statement. Washington, D.C.: The Association, 1983.
3. Association of Pediatric Oncology Nurses. Scope of Practice and Outcome Standards of Practice for Pediatric Oncology Nursing. McLean, Va.: The Association, 1987.
4. Brown J, Ritchie JA. Nurses' perceptions of parent and nurse roles in caring for hospitalized children. Child Health Care 1990; 19:28–36.
5. Brown PG. Families who have a child diagnosed with cancer: What the medical caregiver can do to help them and themselves. Issues Compr Pediatr Nurs 1989; 12:247–260.
6. Bru G. Using the revised APON standards of practice. J Pediatr Oncol Nurs 1990; 7:17–21.
7. Cairns NU, Klopovich P, Hearne E, et al. School attendance of children with cancer. J Sch Health 1982; 52:152–155.
8. Chauvenet AR, Wofford MM. Cures in childhood cancer. Pediatr Rev 1990; 11:311–317.
9. Cleaveland MJ. Stress management for pediatric oncology nurses. J Assoc Pediatr Oncol Nurses 1987; 4:36–37.
10. Coker EB, Schreiber R. The nurse's role in a team conference. Nurs Manage 1990; 21:46–48.
11. Deasy-Spinetta P, Spinetta JJ. Educational issues for children with cancer. Candlelighters 1989; 13:2–7.
12. Ducanis AJ, Golin AK. The Interdisciplinary Health Care Team. Germantown, Md.: Aspen, 1979.
13. Dufour DF. Home or hospital care for the child with end-stage cancer: Effects on the family. Issues Compr Pediatr Nurs 1989; 12:371–383.
14. Elder RG, Bullough B. Nurse practitioners and clinical nurse specialists: Are the roles merging? Clin Nurs Spec 1990; 4:78–84.
15. Fernbach DJ. The role of the family physician in the care of the child with cancer. CA 1985; 35:258–270.
16. Forbes KE, Rafson J, Spross JA, et al. The clinical nurse specialist and nurse practitioner: Core curriculum survey results. Clin Nurse Spec 1990; 4:63–66.
17. Gamis AS, Nesbit ME. Neuropsychologic (cognitive) disabilities in long-term survivors of childhood cancer. Pediatrician 1991; 18:11–19.
18. Gibbons MB. When the dying patient is a child: A challenge for the living. In Hockenberry MJ, Coody DK (eds): Pediatric Oncology and Hematology: Perspectives in Care. St. Louis: CV Mosby, 1986, pp 493–508.
19. Goodell AS. Perceptions of nurses toward parent participation on pediatric oncology units. Cancer Nurs 1979; 2:38–46.
20. Hammond D. Management of childhood cancer. CA 1990; 40:325–326.
21. Hardgrove C, Healy D. The care-through-parent program at Moffitt Hospital, University of California, San Francisco. Nurs Clin North Am 1984; 19:145–160.
22. Hinds PS, Norville R, Anthony L, et al. Establishing pediatric cancer nursing research priorities: A delphi study. J Pediatr Oncol Nurs 1990; 7:101–108.
23. Joint Commission on Accreditation of Healthcare Organizations. Accreditation Manual for Hospitals—1989. USA: The Commission, 1988.
24. Lannering B, Marky I, Lundberg A, et al. Long-term sequelae after pediatric brain tumors: Their effect on disability and quality of life. Med Pediatr Oncol 1990; 18:304–310.
25. Maul-Mellott SK, Adams JN. Childhood Cancer: A Nursing Overview. Boston: Jones & Bartlett, 1987.
26. McCormick D. School re-entry program for oncology patients. J Assoc Pediatr Oncol Nurses 1986; 3:13–17, 25.
27. Monaco GP. Resources available to the family of the child with cancer. Cancer 1986; 58(suppl):516–521.
28. Nason F. Diagnosing the hospital team. Soc Work Health Care 1983; 9:25–45.
29. National Institutes of Health. Diet and Nutrition. NIH publication 88-2038. Bethesda, Md.: National Cancer Institute, 1988.
30. Novack M, Bru G, Davidoff MC. Development of a support group for volunteers in a pediatric oncology setting. J Assoc Pediatr Oncol Nurses 1985; 2:30–35.
31. Peckham VC. Learning disorders associated with the treatment of cancer in childhood. J Assoc Pediatr Oncol Nurses 1988; 5:10–13.
32. Pizzo PA. Cancer and the pediatrician: An evolving partnership. Pediatr Rev 1990; 12:5–6.
33. Poster EC, Betz CL. Survey of sibling and peer visitation policies in Southern California hospitals. Child Health Care 1987; 15:166–171.
34. Richardson AT. Nurses interfacing with other members of the team. In England DA (ed): Collaboration in Nursing. Rockville, Md.: Aspen, 1986, pp 163–185.
35. Rickard KA, Grosfeld JL, Coates TD, et al. Advances in nutrition care of children with neoplastic diseases: A review of treatment, research, and application. J Am Diet Assoc 1986; 86:1666–1676.

36. Riley-Lawless K. School reentry programs. J Pediatr Oncol Nurs 1989; 6:92–93.

37. Russell CA. The team approach: Should we or shouldn't we? Proc Nat Conf Pract Educ Res Oncol Soc Work 1984; 71–73.

38. Saunders RB, Miller BB, Cates KM. Pediatric family care: An interdisciplinary team approach. Child Health Care 1989; 18:53–58.

39. Scharer K. Care for the care-giver. J Assoc Pediatr Oncol Nurses 1988; 5:24.

40. Shah NR. The community physician's involvement in clinical trials and home treatment. Cancer 1986; 58(suppl):504–507.

41. Shelton TL, Jeppson ES, Johnson BH. Family-Centered Care for Children with Special Health Care Needs. Association for the Care of Children's Health, 1987.

42. van Eys J. Medical decisions in the selection of therapy for the child with cancer. Cancer 1986; 58(suppl):454–460.

43. Watson PG. Cancer rehabilitation. Cancer Nurs 1990; 13:2–12.

44. Wellner AM. Psychology. In Valletutti PJ, Christoplos F (eds): Interdisciplinary Approaches to Human Services. Baltimore: University Park, 1977, pp 337–356.

45. Wells RJ. Rehabilitation: Making the most of time. Oncol Nurs Forum 1990; 17:503–507.

INDEX

Note: Page numbers in *italics* refer to illustrations; page numbers followed by (t) refer to tables.

511